HEARING LOSS

Edited by **Sadaf Naz**

Hearing Loss
Edited by Sadaf Naz

Published by InTech
Janeza Trdine 9, 51000 Rijeka, Croatia

Publishing Process Manager Martina Blecic

Technical Editor Teodora Smiljanic

Cover Designer InTech Design Team

Additional hard copies can be obtained from orders@intechopen.com

Hearing Loss, Edited by Sadaf Naz
p. cm.
ISBN 978-953-51-0366-0

Meet the editor

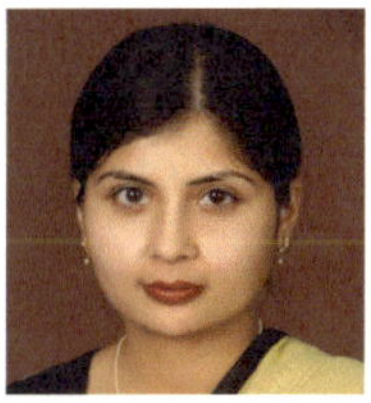

Dr Sadaf Naz obtained her PhD from University of the Punjab, Lahore, where she initiated one of the first studies on determining the genetic underpinnings of hearing loss in Pakistan. After completing different postdoctoral research projects at National Institute on Deafness and other Communication, Disorders, National Institutes of Health, USA, she attained a faculty position at School of Biological Sciences at University of the Punjab, Lahore. Dr. Naz's laboratory studies molecular genetics of different human disorders and the major focus of her research group is identification of genes involved in moderate to severe deafness.

Contents

Preface

Hearing loss affects 278 million people world wide and is one of the most significant health problems. Deafness can be acquired due to environmental insults including injuries and infections. Additionally, about 50 % of hearing loss is genetic and scientists have identified nearly 100 genes implicated in deafness, while many more remain to be identified. This book brings together different topics on our current understanding of hearing loss.

The first section on "Hearing" presents a brief overview about normal hearing as well as the technology and instruments involved in its measurement including audiometry and auditory brainstem response as well as methods to record otoacoustic emissions. Scientists have also investigated the listening scores of audio signals and the psychological impressions related to speech audibility. In the last chapter in this section, the suitability of the Mongolian gerbil is discussed, particularly as a model of structural and functional aspects of age-dependent hearing loss in humans.

The section on "Childhood Hearing loss" provides an overview of parental practices and behaviours related to children with and without hearing loss. The results indicated that the interactions established between mothers and children favour the acquisition and maintenance of social skills. Additionally, early detection of hearing loss and prompt intervention gives children with deafness a chance to develop spoken language comparable to those with normal hearing.

"Injuries & traumas" as cause of hearing loss are the focus of the third chapter in this book. This section includes a report on head injuries in India and the ensuing hearing loss. Symptoms of hearing loss were found in 10% of the patients with head trauma. Sensorineural hearing loss was the most common finding in the affected individuals. Additionally, perforation of the tympanic membrane is reported as a common finding in Nigeria due to trauma to the ear. The next two chapters explore the role of ototoxic agents such as solvents, pesticides and metals, and their interaction with noise in causing hearing loss. Research conducted in human subjects exposed to these chemicals indicates that these agents cause auditory dysfunction. The combined influence of noise and chemical pollutants on hearing loss confirmed the existence of an interaction between physical and chemical factors which influence the alteration of auditory function.

The "Genetics" of hearing loss is discussed in a series of review articles in the next section. An overview is provided of different genes involved in nonsyndromic and syndromic hearing loss and reflects the unparalleled heterogeneity of deafness genes. Different modes of inheritance of deafness are also discussed. The genetics of recessively inherited, moderate to severe and progressive hearing loss in humans is covered in detail. Strategies are described about identification of modifiers of deafness genes. Common craniofacial abnormalities inherited together with hearing loss are discussed in the next chapter. The genes involved in causing Usher syndrome as well as different mouse models for each of these genes are also comprehensively reviewed.

The last section of the book presents the "Treatment" of hearing loss for both genetic and acquired cases of deafness. Cochlear implants are now accepted as the standard of care for children with severe to profound hearing loss. They have allowed many children to attend regular schools, and to develop their language, social and academic skills to levels that exceed those for their peers with severe to profound hearing loss using hearing aids. The efficacy of corticosteroid treatment through the eardrum and into the middle ear to treat various otologic disorders, such as Meniere's disease and sudden sensorineural hearing loss is also reviewed. The last chapter discusses an ancient Chinese technique of acupuncture for treatment of sudden sensorineural hearing loss. The authors' experimentally demonstrate improvement of the hearing loss in more than 20% of the individuals who underwent the treatment. Acupuncture has gained scientific ground after it was experimentally demonstrated that during this process adenosine is released and improves different symptoms in patients. Exactly how acupuncture may help in treating hearing loss remains to be determined.

It is hoped that the research and the reviews on various aspects of hearing loss described in this book will be of benefit to different students and the researchers working actively in this field. The coming years will see accelerated discoveries in many research areas discussed in this book, particularly in genetics of deafness due to the use of massively parallel sequencing technologies to identify disease genes. Therapies based on genetic findings for treatment of hearing loss may also become possible in future.

Ms. Martina Blecic, the publishing process manager, Ms Ana Pantar, editor relations consultant and Ms Nina Dundovic, the technical editor contributed to editing of this book.

Sadaf Naz
School of Biological Sciences,
University of the Punjab, Lahore 54590,
Pakistan

Part 1

Hearing

1

Technology for Hearing Evaluation

Josefina Gutierrez
National Rehabilitation Institute
Mexico

1. Introduction

The hearing system is composed of several components that, by means of a physiological process, break down the broad spectrum of frequencies and intensities of sounds from the environment (speech, music, signals and noise) into frequency components and temporal patterns. These acoustic signals are transmitted to the temporal lobes of the Central Nervous System by electric stimuli to generate the neural message (Salesa et al., 2005). The hearing process utilizes acoustic, mechanical and electrical principles, and in addition analyzes sound waves, removes noise and compares these with signals that have been previously registered in the memory of the subject. In this manner, we are able to know when a person is speaking, when we are hearing a musical note from a violin or a flute, or when a bird is singing.

The auditory system possesses a wide dynamic range for perceiving sounds; humans with normal hearing detect tonal frequencies from 20 Hz to 20 kHz. Acoustic intensity is proportional to sound vibration amplitude. Commonly, sound intensity is measured in terms of decibels as $dB = 10 \log(I/I_0)$, where I_0 is the reference intensity, or equivalently for acoustic pressure, $dB = 20 \log(P/P_0)$, where P_0 is the reference pressure (in Pa). Tonality represents the number of vibrations in time and is measured in cycles/sec or Hz. Timbre characterizes all of the harmonics overheard in a clear sound, allowing differentiation between two sounds with the same tonality and intensity.

The dynamic range at 2-4 kHz, the span between threshold and pain, is approximately 120 dB. The minimum threshold for sound occurs between 2 and 5 kHz and is approximately 20μPa. At the low end of the auditory spectrum, the threshold is 80 dB higher, while at the high end, it is 70 dB higher. Intensity differences of 1 dB can be detected, while frequency differences of 2-3 Hz can be detected at frequencies below 3 kHz (Aitkin, 1990).

Sounds are normally transmitted both by Air conduction (AC), and by Bone conduction (BC). Conduction of sound starts in the pinna or auricle and passes through the external auditory canal on its way to the eardrum, where sounds are amplified to frequencies ranging from 5,000-6,000 Hz at 20 dB. Later, the pressure and strength of the sound wave vibration that reaches the tympanic membrane, particularly of low frequencies of up to 1,500 Hz, are amplified in the middle ear. The acoustic vibration of the sound is thus transformed into a mechanical vibration to be transmitted to the organ of Corti, located in the cochlear duct. The cochlea is a hydromechanical frequency analyzer whose major role is to turn the acoustic signal into a frequency map through which each frequency is assigned to certain groups of receptor cells and their nerve fibers. The cochlear nerve innervates the organ of Corti; it possesses myelinized efferent fibers that carry spatial orientation information from the cochlea to the brain. Efferent signals are amplified and transmitted, frequency discrimination is increased, acoustic otoemissions originate, and mechanical changes produced in the liquid medium of the sound waves are detected (Steele et al., 2000).

Hearing loss can occur at any age. Otorhinolaryngologists, surgeons, and audiologists with assistance technology are readily able to identify different degrees of hearing loss. Children and adults experiencing significant hearing loss suffer specific problems and may need special assistance. Early identification of hearing loss and its treatment is essential for successful speech development, the child's intellectual growth and the adult's social integration.

Hearing impairment is caused by either loss in sensitivity (loss in perceived loudness), loss in the ability to discriminate different speech sounds, or both. Loss of loudness may be due to either increased mechanical impedance between the outer and inner ear or reduced sensitivity of the sensory hearing organ. Loss of the discrimination ability is basically associated with damage to the sensory organ, although other neural structures at higher levels may also be involved.

2. Audiologic evaluation technology

Several subjective and objective methods to assess hearing disorders are available, depending on the individual's age, hearing level and condition type. Among other things, evaluation must be conducted for cochlear integrity, acoustic impedance, and screening of hearing of newborns and infants.

With ever changing technology and new methodologies in healthcare, available for addressing the specific needs of adult and pediatric populations, hearing technology represents not only devices for clinicians' practice, but also devices to meet the high level of need for diagnostic techniques, audiologic rehabilitation, treatment methodologies, and special issues in researching the needs of patients (Montano & Spitzer, 2009).

2.1 Subjective evaluation (technology)

Subjective hearing tests (Miller, 2006) are available for performing a rough estimate of the grade of hearing loss. These tests do not provide a quantitative report of the patient's hearing status, but rather comprise a method with practical clinical value for exploring the cochlea in order to determine location rather than intensity of the damage; results must be evaluated in conjunction with quantitative hearing evaluation. These include the following:

2.1.1 Acumeter

Instrumental acumetry (see Figure 1), which employs the diapason to assess hearing acuity, guarantees limited precision (Marullo et al., 1967). This instrument "tuning fork"produces sounds with frequencies between 16 and 4,096 Hz from octave to octave. This is a U-shaped acoustic resonator that resonates at a specific constant on a frequency-related scale when set to vibrate by striking it against a surface or with an object emitting a pure tone. There are three mean tests:

The Schwabach test determines BC duration. The instrument is placed on the antero-superior region of the mastoid. Normal duration is 20 sec. The Schwabach test makes a comparison between bone conduction of the patient and the examiner. The diapason is placed between the patient and examiner and a sound is created. If the patient can no longer hear the sound even though the examiner can hear it, it is indicative of sensory neural loss; if the examiner stops hearing the sound and the patient continues to hear it, it suggests conductive loss. However, this test is completely dependent on the hearing powers of the examiner. In conduction hypoacusis - the duration is prolonged, while in sensory neural hypoacusis, the duration is shortened.

The Weber test utilizes the low frequency of the instrument (126 Hz), which is placed on vertex. Normally the vibration is heard equally in both ears. This is a common medical test conducted in the physician´s office in which a comparison is made between two hearings. In the first, the base of the tuning fork is applied to the bone and hearing is elicited after this. When the sound is completely inaudible, the vibrating top is brought near the external ear canal. If there is a positive value, it is considered that there is an air-bone gap due to which there is a conductive loss.

The Rinne test employs the diapason as initially placed near the ear to explore aerial conduction and after that, on the mastoid to explore bone conduction. Normally, air conduction is better than bone conduction. With BC/AC=½, the Rinne test is normally positive. In this test, a 512 Hz tuning fork is placed on the forehead of the patient. An ipsilateral conductive hearing loss is occurred if the sound appears to be louder on one side than on the other. A contralateral sensorineural hearing loss may also be determined by use of this test.

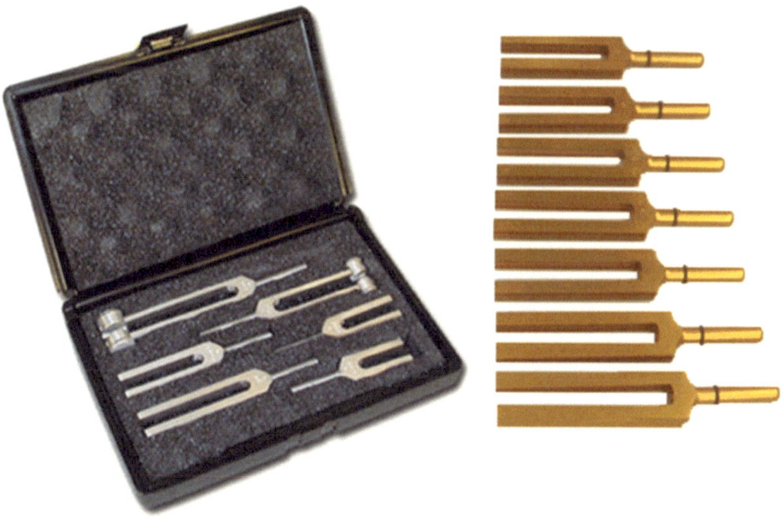

Fig. 1. Set of tuning fork

2.1.2 Speech perception test

This test uses words that the subject hears through headphones and he/she is required to identify them. This test depends on the knowledge of language; it must be adjusted to both adult and pediatric populations. It is categorized according to whether the words are aimed at evaluating detection level ability, syllable, phoneme, word, or sentence perception (Australian Hearing Group, 2001). Additionally, it is designed to provide a useful overview of the key features (e.g., target hearing-impaired group, clinical application) of each of the tests and thereby assists the Audiologist in selecting the appropriate speech perception test/s for the individual patient and the specific clinical situation.

2.1.3 Acoustic reflex test

The acoustic reflex test measures the contraction of the stapedius, a tiny muscle in the middle ear, in response to loud sounds, which occurs under normal conditions when a sufficiently intense sound is presented to the auditory pathway. This muscle contraction causes a stiffening of the ossicular chain, which alters the compliance of the middle ear system. When stimulus presentation and measurement are effected on the same ear by means of the probe tone, this acoustical reflex is referred to as an ipsilateral acoustic reflex. When stimulus presentation and measurement are effected on opposite ears, the reflex is referred to as a contralateral acoustic reflex.

Stimulus tones of varying intensities of 500, 1000, 2000 or 4000 Hz are presented as short bursts. If a change in compliance greater than 0.05ml is detected, a reflex is considered to be present. Because this is an extremely small compliance change, any movement of the probe during the test may produce an artifact (false response). The test result is recorded as Pass/No Response in graphic form (MAICO, 2007). The level of loudness aids in identifying the location of the problem along the auditory pathway.

2.1.4 Scope evaluation

Scope evaluation utilizes a light emitted by an otoscope. The examiner is able to look into the outer and middle ear through a lens on the rear of the instrument and to screen for disease including otitis or infection during regular clinical check-ups. Figure 2 depicts the

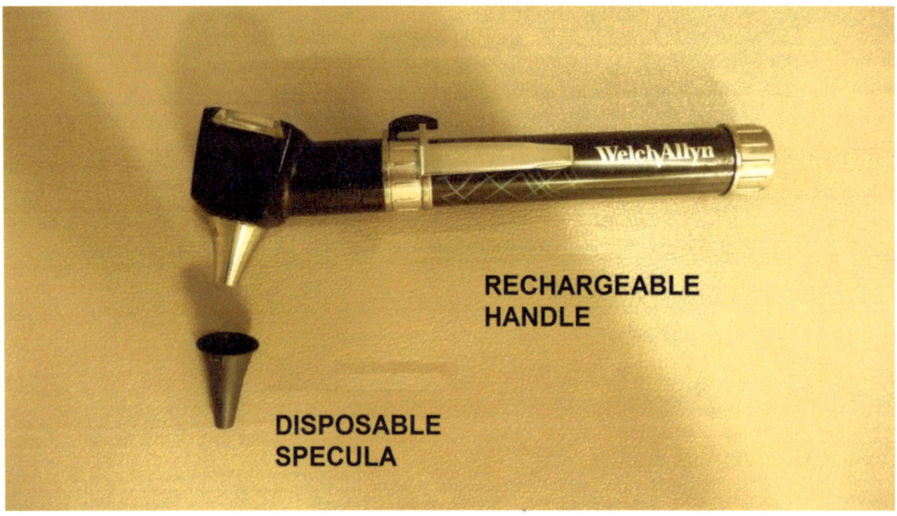

Fig. 2. Welch-Allyn handle otoscope

Welch-Allyn otoscope (Golfain et al., 2008), which is a small hand-held instrument. It has a light that is directed through a funnel-like tip to illuminate the ear canal for examination. The funnel-like tip is called speculum. The specula are disposable and come in sizes for average adult ear canals. The otoscope is powered by a rechargeable battery located in the handle; the handle is detachable and can be plugged into a standard wall outlet for recharging.

2.2 Objective evaluation (technology)

Diagnostic equipment can help to identify different degrees of hearing loss in a more quantitative fashion. There are several techniques that are implemented in medical equipment for screening of hearing. The most widely used initial screen involves a pure-tone, air-conduction hearing test or audiometry, followed by tympanometry, otoacoustic emissions, multilingual speech audiometry, and stem cell evoked potentials.

Hearing testing is conducted in the audiometry testing chamber; a special sound booth is built into this room, which must be constructed based on testing guidance described in the ASTM E336 "Standard Test Method for measurement of Airborne Sound Insulation in Buildings" (ASTM E336-10, 2011). This triangular-shaped booth is designed to ensure that the sound levels inside are sufficiently quiet to permit accurate hearing-threshold measurements. In addition to the sound booth, the examination room possesses several other features designed to reduce sound levels in the room further, as shown in Figure 3. These include sound dampening materials on the interior walls of the examination room and a rubber seal on the exterior door.

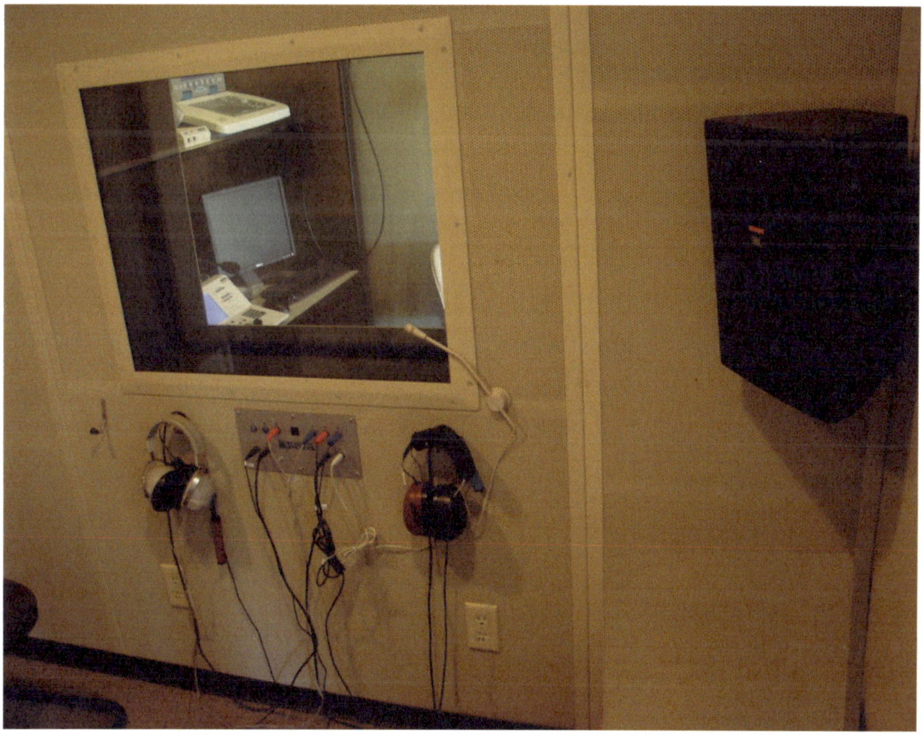

Fig. 3. Anaechoic Chamber for audiometry test.

The testing suite consists of two adjoining rooms: one of single-wall construction, and the other, of double-wall construction. The double portion of the suite is the subject of the noise reduction test that includes the following: 1) generating a high-volume controlled sound field outside the testing chamber; 2) measuring the sound pressure level at the outer wall; 3) measuring the attenuated sound-pressure level of the controlled sound field inside the test chamber, and 4) subtracting internal from the external sound-pressure levels while making corrections for the interior ambient sound pressure level (Acoustic Systems MD, 2000).

2.2.1 Pure-tone audiometry and logoaudiometry

The Audiometry study is used to diagnose the degree and type of hearing loss by determining the faintest tones that a person can hear at selected pitches; the measuring equipment utilized is called audiometer. This device emits a pure tone by means of a fixed-frequency oscillator calibrated at the decibel hearing level (National Health and Nutrition Examination Survey, 2003); frequencies (125-8000 Hz) and intensities (0-110 dB) which can be varied. This unit is controlled by a microprocessor that is sometimes available as a handheld Windows-driven instrument and possesses high accuracy and efficiency (Khandpur, 2005). Such systems can be also employed with bone vibrators to test conductive hearing mechanisms. A pair of headphones is attached, and a test subject feedback button indicates when the subject has heard the sound. On the one hand, audiometry measures hearing thresholds and oral audiometry or logoaudiometry (Aguilera et al., 1997), considered to be a subjective evaluation, is defined by the capacity to evaluate the human speech understanding consists of supplying the patient with words at different energies that aid in recognizing acoustical features and in providing clues concerning the etiology of the hearing loss. On the other hand, audiometry includes supraliminal tests such as SISI, Fowler, Tone Decay, or Békésy, to suggest the sensorineural damage (Ghani, 2005). Figures 4 and 5 ilustrate the SISI and Békésy tests.

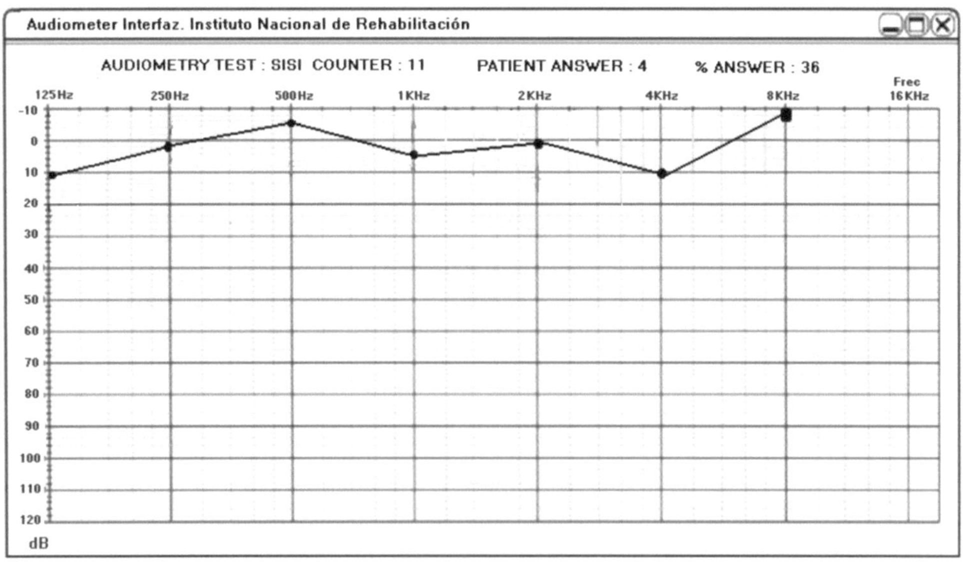

Fig. 4. A patient's SISI Graph with score value (Gutierrez et al., 2009)

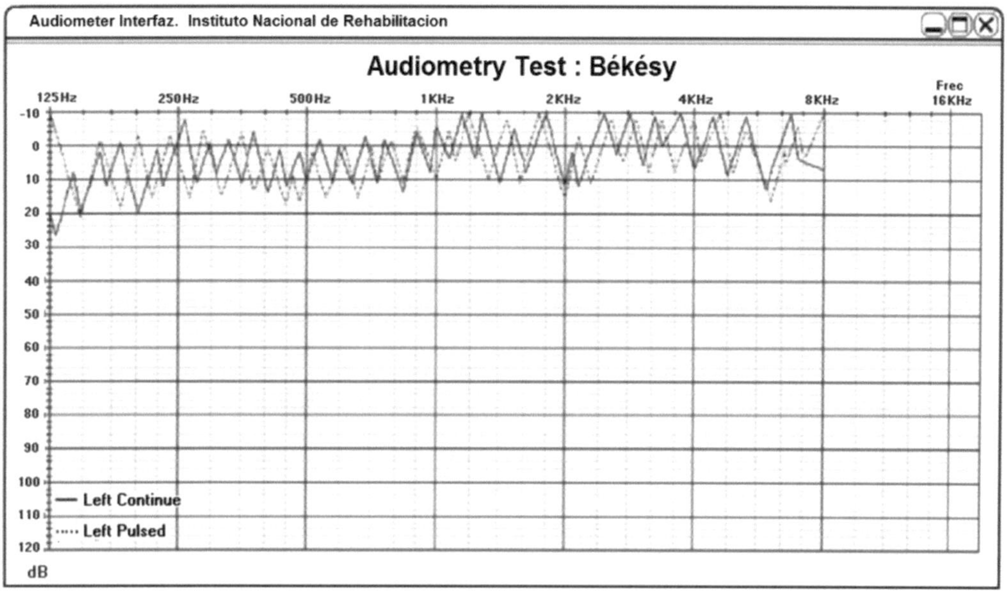

Fig. 5. A patient's Békésy test (Gutierrez et al., 2009)

Generally, an audiometric system controlled by a microprocessor (Penhaker & Kijonka, 2011) is composed of two channels: one for test ear stimulus, and other as a non-test ear masker, as shown in the block diagram of Figure 6.

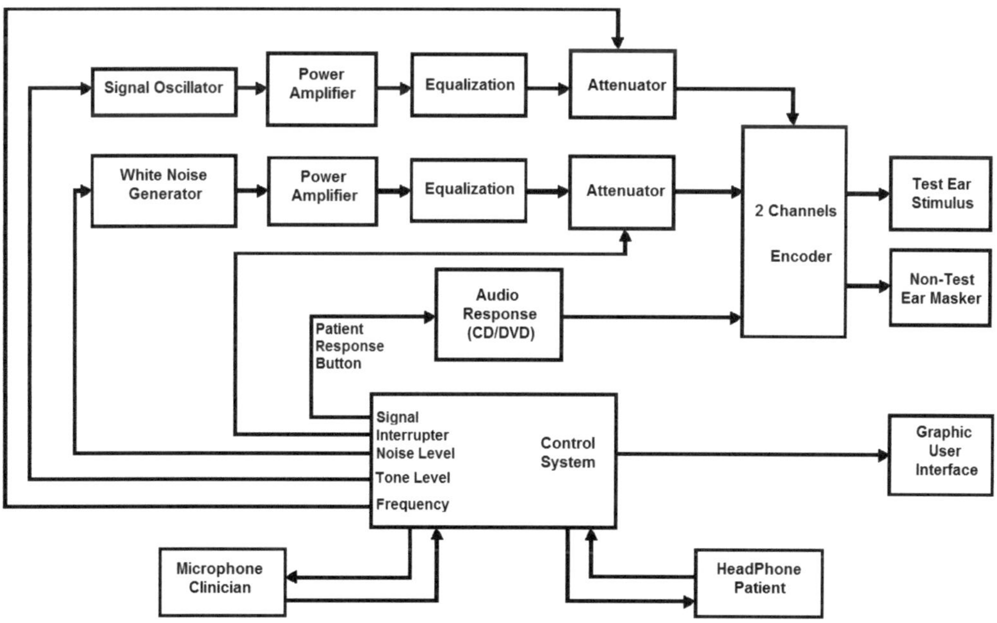

Fig. 6. General block diagram of an audiometer

An audiogram is a chart that depicts the results of the audiometric study; on the x-axis, frequencies are represented in Hz, and on the y-axis, the patient's hearing ability is expressed in dB. Two charts are usually employed: one for the right ear, and one for the left. The right ear is graphed with a circle in red color, the blue color plot the left ear with an X. Symbols and notes should correspond to the recommendations and standards of the American Speech Language Hearing Association (ASHA).

ASHA guidelines for manual pure-tone threshold audiometry (Campbell et al., 2010); these guidelines contain procedures for performing a hearing diagnosis and for monitoring standard pure-tone threshold and include manual air-conduction and bone-conduction, masking. From the inception of modern audiometric technology, staff at the Department of Audiology at the Massachusetts Eye and Ear Infirmary began using an extension of the standard symbols for designating "response at limit" and responses found using speakers (Halpin, 2007). These symbols represent new exploratory developments and are not part of the ASHA standard symbol.

The NOAH-3™ System (Hearing Instrument Manufacturers' Software Association, 2000) is a database that integrates software applications from the several manufacturers of audiologic devices, including Madsen™ (Madsen Electronics, 2004), Amplaid™, Interacustic™, Benson Medical™ . The main purpose of NOAH is to control data exchange from an audiometer to a personal computer, among other applications. The transmitted information is introduced into a database that is manipulated and processed to obtain audiograms, tables, measurements, and statistics, as well as to save and print the patient's study.

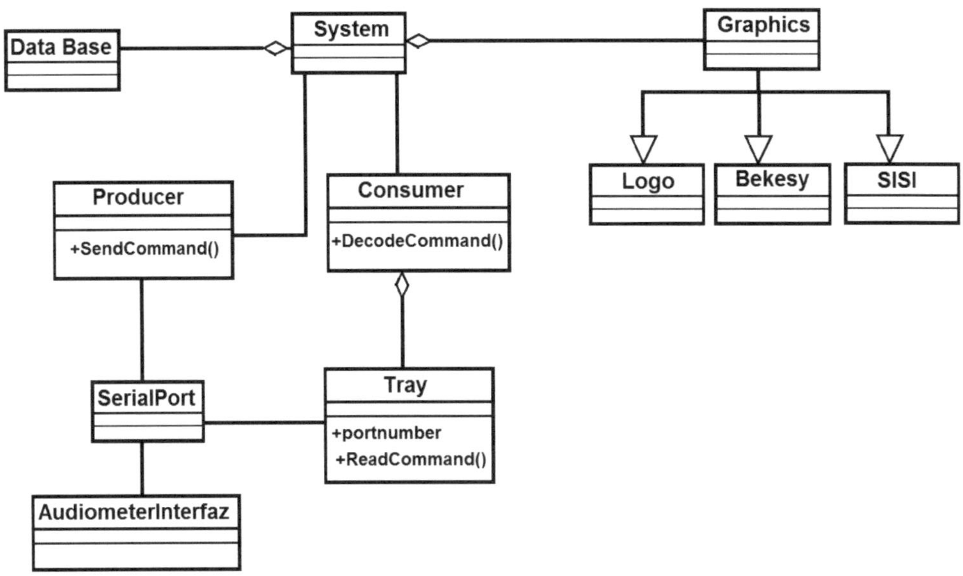

Fig. 7. Overview Producer-Consumer Architecture for the Audiometer Interface.

The NOAH-3™ System does not work with certain special tests (SISI, Békésy) and some audiometers, for example, Madsen™ (Gutiérrez et al., 2009), and it is not possible to transfer data for processing or printing these special tests. When the audiometer is turned off, or when new patient data is introduced, the information of the previous test is lost. There is no database and the hardcopy audiograms are not designed for long term storage because the audiometer has a thermal printer.

This limitation is a problem for the specialist, because he/she needs to store the patient's test data so that this information can be used in clinical and research audiometric protocols. Some authors (Gutiérrez et al., 2009) have described the design and implementation of a communication and graphical module for transmitting, processing, printing, and storing the patient's special audiometric studies as a substitute for the NOAH-3™ System (see Figure 7).

2.2.2 Tympanometry

The Impedance Audiometry or most commonly used Tympanometry, is a magnitude that examines the condition of the middle ear, the status and mobility of the eardrum (tympanic membrane). The equipment produces variations of air pressure in the ear canal by means of a probe measuring the middle ear's acoustic resistance. The secondary purpose of this examination is to evaluate the acoustic reflex pathway which includes the 7th and 8th cranial nerves and the brain stem. Furthermore, tympanometry permits a distinction between sensorineural and conductive hearing loss when results are not apparent via Weber and Rinne testing. It is also helpful in the diagnosis of otitis media by demonstrating the presence of middle-ear effusion. When sound impacts on the eardrum, part of the sound is absorbed and sent via the middle to the inner ear, while the remaining part of the sound is reflected. When the eardrum is inflamed over a long period of time, it can become stiff and heavy and the majority of the sound is reflected; therefore less sound reach the inner ear. Among other things, tympanometery assesses cochlear integrity and evaluates acoustic impedance, i.e., the degree of difficulty that the middle ear and ossicles encounter for the passage of sounds, as a result of the mass, stiffness and ossicular disruption of the auditory system. If there is fluid behind the ear-drum, it will not move back and forth from its resting position when pressure is applied. Tympanometry is thus affected by the mass, mobility, and resistance systems of the external and middle-ear cavities.

The instrument, or tympanometer, applies air pressure to the eardrum and measures the reflected sound. Inside the instrument's probe, a small loudspeaker is installed that emits a tone, typically at 226 Hz, through a tube into the auditory canal in front of the eardrum. The canal's air pressure is altered between +200 and -400 decapascals (dapa), at which the sound strikes the tympanic membrane, causing middle-ear vibration, which in turn results in the perception of hearing. Some of this sound is reflected back and picked up by another tube, which is connected to the microphone inside the probe that receives the sound. Together with a third tube, all three are inserted nearly into the eardrum and are made airtight against outside pressure by the ear tip. A manometer and a pump, which can produce both positive and negative pressure, are connected to tube **C**. Less sound is reflected into the microphone when the eardrum is stiff and the eardrum transmits the majority of the sound via the middle to the inner ear. Highest compliance is normally reached with air pressure that corresponds to the outside pressure. During tympanometric measurement, a continuous change in positive and negative pressure is produced by the instrument's pump in the outer middle auditory canal. This test should not be performed in infants below 7 months of age because the suppleness of the external canal's cartilage may produce misleading results.

Normally, air pressure in the ear canal is the same as ambient pressure. Also, under normal conditions, air pressure in the middle ear is approximately the same as ambient pressure because the Eustachian tube opens periodically to ventilate the middle ear and to equalize pressure. In a healthy individual, maximum sound is transmitted through the middle ear when ambient-air pressure in the ear canal is equal to the pressure in the middle ear.

The general term employed to describe how energy is transmitted through the middle ear is admittance. The impedanciometer measures reflected sound and expresses it in ml as admittance to or compliance with the pressure in daPa, plotting the results on a chart known as a tympanogram, which is illustrated in Figure 8. The maximum compliance occurs when the pressure of the external auditory canal and the middle ear becomes equal. It is only at this pressure that maximal acoustic transmission takes place through the middle ear. Thus, the compliance peak indicates the pressure of the middle ear, implying the efficacy of the Eustachian tube function. The height of the compliance peak indicates the mobility/ stiffness of the tympanic membrane or of the middle-ear cavity.

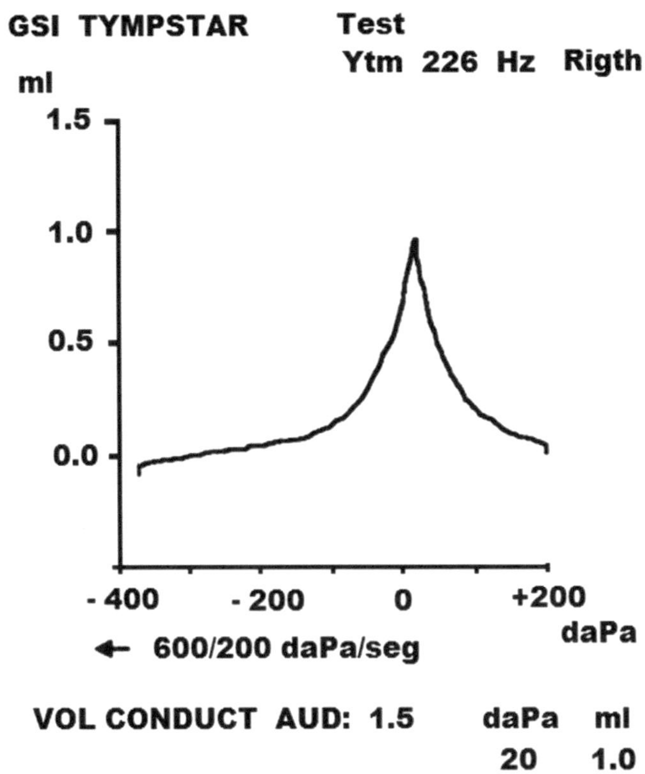

Fig. 8. Tympanogram of a normal subject, their canal's air pressure is altered between +200 and -400 dapa at 226Hz.

This test is not a hearing evaluation, but is rather a measure of energy transmission through the middle ear. It should not be used to assess hearing sensitivity and the results of this test should always be viewed in conjunction with pure-tone audiometry. Figure 9 presents the block diagram of a portable, hand-held tympanometer. Manufacturers, such as Welch Allyn, have marketed the invention registered by Heller et al, (Heller et al., 1987). This instrument has the capacity has the capacity of performing the test and of displaying and storing data.

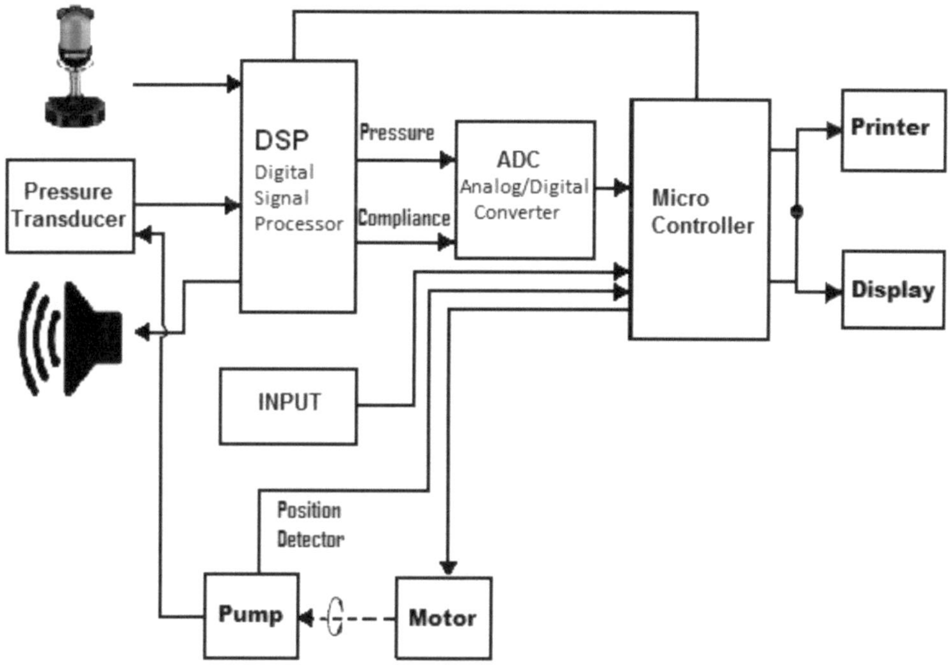

Fig. 9. General block diagram of a hand-held tympanometer.

2.2.3 Otoacoustic emissions

Otoacoustic Emissions (OAE) may occur spontaneously or may be evoked by acoustic stimulation, appearing to originate from within the cochlea and propagating through middle ear structures to the external auditory meatus. OAE are acoustic energy leakages from the biochemical reactions (echoes) of a healthy cochlea that possess a latency of 2-20 msec. If an emission by the cochlea is present, it is likely that hearing is normal at that frequency; those with a hearing loss greater than 25–30 dB usually do not produce these soft sounds. Auditory neuropathy may have OAE even though the hearing loss may be profound.

To measure OAE, the equipment produces a quiet, clicking sound that is emitted by the loudspeaker and OEA is measured with a small probe inserted into the ear canal; recording of the response signal is captured with the aid of a sensitive microphone (Choi, 2011). A number of response epochs must be averaged to improve the signal-to noise ratio (SNR) and produce a clear waveform. Mathematical methods are used for evaluation of the signal, such as Fast Fourier (FF) and Wigner-Ville transforms (WVT), Digital filtering, and Correlation analysis (CA) (Buller, 1997), or Hilbert–Huang transform (HT) for detection of OAE and Time–Frequency Mapping (Janušauskas et al., 2006). The measuring system employed to detect otoacoustic emissions consists of the following several parts, as illustrated in Figure 10: a measuring probe that includes a microphone and loudspeaker; a low-noise preamplifier and amplifier signal; an Analog-to-digital converter (ADC), and Digital Signal Processing (DSP) based on a central processing unit that provides ultra-fast calculation, such as filtering, averaging, FF, WVT, CA or HT in order to obtain otoacoustic emissions response. Additionally, the equipment must be accompanied by the printing and displaying module.

Because the subject being tested is not required to respond, this is an ideal test method for neonates and infants or for those who cannot be evaluated using conventional techniques (Buz & Bower, 2009). OAE are valuable in testing for ototoxicity, detecting blockage in the outer ear canal, as well as the presence of middle-ear fluid and damage to the cochlea outer hair cells.

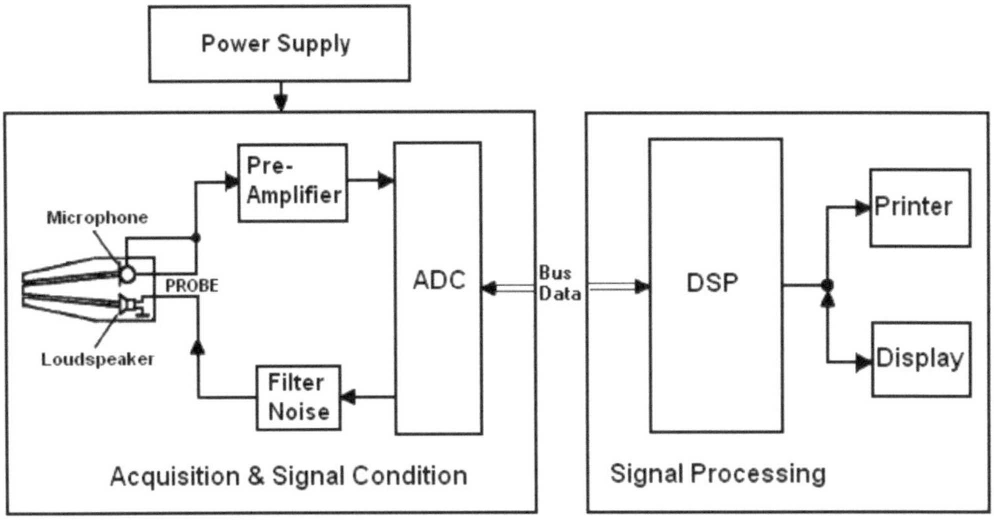

Fig. 10. Block Diagram of the measuring system used to detect OAE

2.2.4 Stem cell evoked potentials

The Vestibular Evoked Myogenic Potential is a test that is frequently performed on patients experiencing dizziness or balance problems. It evaluates additional portions of the inner ear providing a more complete evaluation of the vestibular system which controls balance. Electrodes are placed on the patients head and neck and a loud sound is delivered through inserted earphones. This test is very useful to screen infants and children under 5 years of age for hearing loss.

Auditory Brainstem Response is an electrical potentials activity in the brain that occurs in response to a sound. The test provides information on the cochlea and brain pathways for hearing. Three small disk electrodes are pasted onto the head and neck, and brain wave activity is recorded while the patient listens to a clicking sound. Soft headphones are placed into the patient's ears and quiet clicking sounds are played through the earphones.

Depending on the amount of time elapsing between the "click" stimulus and the auditory evoked response, potentials are classified as early (0-10 msec), middle (11-50 msec), or late

(51-500 msec). Early potentials reflect electrical activity at the cochlea, eighth cranial nerve, and brain-stem levels, while later potentials reflect cortical activity. In order to separate evoked potentials from background noise, a system computer, as shown in Figure 11 (Nicolet™ EMG/PE), analyzes how well the ears respond to the sound by averaging auditory evoked responses at 1,000 to 2,000 clicks at least. Early evoked responses may be analyzed to estimate the magnitude of hearing loss and to differentiate among cochlear, eighth nerve, and brainstem lesions.

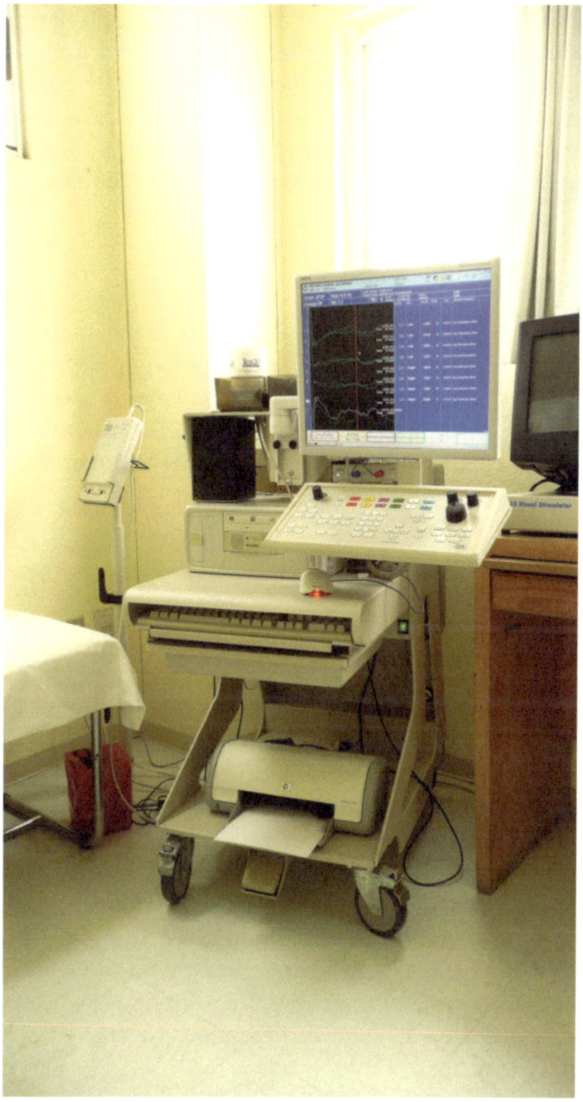

Fig. 11. Evoked Potential/EMG measuring system

For purposes of neonatal screening, only limited auditory evoked potentials or limited evoked otoacoustic emissions are considered medically necessary. Neonates who fail this screening test are then referred for comprehensive auditory evoked response testing or comprehensive otoacoustic emissions. Comprehensive auditory evoked response testing and comprehensive otoacoustic emissions are considered experimental and investigational for neonatal screening because there is a lack of evidence of the value of comprehensive testing in limited auditory evoked potentials or limited otoacoustic emissions for this indication.

2.2.5 Videonystagmography

This technique is used to evaluate the function of the vestibular system; the inner-ear portion may be the cause of any balance or dizziness problems. The instrument records eye movements, most notably involuntary eye movements called nystagmus. Eye movements are recorded by using infrared goggles. There are three evaluations, including: 1) following a light as it moves in different ways; 2) lying flat on the examination table and the subject's moving his/her head left or right, and 3) stimulating the vestibular system with warm and cool air or water.

2.3 Hearing assistance technology

Hearing loss can be categorized according to which part of the auditory system is damaged, the degree or severity of impairment and the configuration or pattern of injury across tones. There are three basic types of hearing loss: conductive hearing loss, sensorineural loss, and mixed hearing loss. Each of these should be approach with assistive devices, such as hearing aids and cochlear implants, so that individual best adapt to managing conversations and take charge of their communication.

2.3.1 Hearing aids

From; tremendous advances in technology of amplification have occurred from the days that ear trumpets and animal horns were used to help to transmit sounds into the ear. A hearing aid is an electroacoustic device that typically fits in or behind the wearer's ear. It is designed to amplify and modulate sound in order to direct the flow of sound into the ear canal, thus enhancing sound quality (Killion, 1997). Hearing aids differ in design, size, ease of handling, volume control, amount of amplification, and the availability of special features such as digitized processing. Their basic functional parts include a microphone to pick up sound and an associated preamplifier, an automatic gain control circuit, a set of active filters, a mixer and power amplifier to make the sound louder, and an output transducer or receiver (a miniature loudspeaker that can be made in integrated form with a field-effect transistor preamplifier) to deliver the amplified sound into the ear. All electronic circuitry is packaged in housing works on a battery. The use of multiple channels in this design provides different compression characteristics for different frequency ranges. Typically, crossover frequencies of the channels and compression characteristics can be adjusted with potentiometers or digital control.

Conventional analog hearing aids are designed for a particular frequency and utilize a fixed or dedicated directional microphone. Although some adjustments are necessary, the aid essentially amplifies all sounds (speech and noise) in the same manner. The directional microphone mode, amplifies sounds from in front more than sounds from other directions. (Berger, 1984).

Analog programmable hearing aids have a microchip that is programed for different listening environments. Program settings depend on the individual's hearing-loss profile, understanding of speech, and range of tolerance for louder sounds (Walden & Walden, 2004). Even with the improvement that analog programmable offer, 25.3% of analog hearing aid users reported that they have a hard time listening in presence of high background noise. Approximately 1% of the users reported difficulty in using the telephone. Examples of environments include quiet conversation in the home, noisy situations such as at a restaurant, or in large areas such as a theater.

In 1996, the Digital signal processing (DSP) chip was introduced into digital programmable hearing aids (Phillips et al., 2007). These hearing aids use digitized sound-processing algorithms to convert sound waves into digital signals. Key benefits of these include improvement in programmability, greater precision in fitting, management of loudness discomfort, control of acoustic feedback, and noise reduction. A processor chip in the aid analyzes the signals to determine whether the sound is noise or speech. It then makes modifications to provide a clear, amplified, distortion-free signal (Clopton & Spelman, 2000).

Digital hearing aids are usually self-adjusting. The digital processing allows for more flexibility in programming the aid. Thus, the sound transmitted matches the patient's specific hearing-loss pattern. This digital technology is more expensive than that of the conventional analog, but it offers many advantages: these generally have a longer life span and may provide better hearing in different listening situations. Some aids can store several programs, i.e., when the listening environment changes, it is possible to change the hearing aid settings. This is usually done by pushing a button on the hearing aid or by using a remote control to switch channels. The aid can be reprogrammed by the Audiologist if the user's hearing or hearing needs change.

Of all of the advances in hearing aid technology in the last several years, perhaps the greatest has been the performance of directional microphones. The use of DSP in hearing aids has opened the door to the many different types of algorithms used in directional microphones. Digital technology offers many options, including automatic, automatic adaptive, multiband automatic adaptive, and, most recently, asymmetric directionality (Kerckhoff, 2008). Each of these options possesses benefits, but some also have limitations and may not prove to be as beneficial to the patient as advertised by hearing aid manufacturers.

Directional microphones were developed in an attempt to improve SNR performance. These microphones can employ different types of polar patterns, some of which have multiple nulls. The fixed directional microphone contains two sound ports and operates by acoustically delaying the signal entering the back microphone port and subtracting this from the signal entering the front port. This creates a null at an azimuth, corresponding to the location where the microphone is least sensitive, and which can be plotted graphically on a polar pattern (Chung, 2004). These patterns are predetermined; thus, the location of sound attenuation always remains the same. Therefore, if the interfering sound is located directly behind the patient, this design acts to attenuate the input level to the hearing aid at the 180° null. If, however, the offending sound arrives from behind but not directly at, 180°, the microphone will be less effective in improving SNR.

Several studies have reported the effectiveness of fixed directional microphones in improving SNR for the hearing aid user by at least 5 dB, (Bilsen et al., 1993). Gravel, Fausel, and Liskow (Gravel et al., 1999) found that children listening with dual microphones achieved a mean improvement of 4.7 dB in SNR when compared with the omnidirectional condition.

Automatic directional microphones were subsequently developed so that patients would not have to bother with manually changing the hearing aid program or setting to the directional microphone mode. Automatic directional microphones utilize an algorithm in which the microphones switch automatically between omnidirectional and directional. Input level, signal location, and SNR are factors that contribute to determining when the microphones switch (Preves & Banerjee, 2008).

The automatic microphone feature works well for patients who do not want to be concerned with manual switching between omnidirectional and directional modes. However, automatic switching can be problematic for patients when the microphone switches but the patient does not prefer switching, or if the switching takes place too rapidly and amplifies unwanted sounds such as a cough or a dog barking (Preves & Banerjee, 2008). The other limitation with automatic directional microphones is that the null is fixed when in the hearing aid is in directional mode. Depending on the location of the noise source and the azimuth of the null in the microphone, there is the possibility that the noise source may not be maximally attenuated.

Although directional microphones have been shown to be successful in the laboratory, there is no guarantee that this success will be achieved in real-life situations for all hearing aid users, due to the difficulty that some persons have in manipulating the hearing aid's controls.

There are four hearing aids styles or configurations. These include the following: the In-the-canal (ITC) style; the In-the-ear (ITE) hearing instruments, which are very easy to operate even if the user has poor dexterity; the behind-the-ear (BTE) style, which is extremely flexible for all hearing loss types, and the Completely-in-the-canal (CIC) style, as depicted in Table 1 (Miller,2006).

HEARING AIDS							
ITC		**ITE**		**BTE**		**CIC**	
Device	User	Device	User	Device	User	Device	User
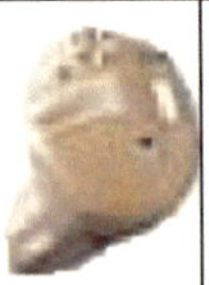	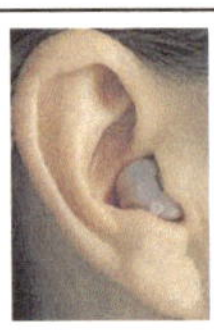	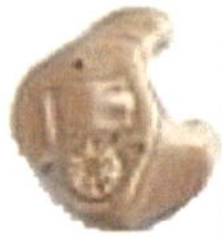	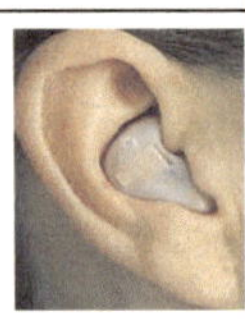	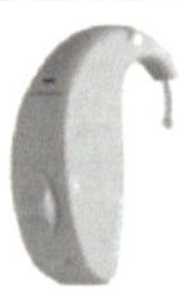	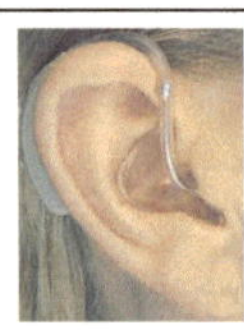	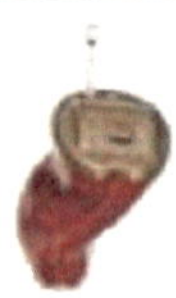	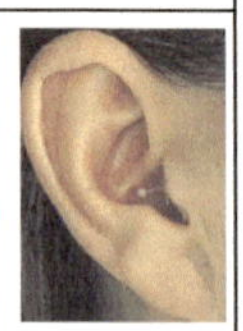

Table 1. Styles of Hearing Aids

There are many manufactures of hearing aids such as Viennatone™, Hansaton™, Bernafon™, Oticon™, Siemens™, Sonic™, Unitron™, and Phonak™. According to the Food and Drug Administration (FDA), the manufacture and sale of hearing aids must meet the following requirements:

1. Dispensers must obtain a written statement from the patient, signed by a licensed physician;
2. A patient aged 18 years or older can sign a waiver for a medical examination, but dispensers must avoid encouraging the patient to waive the medical evaluation requirement;
3. Dispensers must advise patients who appear to have a hearing problem to consult a physician promptly, and
4. FDA regulations also require that an instruction brochure be provided with the hearing aid that illustrates and describes its operation, use, and care.

The FDA Web site that provides standards for hearing aids is at http://www.accessdata.fda.gov/scripts/cdrh/cfdocs/cfStandards/Detail.CFM?STANDARD_IDENTIFICATION_NO=14730

Recent developments in the access to newer forms of wireless transmission and improvements in coupling this technology with hearing aids not only enhance patients' abilities to use telephones or other external devices, but also allow improvement in SNR performance for better speech recognition through noise reduction algorithms.

2.3.2 Cochlear implants

A cochlear implant is a prosthetic inner-ear replacement that provides direct electrical stimulation to the inner ear's auditory nerve, allowing for perception of the sensation of sound. These devices are used for patients with severe-to-profound hearing sensorineural loss who cannot be helped with hearing aids. These implants can benefit patients with bone-conduction thresholds as poor as 65 dB HL. Because of this damage, sound cannot reach the auditory nerve. With a cochlear implant, the damaged hair cells are bypassed and the auditory nerve is electronically stimulated directly (Spitzer, 2010).

Part of the cochlear implant is surgically implanted into the mastoid bone behind the target ear with a titanium screw (osseointegrated material), and a tiny electrode array is inserted into the cochlea at set intervals depending on the number of channels or number of frequency bands to excite (Medical Advisory Secretariat, 2002). The other part of the device is external and includes a microphone, a speech processor, and a transmitter coil.

The signal from the microphone is sent to the speech processor, which comes in two designs. It may be either a BTE model Nucleus Freedom™, which looks like a hearing aid, or a Body-worn device (BWD) that it attached to the belt, for example, the Cordelle II (European Assistive Technology Information Network, 2010), manufactured by Cochlear Deutschland GmbH & Co. KG, as shown in Table 2.

The microphone looks like a BTE hearing aid. It picks up sounds—just as a hearing aid microphone does—and sends these to the speech processor. The speech processor is a computer that analyzes and digitizes the sound signals and sends them to a transmitter worn on the head just behind the ear. The transmitter sends the coded signals to a receiver implanted immediately under the skin. The internal or implanted parts include a receiver and electrodes. The receiver is just under the skin behind the ear. The receiver takes the coded electrical signals from the transmitter and delivers them to the array of electrodes that have been surgically inserted into the cochlea. The electrodes stimulate the fibers of the auditory nerve and sound sensations are perceived. Figure 12 depicts a series of stages of the speech processor of a typical cochlear implant and the associated processing waveforms at each stage (Miller, 2006, as cited in Loizou, 1998).

COCHLEAR IMPLANTS			
BTE		BMD	
Device	User	Device	User
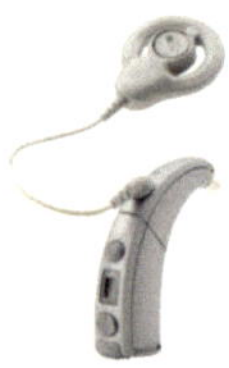	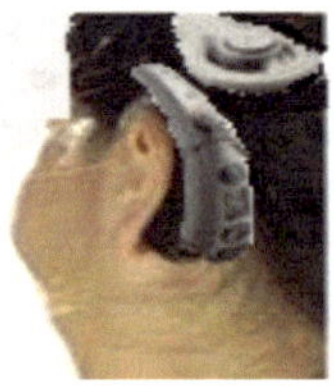	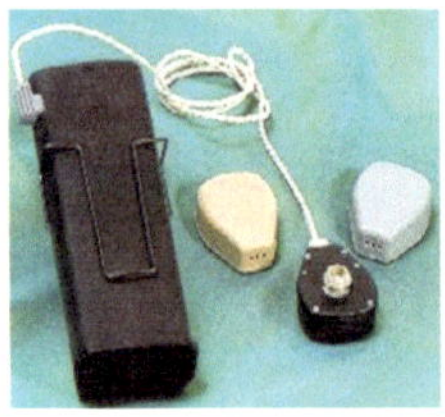	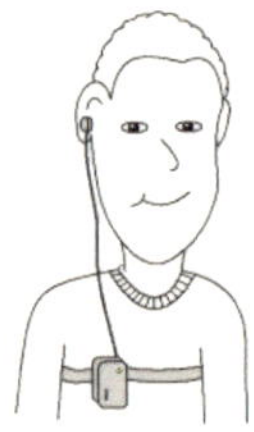

Table 2. Styles of Cochlear Implants.

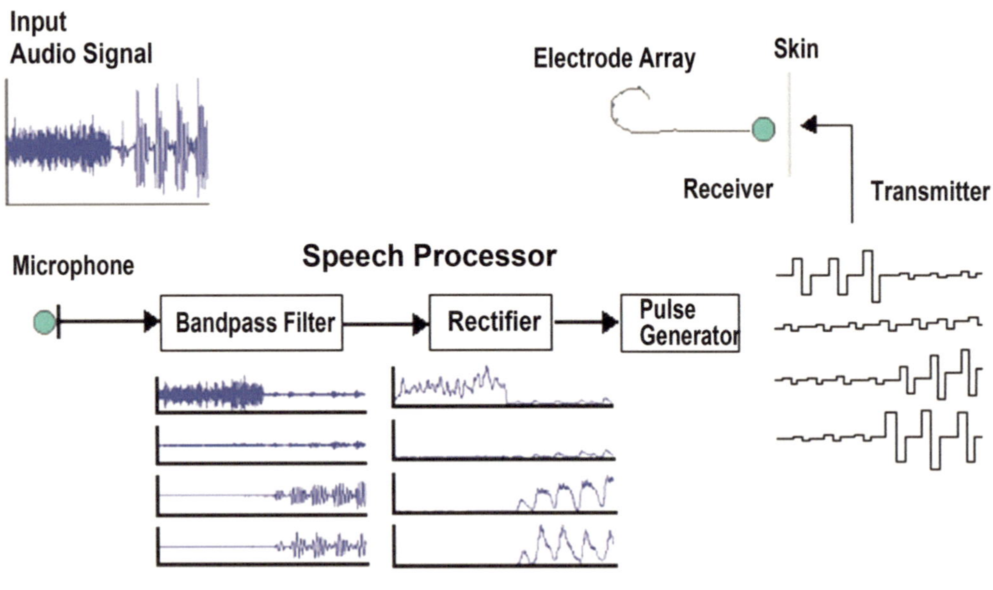

Fig. 12. Block Diagram of a typical cochlear implant and processing waveforms

2.4 Hearing Assistive Technology Systems

Other devices are employed to assist individuals with hearing impairment who have not previously experienced benefit with hearing aids or cochlear implants alone. Hearing assistive technology systems (HATS) are devices that can help patients function better in their day-to-day listening and communication situations. HATS can be used with or without hearing aids or cochlear implants to make hearing easier—and thereby reduce stress and fatigue. HATS must be directed toward resolving any one of the following situations: distance; noise, or reverberation that can create listening problems (Medical Services Advisory Committee, 2010).

2.4.1 FM systems

FM systems operate on special frequencies. A receiver worn around the neck transmits sound to the hearing aid. The sound comes from a transmitter microphone used by a speaker, although in many public places, the transmitter is built into the general sound system.

Because of their flexibility, mobility, and sturdiness, these systems are among the most commonly used HATS. Studies have shown that FM systems have the best results when implementation is carried out early in the amplification-fitting or cochlear-implant process. Also, infrared wireless headset are available for television listening and interface. However, there are other systems, denominated sound-field systems, which assist listening for all of the children in the classroom. The teacher speaks into a microphone transmitter and his/her voice is projected through speakers mounted around the classroom.

2.4.2 High-frequency hearing loss

Newer devices, such as the BAHA™ system manufactured by Entific Medical (Medical Advisory Secretariat, 2002) have been developed for patients diagnosed with unilateral profound sensorineural hearing loss, also referred to as single-sided deafness. Other devices have been designed for patients exhibiting severe high-frequency transposition hearing loss and comprise self-learning features on hearing aids and cochlear implants that allow integrate of actual measurements. Finally, an infrared wireless headset is used with television for listening at a higher volume than others sitting in the same room. Bluetooth interface allows persons to hear telephone conversations more easily, amplifying any devices that employ this technology.

3. Conclusion

The present section provided a brief guide on equipment for diagnosis of deafness and hearing assistive technology.

Although, audiology equipment for evoked potentials and otoacoustic emissions provides highly relevant information deriving from hearing damage, in future, new technological developments should be directed toward improving the hearing test. The research will continue to study algorithms for more accurate, physically realistic modeling of the cochlea, which should assist in the process of diagnosing local inner-ear problems.

Audiometers, Tympanometers and other electronic equipment for hearing diagnosis must be designed taking into account specific data formats, communication protocols and interoperability standards, as such HL7 (Health Level Seven) to send data from audiology equipment to electronic medical record, then it is possible to share and use data for research and clinical propose.

Potential areas for improving hearing aids and cochlear implants include frequency response by analyzing sound across several bands, enhancing the signal-to-noise ratio with adaptive filtering, installing additional detectors for monitoring the environment. Subsequently applying average algorithms to turn the acoustic signal into a frequency map and for the application of noise reduction while maintaining high gain in bands in which speech is detected., will improve speech understanding in noise.

For patient with nerve deafness, one goal is to restore hearing with cochlear electrode implants in order to stimulate the nerve endings directly. However, despite electrode stimulation of nerves at the correct place along the cochlea, the perception of high frequency has not been achieved to date.

Finally, the research on FM and infrared systems, Bluetooth adaptors, and other novel communication techniques and devices continues for helping patient to achieve greater comfort, higher satisfaction-of-fit and less fatigue, when he/she is exposed to a noisy environment

4. Acknowledgment

We thank the staff of the Department of Biomedical Engineering as well as that of the Audiology and Electrodiagnosis Services for the support received in the collection of information.

5. References

Acoustic Systems MD. (2000). International. Audiometric Testing Suites Field Performance Verification, Instruction Manual, pp.(2)

Aguilera, S.; Pescador, F.; Godino, JI. & Novillo R. (1997). Improvement of a Spanish Speech Processing System. In: *Advancement of Assistive Technology*, Anogianahis G., Bühler CH. & Soede M., pp.(115-119), IOS Press Ohmsha, ISBN:9051993617

Aitkin, L. (1990). *The Auditory Cortex: Structural and Functional Bases of Auditory Perception*, Chapman and Hall, ISBN:04123249039780412324901, London; New York

ASTM E336 - 10. (2011). Standard Test Method for Measurement of Airborne Sound Attenuation between Rooms in Buildings, available from: http://www.astm.org/Standards/E336.htm

Australian Hearing Group. (2001). Manual of Speech Perception. National Acoustic Laboratories, pp. (10-32), available from: http://www.nal.gov.au/dvd-cd-report_tab_manual-of-speech-perception.shtml

Berger, KW. (1984). The hearing aid, its operation and development, In: *The Hearing Aid. 3rd* ed. Thieme Medical Publishers, ISBN:0387955836

Bilsen, F.; Soede, W. & Berkhout, A. (1993). Development and assessment of two fixed-array microphones for use with hearing aids. *Journal of Rehabilitative Research Dev*, Vol. 3, No.1, pp.(73–81), ISSN:0748-711

Buller, G. & Saβ, T. (1997). Implementing a Signal Processing Subsystem to Detect Stimulated Otoacoustic Emissions Using the TMS320C31 DSP. Texas Instrument., pp.(9-15), USA

Buz, A. & Bower, Ch. (2009). Hearing Assessment in Infants and Children: Recommendations Beyond Neonatal Screening. *Pediatrics* Vol. 12, No.1, (September 2009), pp.(40-52), ISSN: 0031-4005

Campbell, J.; Graley, J.; Meinke, D.; Vaughan, L.; Aungst, R. & Madison, T. (2010). Guidelines for Manual Pure-Tone Threshold Audiometry, In: ASHA Main Page, 2011, Available from: http://www.asha.org/docs/html/GL2005-00014.html

Choi, Y. (2011). Method and Apparatus for Measuring Otoacoustic Emission. Patent Application Publication, No. US2011/0166806A1, (Jul 7, 2011), pp.(1-12), available from: patents.com/us-20110166806.html

Chung, K. (2004). Challenges and recent developments in hearing aids: Part I. Speech understanding in noise, microphone technologies and noise reduction algorithms. Trends in Amplification, Vol. 1 No. 1, pp.(83–124), ISSN:1084-7138

Clopton, B. & Spelman F. (2000). Auditory System, In: *The Biomedical Engineering Handbook*, Bronzino, J., pp. (83-95), CRC IEEE PRESS, ISBN: 0-8493-0461-X, Boca Raton Florida USA

European Assistive Technology Information Network. (2010). Assistive Technology Products. EASTIN Group. Available from: http://www.eastin.eu/en-GB/searches/products/detail/database-rehadat/product-897460

Ghani, J.; Ellermeier, W. & Karin Zimmer K. (2005). A test battery measuring auditory capabilities of listening panels, *Proceedings of Forum Acusticum*, ISSNs: 1610-1928, Budapest, Hungary, (August 29 - September 2 2005)

Goldfain, E.; Slawson, S.; Andreassen, E.; Kuiper, C.; Staples, E. & Lia R. (2008). Otoscope. United States Patent No. 7399275, pp.(1-13), available from: http://patents.justia.com/2008/index.html

Gravel, J., Fausel, N., & Liskow, C. (1999). Children's speech recognition in noise using omnidirectional and dual microphone hearing aid technology. *Ear and Hearing*, Vol. 20, No. 1, pp.(1–11), ISSN:01960202

Gutiérrez, J.; Barraza, FE.; Guadarrama, A.; Núñez, MA.; Delgado, RE. & Gutiérrez, I. (2009) Communication Interface and Graphic Module for Audiometry Equipment. *Biomedical Instrumentation & Technology*. Vol. 43, No. 6, (December, 2009), pp.(484-488), ISSN: 0899-8205-43.6.484

Halpin, C. (2007). Something new for the audiogram: Alternative symbol developed for response at limit. *The ASHA Leader,* (2007, Jan. 23), Vol. 12 No 1, pp.(5-19)

Heller, J.; Kugler, A.; Longacre, A. & Williams, D. (August 25, 1987). Tympanometer Portatil. United States Patent No. 4688582, available from: es.patents.com/us-4688582.html

Hearing Instrument Manufacturers' Software Association. (2000). NOAH System Software In: User´s NOAH Manual, HIMSA, pp.(6-25) Version 3. A/S

Janušauskas, A.; Maroza, V. & Lukoševicius A. (2006). The Hilbert–Huang Transform for Detection of Otoacoustic Emissions and Time–Frequency Mapping, *Informatica*, Vol. 17, No. 1, (March 2006), pp.(25–38), ISSN:0868-4952

Kerckhoff, J.; Listenberger, J. & Valente, M. (2008). Advances in Hearing Aid Technology. *Communication Science and Disorders*, Vol. 35, pp.(102–112), ISSN:1092-5171

Khandpur, R.S. (2005). *Biomedical Instrumentation Technology and Applications,* Ed. McGrawHill, ISSN: 0071447849 9780071447843, New York USA

Killion, MC. (1997). Hearing aids: Past, present, future and moving toward normal conversation in noise. *British Journal of Audiology,* Vol. 31, No. 3, (October 1997), pp.(141–148), ISSN:0300-5364

Loizou, PC. (1998). Introduction to cochlear implants. *IEEE Signal Processing Mag,* ISSN:0739-5175, (September 1998), pp.(101–130)

Madsen Electronics. (2004). 922Orbiter In: *Operation Manual of Clinical Audiometer*. MADSEN, pp.(102-105), Version 2.X. Part No.7-26-110, Doc. No. 7-26-1100/0, Copenhagen, Denmark

MAICO. (2007). Operating Instructions Race Car Tympanometer. 1162-0703 Rev A, pp.4-15.

Marullo, T.; Mazza, G. & Bianchi, F. (1967). Evaluation of vocal acumetry. *PubMed:* 5612940, Vol. 43 No. 4, (August 1967), pp.(217-243),ISSN:0899-8205

Medical Advisory Secretariat. (2002). Bone anchored hearing aid: an evidence based analysis. Ontario Health Technology Assessment Series Vol. 2, No.3

Medical Service Advisory Committe. (2010). Middle ear implant for sensorineural, conductie and mixed hearing losses, Cormmonwalth of Australia, (November, 2010), ISBN: 978-1-74241-348-8

Miller, G. (2006). *Sensory Organ Replacement and Repair,* (1st Edition), Ed Morgan & Claypool Publishers' Series, ISBN:1598290630, San Rafael, CA USA

Montano, J. & Spitzer, J. (2009). *Adult Audiologic Rehabilitation,* Ed Plural Publishing, ISBN: 9781597562508, San Diego, CA USA

National Health and Nutrition Examination Survey. (2003). Audiometry Procedures Manual, (January 2003), pp.(2.1-2.55)

Penhaker, M. & Kijonka J. (2011). Audiometry for Teaching Experiment in PowerLabSystems, In: Electrical Power Systems and Computers, Xiaofeng W, pp.(831-838), Springer-Verlag, ISBN:978-3-642-21746-3, Berlín

Phillips, W.; Knight, L.; Caldwell, N. & Warrington, J. (2007). Policy through procurement—The introduction of digital signal process (DSP) hearing aids into the English NHS. *Health Policy,* Vol. 4, No. 1, pp.(77–85), ISSN:0168-8510

Preves, D. & Banerjee, S. (2008). Hearing aid instrumentation signal processing and electroacoustic testing. In: *Audiology treatment,* Valente, M.; Hosford-Dunn, H. & Roeser, R., pp.(1–35), Thieme Medical, New York USA, ISBN:978-3-13

Salesa, E.; Bonavida, A. & Perelló, J. (2005). *Tratado de Audiología,* (1a Edición), Elsevier-Masson., ISBN: 844581554-7, Madrid España

Spitzer, JB. (2010) Implantable Devices for Rehabilitation of Persons with Hearing Loss. In : *Implantable Technologies. Seminars in Hearing,* Spitzer JB., pp.(3-6), Thieme-Stratton, New York USA, ISSN:0734-0451

Steele, CH.; Baker, G.; Tolomeo, J. & Zetes-Tolomeo D. (2000). Cochlear Mechanics, In: *The Biomedical Engineering Handbook,* Bronzino, J., pp. (581-594), CRC IEEE PRESS, ISBN 0-8493-0461-X, Boca Raton Florida USA

Walden, T. & Walden, B. (2004). Predicting success with hearing aids in everyday living. *Journal of the American Academy of Audiology,* Vo. 15, No. 5, pp. (342–352), ISSN:1050-0545

2

Contralateral Suppression of Otoacoustic Emissions: Working Towards a Simple Objective Frequency Specific Test for Hearing Screening

Nikolaus E. Wolter[1], Robert V. Harrison[2] and Adrian L. James[3]
[1]*Department Otolaryngology, Head and Neck Surgery, University of Toronto*
[2]*Hospital for Sick Children, Department of Otolaryngology – Head and Neck Surgery, Department of Neurosciences and Mental Health, University of Toronto*
[3]*Hospital for Sick Children, Department of Otolaryngology – Head and Neck Surgery, University of Toronto*
Canada

1. Introduction

Hearing loss affects all demographics regardless of geographical location or age. In a similar fashion to how hearing loss can isolate post-lingualy deaf adults, hearing loss in the pediatric population has profound detrimental effects despite the richness of the deaf culture. A complete discussion of the adverse effects of hearing loss must include discussion of this important component of the deaf and hearing impaired population. The World Health Organization defines "disabling hearing impairment" in children under the age of 15 years as an unaided hearing threshold level in the better ear of 31 dB HL or more using pure tone averages at 0.5, 1, 2 and 4 kHz. The prevalence of childhood hearing loss is 1.2 to 1.7 cases per 1000 live births and the prevalence increases up to 6 years of age as a result of meningitis, delayed onset of genetic hearing loss, or delayed diagnosis (Kral & O'Donoghue, 2010). In the majority of cases of childhood hearing loss is congenital with a smaller proportion being progressive or acquired (A. Davis & Wood, 1992; A. Davis et al., 1997).The prevalence is greater still in developing countries because of lack of immunization, exposure to ototoxic drugs, and consanguinity (Kral & O'Donoghue, 2010). Profound hearing loss (hearing loss > 90 dB) has far-reaching, lifelong consequences in children (Kral & O'Donoghue, 2010). Andrej *et al.* report that there can be a restriction in learning and literacy as a result of the lack of development of spoken language with its impact on daily communication (Kral & O'Donoghue, 2010; Marschark & Wauters, 2008). This in turn has been shown to substantially compromise educational achievement and employment opportunity later in life (Allen, 1986; A. Davis et al., 1997; Schroeder et al., 2006; Thompson et al., 2001; Wake, Hughes, Poulakis, Collins, & Rickards, 2004a). The detrimental effects of profound hearing loss in children are summarized in Table 1. Unless children are afforded opportunities to develop language, deaf children can fall behind their hearing peers in communication, cognition, literacy and psychosocial development (Holden-Pitt & Albertorio, 1998).

Speech and language development
Academic achievement
Social-emotional development
Childhood behavioral problems
Comprised employment opportunities in later life
Self-perceived health status

*(Allen, 1986; A. Davis et al., 1997; Kral & O'Donoghue, 2010; Marschark & Wauters, 2008; Schroeder et al., 2006; Thompson et al., 2001; Wake, Hughes, Poulakis, Collins, & Rickards, 2004a)

Table 1. Detrimental Effects of Profound Hearing Loss in Childhood*

The widespread use of universal neonatal hearing screening has been established based on the growing body of evidence that early detection of hearing loss leads to early aural rehabilitation (Kennedy, McCann, Campbell, Kimm, & Thornton, 2005). Multiple studies have demonstrated the deleterious effect of bilateral hearing loss on speech and language development (Allen, 1986; A. Davis et al., 1997; Thompson et al., 2001; Wake, Hughes, Poulakis, Collins, & Rickards, 2004b). However if caught early, the effects of hearing loss are somewhat mitigated. Yoshinaga-Itano *et al.* reported on the ability of early detection of hearing loss to improve language development as measured by standardized testing (Yoshinaga-Itano, Sedey, Coulter, & Mehl, 1998; Yoshinaga-Itano, 2003). Children enrolled into language programs at earlier ages have improved vocabulary and verbal reasoning skills on standardized tests at 5 years of age (Moeller, 2000) Opponents to Universal screening cite the great cost of such widespread screening as well as efficacy in earlier years. From a pragmatic, fiduciary perspective, a cost-effectiveness study has shown that as a result of special education needs, failure to detect severe-to-profound hearing loss can cost the educational system approximately $38 000 - 240 000 (USD) per child over their educational lifetime (Mohr et al., 2000). It would seem then that detecting these children would offset a significant amount of the cost. Furthermore, in areas that have adapted a Universal Newborn Hearing protocol, detection of congenital hearing loss has nearly doubled since its introduction (Choo & Meinzen-Derr, 2010).

It is clear that the early detection of hearing loss has strong developmental, psychosocial and societal implications as well. Therefore, in 2007 the American Academy of Pediatrics' Joint Committee on Infant hearing endorsed the early detection of hearing loss with an aim at early intervention to improve linguistic competence and literary development (Busa et al., 2007). They recommended that all infants should be screened prior to 1 month of age. Children identified with hearing loss by screening should have a comprehensive audiological assessment by 3 months of age. After audiological assessment, children with confirmed hearing loss should receive appropriate intervention by dedicated hearing loss health care and education professionals not later than 6 months of age. Children with risk factors for hearing loss (a summary of commonly cited risk factors can be found in Table 2.) should be followed by on-going surveillance starting at 2 months of age. Unfortunately in many centers the "lost to follow up" rates approach 40% of infants who do not pass their infant screening (Choo & Meinzen-Derr, 2010). All centers must work diligently to ensure children who fail their hearing screen are referred appropriately to maximize their potential and mitigate the lifelong effects of hearing loss. The following sections will provide an overview of existing neonatal hearing screening tests and use of the medial olivocochlear system as a potential new screening method.

Craniofacial syndromes: Crouzon disease, Klippel-Feil syndrome, and Goldenhar syndrome
Syndromes known to be associated with sensorineural hearing loss: Brancho-oto-renal syndrome, Pendred syndrome, Wardenburg syndrome, Treacher-Collins, Stickler syndrome, Usher syndrome
Neurodegenerative disorders: Hunter syndrome, Friedrich's ataxia, Charcot-Marie-Tooth syndrome
Trauma
Extracorporeal membrane oxygenation
Chemotherapy
Consanguinity
Family history of hearing loss
Neonatal hyperbilirubinemia
Neonatal intensive care unit admission for > 5 days
Infection and neonatal sepsis: CMV, measles, mumps, rubella, *H influenzae* type b, and childhood meningitis, toxoplasmosis, herpes, syphilis, bacterial meningitis
Genetic mutations

*(Busa et al., 2007; Manchaiah, Zhao, Danesh, & Duprey, 2011)

Table 2. Risk factors for childhood hearing loss*

2. Existing neonatal hearing tests

The difficulty of testing young individuals using subjective methods has lead to the development of hearing testing based on objective methods such as otoacoustic emissions and auditory brainstem response testing (James, 2011; Thompson et al., 2001).

2.1 Auditory evoked potentials

Measurement of auditory evoked potentials (AEP) has been possible since the 1960s. AEPs represent electrical activity occurring along the length of the auditory pathway. They are typically described by their latency from the onset of the auditory stimulus: early (0 to 15 milliseconds), middle (15 to 100 milliseconds) and late (100 to 500 milliseconds). Auditory brainstem responses (ABR) appear to be the most clinically useful early latency AEPs for detecting hearing loss in newborns and infants (Hecox 1974). Hecox *et al.* first speculated on the use of Auditory Brainstem Responses (ABR) as an objective method of assessing infant hearing in 1974 (Hecox & Galambos, 1974). Measurement of ABR makes use of the summation of action potentials from the cochlear nerve to the inferior colliculus of the midbrain in response to a click stimulus applied to the test ear. Since that time the use of ABR has become a widely accepted method to assess auditory function and hearing sensitivity. The commonly cited advantages and disadvantages of ABR are summarized in Table 3.

Screening ABR utilizes a click or tone pip stimulus presented via a headphone or a transducer inserted into the subject's ear. Click stimuli are commonly used and make use of a broad range of frequencies (1 - 6 kHz) but do not provide information about hearing in lower frequencies (Jacobson & Jacobson, 2004) . If necessary, tone pips can be used to acquire frequency specific information (Jacobson & Jacobson, 2004). The subject is prepared with three surface electrodes placed on the forehead and both mastoids or earlobes. The electrodes detect click or tone pip-induced action potentials that are generated in the cochlea. The signal is transmitted from along the cochlear nerve from the cochlear nucleus to the inferior colliculus. The amplitude of the action potential is measured in microvolts and averaged. The averaged potential is then plotted against time to create a waveform with characteristic peaks labeled I-VII (Table 4). Only waves I and II correspond to true action potentials. Waves III-VII are thought to represent post-synaptic activity in the major brainstem auditory centres. Given the necessity of electrode placement and duration of approximately 15 minutes, sedation is often required (Kral & O'Donoghue, 2010). The morphology and latency of the wave form is compared to a normal wave form and a pass or fail result is generated. The sensitivity of ABR is generally quoted as 84-100% and the specificity is 99.7% (A. Davis et al., 1997; Hall, Smith, & Popelka, 2004; Llanes & Chiong, 2004).

2.2 Otoacoustic emissions

Initially hypothesized in 1948 by the theoretical physicist Thomas Gold and later confirmed by Kemp in 1978, Otoacoustic emissions (OAE) now provide an important non-invasive method of auditory testing (Gold, 1948; Kemp, 1978b). OAEs are acoustic signals generated by the activity of the outer hair cells of the cochlea that occur during normal hearing. Control of outer hair cell activity is intimately linked with the olivocochlear pathway and will be discussed further in later sections. In brief, the mechanical energy generated by the outer hair cells propagates backward to the tympanic membrane. Movements of the tympanic membrane in turn produce acoustic signals that can be detected by an extremely sensitive microphone placed in the external ear canal. The presence of OAEs demonstrates the presence of functional outer hair cells suggesting the presence of a cochlea which forms the basis of this screening method. Testing of OAEs is simple and efficient requiring approximately 10 minutes. Sensitivity and specificity of OAE testing for hearing impairment ranges from 76.9-98% and 90% respectively (A. Davis et al., 1997; Llanes & Chiong, 2004; Thompson et al., 2001).

Different types of OAE can be detected but only some are useful in hearing testing (Saurini, Nola, & Lendvai, 2004). Spontaneous OAEs are obtained without any acoustic simulation. They are narrow band signals present in 40-70% of normal ears. Evoked OAEs are stimulated by acoustic signals and comprise a range of subtypes. Sustained frequency OAEs are obtained by continuous acoustic stimuli and are found in approximately 94% of people. Their measurement is typically complex and is not used very often. Transient OAEs are stimulated by clicks or tone bursts. Distortion Product OAEs (DPOAE) are produced in response to the simultaneous presentation of two stimuli and can be found in up to 98% of normal hearing individuals. As suggested by the name, stimuli for DPOAE consist of the combination of two stimuli that vary by frequency (f_1 and f_2) and intensity (L_1 and L_2). Varying the relationship of f_1 and f_2 and L_1 and L_2 determine the frequency response. Achieving an optimal response is usually obtained by setting L_1 equal or greater than L_2 e.g.

65 and 55 dBL SPL respectively are commonly used. Responses are usually the most robust when recorded at the frequency $2f_1$-f_2. Transient OAE testing applies a brief click to the test ear to elicit the hair cell response. As such, Transient OAE measurement lacks frequency specificity (Jacobson & Jacobson, 2004). Conversely, stimulus tones used in DPOAE testing combine frequency stimuli in a predictable way that can measure specific regions of the cochlea allowing frequency specific testing (Jacobson & Jacobson, 2004). While OAEs have been widely adapted for newborn hearing screening programs, they are still only surrogate markers for hearing. Their presence indicates normal function of the outer hair cell, middle ear and ear canal. As such, conditions such as auditory neuropathy, cochlear nerve hypoplasia or inner hair cell anomalies can be missed and may lead to delay in diagnosis and initiation of aural rehabilitation.

	Advantage	**Disadvantage**
Otoacoustic Emissions	Simple administration - minimal training required	Only asses outer hair cell function
	Cost-effective	Debris or fluid in the external ear may affect results
	Results are immediately available	Failure rates are high during first 24 hours after birth
	Average screening time is less than ABR	No use in fluid filled middle ear
		Requires quiet environment
		Sensitivity - may fail to detect infants with very mild hearing loss or central auditory pathologies
Automated auditory brainstem response	Assess greater extent of auditory system	Requires more operator knowledge than ABR
	Requires no interpretation by the screener	ABR may be susceptible to electrical interference
	ABR results are less affected by middle ear or external ear debris than OAEs	Sensitivity - may fail to detect Infants with very mild hearing loss
	Results are immediately available	Requires long period of time
	May detect neural or central auditory pathologies	Cost
		May take longer in noisy environment
		Patient must be sleeping
		Potential for electrical and noise artifact

Table 3. Advantages and Disadvantages of Existing Hearing screening methods

Wave I	**Action potential arising from afferent activity of cochlear nerve entering internal auditory canal**
Wave II	**Action potential arising from proximal cochlear nerve entering brainstem**
Wave III	**Arise from second order neurons beyond the cochlear nerve in the cochlear nucleus**
Wave IV	**Arise from third order neurons located in the superior olivary complex**
Wave V	**Multiple anatomic origins postulated in the vicinity of the inferior colliculus**
Wave VI	**Arise from medial geniculate body**
Wave VII	**Arise from medial geniculate body**

Table 4. Characteristic auditory brainstem response waves

3. Auditory neuropathy spectrum disorder (ANSD)

One disorder that continuously eludes the new born hearing screen is ANSD. ANSD represents a range of hearing disorders of variable severity which present with pure tone hearing thresholds that may be low or approach normal, but underestimate the subject's perception of hearing difficulty. Included within the spectrum are inner hair cell anomalies, neuropathy of the auditory nerve, disruption of the olivocochlear response (OCR), and brainstem dysfunction that can be secondary to kernicterus (Amatuzzi et al., 2001; Berlin et al., 2005; Harrison, 1998; Hood & Berlin, 2001; Shapiro, 2003; Starr, Picton, Sininger, Hood, & Berlin, 1996; Yasunaga et al., 1999).The unifying feature of ANSD diseases are a characteristic finding of abnormal ABR waveforms in the presence of normal OAE and/or cochlear microphonic (CM). Middle ear muscle reflexes and the olivocochlear reponse are also absent. These findings are suggestive of persistent outer hair cell activity but lack of a normal afferent auditory pathway and as such would be missed by currently employed screening methods (Manchaiah et al., 2011). Accurate diagnosis is hampered by the lack of a simple commercially available test for OCR function but typically the diagnosis can be assumed from OAE and ABR results alone.

Etiologies of ANSD that have been identified include polyneuropathy (especially in adults), perinatal anoxia and hypoxia, and hyperbilirubinaemia, congenital brain anomalies, ototoxic drug exposure, and genetic factors. An estimated 40% of cases have an underlying genetic basis, which can be inherited in both syndromic and non-syndromic conditions (Harrison, 2001; Manchaiah et al., 2011; Nadol Jr, 2001; Starr et al., 1996).

Treatment options in ANSD include auditory verbal therapy, cued speech, hearing aids and cochlear implantation (Cone-Wesson, Rance, & Sininger, 2001; Rance & Barker, 2008a; Hood & Berlin, 2001). Prognostication and predicting treatment outcome is difficult and varies depending on origin. Some forms of neonatal ANSD can show significant spontaneous improvement (Attias & Raveh, 2007; Rance & Barker, 2008b). As such determination of patient who will benefit from hearing aids or cochlear implantation is difficult (Raveh, Buller, Badrana, & Attias, 2007). The development of improved testing techniques that can be used to diagnose, characterize, and differentiate between the numerous diseases that make up this spectrum may allow patients to be treated earlier.

4. The olivocochlear pathway

4.1 Neuroanatomy and physiology

Cochlear function including the sensitivity and frequency tuning of the peripheral auditory system is influenced by incoming acoustic stimuli but also higher cochlear function. The olivocochlear pathway is a neural pathway which innervates cochlear outer hair cells (OHC), linking the superior olivary complex to the cochlea. Further insights into this pathway may improve our ability to screen for various forms of hearing loss such as ANSD.

The olivocochlear neural pathway is comprised of efferent neurons that travel from the superior olivary complex in the brainstem to cochlear hair cells. First described in 1946, Rasmussen (Rasmussen, 1946) traced the neural fibres from the floor of the fourth ventricle, along the inferior and superior vestibular nerves, then into the cochlear nerve in the bundle of Oort (the vestibulocochlear anastomosis). Later he confirmed passage of the pathway into the cochlea and named it the olivocochlear bundle (Rasmussen, 1953). This neural pathway, the olivocochlear efferent pathway, is now thought to play an important role in the olivocochlear reflex. There appear to be two forms of olivocochlear efferent fibres, medial olivocochlear (MOC) and lateral olivocochlear (LOC) efferents. The majority are the thin, unmyelinated fibres of the LOC system arising from the lateral superior olive and travel via the vestibular nerve to the cochlea where they innervate the auditory nerve supplying the inner hair cells (Kimura & Wersäll, 1962; Warr, 1975). While the LOC system received contributions from both sides of the brainstem, the majority of fibres innervate the ipsilateral cochlea (Guinan Jr, 2006). Thick, myelinated neurons of the MOC pathway originate in the medial part of the superior olivary complex. A portion of fibres cross the midline to the contralateral cochlea while others project to the ipsilateral cochlea both via the vestibular nerves (Guinan Jr, 2006). Within the cochlea the MOC fibres innervate the outer hair cells; this is referred to as the medial olivocochlear system (MOCS). The MOCS is innervated by ascending and descending neural pathways. Descending innervations arises from the inferior colliculus and auditory cortex (Mulders & Robertson, 2000a; Mulders & Robertson, 2000b).

Ascending innervation arises predominantly from the contralateral cochlea, by way of inter-neurons which cross the brainstem from cochlear nucleus to the olivary complex (Brown, Venecia, & Guinan, 2003; Morest, 1973; Ye, Machado, & Kim, 2000). The majority of MOCS fibres cross back over the midline to innervate the cochlea from which innervation is received (Azeredo et al., 1999; M. Liberman & Brown, 1986). A smaller proportion of MOCS fibers do not travel back across the brainstem and therefore innervate the cochlea on the same side. As they are stimulated by signals from the contralateral ear they provide a mechanism by which stimulation of one ear can influence the detection of acoustic signals by the other ear (Azeredo et al., 1999; Warren III & Liberman, 1989a).

4.2 Physiology of the olivocochlear pathway

Despite decades of investigation since the discovery of the olivocochlear pathway, understanding of its purpose remains somewhat speculative (Rasmussen, 1946). Proposed roles include protection against noise-induced hearing loss, enhancement of discrimination of sound in noise, or a role predominantly during development of the auditory pathway (Micheyl, Khalfa, Perrot, & Collet, 1997; Rajan & Johnstone, 1988; Walsh, McGee, McFadden, & Liberman, 1998).

There are a few studies of inter-cochlear interaction in humans which are consistent with MOCS functioning to reduce sensitivity of the cochlea to auditory stimuli. For example, contralateral pure tone stimulation causes a reduction of compound action potentials (Folsom & Owsley, 1987). Contralateral narrow band noise causes a 'negativation' of the summating potential response to ipsilateral tone bursts (i.e. the negative amplitude of summating potential increases) (Innitzer & Ehrenberger, 1977). There are indications that cortical function (e.g. visual or auditory attention tasks) influences olivocochlear activity via descending neural pathways (Froehlich, Collet, & Morgon, 1993; Maison, Durrant, Gallineau, Micheyl, & Collet, 2001).

Much more information on olivocochlear function has come from electrophysiological studies in animal models. Various investigations have supported the conclusion that MOCS activity turns down the gain of the cochlear amplifier (Siegel & Kim, 1982). The cochlear amplifier is an active process within the cochlea in which motor activity of OHCs increases sensitivity of the cochlea, by amplification of the basilar membrane motion induced by acoustic energy. With electrical stimulation of the olivocochlear bundle (OCB) in the floor of 4th ventricle, the amplitude of the compound action potential of the auditory nerve induced by auditory stimuli is reduced (Galambos, 1956; Nieder & Nieder, 1970; Wiederhold & Peake, 1966). In this way, the threshold of the auditory nerve can be increased by as much as 25dB an effect referred to as the 'level shift' (Galambos, 1956). By using focal simulation near the cell bodies of olivocochlear fibers, it has been shown that MOCS mediates this effect (i.e., via action on OHCs), rather than LOCS (Gifford & Guinan Jr, 1987). Electrical stimulation of the OCB increases the cochlear microphonic and causes a decrease in the electrical impedance of scala media of the guinea pig (Mountain, Daniel Geisler, & Hubbard, 1980). These changes are considered to be due to hyperpolarization of outer hair cells (Art, Fettiplace, & Fuchs, 1984; Mountain et al., 1980). Thus electrical stimulation of MOCS suppresses OHC activity so dampening basilar membrane motion and reducing cochlear amplification. This has an indirect effect on IHC activity, as demonstrated by the level shift.

Contralateral acoustic stimulation (CAS) has been found to elicit similar effects to electrical stimulation of the MOCS. This was first reported by Fex, who found that CAS increased the cochlear microphonic (Fex, 1962). Recording from the round window in cats, Liberman showed that the compound action potential generated by ipsilateral tone pips was suppressed by contralateral noise or tones. Sectioning of the olivocochlear bundle in the floor of 4th ventricle or in the inferior vestibular nerve abolished this contralateral suppression effect (M. C. Liberman, 1989; Warren III & Liberman, 1989b). Such studies clearly show that the MOCS is stimulated by ascending signals from the auditory pathway.

Descending neural pathways also contribute to the MOCS. This has been shown in humans by increased MOCS activity when attention is focused on acoustic signals (Maison, Micheyl, & Collet, 2001). Animal studies have shown that electrical stimulation of the inferior colliculus increases MOCS activity (Mulders & Robertson, 2000a; Scates, Woods, & Azeredo, 1999). Axonal transport studies also suggest that MOCS neurons are innervated directly by neurons arising in the auditory cortex (Mulders & Robertson, 2000b). Though giving insight into olivocochlear activity electrophysiological studies have many limitations (Collet et al., 1990). Sectioning experiments, especially at the level of the floor of 4th ventricle, are imprecise and are not fully selective for efferents (though their effectiveness has been carefully demonstrated (M. C. Liberman, 1989; Warren III & Liberman, 1989b)). Electrical stimuli provide global stimulation, and in the floor of the 4th ventricle may simulate both crossed and uncrossed medial efferents that loop close to the midline (however, the LOCS is probably less easily stimulated this way as its fibers are unmyelinated). The main disadvantage with electrical stimulation is that it does not necessarily reflect normal cochlear input/output activity. Stimulation is often at supraphysiological levels, and provides unnatural synchronization and frequency of stimulation. Results can be confounded by stimulation artifact. Also neither sectioning nor electrical stimulation can be applied to humans, which limits extrapolation of findings from the animal models. The opportunity to study the MOCS non-invasively in animal models and humans was facilitated by the discovery of otoacoustic emissions (OAEs) (Kemp, 1978a).

The function of the LOCS is not well understood. Some groups have proposed a role in providing "binaural balance" for sound localization has been proposed (Darrow, Maison, & Liberman, 2006; Guinan Jr, 2006). Studies to confirm this hypothesis are still needed.

5. New technology

5.1 Frequency specificity in the Medial Olivocochlear System (MOCS)

It is now well established that the sensitivity and frequency tuning of the peripheral auditory system is influenced by the cochlear efferent neural pathways (Guinan Jr, 2006). Activation of the MOCS by acoustic stimulation of the contralateral ear has been shown to suppress sensitivity of the cochlea, for example by reduction in cochlear nerve action potential amplitude (Fex, 1962). It is considered that this effect is mediated by suppression of the cochlear amplifier effect of OHC activity (Siegel & Kim, 1982). It is likely that relatively specific stimulus conditions are required for efferents to play a role in hearing (M. C. Liberman, 1988), but despite intensive investigation, the nature of this role remains unclear. Further assessment of how the MOCS is activated by different stimuli should improve understanding of this issue (Maison, Micheyl, Andéol, Gallégo, & Collet, 2000).

Tonotopicity of the MOCS has been clearly demonstrated in recordings from single olivocochlear fibers in the cat and guinea pig (Brown, 1989; Cody & Johnstone, 1982; M. Liberman & Brown, 1986). In these studies, efferent neural tuning curves were derived by measuring firing rate in response to contralateral tones of different frequency, and were found to have a shape and sharpness similar to cochlear afferent tuning curves. In addition, horseradish peroxidase injection was used to reveal the projection of some fibers, and in all cases they terminated on OHCs at a cochlear position where afferent neurons have a characteristic frequency (CF) similar to that measured in the cochlear efferent.

Frequency specificity of MOCS activity can also be detected when recording the response of inner hair cells and auditory nerve fibers to acoustic stimulation. For example in cats, the response of single cochlear afferent fibers to tone pips is suppressed by simultaneously applying tone pips to the contralateral ear. This suppression is maximal when the contralateral tone is similar to the characteristic frequency of the afferent fiber (Murata, Tanahashi, Horikawa, & Funai, 1980; Warren III & Liberman, 1989a; Warren III & Liberman, 1989b). Similarly, when recording the compound action potential induced by tone pips with a round window electrode, maximum suppression is induced by contralateral tone pips of similar frequency (M. C. Liberman, 1989).

As OAEs are generated by OHC activity, they may provide a more direct and non-invasive insight into the effect of the MOCS on its target cells than neural recordings. In human subjects, suppression of spontaneous OAEs is maximal with a CAS tone at a frequency close to the spontaneous OAE (Mott, Norton, Neely, & Bruce Warr, 1989). In addition to suppression, a frequency shift of spontaneous OAEs is caused by CAS and interestingly this is maximal with a CAS about 3/8 to 1/2 octaves below the spontaneous OAE frequency. OAEs evoked by tone pips can be suppressed by contralateral narrow band noise, suppression being maximal with CAS frequencies close to the frequency of the tone pip (Veuillet, Collet, & Duclaux, 1991).

Contralateral suppression of OAEs has not been widely used to investigate MOCS frequency specificity in animal models. A systematic study in the barn owl produced frequency response functions in which DPOAE suppression was plotted as a function of CAS frequency (Manley, Taschenberger, & Oeckinghaus, 1999). This showed maximal suppression with CAS similar to primary frequencies. Extrapolation of these findings to other models is limited by the variability of DPOAE levels and the additional types of efferent fiber which are present in birds.

The purpose of the present study was to investigate the frequency specificity of the MOCS in the chinchilla. In this species there has been a report of difficulty in detecting MOCS change in response to contralateral stimulation (Azeredo et al., 1999). On the other hand, electrical stimulation of the olivocochlear bundle in the floor of the fourth ventricle elicits OAE suppression (Siegel & Kim, 1982). In our present study, the suppressive effect on DPOAEs of contralateral pure tone stimuli is investigated with real-time recording of the DPOAE.

5.1.1 Materials and methods

5.1.1.1 Animals

Ten anaesthetized adult chinchillas (Chinchilla laniger) weights 505 - 725 g were studied. The anesthetic regime was intra-peritoneal Ketamine 15mg/kg (Ketamine Hydrochloride U.S.P. 100mg/ml, Ayerst Laboratories, Ontario), Xylazine 2.5mg/kg (Xylazine 20mg/ml, Bayer Inc., Toronto), and Atropine 0.04mg/kg (Atropine Sulfate 0.5mg/ml, MTC Pharmaceuticals, Ontario). Recordings were started 15 minutes after induction of anesthesia. A second dose of anesthetic was given 45 minutes later (intra-peritoneal Ketamine 8mg/kg,

Xylazine 1.3mg/kg). Five animals were studied twice, typically with an interval of >4 weeks between recording sessions. Thus in total, 15 recording sessions were completed. All studies were approved by the local Animal Care Committee, following the guidelines of the Canadian Council on Animal Care.

5.1.1.2 Real time DPOAE measurement

DPOAEs were measured in real time with a Vivo 600 DPR device (Vivosonic Inc., Toronto, ON). In contrast to conventional OAE techniques which employ signal averaging to extract the signal from noise, this technique uses digital filtering and signal modeling. The continuous real-time signal is ideally suited to the detection of changes in OAE amplitude, such as those produced by contralateral stimuli (James et al., 2005). Primary frequencies were set at f_2/f_1= 1.22 for values of f_2 between 1.6 and 8.0 kHz, with intensities of L_1 = 70dB and L_2 = 65dB. DPOAEs were measured at $2f_1$-f_2. The OAE probe, in a conforming soft plastic cuff, was inserted into the external auditory meatus by straightening the soft tissues to allow the probe to abut the lateral aspect of the bony meatus (approximately 13mm from the tympanic membrane). Multiple recordings of up to three minutes duration were made in each session. All recordings were made in a sound-attenuating booth. The DPOAE probe was calibrated in the ear canal by the device and calibration confirmed in a 2ml coupler using an SR760 FFT Spectrum Analyzer (Stanford Research Systems, Sunnyvale, CA) and a precision CR: 511D Acoustic Calibrator (Cirrus Research plc, North Yorkshire, U.K.).

5.1.1.3 Contralateral stimulus

An intermittent pure tone stimulus was applied to the contralateral ear using an ER-2 transducer with a foam ear-insert (Etymotic Research Inc., IL). 60 different CAS frequencies were tested between 0.6 – 17 kHz. Sweep direction from high to low, or low to high frequency of contralateral stimulation was changed between sweeps to control for any gradual drift in DPOAE level that might occur during a recording period. CAS intensity was set at 50 dB SPL as a previous study had shown the threshold for a response to be around 30dB SPL while acoustic cross talk occurred at intensities of ≥70 dB SPL (using noise floor measures and recordings in cadaveric chinchilla). Stimulus duration was set at 0.5s with rise / fall times of 4 ms. The interval between stimuli was long enough to allow DPOAE levels to return to pre-stimulus levels (typically > 300ms longer than CAS duration).

5.1.1.4 Analysis of results

DPOAE signals were recorded in real time, and level changes occurring in synchrony with contralateral stimulation were noted. Subsequent analysis was performed on the recorded real time trace and on averaged data, using VivoAnalysis software (Vivosonic Inc., ON), based on LabVIEW 5.1 data acquisition software (National Instruments, TX). Averaging was synchronized with the start of the CAS and was used to smooth the data and remove non-synchronous or spontaneous variation in the DPOAE signal. Averaged data were used to measure the magnitude of the DPOAE response to CAS from the baseline (no contralateral stimulation condition) to maximum OAE change (i.e. at asymptotic level). Frequency response curves to indicate tuning of contralateral suppression were plotted with magnitude of suppression (dependent variable) versus frequency of CAS tone (independent variable).

5.1.2 Results

DPOAEs were successfully recorded in real time in all animals. DPOAE levels were stable for the duration of the experiments, though they tended to fall gradually around 2 - 4 dB/hr. Figures 1 through 5 demonstrate DPOAE suppression data progressing from the initial real time signal, to the averaged waveform, and finally ideal curve fitting to the contralateral frequency response function.

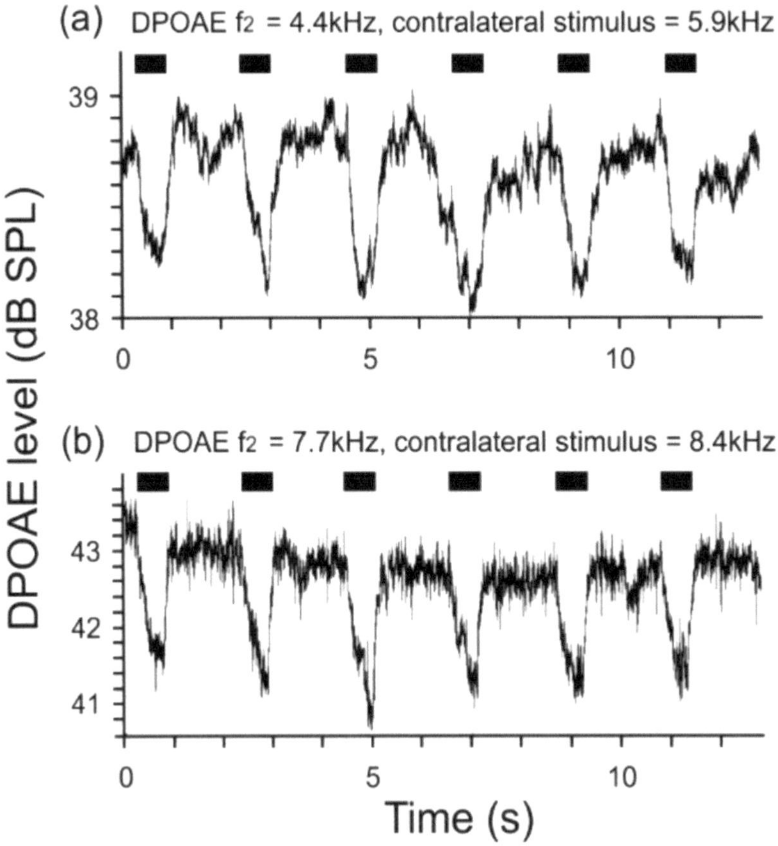

Fig. 1. Typical example of contralateral suppression of real time DPOAE signals in chinchilla: (a) DPOAE at f_2 = 4.4 kHz, contralateral acoustic stimulation = 5.9 kHz at 50dB SPL; (b) DPOAE at f_2 = 7.7 kHz, contralateral acoustic stimulation = 8.4 kHz at 50 dB SPL. (Stimulus duration = 550ms, marked by horizontal black bar).

Figure 1 shows examples of real time recordings of DPOAE suppression. Panel 1a shows variation in DPOAE level at f_2 = 4.4 kHz over a twelve second period during six periods of CAS at 5.9 kHz (marked by horizontal bar). Suppression of 0.5 dB from the baseline level of 38.8 dB SPL occurs with each CAS. In panel 1b, a DPOAE at f_2 = 7.7 kHz is suppressed by 1.2 dB by CAS of 8.4 kHz. The suppression response was sometimes smaller than the spontaneous signal variation so was not always readily visible in real-time. However, by averaging the raw real-time data in synchrony with the onset of CAS, suppression could usually be detected.

Typical examples of averaged DPOAE suppression responses are shown in figure 2. Here the DPOAE measured is at f_2 = 4.4 kHz, with contralateral suppression stimuli between 2.8 and 6.7 kHz. In this series, suppression is greatest (0.8 dB) with contralateral stimulations at 4.5 kHz, but is only half this value when contralateral stimulation is at 2.8 kHz or 6.7 kHz, indicating the frequency dependence of DPOAE suppression.

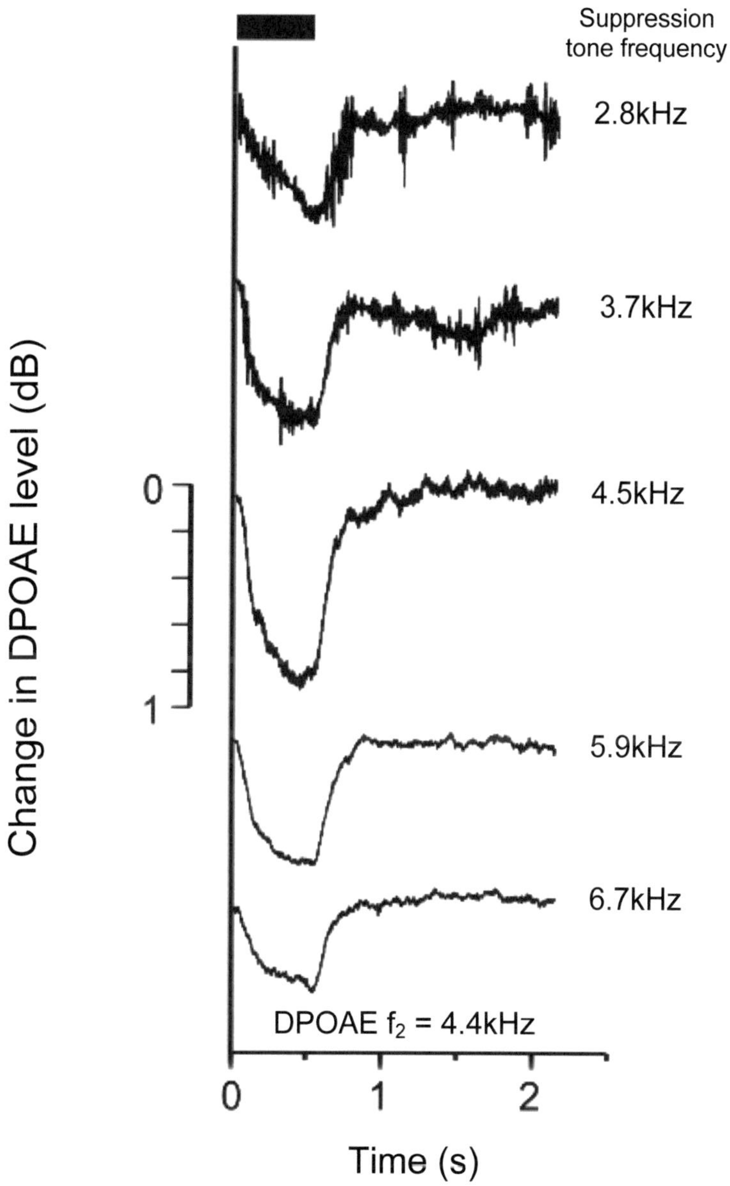

Fig. 2. Averaged DPOAE signal from 20s recording periods, synchronized with onset of contralateral stimulus. (DPOAE at f_2 = 4.4 kHz; contralateral acoustic stimulation at frequencies of 2.8 - 6.7 kHz (550ms duration, as black bar).

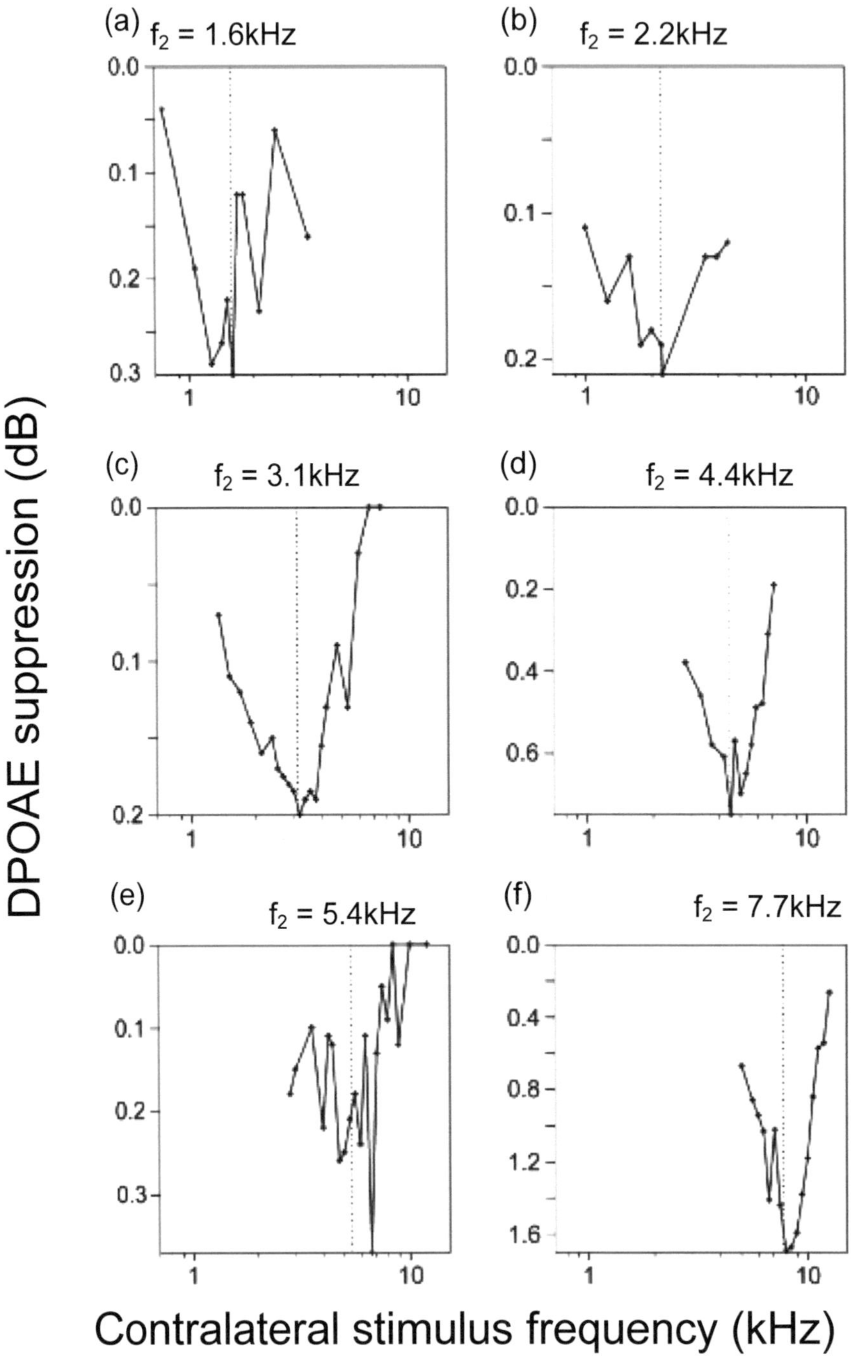

Fig. 3. DPOAE suppression plotted against contralateral stimulation frequency. Panels a – f show suppression response measured from single animal recordings at DPOAE frequencies ranging from f_2 of 1.6 kHz to 7.7 kHz.

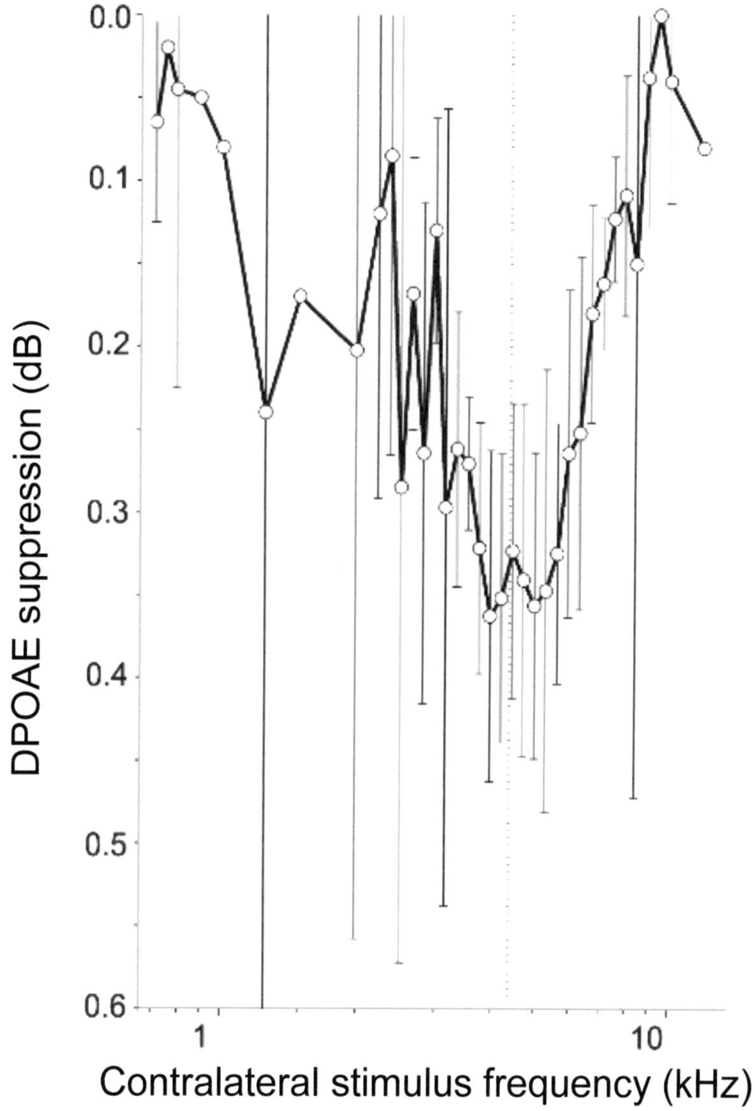

Fig. 4. Contralateral suppression frequency response curve for DPOAE of $f_2 = 4.4$ kHz (marked by vertical dotted line), derived from pooling data from 8 animals. Bars show 95% confidence intervals.

The frequency response function for $f_2 = 4.4$ kHz in figure 4 was derived from 22 recordings in eight animals. Mean suppression was plotted against CAS frequency. The large 95% confidence intervals reflect the variability of response in different experiments. However, as in figure 3, the curve peaks near the f_2 frequency (dotted line).

In figure 3, magnitude of contralateral suppression is plotted against CAS frequency for six different DPOAE frequencies. The curves peak close to the f_2 value (marked by the dotted line) but typically peak suppression magnitude occurs at a frequency slightly higher than f_2.

In an attempt to reduce the variability of the response between recordings and to obtain finer details on the shape of the frequency response, repeated measures from CAS close to f_2 were made in successive recordings in one chinchilla. The results are shown in figure 5. Even within this single recording period in an individual animal, variability (up to 0.15dB) can be seen in successive sweeps. No repeatable notches in the curve were visible.

As illustrated in figure 5 by the continuous line, the general shape of the DPOAE suppression tuning can be characterized by fitting a regression curve to the data. In figure 6, the same regression function is plotted for four values of f_2 between 3.1 - 7.7 kHz using data combined from multiple recordings. The responses are asymmetric with a tendency to drop off more steeply at values of CAS greater than f_2. Small suppression responses can be obtained by CAS tones more than one octave lower than the f_2 frequency.

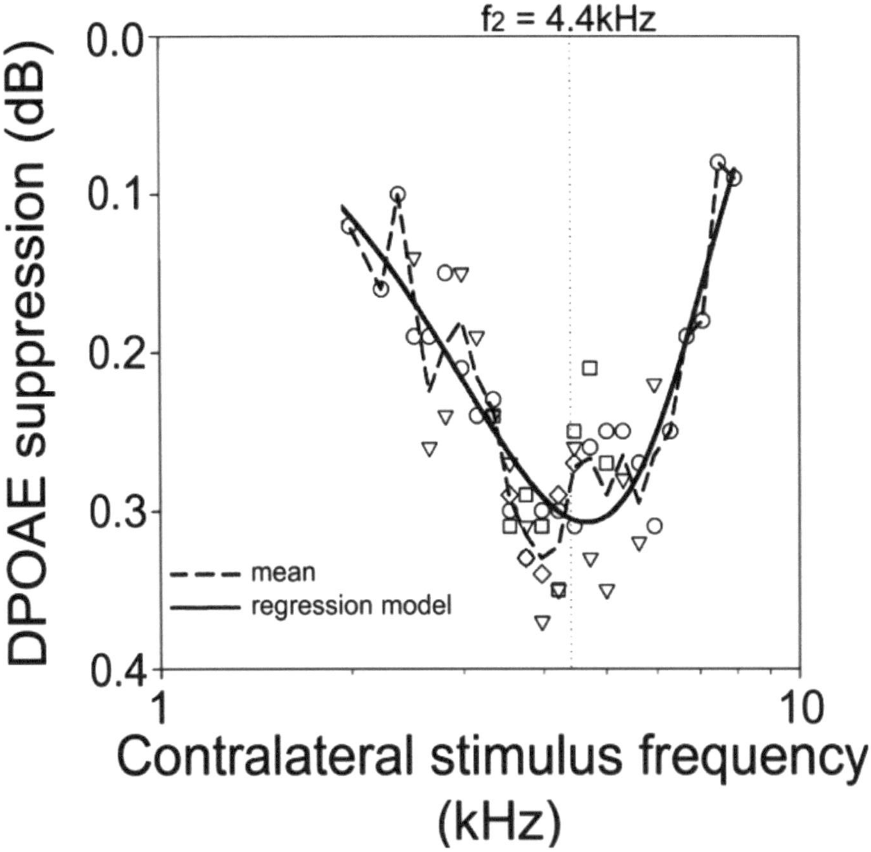

Fig. 5. Contralateral suppression frequency response curve for DPOAE of f_2 = 4.4 kHz derived from one subject. Dashed line is mean value. Solid line is regression curve (Weibull).

In figure 7, the suppression curves of fig. 6 are plotted on a normalized amplitude scale. The curves are broadly tuned and thus there is considerable overlap. The tuning of suppression curves for high frequency DPOAEs is narrower than at lower frequencies. The (half-amplitude) bandwidth values for suppression curves at 3.1, 4.4, 5.4, 6.6, and 7.7 kHz (f_2) are, respectively, 1.7, 1.8, 1.4, 1.15, and 1.3 octaves.

DPOAE suppression was seen in all animals with contralateral pure tone stimulation. On rare occasions, CAS induced an increase in DPOAE level. This occurred at f_2 = 2.2 kHz in one chinchilla and at f_2 = 6.6 and 7.7 kHz in another. The maximum response occurred with a contralateral tone at or just below the frequency of f_2. These data were excluded from analysis as they may represent a different process.

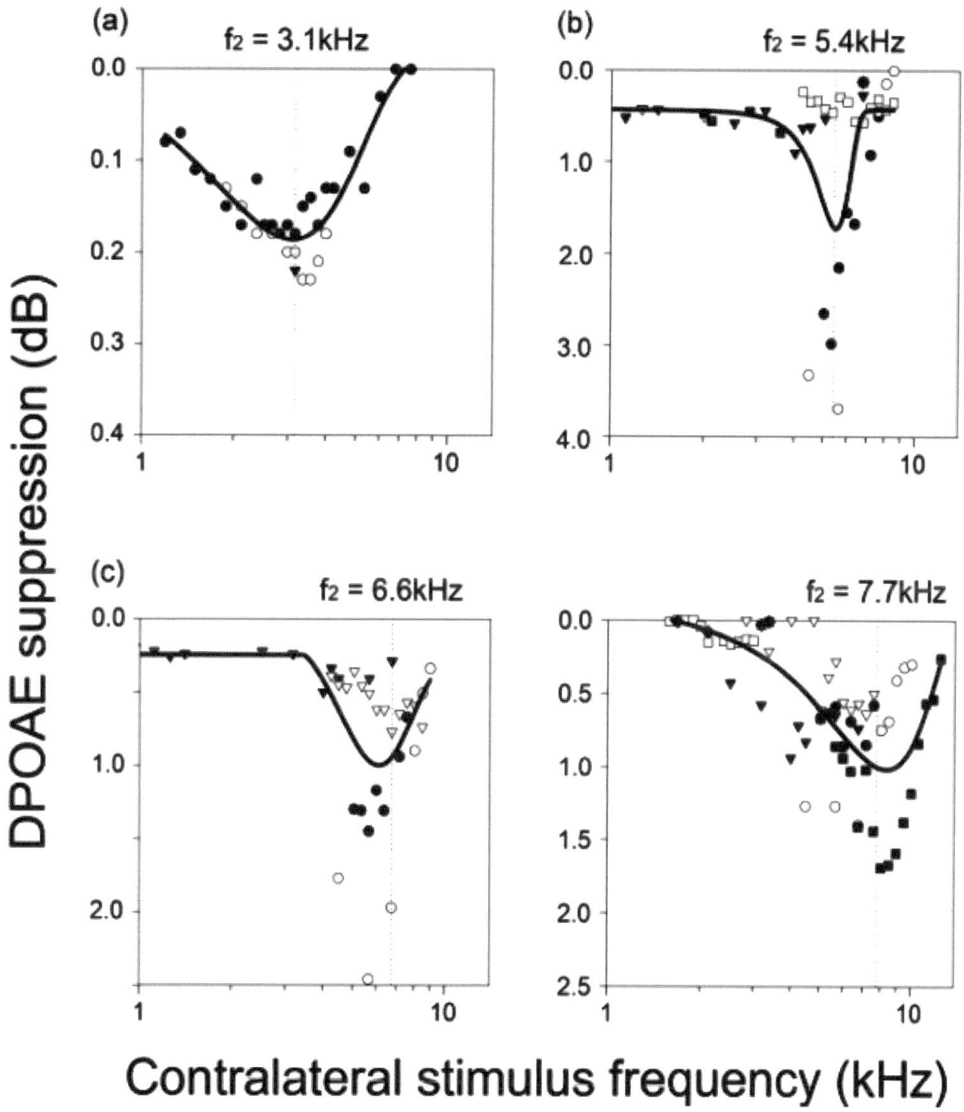

Fig. 6. Regression functions (Weibull) of DPOAE suppression frequency response curves for four values of f_2 between 3.1 and 7.7 kHz. Curves are plotted on an absolute dB suppression scale.

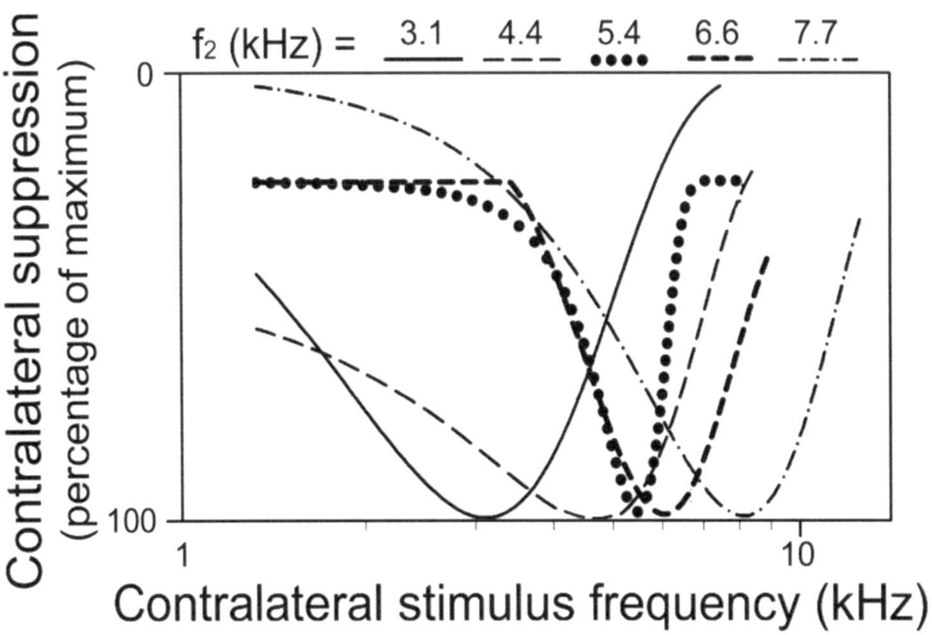

Fig. 7. DPOAE suppression frequency response curves (Weibull regressions) for f_2 values between 3.1 and 7.7 kHz, plotted on a normalized suppression scale (data from figs 4 and 6).

5.1.3 Discussion

This study demonstrates that suppression of DPOAEs by contralateral pure tones can be detected in the chinchilla with real time recording. DPOAE suppression is greatest when using contralateral stimulation tones close to primary tone f_2. This tonotopic response is consistent with other investigations of frequency specificity in the MOCS pathway (Chery-Croze, Moulin, & Collet, 1993; Cody & Johnstone, 1982; M. C. Liberman, 1989; Murata et al., 1980; Robertson, 1984; Robertson & Gummer, 1985; Veuillet et al., 1991; Warren III & Liberman, 1989a; Warren III & Liberman, 1989b). Unlike observations in human subjects, we did not observe any dips in fine structure DPOAEs to account for differences in the magnitude of suppression at different values of f_2 or between chinchillas (Wagner, Heppelmann, Müller, Janssen, & Zenner, 2007).

Measurement of contralateral frequency tuning of MOCS fibers has revealed narrow band tuning equivalent in sharpness to cochlear afferent neurons (Brown, 1989; M. Liberman & Brown, 1986; Robertson, 1984). The final, divergent innervation pattern of MOCS fibers at the OHC level appears to degrade this cochleotopicity (or frequency tuning) by a factor of 4-5 from 0.33 octaves (the approximate bandwidth of auditory afferents) to about 1.7 octaves for f_2 = 3.1kHz and 1.3 octaves for f_2 = 7.7kHz. The difference in tuning likely rests with the divergent OHC innervation by the MOCS fibers. Neural tracing studies in guinea pig have shown MOCS fibers innervating 15 -61 OHCs (Brown, 1989). In the cat, individual cochlear efferents contact 23 - 84 OHCs spanning 0.55-2.8mm (M. Liberman & Brown, 1986). Thus although tuning in the efferent fibers themselves appears to be as sharp as afferent tuning, the effect of individual fibers on the organ of Corti will be much less precise.

MOCS frequency tuning has been assessed in the cat by recording changes in single afferent fiber activity during CAS. Suppression of afferent firing rate is maximal with a CAS of similar frequency to the characteristic frequency of the afferent fiber (Warren III & Liberman, 1989a; Warren III & Liberman, 1989b)). Tuning of this form of contralateral suppression was asymmetric, falling off more sharply at CAS frequencies above characteristic frequency, and were much less sharp than afferent tuning. Tuning tended to be sharper at higher frequencies. These observations in the cat are consistent with the contralateral DPOAE suppression tuning reported here for the chinchilla, where bandwidths for curves at 6.6 and 7.7 kHz (f_2) are 1.15 and 1.3 octaves respectively, but are 1.7 and 1.8 octaves at 3.1 and 4.4 kHz.

As shown by others, the primary tones used to generate DPOAE stimulate the MOCS and so cause ipsilateral DPOAE suppression (Guinan, Backus, Lilaonitkul, & Aharonson, 2003; M. C. Liberman, Puria, & Guinan Jr., 1996). It can be expected that the primary tones would suppress cochlear function in the contralateral ear by MOCS activation, with the same broad frequency tuning that we have observed. Given that the magnitude of contralateral suppression of DPOAE is dependent upon intensity of the contralateral stimulus (A. James, Mount, & Harrison, 2002), a hypothetical outcome would be a notch in the frequency response curve at the primary frequencies, f_1 and f_2. This has been observed at f_1 in the barn owl but despite thorough investigation at one frequency (f_2 = 4.4kHz, figure 5), we were unable to demonstrate this phenomenon in the chinchilla (Manley et al., 1999).

As in other studies, recordings were completed under anesthesia with ketamine and xylazine. This does reduce the magnitude of contralateral suppression of DPOAE and other measures of olivocochlear function but facilitates recording by providing stable recording conditions, with less behavioral noise and movement artifact (Cazals & Huang, 1996; da Costa, Erre, de Sauvage, Popelar, & Aran, 1997; Harel, Kakigi, Hirakawa, Mount, & Harrison, 1997). We have not investigated the effect of anesthesia on tuning sharpness.

As mentioned previously the exact function of the medial olivo-cochlear system remains speculative. Because of the predominantly inhibitory effect seen on outer hair cell function, improved detection of sound in noise or a protective effect have been hypothesized. Any role postulated for the contralateral suppression response should take into account the relatively slow dynamic of this reflex, being of the order of 26ms in chinchilla and 45ms in humans (James, Harrison, Pienkowski, Dajani, & Mount, 2005). The presence of a response from low intensity contralateral stimuli suggests the function of this system is less likely a protective one, but more to do with frequency tuning of the afferent neural responses via efferent effects on OHC motility. The efferent system may function as a gain control with a long time-constant, equalizing sensitivity between the ears. The optimal condition for detecting inter-aural timing or intensity differences would perhaps be when the two ears have equivalent function. In this respect, the medial contralateral efferent system may also have a role in "balancing" the ears such as to improve the accuracy of these binaural sound localization tasks.

6. Conclusions

Objective tests such as OAE and ABR are widely used in hearing screening programs and have lead to great advances in the early detection and rehabilitation of neonatal hearing loss. However these tests do not provide a quick and easy means for assessing hearing threshold at different frequencies, indeed the presence of OAE does not even guarantee the presence of normal hearing. An objective frequency specific test of hearing ability would have widespread advantages, not just for neonatal testing but in many circumstances in all age groups.

In the present study we have demonstrated frequency specificity in contralateral suppression using a chinchilla model. The majority of studies shedding light onto the function of the MOCS have been derived from animal experiments. However, there is enough data in human studies to suggest that the human efferent system is qualitatively similar (Guinan Jr, 2006; James, 2006). We have shown previously that contralateral suppression of DPOAE can be assessed in real time in babies and adults (James et al., 2005) and can be used to test hearing very effectively in neonates (James, 2011). We have shown that this technique can distinguish between middle ear muscle reflexes and the OCR in an animal model (Wolter, Harrison, & James, 2011) and here show that it can be used to assess hearing threshold in a frequency specific manner. We envisage many clinical applications of this technique including the diagnosis and assessment of ANSD and more accurate hearing screening in neonatal and elderly populations.

7. References

Allen, T. E. (1986). Patterns of academic achievement among hearing impaired students: 1974 and 1983. In K. A. Schildroth A (Ed.), *Deaf children in america* (pp. 161-206) San Diego: College-Hill Press.

Amatuzzi, M. G., Northrop, C., Liberman, M. C., Thornton, A., Halpin, C., Herrmann, B., et al. (2001). Selective inner hair cell loss in premature infants and cochlea pathological patterns from neonatal intensive care unit autopsies. *Archives of Otolaryngology- Head and Neck Surgery, 127*(6), 629.

Art, J., Fettiplace, R., & Fuchs, P. (1984). Synaptic hyperpolarization and inhibition of turtle cochlear hair cells. *The Journal of Physiology, 356*(1), 525.

Attias, J., & Raveh, E. (2007). Transient deafness in young candidates for cochlear implants. *Audiology and Neurotology, 12*(5), 325-333.

Azeredo, W. J., Kliment, M. L., Morley, B. J., Relkin, E., Slepecky, N. B., Sterns, A., et al. (1999). Olivocochlear neurons in the chinchilla: A retrograde fluorescent labelling study. *Hearing Research, 134*(1-2), 57-70.

Berlin, C. I., Hood, L. J., Morlet, T., Wilensky, D., St. John, P., Montgomery, E., et al. (2005). Absent or elevated middle ear muscle reflexes in the presence of normal otoacoustic emissions: A universal finding in 136 cases of auditory neuropathy/dys-synchrony. *Journal of the American Academy of Audiology, 16*(8), 546-553.

Brown, M. (1989). Morphology and response properties of single olivocochlear fibers in the guinea pig. *Hearing Research, 40*(1-2), 93-109.

Brown, M., Venecia, R. K., & Guinan, J. (2003). Responses of medial olivocochlear neurons. *Experimental Brain Research, 153*(4), 491-498.

Busa, J., Harrison, J., Chappell, J., Yoshinaga-Itano, C., Grimes, A., Brookhouser, P. E., et al. (2007). Year 2007 position statement: Principles and guidelines for early hearing detection and intervention programs. *Pediatrics, 120*(4), 898-921.

Cazals, Y., & Huang, Z. (1996). Average spectrum of cochlear activity: A possible synchronized firing, its olivo-cochlear feedback and alterations under anesthesia. *Hearing Research, 101*(1-2), 81-92.

Chery-Croze, S., Moulin, A., & Collet, L. (1993). Effect of contralateral sound stimulation on the distortion product 2f1-f2 in humans: Evidence of a frequency specificity. *Hearing Research, 68*(1), 53-58.

Choo, D., & Meinzen-Derr, J. (2010). Universal newborn hearing screening in 2010. *Current Opinion in Otolaryngology & Head and Neck Surgery, 18*(5), 399.

Cody, A., & Johnstone, B. (1982). Acoustically evoked activity of single efferent neurons in the guinea pig cochlea. *The Journal of the Acoustical Society of America, 72*, 280.

Collet, L., Kemp, D. T., Veuillet, E., Duclaux, R., Moulin, A., & Morgon, A. (1990). Effect of contralateral auditory stimuli on active cochlear micro-mechanical properties in human subjects. *Hearing Research, 43*(2-3), 251-261.

Cone-Wesson, B., Rance, G., & Sininger, Y. (2001). For patients with auditory neuropathy. In Y. S. Sininger, & A. Starr (Eds.), *Auditory neuropathy: A new perspective on hearing disorders* (pp. 233). San Diego: Singular Pub Group.

da Costa, D. L., Erre, J. P., de Sauvage, R. C., Popelar, J., & Aran, J. M. (1997). Bioelectrical cochlear noise and its contralateral suppression: Relation to background activity of the eighth nerve and effects of sedation and anesthesia. *Experimental Brain Research, 116*(2), 259-269.

Darrow, K. N., Maison, S. F., & Liberman, M. C. (2006). Cochlear efferent feedback balances interaural sensitivity. *Nature Neuroscience, 9*(12), 1474.

Davis, A., & Wood, S. (1992). The epidemiology of childhood hearing impairment: Factors relevant to planning of services. *British Journal of Audiology, 26*(2), 77-90.

Davis, A., Bamford, J., Wilson, I., Ramkalawan, T., Forshaw, M., & Wright, S. (1997). A critical review of the role of neonatal hearing screening in the detection of congenital hearing impairment. *Health Technology Assessment (Winchester, England), 1*(10), i-iv, 1-176.

Fex, J. (1962). Auditory activity in centrifugal and centripetal cochlear fibres in cat. A study of a feedback system. *Acta Physiologica Scandinavica.Supplementum, 189*, 1-68.

Folsom, R. C., & Owsley, R. M. (1987). N1 action potentials in humans: Influence of simultaneous contralateral stimulation. *Acta Oto-Laryngologica, 103*(3-4), 262-265.

Froehlich, P., Collet, L., & Morgon, A. (1993). Transiently evoked otoacoustic emission amplitudes change with changes of directed attention. *Physiology & Behavior, 53*(4), 679-682.

Galambos, R. (1956). Suppression of auditory nerve activity by stimulation of efferent fibers to cochlea. *Journal of Neurophysiology, 19*(5), 424.

Gifford, M. L., & Guinan Jr, J. J. (1987). Effects of electrical stimulation of medial olivocochlear neurons on ipsilateral and contralateral cochlear responses. *Hearing Research, 29*(2-3), 179-194.

Gold, T. (1948). Hearing. II. the physical basis of the action of the cochlea. *Proceedings of the Royal Society of London.Series B, Biological Sciences*, , 492-498.

Guinan Jr, J. J. (2006). Olivocochlear efferents: Anatomy, physiology, function, and the measurement of efferent effects in humans. *Ear and Hearing, 27*(6), 589.

Guinan, J. J., Backus, B. C., Lilaonitkul, W., & Aharonson, V. (2003). Medial olivocochlear efferent reflex in humans: Otoacoustic emission (OAE) measurement issues and the advantages of stimulus frequency OAEs. *JARO-Journal of the Association for Research in Otolaryngology, 4*(4), 521-540.

Hall, J. W., Smith, S. D., & Popelka, G. R. (2004). Newborn hearing screening with combined otoacoustic emissions and auditory brainstem responses. *Journal of the American Academy of Audiology, 15*(6), 414-425.

Harel, N., Kakigi, A., Hirakawa, H., Mount, R. J., & Harrison, R. V. (1997). The effects of anesthesia on otoacoustic emissions. *Hearing Research, 110*(1-2), 25-33.

Harrison, R. V. (1998). An animal model of auditory neuropathy. *Ear and Hearing, 19*(5), 355.

Harrison, R. V. (2001). Models of auditory neuropathy based on inner hair cell damage. In Y. S. Sininger, & A. Starr (Eds.), (pp. 51–66). San Diego: Singular.

Hecox, K., & Galambos, R. (1974). Brain stem auditory evoked responses in human infants and adults. *Archives of Otolaryngology- Head and Neck Surgery, 99*(1), 30.

Holden-Pitt, L., & Albertorio, J. (1998). Thirty years of the annual survey of deaf and hard-of-hearing children & youth: A glance over the decades. *American Annals of the Deaf, 143*(2), 72-76.

Hood, L. J., & Berlin, C. I. (2001). In Sininger Y. S., Starr A. (Eds.), *Auditory neuropathy (auditory dys-synchrony) disables efferent suppression of otoacoustic emissions*. San Diego: Singulair.

Innitzer, J., & Ehrenberger, K. (1977). The influence of contralateral acoustic stimulation on the summating potential in the human cochlea. [DER EINFLUSS KONTRALATERALER BESCHALLUNG AUF DAS SUMMATIONSPOTENTIAL DER MENSCHLICHEN KOCHLEA] *Laryngologie Rhinologie Otologie, 56*(11), 921-924.

Jacobson, J., & Jacobson, C. (2004). Evaluation of hearing loss in infants and young children. *Pediatric Annals, 33*(12), 811-821.

James, A. L. (2006). *Real time measurement of distortion product otoacoustic emissions in the assessment of the olivocochlear contralateral reflex.* Unpublished

James, A. L. (2011). The assessment of olivocochlear function in neonates with real-time distortion product otoacoustic emissions. *The Laryngoscope, 121*(1), 202-213.

James, A. L., Harrison, R. V., Pienkowski, M., Dajani, H. R., & Mount, R. J. (2005). Dynamics of real time DPOAE contralateral suppression in chinchillas and humans dinámica de la supresión contralateral de las DPOAE en tiempo real en chinchillas y humanos. *International Journal of Audiology, 44*(2), 118-129.

James A. L., Mount, R., & Harrison, R. (2002). Contralateral suppression of DPOAE measured in real time. *Clinical Otolaryngology & Allied Sciences, 27*(2), 106-112.

Kemp, D. T. (1978a). Stimulated acoustic emissions from within the human auditory system. *Journal of the Acoustical Society of America, 64*(5), 1386-1391.

Kemp, D. T. (1978b). Stimulated acoustic emissions from within the human auditory system. *Journal of the Acoustical Society of America, 64*(5), 1386-1391.

Kennedy, C., McCann, D., Campbell, M. J., Kimm, L., & Thornton, R. (2005). Universal newborn screening for permanent childhood hearing impairment: An 8-year follow-up of a controlled trial. *The Lancet, 366*(9486), 660-662.

Kimura, R., & Wersäll, J. (1962). Termination of the olivo-cochlear bundle in relation to the outer hair cells of the organ of corti in guinea pig. *Acta Oto-Laryngologica, 55*(1-6), 11-32.

Kral, A., & O'Donoghue, G. M. (2010). Profound deafness in childhood. *New England Journal of Medicine, 363*(15), 1438-1450.

Liberman, M. C. (1988). Response properties of cochlear efferent neurons: Monaural vs. binaural stimulation and the effects of noise. *Journal of Neurophysiology, 60*(5), 1779.

Liberman, M. C. (1989). Rapid assessment of sound-evoked olivocochlear feedback: Suppression of compound action potentials by contralateral sound. *Hearing Research, 38*(1-2), 47-56.

Liberman, M., & Brown, M. (1986). Physiology and anatomy of single olivocochlear neurons in the cat. *Hearing Research, 24*(1), 17-36.

Liberman, M. C., Puria, S., & Guinan Jr., J. J. (1996). The ipsilaterally evoked olivocochlear reflex causes rapid adaptation of the 2f1-f2 distortion product otoacoustic emission. *Journal of the Acoustical Society of America, 99*(6), 3572-3584.

Llanes, E. G. D. V., & Chiong, C. M. (2004). Evoked otoacoustic emissions and auditory brainstem responses: Concordance in hearing screening among high-risk children. *Acta Oto-Laryngologica, 124*(4), 387-390.

Maison, S., Durrant, J., Gallineau, C., Micheyl, C., & Collet, L. (2001). Delay and temporal integration in medial olivocochlear bundle activation in humans. *Ear and Hearing, 22*(1), 65.

Maison, S., Micheyl, C., Andéol, G., Gallégo, S., & Collet, L. (2000). Activation of medial olivocochlear efferent system in humans: Influence of stimulus bandwidth. *Hearing Research, 140*(1-2), 111-125.

Maison, S., Micheyl, C., & Collet, L. (2001). Influence of focused auditory attention on cochlear activity in humans. *Psychophysiology, 38*(1), 35-40.

Manchaiah, V. K. C., Zhao, F., Danesh, A. A., & Duprey, R. (2011). The genetic basis of auditory neuropathy spectrum disorder (ANSD). *International Journal of Pediatric Otorhinolaryngology, 75*(2), 151-158.

Manley, G. A., Taschenberger, G., & Oeckinghaus, H. (1999). Influence of contralateral acoustic stimulation on distortion-product and spontaneous otoacoustic emissions in the barn owl. *Hearing Research, 138*(1-2), 1-12.

Marschark, M., & Wauters, L. (2008). Language comprehension and learning by deaf students. *Deaf Cognition: Foundations and Outcomes,* , 309–350.

Micheyl, C., Khalfa, S., Perrot, X., & Collet, L. (1997). Difference in cochlear efferent activity between musicians and non-musicians. *Neuroreport, 8*(4), 1047.

Moeller, M. P. (2000). Early intervention and language development in children who are deaf and hard of hearing. *Pediatrics, 106*(3), e43.

Mohr, P. E., Feldman, J. J., Dunbar, J. L., McConkey-Robbins, A., Niparko, J. K., Rittenhouse, R. K., et al. (2000). The societal costs of severe to profound hearing loss in the united states. *International Journal of Technology Assessment in Health Care, 16*(4), 1120-1135.

Morest, D. (1973). Auditory neurons of the brain stem. *Advances in Oto-Rhino-Laryngology, 20*, 337.

Mott, J. B., Norton, S. J., Neely, S. T., & Bruce Warr, W. (1989). Changes in spontaneous otoacoustic emissions produced by acoustic stimulation of the contralateral ear. *Hearing Research, 38*(3), 229-242.

Mountain, D. C., Daniel Geisler, C., & Hubbard, A. E. (1980). Stimulation of efferents alters the cochlear microphonic and the sound-induced resistance changes measured in scala media of the guinea pig. *Hearing Research, 3*(3), 231-240.

Mulders, W., & Robertson, D. (2000a). Effects on cochlear responses of activation of descending pathways from the inferior colliculus. *Hearing Research, 149*(1-2), 11-23.

Mulders, W., & Robertson, D. (2000b). Evidence for direct cortical innervation of medial olivocochlear neurones in rats. *Hearing Research, 144*(1-2), 65-72.

Murata, K., Tanahashi, T., Horikawa, J., & Funai, H. (1980). Mechanical and neural interactions between binaurally applied sounds in cat cochlear nerve fibers. *Neuroscience Letters, 18*(3), 289-294.

Nadol Jr, J. B. (2001). Primary cochlear neuronal degeneration. *Auditory Neuropathy: A New Perspective on Hearing Disorders,* , 99–140.

Nieder, P. C., & Nieder, I. (1970). Crossed olivocochlear bundle: Electrical stimulation enhances masked neural responses to loud clicks. *Brain Research, 21*(1), 135-137.

Rajan, R., & Johnstone, B. (1988). Binaural acoustic stimulation exercises protective effects at the cochlea that mimic the effects of electrical stimulation of an auditory efferent pathway. *Brain Research, 459*(2), 241-255.

Rance, G., & Barker, E. J. (2008a). Speech perception in children with auditory neuropathy/dyssynchrony managed with either hearing aids or cochlear implants. *Otology & Neurotology, 29*(2), 179.

Rance, G., & Barker, E. J. (2008b). Speech perception in children with auditory neuropathy/dyssynchrony managed with either hearing aids or cochlear implants. *Otology & Neurotology, 29*(2), 179.

Rasmussen, G. L. (1946). The olivary peduncle and other fiber projections of the superior olivary complex. *The Journal of Comparative Neurology, 84*(2), 141-219.

Rasmussen, G. L. (1953). Further observations of the efferent cochlear bundle. *The Journal of Comparative Neurology, 99*(1), 61-74.

Raveh, E., Buller, N., Badrana, O., & Attias, J. (2007). Auditory neuropathy: Clinical characteristics and therapeutic approach. *American Journal of Otolaryngology, 28*(5), 302-308.

Robertson, D. (1984). Horseradish peroxidase injection of physiologically characterized afferent and efferent neurones in the guinea pig spiral ganglion. *Hearing Research, 15*(2), 113-121.

Robertson, D., & Gummer, M. (1985). Physiological and morphological characterization of efferent neurones in the guinea pig cochlea. *Hearing Research, 20*(1), 63-77.

Saurini, P., Nola, G., & Lendvai, D. (2004). Otoacoustic emissions: A new method for newborn hearing screening. *European Review for Medical and Pharmacological Sciences, 8*, 129-133.

Scates, K. W., Woods, C. I., & Azeredo, W. J. (1999). Inferior colliculus stimulation and changes in 2f1-f2 distortion product otoacoustic emissions in the rat. *Hearing Research, 128*(1-2), 51-60.

Schroeder, L., Petrou, S., Kennedy, C., McCann, D., Law, C., Watkin, P. M., et al. (2006). The economic costs of congenital bilateral permanent childhood hearing impairment. *Pediatrics, 117*(4), 1101.

Shapiro, S. M. (2003). Bilirubin toxicity in the developing nervous system. *Pediatric Neurology, 29*(5), 410-421.

Siegel, J. H., & Kim, D. (1982). Efferent neural control of cochlear mechanics? olivocochlear bundle stimulation affects cochlear biomechanical nonlinearity. *Hearing Research, 6*(2), 171-182.

Starr, A., Picton, T. W., Sininger, Y., Hood, L. J., & Berlin, C. I. (1996). Auditory neuropathy. *Brain, 119*(3), 741.

Thompson, D. C., McPhillips, H., Davis, R. L., Lieu, T. A., Homer, C. J., & Helfand, M. (2001). Universal newborn hearing screening. *JAMA: The Journal of the American Medical Association, 286*(16), 2000.

Veuillet, E., Collet, L., & Duclaux, R. (1991). Effect of contralateral acoustic stimulation on active cochlear micromechanical properties in human subjects: Dependence on stimulus variables. *Journal of Neurophysiology, 65*(3), 724-735.

Wagner, W., Heppelmann, G., Müller, J., Janssen, T., & Zenner, H. -. (2007). Olivocochlear reflex effect on human distortion product otoacoustic emissions is largest at frequencies with distinct fine structure dips. *Hearing Research, 223*(1-2), 83-92.

Wake, M., Hughes, E. K., Poulakis, Z., Collins, C., & Rickards, F. W. (2004a). Outcomes of children with mild-profound congenital hearing loss at 7 to 8 years: A population study. *Ear and Hearing, 25*(1), 1.

Wake, M., Hughes, E. K., Poulakis, Z., Collins, C., & Rickards, F. W. (2004b). Outcomes of children with mild-profound congenital hearing loss at 7 to 8 years: A population study. *Ear and Hearing, 25*(1), 1.

Walsh, E. J., McGee, J. A., McFadden, S. L., & Liberman, M. C. (1998). Long-term effects of sectioning the olivocochlear bundle in neonatal cats. *The Journal of Neuroscience, 18*(10), 3859.

Warr, W. B. (1975). Olivocochlear and vestibular efferent neurons of the feline brain stem: Their location, morphology and number determined by retrograde axonal transport and acetylcholinesterase histochemistry. *The Journal of Comparative Neurology, 161*(2), 159-181.

Warren III, E. H., & Liberman, M. C. (1989a). Effects of contralateral sound on auditory-nerve responses. I. contributions of cochlear efferents. *Hearing Research, 37*(2), 89-104.

Warren III, E. H., & Liberman, M. C. (1989b). Effects of contralateral sound on auditory-nerve responses. II. dependence on stimulus variables. *Hearing Research, 37*(2), 105-122.

Wiederhold, M. L., & Peake, W. T. (1966). Efferent inhibition of auditory-nerve responses: Dependence on acoustic-stimulus parameters. *Journal of the Acoustical Society of America,*

Wolter, N. E., Harrison, R. V., & James, A. L. (2011). Investigation of olivocochlear and middle ear muscle reflexes with contralateral suppression of DPOAEs in real time [Abstract]. *Triological Society Eastern Section Annual Resident Competition - Podium Presentation,*

Yasunaga, S., Grati, M., Cohen-Salmon, M., El-Amraoui, A., Mustapha, M., Salem, N., et al. (1999). A mutation in OTOF, encoding otoferlin, a FER-1-like protein, causes DFNB9, a nonsyndromic form of deafness. *Nature Genetics, 21*(4), 363-369.

Ye, Y., Machado, D., & Kim, D. (2000). Projection of the marginal shell of the anteroventral cochlear nucleus to olivocochlear neurons in the cat. *The Journal of Comparative Neurology, 420*(1), 127-138.

Yoshinaga-Itano, C. (2003). Universal newborn hearing screening programs and developmental outcomes. *Audiological Medicine, 1*(3), 199-206.

Yoshinaga-Itano, C., Sedey, A. L., Coulter, D. K., & Mehl, A. L. (1998). Language of early- and later-identified children with hearing loss. *Pediatrics, 102*(5), 1161.

3

A Prediction Method for Speech Audibility Taking Account of Hearing Loss Due to Aging Under Meaningless Noise

Takahiro Tamesue
Organization for Academic Information, Yamaguchi University
Japan

1. Introduction

Securing good transmission characteristics for speech information and achieving a comfortable sound environment in buildings used by a great variety of people in public city spaces, to say nothing of spaces used for intellectual or mental work such as schools and offices, comprise two of the most important problems of environmental design. A common method for evaluating listening scores and psychological impressions for audio signal has been discussed previously (Tamesue T. et al., 2003). However, this research paid attention only to subjects in their twenties with normal hearing, and as a result the relationships between the frequency characteristics of hearing loss due to factors such as aging and the listening scores for audio signals and the psychological impressions related to speech audibility were not considered. Taking this into consideration, this chapter considers how the listening scores of audio signals and the psychological impressions for speech audibility change while taking into account the effects of hearing loss due to factors such as aging. Specifically, frequency filters for simulating hearing loss are first prepared. Next, psychological listening experiments are conducted in which both the audio signal and the noise passing through the above-mentioned filters are transmitted to subjects with normal hearing. Using the observed experimental data, the relationships between the weight-mean spectral distance (Tamesue T. et al., 2003) and the listening scores of the audio signals and psychological impressions with respect to speech audibility are investigated. Next, based on these relationships, problems associated with the prediction of listening scores and psychological impressions with respect to speech audibility are discussed.

2. Outline of psychological listening experiment I

Psychological listening experiment I was conducted to establish the regression models of the listening scores of the audio signal and the psychological impressions related to speech audibility. The outline of the indoor experiment is as follows.

2.1 Location

The experiment was conducted in a simple soundproof room on campus having the following dimensions: length 5.1 m, width 3.3 m, and height 2.2 m. The sound pressure level of the background noise was about 37 dB. The sound pressure level in this chapter is the value measured by a sound level meter with FLAT response. The A-weighted sound pressure level was about 21 dB(A).

2.2 Subjects

A total of 8 students, 7 male and 1 female, all in their 20s with normal hearing, participated in the psychological listening experiment.

2.3 Presented sound

2.3.1 Audio signal

A monosyllable list (a list containing 50 monosyllables) from a CD originally designed for the evaluation and fitting of hearing aids (TY-89) (Yonemoto K., 1995) was used. The maximum band levels of speech were measured with a real-time octave-band analyzer. Maximum band levels were adopted as the band levels of the speech peaks. The over-all sound pressure level of the speech peaks was about 62 dB.

2.3.2 External noise

The external noise consisted of band-limited pink noise with frequency bandwidth [44, 11,300] Hz. The sound pressure level in each subject's ears was adjusted to 44, 47, 50, 53, 56, 59, 62, 65, 68, 71, 74, and 77 dB.

It is well known that hearing acuity declines with age. Moreover, several studies have reported on the frequency characteristics of hearing loss associated with aging (ISO7029, 1984) (Yokouchi Y., 1967) . Taking into account the frequency characteristics of such hearing loss (Yokouchi Y., 1967), both the audio signal and noise were passed through frequency filters A, B, C, and D to simulate hearing loss experienced by individuals in their 20s, 50s, 70s and 80s based on their 20s. The frequency characteristics of the filters are shown in Figure 1. There is a tendency for the overall sound pressure level to decrease and for the higher frequency to attenuate in the following order: A, B, C, D.

2.4 Measurement of listening scores and psychological impressions

Both the audio signal and noise were presented to the eight subjects through two speaker boxes to allow assessment of the listening scores of the audio signal and the psychological impressions associated with speech audibility while listening to the audio signal. It was confirmed prior to the experiment that there was no difference in the sound pressure levels at the subjects' ears. To quantify the psychological evaluation of speech audibility, various psychological evaluation scales for audio signals were considered. For this experiment, the seven categorized psychological impressions A_i $(i = 1, 2, ..., 7)$ of speech audibility (Nakajima T. et al., 1984) were adopted:

A_1: Very inaudible
A_2: Quite inaudible
A_3: Slightly inaudible
A_4: Medium
A_5: Slightly audible
A_6: Quite audible
A_7: Very audible

The eight subjects participated simultaneously in the psychological listening experiment. They listened to the audio signal and completed a response sheet asking them to report exactly what they had heard. In addition, they performed the above psychological evaluation, i.e., A_i $(i = 1, 2, ..., 7)$, related to speech audibility. This operation was then carried out with the same subjects for an external noise condition as well. The subjects were given sufficient rest to avoid fatigue.

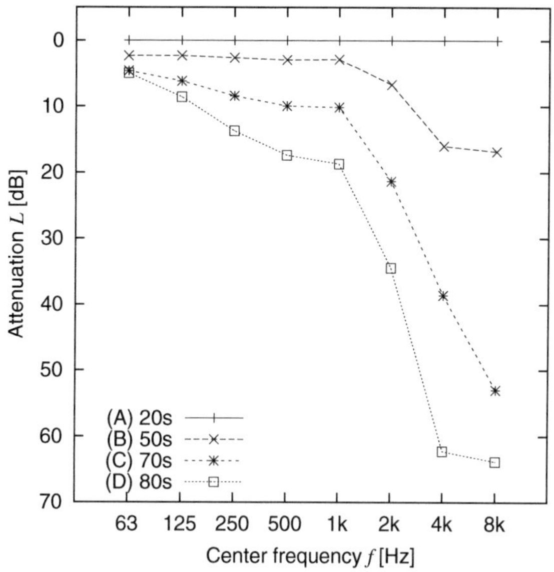

Fig. 1. Frequency characteristics of simulated hearing loss by filter (A: 20s, B: 50s, C: 70s, D: 80s)

3. Relationships between index and listening scores / psychological impressions

3.1 Index for evaluating listening scores and psychological impressions

In our previous research (Tamesue T. et al., 2003), the most useful indexes for evaluating the listening scores of audio signals and psychological impressions as they relate to speech audibility under conditions of meaningless steady noise while listening to an audio signal were investigated. The results indicated that weighted-mean spectral distance $WSPD$ was the most useful target index. We therefore used the same index in this study. $WSPD$ was calculated as follows:

$$WSPD = \sum_{i=1}^{8} a_i[L_S(f_i) - L_N(f_i)] \tag{1}$$

where a_i denotes the weight considered to be percentages of 20 frequency bands(Kryter KD., 1962) that contribute equally to speech intelligibility. These are included in octave bands with center frequency f_i (f_1 = 63, f_2 = 125, $\cdots$, f_8 = 8000 Hz), and are shown as follows:

$$\begin{array}{llll} a_1 = 0.000000 & a_2 = 0.000000 & a_3 = 0.063794 & a_4 = 0.140096 \\ a_5 = 0.226255 & a_6 = 0.319855 & a_7 = 0.227360 & a_8 = 0.022640 \end{array} \tag{2}$$

$L_S(f_i)$ denotes the band level with center frequency f_i (f_1 = 63, f_2 = 125, $\cdots$, f_8 = 8000 Hz) of the speech peaks. In this, the maximum band levels of the audio signal, measured by a sound level meter (RION, type NL-22) along with a real-time octave-band analyzer (RION, type NX-22RT) with FAST dynamic response for 180 seconds, are adopted as the band levels of the speech peaks. $L_N(f_i)$ denotes the band level with center frequency f_i of the noise. These band levels were measured by the real-time octave-band analyzer built into the sound level meter with FAST dynamic response.

3.2 Relationship between $WSPD$ and the listening score of the audio signal

The subjects noted the monosyllables exactly as they heard them, as described in **2.4**. The number of correct answers given by each subject was assessed, with the listening score for the audio signal being defined as the percentage of correct monosyllables from the total (50). Using the observed data obtained during psychological listening experiment I, the relationship between $WSPD$ and the listening scores of the audio signal were examined. In order to understand this relationship, the following models describing the regression between them were adopted.

Linear function:

$$y = ax + b \tag{3}$$

Logistic function:

$$y = \frac{k - c}{1 + a\exp(-bx)} + c \tag{4}$$

Gomperz function:

$$y = (k - c)\exp(-\exp(-a(x - b))) + c \tag{5}$$

In each case both the audio signal and noise passed through one of the frequency filters, A, B, C, or D, and the relationship between $WSPD$ and the listening score of the audio signal was calculated. These results are shown in Figure 2. The lines in the figure indicate the regression line as selected by AIC (Akaike H., 1974).

Here, the expressions are represented by eqn.(5). This figure reveals the following: when the value of $WSPD$ decreased, the listening score of the audio signal approached 0. This indicates that when there is a larger level of hearing loss, the listening score of the audio signal clearly decreases.

3.3 Relationship between $WSPD$ and psychological impressions related to speech audibility

The relationships between $WSPD$ and the psychological impressions related to speech audibility were investigated using frequency filters A, B, C, D in the same way as the above investigation of the listening scores of the audio signal. Figure 3 shows the results of the regression models represented by eqn.(5), which was found to be the most suitable. In Figure 3, when the value of $WSPD$ decreased, the psychological impression related to speech audibility approached A_1. This indicates that the psychological impression related to speech audibility decreases with a reduction of hearing acuity.

4. Outline of psychological listening experiment II

Psychological listening experiment II was conducted to compare the observed values of the listening scores of the audio signal and the psychological impressions related to speech audibility with the predicted values. This experiment was conducted as follows.

4.1 Subjects

A total of 24 students, 20 male and 4 female, all in their 20s with normal hearing, participated in psychological listening experiment II. These subjects were different from the subjects who participated in psychological listening experiment I.

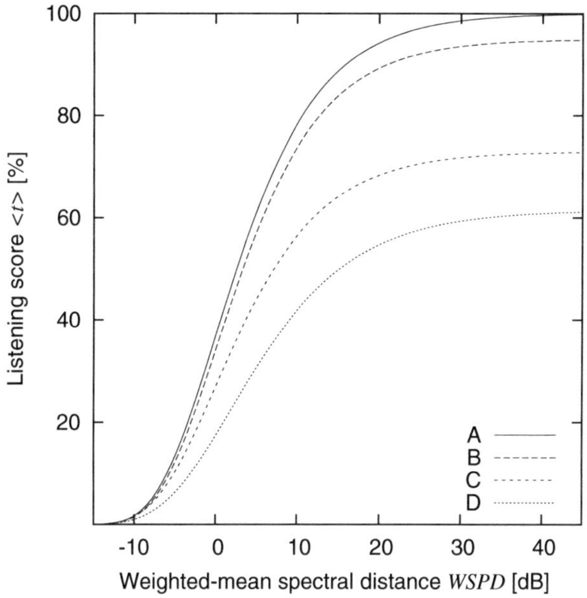

Fig. 2. Relationship between the listening score of the audio signal and the weighted-mean spectral distance (A: 20s, B: 50s, C: 70s, D: 80s)

4.2 Location

The experiment was conducted in a soundproof room on campus having the following dimensions: length 3.0 m, width 3.0 m, and height 1.9 m. The sound pressure level of the background noise was about 36 dB. The A-weighted sound pressure level was about 20 dB(A).

4.3 Audio signal

The same audio signal used in psychological listening experiment I

4.4 External noise

In order to best simulate an actual noise environment, various realistic external noises that contained many frequency components were used. The following two noises were adopted as examples of steady noise.

(a) Voice noise
A voice noise from a CD originally designed for the evaluation and fitting of hearing aids (TY-89) was used. The sound pressure level was adjusted to 57, 62, and 67 dB.

(b) Road traffic noise
This consisted of pink noise whose power spectrum closely resembled that of actual road traffic noise. The sound pressure level was adjusted to 57, 62, and 67 dB.

The following three noises were adopted as examples of a typical irregular fluctuating noise.

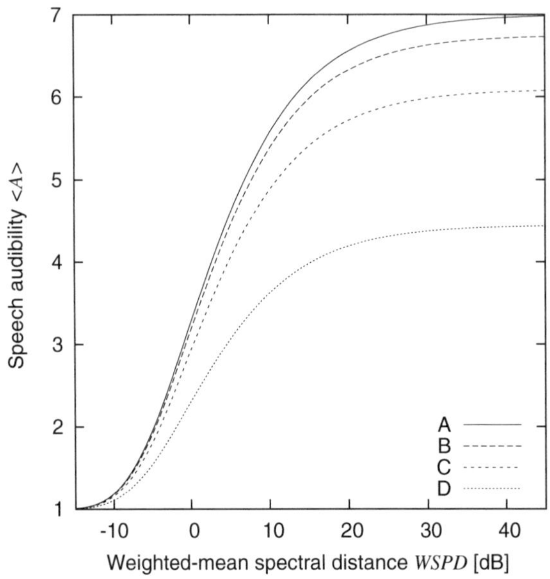

Fig. 3. Relationship between the psychological impressions related to speech audibility and weighted-mean spectral distance (A: 20s, B: 50s, C: 70s, D: 80s)

(c) Non-stationary road traffic noise
Actual road traffic noise under interrupted traffic flow conditions, recorded in advance for approximately two hours at the side of a road. The equivalent continuous sound pressure level was adjusted to 62 and 67 dB.

(d) Stationary road traffic noise
Actual road traffic noise under uninterrupted traffic flow conditions obtained from the "Audio/Acoustics Technical CD for Professional Use." The equivalent continuous sound pressure level was adjusted to 62 and 67 dB.

(e) Aircraft noise
Actual aircraft noise during take off obtained from the "Audio/Acoustics Technical CD for Professional Use." The equivalent continuous sound pressure level was adjusted to 62 and 67 dB.

In addition, the following condition for predicting the listening score of the audio signal and psychological impressions related to speech audibility was used.

(f) No external noise

Similar to psychological listening experiment I, both the audio signal and the noise were passed through frequency filters A, B, C, and D.

4.5 Measurement of listening scores and psychological impressions

The specific method of measurement of the listening score of the audio signal and psychological impressions related to speech audibility was the same as that used in psychological listening experiment I.

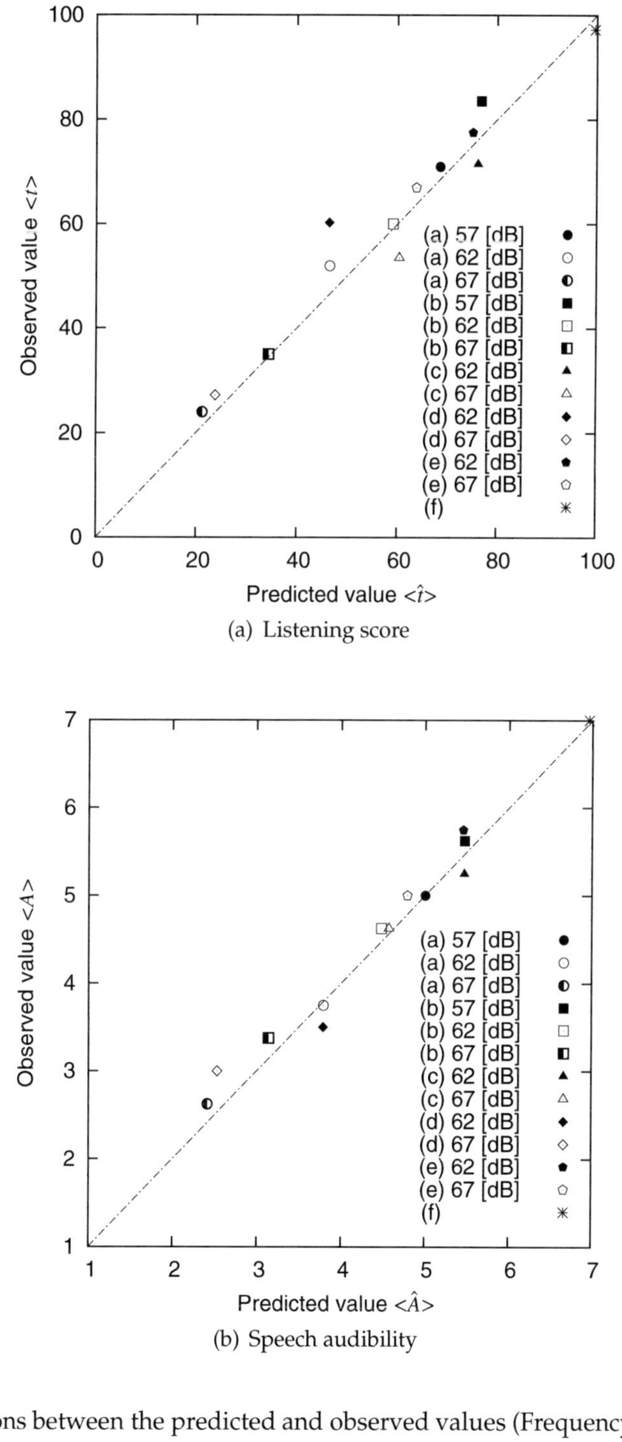

(a) Listening score

(b) Speech audibility

Fig. 4. Comparisons between the predicted and observed values (Frequency filter: A)

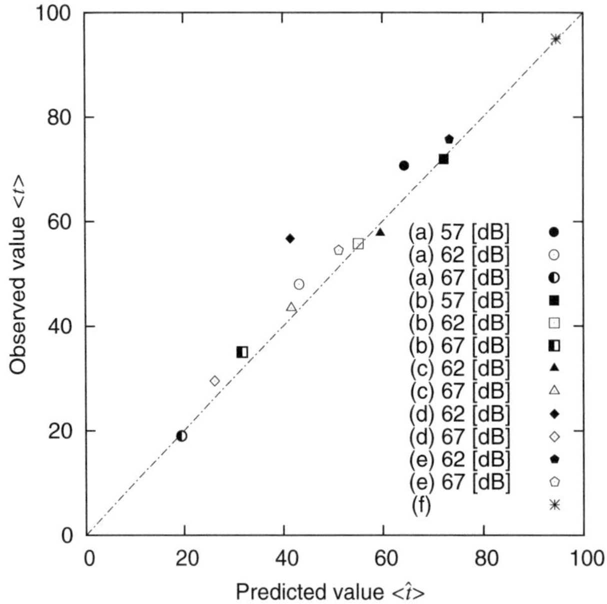

(a) Listening score

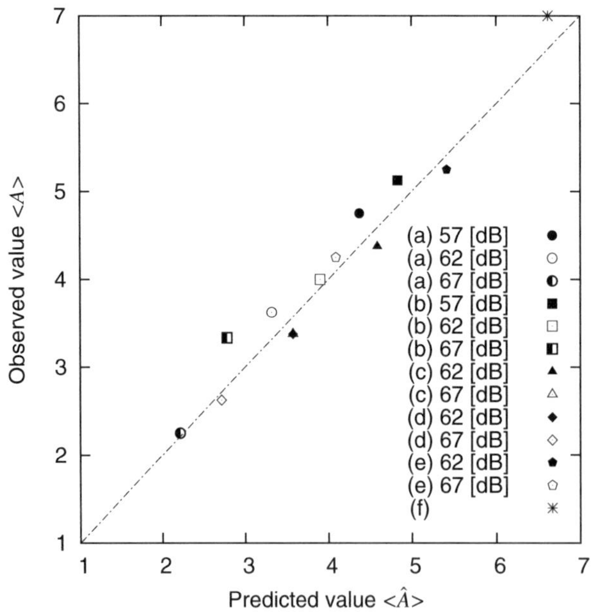

(b) Speech audibility

Fig. 5. Comparisons between the predicted and observed values (Frequency filter: B)

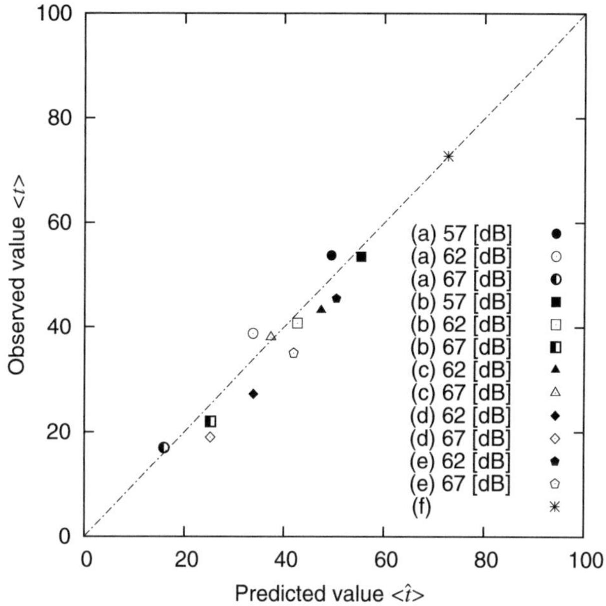

(a) Listening score

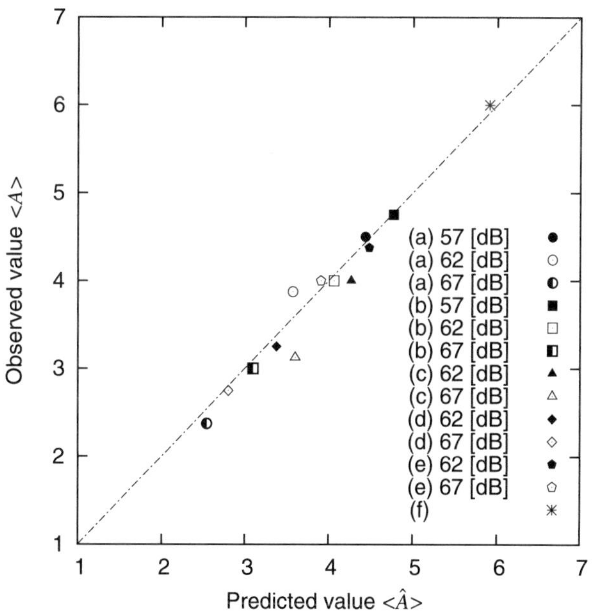

(b) Speech audibility

Fig. 6. Comparisons between the predicted and observed values (Frequency filter: C)

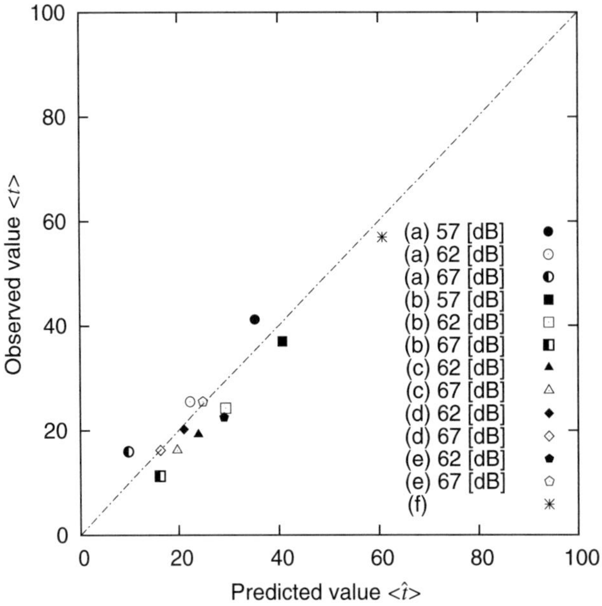

(a) Listening score

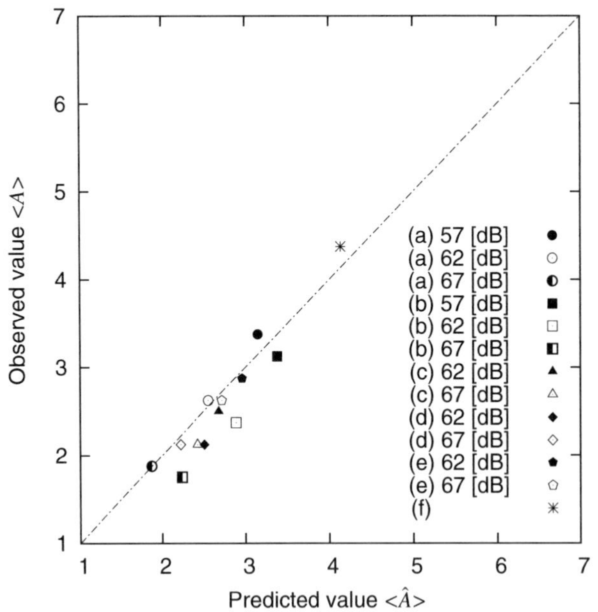

(b) Speech audibility

Fig. 7. Comparisons between the predicted and observed values (Frequency filter: D)

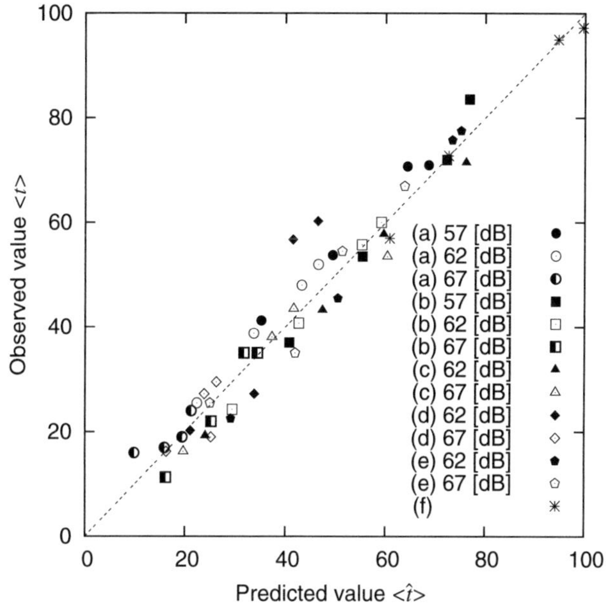

(a) Listening score

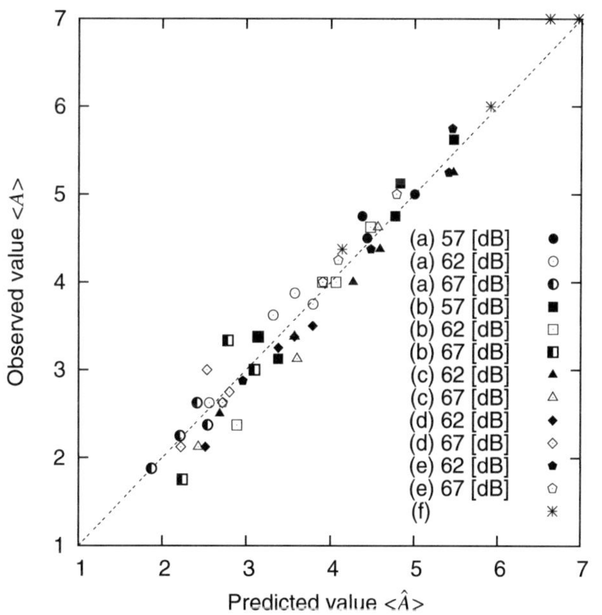

(b) Speech audibility

Fig. 8. Comparisons between the predicted and observed values

5. Prediction of listening scores and psychological impressions

Employing the regression model shown in Figures 2 and 3, it was predicted that the listening scores of the audio signal and the psychological impressions related to speech audibility would change depending on actual noise environment . The subjects were exposured to the meaningless steady or fluctuating noise, with various power spectral level forms and sound pressure levels.

The value of $WSPD$ were calculated for each noise condition (a) and (b). Using Figures 2 and 3, the theoretical predicted values of the listening scores of the audio signal were estimated for each noise condition (a) and (b). These were compared with the values obtained directly from the recorded data in psychological listening experiment II. As an example of the predictin results, comparisons between the predicted and observed values of the listening score of the audio signal when using frequency filter A, which simulated the hearing loss experienced by individuals in their 20s, are shown in Figure 4(a). It can be seen from this figure that the predicted results are consistent with the observed values. In addition, the results from using frequency filter B, C, and D, which simulated the hearing loss experienced by individuals in their 50s, 70s, and 80s, are shown in Figure 5(a), Figure 6(a) and Figure 7(a). The predicted values are in good agreement with the observed values shown in these figures, which become smaller than those in Figure 4(a). Finally, Figure 8(a) shows the results for all of the frequency filters (A, B, C, and D). Since the predicted values are in good agreement with the observed values, both the validity and the applicability of the proposed method were confirmed experimentally.

With respect to the psychological impressions associated with speech audibility, the theoretical predicted values were calculated for each of the noise conditions (a) and (b) using the regression models. As examples of the results, comparisons between the predicted and observed values of the psychological impressions associated with speech audibility when using frequency filters A, B, C, and D are shown in Figures 4(b), 5(b), 6(b) and 7(b), respectively. In these figures, a high level of consistency can also be seen between the predicted and observed values. Figure 8(b) shows the results for all of the frequency filters (A, B, C, D). Since the predicted values are in good agreement with the observed values similar to the listenig scores of audio signal, reasonable results were obtained.

Since $WSPD$ is reflected in the mutual relationship between the spectral level of the speech peaks and that of noise, which is limited to steady noise with no fluctuations in sound pressure level or frequency components, it is not reasonable to evaluate the listening scores of the audio signal or the psychological impressions related to speech audibility in an actual noise environment where the sound pressure levels and frequency components of noise show an irregular fluctuation over time.

Thus, here we introduce the new index as instantaneous spectral distance $ISPD$, which reflects the relationship between the spectral level of the speech peaks and that of noise within a short time scale based on the $WSPD$. $ISPD$ can be calculated as follows:

$$ISPD = \sum_{i=1}^{8} a_i [L_S(f_i) - L_N^{'}(f_i)] \quad (6)$$

where a_i and $L_S(f_i)$ are the same as those of eqn.(1). $L'_N(f_i)$ denotes the band level with center frequency f_i (f_1 = 63, f_2 = 125, $\cdots$, f_8 = 8000 Hz) of the noise within a short time scale, measured with FAST dynamic response and a sampling frequency of 10 Hz.

When the sound pressure levels and frequency components of noise show an irregular fluctuation over time, $ISPD$ is a random variable. If regression models $f_t(ISPD)$ and $f_A(ISPD)$ of the listening score of the audio signal and psychological impressions associated with speech audibility (based on $ISPD$) and a probability density function $p(ISPD)$ on $ISPD$ are known, the averages of the listening scores of the audio signal and psychological impressions related to speech audibility can be calculated as follows:

$$< * > = \int_D f_*(ISPD)p(ISPD)dISPD \quad (D = [-40, 40] \text{ dB}) \tag{7}$$

where * denotes t and A in the case of the listening scores of the audio signal and psychological impressions associated with speech audibility.

Here, the regression model to the listening score of audio signal and psychological impression for speech audibility based on $ISPD$, and the probability density function of $ISPD$ for each noise condition were employed. From a practical point of view, $f_t(WSPD)$, shown in Figure 2, and $f_A(WSPD)$, shown in Figure 3, were adopted as $f_t(ISPD)$ and $f_A(ISPD)$.

The probability distribution was obtained for each presented sound of the psychological listening experiment. Figures 9 and 10 show examples of the results in the case of noise **(c)**(62 dB) using frequency filter A, B, C, and D (which simulated the hearing loss experienced by individuals in their 20s, 50s, 70, 80s), respectively. Comparing these figures, it can be seen that probability distribution is translated in the direction of a higher level, and the spread of the values of $ISPD$ is relatively small, caused by hearing loss due to factors such as aging.

The predicted values of the listening score of the audio signal were calculated from eqn.(7) with the probability distribution obtained for each fluctuating noise condition. As an example of these results, comparisons between the predicted and observed values of the listening scores of the audio signal for each of the fluctuating noise conditions (c), (d), and (e) when using frequency filter A are shown in Figure 4(a). Even in an actual noise environment, the predicted values are in good agreement with the observed values. The results obtained when using frequency filter B, C, and D are shown in Figure 5(a), Figure 6(a), and Figure 7(a), respectively. Finally, the results from using all of the frequency filters (A, B, C, D) are shown in Figure 8(a). Since the predicted values of the listening score of audio signal by use of $ISPD$ are in good agreement with the observed values, both the validity and the applicability were confirmed in fluctuating noise environment.

In addition, the predicted values of the psychological impressions associated with speech audibility were calculated for each of the fluctuating noise conditions of (c), (d), and (e) using eqn.(7). Comparisons between the predicted and observed values of the psychological impression associated with speech audibility when using frequency filters A, B, C, and D are shown in Figures 4(b), Figure 5(b), Figure 6(b), and Figure 7(b), respectively. The results from using all of the frequency filters (A, B, C, D) are shown in Figure 8(b). Even the predicted values of the the psychological impressions associated with speech audibility by use of $ISPD$ are in good agreement with the observed values. It is possible to predict a psychological impressions associated with speech audibility as a whole over a long period of time, after a certain amount of exposure to noise.

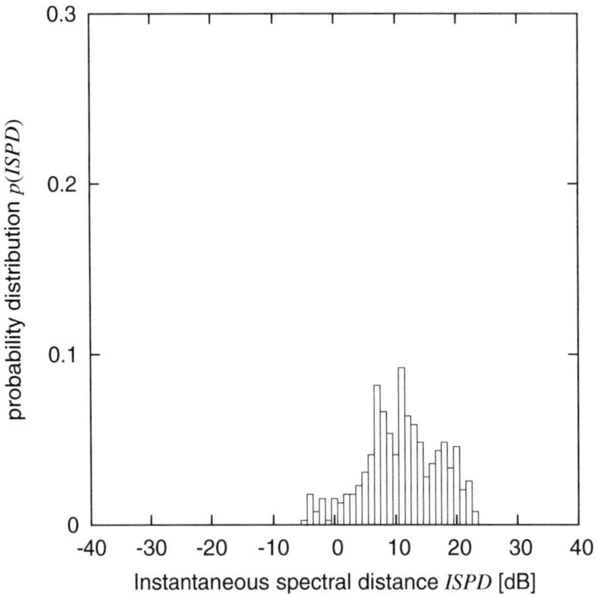

(a) Frequency filter: A

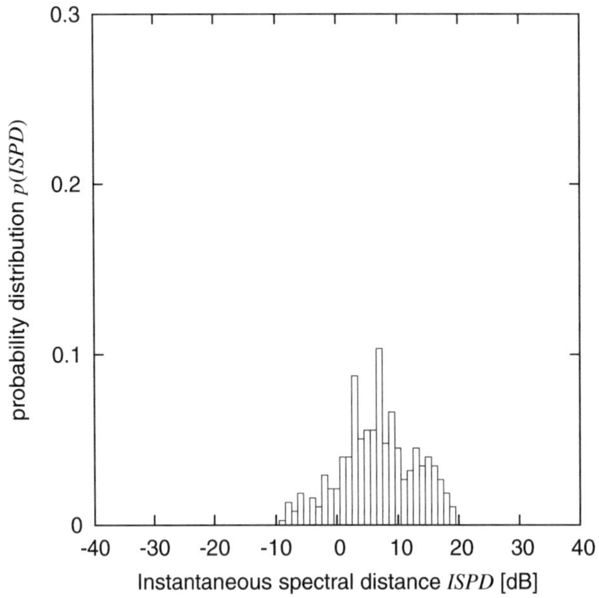

(b) Frequency filter: B

Fig. 9. Probability distribution on instantaneous spectral distance ((c) 62 dB)

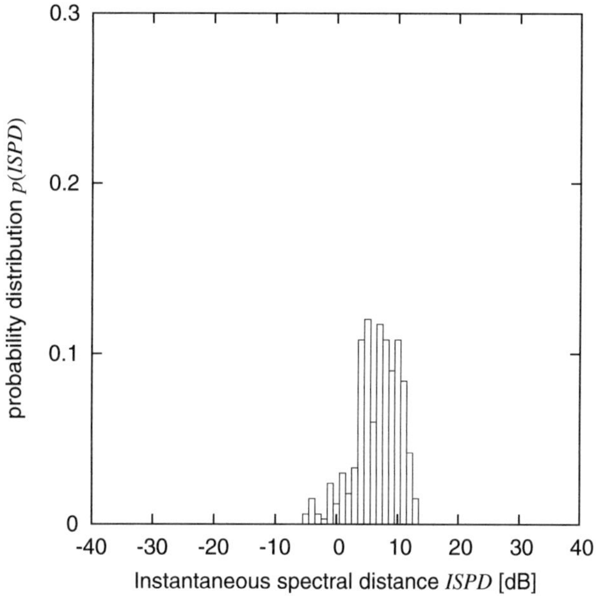

(a) Frequency filter: C

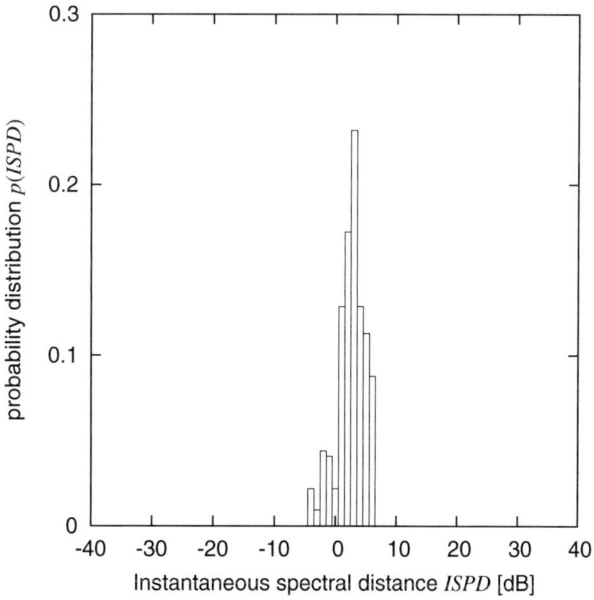

(b) Frequency filter: D

Fig. 10. Probability distribution on instantaneous spectral distance ((c) 62 dB)

6. Conclusion

This investigated how the listening scores of an audio signal and the psychological impressions related to speech audibility when listening to the audio signal under conditions of meaningless steady or fluctuating noise change when the frequency characteristics of hearing loss related to aging are taken into account. Specifically, psychological listening experiments by subjects with normal hearing were performed using artificial hearing impairments (frequency filters) that simulated hearing loss. Using the observed data obtained in psychological listening experiments, the relationships between $WSPD$ and the listening scores of an audio signal and the psychological impressions related to speech audibility were established using regression models. Further, the effect of hearing loss due to factors such as aging on the listening scores of the audio signal and the psychological impressions related to speech audibility was predicted from the above relationships. Since the predicted values are in good agreement with the observed values, both the validity and the applicability of the proposed method were confirmed experimentally, and reasonable results were obtained.

Future studies should examine the following aspects of this research.

(1) Since the current study was limited to subjects with normal hearing who experienced artificial hearing impairment with frequency filter-simulated hearing loss, the applicability of the same method to situations where the subjects are actually hearing impaired persons should be confirmed. However, comparing the available data on hearing impaired persons with the results of our simulations of hearing impairment in this study, we can conclude that our study provides fundamental data to aid in determining whether the results of such psychological listening experiments conducted using normal-hearing subjects who experience artificial hearing impairment are as valid as those conducted on hearing-impaired subjects.

(2) Decreasing pure-tone audiometric thresholds were employed as hearing loss with increasing age. However, it is still necessary to consider other factors, such as loss of frequency selectivity and reduced temporal resolution in peripheral auditory deterioration.

7. References

Tamesue T. ; Yamaguchi S.; Saeki T. Psychological impressions and listening score while listening to audio signal under meaningless steady noise. *Applied Acoustics* Vol.64, No.4, 443-457.

Yonemoto K. Characteristics of CD for the evaluation of fitting condition with hearing aids (TY-89). *Journal of Otolaryngology, Head and Neck Surgery* Vol.11, No.9, 1395-1401.

ISO7029.Threshold of hearing by air conduction as a function of age and sex for otologically normal persons. 1984.

Yokouchi Y. Studies on the physiological hearing loss by age. *Nippon Jibiinkoka Gakkai Kaiho* Vol.67, No.9, 1307-1312.

Nakajima T. ; Maeda S. The application of speech transmission index (STI) as a measure of Japanese speech audibility. *Proceedings of the Research Committee Meeting on Architectural Acoustics of the Acoustical Society of Japan* No.AA-84-30, 1-8, 1984.

Kryter KD. Method for the calculation and use of the articulation index. *The Journal of the Acoustical Society of America* Vol.34, No.11,1692-1697, 1962.

Akaike H. A new look at the statistical model identification. *IEEE Transactions on Automatic Control* Vol.AC-19, No.6, 716-723, 1974.

4

The Mongolian Gerbil as a Model for the Analysis of Peripheral and Central Age-Dependent Hearing Loss

Gleich Otto and Strutz Jürgen
University of Regensburg
Germany

1. Introduction

Age-dependent hearing loss involves pathological changes affecting the peripheral as well as the central auditory system. The Mongolian Gerbil is a rodent with an average life span of 3-4 years, which shows, in contrast to mice and rats, sensitive hearing in the frequency range that is important for human communication. Consequently, gerbils have been used to study structural and functional aspects of age-dependent hearing loss at the level of the cochlea and auditory brain stem nuclei. In addition, age-dependent changes in behavioural performance have been characterised for different auditory tasks. We have also analysed the effect of certain drugs on impaired temporal processing in old gerbils. The data from gerbils contribute to a framework that helps to better understand the mechanisms contributing to age-dependent hearing loss and may lead to new pharmacotherapeutic strategies for the treatment of age-dependent central hearing loss.

2. Gerbils as model organism

Like mice and rats, gerbils are small rodents. Henceforth, when we use the term gerbil, we refer to the species *Meriones unguiculatus*. The natural range of distribution of this species is Mongolia and the adjacent regions of Siberia and China. The first description of the species was by Milne Edwards in 1867 (Milne-Edwards, 1867). The history of the "laboratory gerbil" has been summarised by Stuermer et al. (2003). Briefly, a small group of 20 wild pairs were originally collected in 1935 during a Japanese expedition to Mongolia and subsequently bred in Japan. In 1954, eleven pairs from this Japanese colony were sent to Tumblebrook Farm in New York. Offspring of the Tumblebrook Farm breeding colony have subsequently been distributed worldwide and are used as models for different lines of research. A search for the term "gerbil" in combination with the terms "hearing", "ear" and "auditory" on Sept. 7th 2011 in the PubMed database lists 1405 publications, illustrating that gerbils have become an important model in auditory research.

The sensitivity of gerbils at low frequencies important for speech perception is similar to that of humans, while thresholds of rats and mice are much higher for frequencies below 4 kHz (Fig. 1). Thus, gerbils appear to be a better model than mice and rats to study aspects of age-dependent hearing loss that affect communication and speech perception in older human subjects. Gerbils have been suggested as a particularly suitable model for research on diverse aspects of ageing, including audition (Cheal, 1986). Here we will review the studies of age-dependent changes in the auditory system of gerbils.

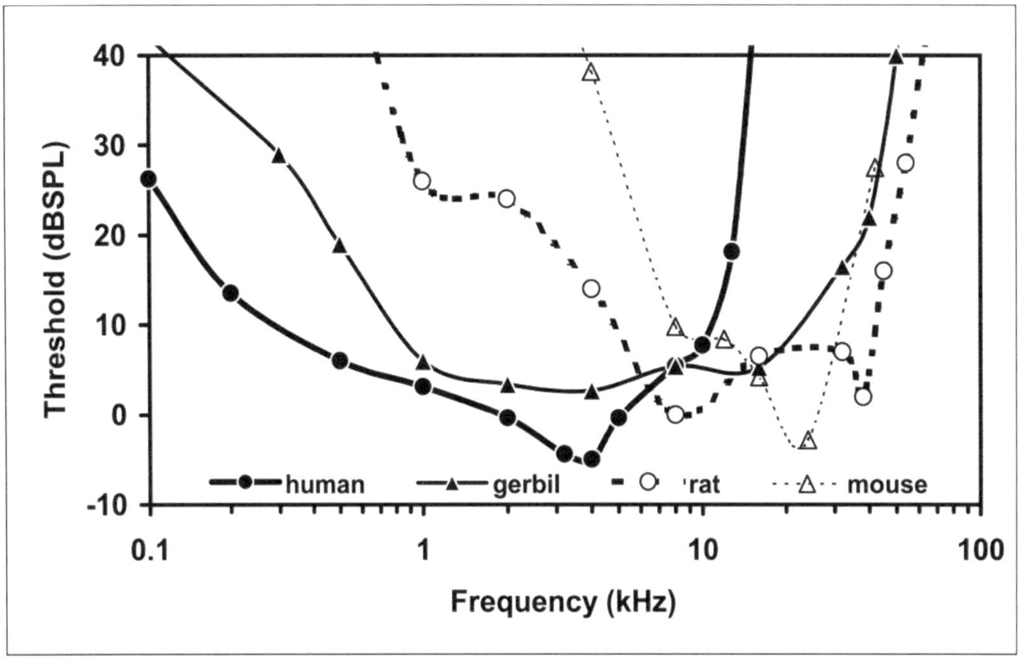

Fig. 1. Audiograms from human, gerbil, rat and mouse

The human audiogram (filled circles, thick continuous line; Zwicker & Fastl, 1990) shows the lowest thresholds at low frequencies. The gerbil audiogram (filled triangle, black continuous line; Ryan, 1976) is similar to the human audiogram, but the hearing range of gerbils extends to frequencies above 20 kHz. Compared to human and gerbil, thresholds of rat (open circles, thick dotted line; Kelly & Masterton, 1977) and mouse (open triangles, thin dotted line; Radziwon et al., 2009) are much higher for frequencies below 4 kHz.

3. The cochlea

Comparative studies (Webster & Plassmann, 1992) show that the low-frequency hearing in gerbils is associated with adaptations of the middle ear (e.g. large middle ear cavities that facilitate the transmission of low frequencies to the inner ear) and of the basilar membrane (e.g. increased width compared to other small rodents).

3.1 Activity of single auditory nerve fibres

Analysis of auditory nerve fibre activity provides information about sound processing in the cochlea. A reference species, in which auditory nerve fibre function has been studied in much detail, is the cat (Kiang, 1965). In a comparative analysis of gerbil auditory nerve fibre activity, Schmiedt (1989) demonstrated a good correspondence with data from the cat and suggested that this "implies the presence of fundamental mechanisms that are common to mammalian auditory systems", making the gerbil a useful model for hearing loss in ageing studies.

In addition to normative data gathered using young gerbils, several studies have also analysed auditory nerve fibre activity in gerbils older than 1 year. In auditory nerve fibres of quiet aged three-year-old gerbils, Schmiedt et al. (1990) found that thresholds were elevated by 20-30 dB at the tip (characteristic frequency, CF) of the tuning curves, while the low frequency tails were much less affected, resulting in a reduced tip-to-tail ratio. Measures of frequency selectivity, like Q_{10dB} and Q_{40dB} (Hellstrom & Schmiedt, 1996), were similar for young and old gerbils in fibres with CFs below 4 kHz, while auditory nerve fibres with higher CFs were on average less sharply tuned in old gerbils. A comparison of rate-level functions (the discharge rate of auditory nerve fibres plotted as a function of stimulus level) at CF in old and young gerbils showed that these functions in old gerbils were shifted to higher levels, consistent with elevated thresholds of auditory nerve fibres. However, the slopes of functions in the dynamic range region between threshold and saturation of old gerbils were at least as steep as those from young gerbils. The distributions of spontaneous rates in large samples of auditory nerve fibres from young and old gerbils were similar for fibres with CFs below 6 kHz, while the proportion of low spontaneous rate fibres with CFs above 6 kHz was only 30% in old gerbils, compared to 60% in young gerbils (Schmiedt et al., 1996). Fibres with low spontaneous activity typically have higher thresholds and larger dynamic ranges compared to fibres with high spontaneous rates (Winter et al., 1990). Thus, a loss of the contribution of auditory nerve fibres with low spontaneous rate may affect processing of supra-threshold signals and contribute to a decreased ability to understand speech in noise.

3.2 The compound action potential (CAP)

Although single-fibre recordings provide much information, the amount of data that can be generated in an individual gerbil, especially in aged animals, is limited. An alternative to evaluate the state of the cochlea is the compound action potential (CAP), an electrical signal that is generated by the synchronised population response of the auditory nerve fibres to the onset of a signal (Hellstrom & Schmiedt, 1996).

3.2.1 CAP threshold and growth with stimulus intensity

By plotting CAP thresholds across a range of test frequencies, Hellstrom & Schmiedt (1990) compared CAP audibility curves of young and old gerbils and found a varying degree of frequency-specific threshold elevation in old gerbils. Compared to young gerbils, the inter-animal variability of thresholds was much higher in old gerbils for frequencies above 3 kHz. Below 3 kHz, old gerbils showed an average of less than 20 dB threshold elevation, while the difference increased at higher frequencies to more than 30 dB. The growth of the peak-to-peak CAP amplitude with increasing level of the tone pip was considerably reduced in old gerbils and a quantitative analysis confirmed that the slopes of the CAP input-output functions were significantly reduced for test frequencies between 1 and 8 kHz. While the elevated CAP thresholds in old gerbils reflect the elevated thresholds at the tip of the tuning curve in recordings from auditory nerve fibres (Schmiedt et al., 1990), the reduced slope of the CAP growth functions in old gerbils was not reflected in the rate-level functions of auditory nerve fibres (Hellstrom & Schmiedt, 1991). Given that the slopes of rate-level functions of auditory nerve fibres did not differ between young and old gerbils, Hellstrom & Schmiedt (1990, 1991) argued that a loss of auditory nerve fibres and spiral ganglion cells and a loss of synchrony of the auditory nerve fibre population response could result in reduced CAP amplitudes in old gerbils.

3.2.2 CAP measure of cochlear frequency selectivity

CAP measurements have also been conducted to compare cochlear frequency selectivity of young and old gerbils (Hellstrom & Schmiedt, 1996). A forward masking paradigm was used to determine masked CAP tuning curves at probe frequencies between 1 and 16 kHz. Briefly, a probe of a given frequency was presented 10-15 dB above the CAP threshold, eliciting a robust CAP response. The response to the probe was masked by a 60 ms tone burst that was presented 5 ms before the probe. The masked CAP tuning curve was obtained by plotting the masker level that just suppressed the response to the probe as a function of masker frequency. The masked CAP tuning curves share many characteristics with auditory nerve fibre tuning curves. The elevation of threshold at the tip of single fibre tuning curves in old gerbils (Schmiedt et al., 1990), especially at higher frequencies, was also evident in masked CAP tuning curves. In addition, the loss of frequency selectivity in auditory nerve fibres with characteristic frequencies above 4 kHz in old gerbils was paralleled by a corresponding loss of frequency selectivity in the masked CAP tuning curves (Hellstrom & Schmiedt, 1996).

3.3 Distortion product otoacoustic emissions (DPOAE)

Distortion product otoacoustic emissions (DPOAE) characterise the function of outer hair cells that are the central element of the "cochlear amplifier". They can be used to determine the sensitivity of the cochlea and to construct audiograms (Janssen et al., 2006). Eckrich et al. (2008) measured DPOAE audiograms of "laboratory" gerbils and gerbils that had been caught in the wild and bred for 6-7 generations in captivity. While thresholds of "wild" gerbils remained stable across age, thresholds of 15-28 month old, domesticated gerbils were increased at 2 kHz (6 dB), between 8 and 20 kHz (6-11 dB) and above 44 kHz (6-12 dB), when compared to the thresholds of 3 and 6 month old, domesticated gerbils. For the most basal test frequencies above 50 kHz, threshold elevation of more than 6 dB was present in the 9 and 12 month old, domesticated gerbils. Eckrich et al. (2008) suggested that elevated DPOAE thresholds in the older gerbils may have been caused by a loss of the endocochlear potential and/or a loss of outer hair cells.

3.4 Age-dependent hair cell loss

The loss of hair cells is one mechanism that causes hearing loss. Cytocochleograms are plots of the proportion of missing and abnormal hair cells as a function of the position along the cochlea. When the cochlear place-frequency map is known, frequency specific hearing loss can be directly correlated with hair cell loss. Tarnowski et al. (1991) performed such a comparison of cytocochleograms and CAP thresholds in 16 old gerbils raised in a low-noise environment. In their sample, they found a substantial inter-animal variation of threshold shift and hair cell loss and defined 3 groups based on the degree of hair cell loss. In 6 animals with minimal hair cell loss (5-8%), only outer hair cells were missing, predominantly in the apical turn and to a lesser degree in the extreme basal turn. This group of animals showed the least degree of threshold elevation (0-25 dB). Eight animals with a moderate degree of hair cell loss (8-14%) showed, on average, higher degrees of threshold shift (5-55dB). Outer hair cell loss was more pronounced at the apex, but was also present towards the base of the cochlea. In 2 gerbils, 41-54% of the hair cells, predominantly outer and to a lesser degree inner hair cells, were missing. The hair cell loss in this group was associated with more than 50 dB hearing loss. In addition to hair cell loss, a varying proportion of outer hair cells in the low-frequency (apical) region of old gerbils appeared grossly abnormal with a spherical shape and larger diameters. These cells were located between normally appearing outer hair cells. No such abnormalities were found in young animals. Although the degree of hair cell loss was associated with the degree of threshold shift in the 3 groups, the pattern of hair cell loss did not correlate with the frequency-dependent CAP threshold shifts along the cochlea. Loss of outer hair cells at the apex was found without corresponding threshold shifts for frequencies below 3 kHz. Above 4 kHz, threshold shift was present without a loss of outer hair cells in the corresponding frequency region. These data demonstrate that cytocochleograms cannot predict the frequency-specific CAP threshold shifts in old gerbils raised in a low noise environment.

3.5 Pathology of non-sensory cells in the organ of Corti and Reissner's membrane

Adams & Schulte (1997) expanded the analysis of cochlear pathology in old gerbils to the non-sensory cells of the organ of Corti and Reissner's membrane. In addition to the loss and pathology of hair cells, they observed pathological changes to pillar cells in regions where outer hair cells had been lost. Compared to young gerbils, where the cells forming Reissner's membrane appeared uniformly distributed, gerbils older than 2 years showed a formation of cell clusters mixed with regions of lower cell density. However, this rearrangement of cells in Reissner's membrane appeared to not be related to hearing loss. In summary, Adams & Schulte (1997) emphasised the discrepancy between the frequencies affected by hearing loss and the position of cell pathology along the cochlea.

3.6 Spiral ganglion cells and auditory dendrites

Keithley et al. (1989) compared the density of spiral ganglion cells in young and old gerbils. The mean ganglion cell density averaged along the whole cochlea was 1106 cells/mm^2 for 4 gerbils with an age of 2 months. Compared to the mean of these young gerbils, the density decreased to 86% and 83% in 5 animals aged 24-30 months and in 3 animals aged 36-42 months respectively, though the difference between the young animals and the 2 groups of old animals was not significant in this sample. When they compared mean spiral ganglion cell density for separate half turns of the cochlea, a significant reduction that varied between 16 and 55% in the two groups of old gerbils with reference to the 2 month old animals was only found for the most basal position (80-90% from the apical end, corresponding to frequencies above 20 kHz). Overall, the loss of spiral ganglion cells was limited and predominantly affected high frequencies.

Based on a small sample that precluded statistical analysis, Suryadevara et al. (2001) suggested a slightly decreased number of auditory dendrites per inner hair cell in old gerbils. Their data in young gerbils showed a gradient of auditory nerve fibre dendrite diameter within the osseous spiral lamina, with increasing diameter from the scala vestibuli to the scala tympani side. With decreasing endocochlear potential (EP) in old gerbils, this gradient disappeared due to fewer large diameter fibres found near scala tympani. In addition, the cross-sectional area of spiral ganglion cells decreased with decreasing EP. Thus, decreasing EP was associated with a loss or shrinkage of large diameter auditory nerve fibre dendrites and a reduction of the size of spiral ganglion cells.

Rüttiger et al. (2007) found an age dependent reduction of BDNF mRNA expression in high frequency spiral ganglion cells. In contrast, BDNF protein expression was preserved in the cochlear ganglion cells of old gerbils but declined in their central and peripheral processes.

3.7 The endocochlear potential and pathology related to endolymph homeostasis

The sensitivity of the mechano-electrical transduction by hair cells in the mammalian cochlea depends on the endocochlear potential (EP) in scala media (Wangemann, 2006). The positive EP (80-100 mV) together with the negative intracellular potential of hair cells is the driving force (battery) of sensory transduction. The important contribution of the EP to the sensitivity of the cochlea was demonstrated in experiments, where a reduction of the endocochlear potential by the application of furosemide was associated with threshold shifts in single auditory nerve fibres in cat (Sewell, 1984).

3.7.1 Age-dependent loss of the endocochlear potential

Several studies in gerbils have shown that the EP, on average, declines with age and inter-animal variability of the EP in old gerbils becomes much higher compared to young gerbils (Gratton et al., 1996, 1997a; Schmiedt, 1983, 1996; Schulte & Schmiedt, 1992). The EP in young gerbils (Schmiedt, 1983) was highest at the base, determined through the round window (92 mV), and slightly lower at more apical locations (76-81 mV); the reduction of the mean EP determined in 3 year old gerbils relative to the means obtained in young gerbils was more pronounced at the base (40 kHz region: 31 mV) and the apex (0.5 kHz region: 27 mV) as compared to the intermediate parts of the cochlea (2 kHz region: 19 mV; 16 kHz region: 23 mV). The loss of the EP and threshold shifts in old gerbils were not related to each other in a direct and simple way. The pattern of CAP threshold shift from low to high frequencies differed from the pattern of EP loss. In addition, the plots of CAP threshold shift as a function of EP shift (Schmiedt, 1983) demonstrate no correlation for young and 30 month old gerbils, despite a variation of the EP over a 40-60 mV range. Only the data from 3 year old gerbils indicated some correlation between CAP threshold and EP, although the scatter in the data was large. Overall, a linear regression analysis suggested that the variation of EP in 3 year old gerbils accounts for 31% of the variation in CAP thresholds (Schmiedt, 1983). The reduction of the mean EP was not associated with a mean loss of potassium concentration in the endolymph of old gerbils and the "effects of age are primarily on EP generation, and not on the chemical potential of K_e^+" between endolymph and perilymph (Schmiedt, 1996).

3.7.2 Histological changes in the stria vascularis and the spiral ligament

The stria vascularis (SV) plays a central role in the generation of the EP (Wangemann, 2006). Age-dependent changes in the microvasculature that might lead to ischemia and affect SV function have been the focus of several studies (Gratton & Schulte, 1995; Gratton et al., 1996, 1997b; Sakaguchi et al., 1997a, 1997b; Thomopoulos et al., 1997). Gratton & Schulte (1995) described small regions at the apical and basal ends of the SV that were devoid of capillaries in gerbils as young as 5-10 months. With increasing age, loss of capillaries progressed from both ends towards the middle of the cochlea. Gerbils older than 33 months showed a normal pattern of strial vascularisation only in the mid-region of the cochlea. In the regions of capillary loss, strial atrophy was observed with missing marginal cells and "clumps of pigment" in remaining cells. Gratton et al. (1996) found a significant correlation between the proportion of the SV with normal vascularisation and the EP. However, due to the large inter-animal variability of both parameters, the correlation coefficient indicated that SV pathology explained only up to 37% of the EP variation.

In addition to loss of vascularisation and atrophy of the SV, different types of fibrocytes in the spiral ligament of old gerbils are also affected. Spicer & Schulte (2002) suggested that vacuolisation of type II fibrocytes in regions of old cochleae that show no strial atrophy can be regarded as an early event in the development of strial pathology. Regions with apoptotic or necrotic type II fibrocytes were associated with moderate degeneration of SV, while regions with a complete absence of type II fibrocytes showed advanced SV atrophy. Also, type IV and V fibrocytes showed vacuolisation in old gerbils, while type I fibrocytes did not. Thus, vacuolisation was found in Na,K-ATPase positive fibrocyte types II, IV and V, but not in negative type I fibrocytes. Unfortunately the hearing status was not known and could not be directly correlated with the degree of structural changes in these specimen. Based on their data, Spicer & Schulte (2002) put forward the hypothesis that, within the potassium recycling pathway, impaired secretion of potassium into the endolymph by strial marginal cells could reduce the flow of potassium towards the stria and lead to potassium accumulation and the development of vacuoles in Na,K-ATPase positive fibrocytes. They proposed that dysfunction of marginal cells is the first step leading to fibrocyte pathology and strial degeneration.

3.7.3 Changes in enzymes regulating potassium homeostasis

Spicer et al. (1997) compared the Na,K-ATPase-immunoreactivity (an ion exchange enzyme that uses ATP to pump 3 sodium ions out of the cell in exchange for 2 potassium ions that are pumped into the cell) in the lateral wall and SV of young and old gerbils. Immunostaining in cochleae of old gerbils was more variable than in young gerbils. Old animals showed strial atrophy and no Na,K-ATPase immunoreactivity at the apex, best preservation of SV and immunoreactivity in the middle, and atrophy of SV and loss of immunoreactivity at the base of the cochlea. Immunoreactivity in type II, IV and V fibrocytes of old gerbils decreased less than expression in the adjacent SV, although complete SV degeneration was also associated with loss of immunoreactivity in fibrocytes. The observation that a loss of Na,K-ATPase immunoreactivity in fibrocytes of the spiral ligament appeared to lag behind the loss of staining in the SV supports the suggestion that changes in fibrocytes occur secondarily to alterations in the SV. Sakaguchi et al. (1998) found that age-dependent changes in the expression of the Na-K-Cl co-transporter closely paralleled those reported for the Na,K-ATPase.

Schulte & Schmiedt (1992) determined the Na,K-ATPase immunoreactive volume of the SV from immunostained cochlear sections. A plot of the EP as a function of the normalised SV volume showed a group of 4 old gerbils with an EP below 20 mV where the SV volume was reduced by more than 70%. In another group of 9 old gerbils, EP varied between 50 and 80 mV with an associated loss of the SV volume between 20% and 70%. Thus, a reduction of the SV volume expressing Na,K-ATPase by up to 70% was associated with only a small loss of the EP. Only when the loss of Na,K-ATPase expressing SV volume increased beyond 70% did the EP show an abrupt break down: the EP appeared tolerant to a relatively large loss of Na,K-ATPase. Consistent with a mean reduction of the Na,K-ATPase immunoreactive volume of SV, the activity of this enzyme was reduced in the lateral wall of old as compared to young gerbils (Gratton et al., 1995) and a low level of Na,K-ATPase activity was associated with a low EP (Gratton et al., 1997b).

Spicer & Schulte (1998) proposed a medial pathway for the recycling of potassium released by inner hair cells. In old gerbils, in contrast to the SV and the lateral wall, fibrocytes of the spiral limbus showed unaltered or upregulated Na,K-ATPase immunoreactivity. In addition, interdental cells remained immunoreactive in cochleae with SV atrophy. Based on these observations, Spicer & Schulte (1998) suggested a normal function of inner hair cells in old gerbils with strial atrophy (although the hearing status of the specimen they analysed was not known). Potassium released by inner hair cells can be recycled into the endolymph by the medial pathway via the remaining Na,K-ATPase immunoreactive limbal fibrocytes and interdental cells.

3.8 The gerbil as a model of strial or metabolic presbyacusis

The data discussed above describe a wide range of age-dependent pathologies of the gerbil cochlea. In summary, they suggest that loss of EP due to pathology of the SV and the lateral wall are the main factors that contribute to the threshold shifts observed in auditory nerve fibres and the CAP in old gerbils. This pattern resembles the category of strial atrophy in humans (Schuknecht & Gacek, 1993).

The loss of sensitivity was most pronounced at the tip of single-fibre tuning curves (Schmiedt et al., 1990) and in masked CAP tuning curves (Hellstrom & Schmiedt, 1996) of old gerbils and led to a decreased tip-to-tail ratio of the tuning curves. These changes are similar to the effects of a reduced EP on single-fibre tuning curves in cat (Sewell, 1984). Consequently, Hellstrom & Schmiedt (1996) proposed that "the quiet-aged gerbil can be used as a model for an intact hair-cell system coupled to a chronically lowered EP". This view was supported by a subsequent study where changes of cochlear function due to a reduction of the EP by chronic furosemide application to the round window in young gerbils resembled those found in quiet-aged, old gerbils (Lang et al., 2010). Schmiedt (1983) proposed the "dead battery theory" and reported that increasing the EP by current injection into scala media in an old animal with an initial EP of 41 mV was associated with increased CAP amplitude and a 20 dB reduction of CAP threshold.

In summary, cochlear sensitivity in quiet-aged gerbils declines on average with a high degree of inter-animal variability. The loss of EP due to degeneration of the SV appears to be the main reason for decreased sensitivity in old gerbils, while loss of hair cells and auditory nerve fibres appear less important. Consequently, gerbils are a useful model of human strial or metabolic cochlear presbyacusis.

4. The auditory brainstem nuclei

An overview of the auditory pathway is summarised in Strutz (1991) and Schwartz (1991). The central processes of the auditory nerve fibres enter the brain through the internal auditory meatus. Each fibre bifurcates when it enters the cochlear nucleus and sends an ascending branch to the antero-ventral (AVCN) and a descending branch through the postero-ventral (PVCN) to the dorsal (DCN) cochlear nucleus. All auditory nerve fibres terminate in the cochlear nucleus. Neurons of the ventral cochlear nucleus (VCN) predominantly project to the ipsi- and contra-lateral nuclei of the superior olivary complex. The neurons of the DCN project primarily to the contra-lateral, and to a lesser degree, to the ipsi-lateral inferior colliculus (IC). The medial nucleus of the trapezoid body (MNTB) receives input from the contra-lateral VCN and projects primarily to the ipsi-lateral medial (MSO) and lateral (LSO) nuclei of the superior olive. MSO and LSO also receive input from the ipsi- and contra-lateral VCN. MSO neurons project almost exclusively to the ipsi-lateral IC and send collaterals to the dorsal nucleus of the lateral lemniscus. The LSO projects to the ipsi- and contra-lateral IC.

4.1 The auditory brainstem response (ABR)

The auditory brainstem response (ABR), recorded from needle electrodes placed behind the ear and the vertex, reflects the synchronised neural activity to the onset of a stimulus. It is less invasive than single-fibre and CAP recordings for evaluating hearing status. Short tone-pips elicit a typical ABR waveform in gerbils with peaks occurring at characteristic latencies. They have been termed i (1-2 ms), ii-iii (2-3.5 ms) and iv (4-5 ms) and can be homologised with the human ABR waves I (generated by the auditory nerve), III (generated by the cochlear nucleus or the MNTB) and V (generated by the lateral lemniscus and IC; Boettcher et al., 1993a).

4.1.1 Age-dependent changes of ABR thresholds

Age-related hearing loss in gerbils was first reported by Henry et al. (1980), showing 15-20 dB threshold elevation for frequencies between 1 and 32 kHz in 2 year old as compared to 3 month old gerbils. Mills et al. (1990) derived ABR thresholds for gerbils between 8 and 36 months of age that were raised in a low-noise environment. Thresholds in 3 year old gerbils varied over a wide range; some old animals showed no or only small threshold elevation compared to young controls, while some old gerbils had more than 50 dB hearing loss. Hearing loss was less than 10 dB in a group of 19 month old gerbils, increased to 10-20 dB at 2 years and further progressed with age. Mean threshold shift at 3 years was approximately 20 dB for the 1-4 kHz range and 25-30 dB for higher frequencies. Threshold shift determined by ABR and CAP measurements in 3 year old gerbils showed a good correspondence.

4.1.2 Age-dependent changes of ABR growth functions

Boettcher et al. (1993a) compared wave ii-iii and wave iv ABR input-output functions of young and old gerbils. The plots of wave ii-iii and iv amplitude as a function of the tone pip level showed a reduction in old as compared to young gerbils that was not directly related to threshold. This was seen through the response amplitude of the best old gerbils with near normal thresholds being greatly reduced at high stimulus levels, especially for the lower test frequencies. The reduction in response amplitude to high stimulus levels was more pronounced at lower test frequencies, while ABR threshold elevation was more pronounced at the higher test frequencies. As a consequence of the reduced ABR response amplitudes, the slopes of the ABR growth functions were also reduced in old gerbils. Boettcher et al. (1993a) discussed that a loss of spiral ganglion cells could lead to a similar reduction in CAP and ABR amplitudes. However, Keithley et al. (1989) reported a significant reduction in spiral ganglion cell density only for the most basal portion of the cochlea (20 kHz region), while the reduction of ABR response amplitude in old gerbils appeared more pronounced at frequencies ≤ 4 kHz. In addition to ganglion cell loss, ABR response amplitude may be affected by a reduction of the EP or a reduction in the degree of synchronisation of the response across the population of auditory neurons. The reduction of ABR amplitude was prominent in old gerbils and largely independent of threshold elevation (Boettcher, 2002a).

4.1.3 Age-dependent changes of ABR response latencies

Boettcher et al. (1993b) compared wave i, ii and iv response latency between young and old gerbils with different degrees of threshold shift. In the group of normal hearing old gerbils, they found no increase in response latency. Instead, response latency appeared reduced at 8 and 16 kHz for wave i and ii and at all frequencies for wave iv. The reduction was small for wave i and increased for wave iv, resulting in reduced i-iv intervals in normal hearing old as compared to young gerbils. In gerbils with hearing loss, ABR latencies were prolonged at low stimulus levels and normal at high stimulus levels for wave i and ii. Response latency for wave iv in old gerbils with hearing loss was increased for all stimulus levels at 1 and 2 kHz and appeared normal at higher frequencies. Boettcher et al. (1993b) suggested that the decreasing latency along the auditory pathway in normal hearing old gerbils does not reflect changes originating in the periphery, but could rather reflect age-dependent changes in the central auditory system (e.g. loss of inhibition).

4.1.4 The effect of low- and high-pass maskers on ABR thresholds

ABR measurements have also been used to characterise masking of the response to tone pips by continuous low-pass (< 1 kHz) and high-pass (> 8 kHz) noise-maskers presented at an overall level of 80 dBSPL in young and old gerbils (Boettcher et al. 1995). Threshold shifts for the high-pass masker were similar for young and old gerbils. The shift of the quiet threshold in old gerbils was correlated with the shift of the masked threshold (relative to the mean quiet and masked threshold of young gerbils respectively) for 2 kHz and 4 kHz. For the low-pass masker, old gerbils, especially those with low ABR thresholds in the quiet condition, showed excessive masking compared to young gerbils. Threshold shift in old gerbils in the quiet condition was not correlated with the shift in the presence of the low-pass masker. These data suggest excess upward spread of masking in old as compared to young gerbils: the low-pass masker affected or spread to more basal (higher frequency) cochlear regions in old gerbils, even when ABR thresholds in quiet were near normal.

4.1.5 The interaction of age and acoustic trauma analysed by ABR thresholds

The interaction of noise-induced and age-dependent hearing loss has been analysed by ABR threshold measurements in gerbils (Boettcher, 2002b; Mills et al., 1997). Anaesthetised gerbils were exposed monaurally to a 3.5 kHz tone with 113 dBSPL for 1 hour. Pilot experiments had shown that this exposure was associated with a permanent threshold shift around 20 dB in the 4-8 kHz region (Mills et al., 1997).

In the first study (Mills et al., 1997), pre-exposure thresholds for both ears were determined in 18 month old gerbils. Thresholds for the exposed and the non-exposed ears were re-evaluated six weeks (age 19-20 months) after the exposure and at an age of 3 years. Pre-exposure thresholds at the age of 18 months were similar for both ears. Six weeks following the exposure, thresholds of the unexposed ears were similar to pre-exposure thresholds while thresholds of the exposed ears were clearly elevated at 4 and 8 kHz. Comparing the pre-exposure thresholds determined at an age of 18 months and thresholds at 3 years of age for the unexposed ears in this sample showed a relatively small age-dependent increase of 10-13 dB across the whole frequency range (this sample had excellent high frequency hearing compared to data previously presented in Mills et al., 1990). The threshold difference between exposed and unexposed ears was 15 and 12 dB for 4 kHz and 8 kHz 6 weeks following exposure and decreased to 11 and 6 dB in 3 year old gerbils. The additional age-dependent threshold loss in the exposed ear was smaller than in the unexposed ear.

In the second study (Boettcher, 2002b), ABR thresholds were determined for groups of 6-8 and 34-38 month old gerbils before and 30 days following sound exposure to evaluate the effect of age on the susceptibility to acoustic trauma. Pre-exposure thresholds of the 17 old gerbils in this study were exceptionally low, and were only 5-9 dB higher than pre-exposure thresholds of 17 young gerbils across the frequency range tested. Threshold shift (elevation above pre-exposure threshold) induced by the sound exposure was very similar for both age groups below 16 kHz. It was 6 dB or less at 1 and 2 kHz and 15-18 dB at 4 and 8 kHz. Only at 16 kHz was the threshold loss in old gerbils (17dB) higher than in young (9 dB) gerbils. Thus, except for the high frequency region, susceptibility to acoustic trauma in relatively normal hearing old gerbils was not higher than in young gerbils.

4.1.6 ABR and CAP for characterising auditory temporal resolution

Boettcher et al. (1996) analysed the CAP and ABR responses to two successive 50 ms broadband noise pulses at 60 and 80 dBSPL as a function of the time interval (gap; 2, 4, 8, 16 and 32 ms) between the two noise pulses in young and old gerbils. This design corresponds to the gap detection paradigm in psychoacoustic studies, where the duration of the smallest detectable gap is used as a measure of auditory temporal resolution. The CAP and ABR analysis compared the onset responses to the first and second noise pulse as a function of gap duration. ABR thresholds for tone pips between 1 and 16 kHz were elevated by 10-15 dB in the group of 10 old (33-38 months) as compared to 9 young (4-8 months) gerbils, indicating only a moderate degree of peripheral hearing loss. Consistent with previous CAP (Hellstrom & Schmiedt, 1990) and ABR (Boettcher et al., 1993a) studies, the amplitudes of the potentials evoked by the noise bursts were reduced in old gerbils. In both age groups, the response amplitude to the onset of the second noise pulse decreased with decreasing gap duration, while the response amplitude to the first pulse was independent of gap duration. To compare the recovery of the response with increasing gap duration between the two age groups, despite the reduced response amplitude in old gerbils, the ratio of the response to the second burst divided by the response to the first burst was used. The ratio was smallest for the 2 ms gap duration. For the CAP, the response to the onset of the second noise pulse for the 32 ms gap had not fully recovered and the ratio was around 0.6 in young and old gerbils. Recovery of ABR wave ii and iv functions with increasing gap duration was more complete as compared to the CAP in young and old gerbils. The comparison of amplitude ratio as a function of gap duration showed no clear systematic difference between both age groups. Thus, despite an absolute difference of response amplitude, the recovery of the response amplitude to the second noise burst with increasing gap duration was similar in young and old gerbils.

The latency for the first noise pulse in the CAP and ABR responses was very similar in young and old gerbils, despite the elevated ABR thresholds to tone pips and the reduced response amplitudes in old gerbils. For the CAP, response latency to the second noise pulse was very similar in old and young gerbils and showed only a small decrease ($\approx$ 0.1 ms) with increasing gap duration. In contrast to the CAP, response latency to the second noise burst showed a higher degree of variation with gap duration for wave ii ($>$ 0.2 ms) and for wave iv ($>$ 0.28 ms). Compared to young gerbils, the response latency of ABR wave ii was elevated for the 2 ms gap and that of wave iv for the 2 and 4 ms gaps in old gerbils. The variation of response latency as a function of gap duration did not differ between young and old gerbils for the CAP. Thus, while response latencies at the level of the cochlea (CAP) did not differ between age groups, the elevated latencies for short gaps in the ABR response (most pronounced for wave iv) argue for altered processing at the brainstem level that is not related to peripheral deficits. Boettcher et al. (1996) proposed that the latency shifts at the level of the brainstem without corresponding shifts in the periphery could be related to a loss of inhibition in the central auditory pathway of aged subjects.

4.2 Structural changes

"Healthy" ageing is associated with shrinkage of the brain that is predominantly due to shrinkage of neurons, loss of synapses, reduction of synaptic spines, reduction of the length of myelinated axons and, to a lesser degree, loss of neurons (Fjell & Waldhovd, 2010). The pattern of age-dependent structural changes varies greatly between different brain regions. In the following, we will present data on age-dependent changes of auditory brainstem nuclei in the gerbil.

4.2.1 The cochlear nucleus (CN)

Spongiform lesions begin to develop in the CN of young gerbils at the age of a few weeks or months and increase in size and number as the gerbil reaches 1-2 years of age (Czibulka & Schwartz, 1991; McGinn & Faddis, 1987; Ostapoff & Morrest, 1989; Statler et al., 1990). Lesions first become prominent in the PVCN and auditory nerve root and can spread to the deep layer of DCN and the caudal region of AVCN. In 1-2 year old gerbils, microcysts also developed in the superior olive, including LSO, the lateral lemniscus and ventral IC, while other non-auditory regions of the brain remained free of lesions (Ostapoff & Morest, 1989). Using immunostaining with antibodies against GFAP and S100, Czibulka & Schwartz (1993) concluded that up to 80% of the microcysts arise from astrocytes and only few lesions occur in dendrites or axons. In contrast, based on ultrastructural analysis and immunostaining with antibodies to MAP2, GFAP and S100, Faddis & McGinn (1997) concluded that their data "did not support a major role for astrocytes in lesion formation", and transmission electron microscopy revealed only 8% of the lesions in association with myelinated axons. Thus the contribution of glia and neurons to the formation of microcysts is currently not resolved.

McGinn & Faddis (1987) showed that ligature of the external auditory ear canal in 12 day old gerbils before the onset of hearing suppressed the development of the lesions. Gerbils kept in acoustic isolation between 1 and 3 months of age developed fewer lesions compared to controls exposed to 74-80 dB ambient noise (McGinn et al., 1990). Czibulka & Schwartz (1991) found that the number and size of microcysts decreased between 1 and 3 years of age and the degree of lesions in old gerbils was related to hearing status: the number and the size of lesions were largest in the normal hearing old gerbils, while hearing loss was associated with smaller and fewer lesions. Thus, the activity of auditory nerve fibres terminating in the CN is an important factor for the formation of spongiform lesions and it has been suggested that lesions may be the result of excitotoxicity due to transmitter release by the auditory nerve fibres (Czibulka & Schwartz, 1991; McGinn et al., 1990; Faddis & McGinn, 1997). However, it remains an enigma why lesions are prominent in PVCN, yet typically spare AVCN, which also receives massive input from auditory nerve fibres. Possible functional consequences of spongiform lesions in old gerbils are not yet known.

In addition to spongiform lesions, evidence for neuronal degeneration in the CN was observed by electron microscopy (Ostapoff & Morest, 1989) and through use of amino-cupric silver impregnation (McGinn & Faddis, 1998). Czibulka & Schwartz (1991) found a significant reduction in the size of PVCN neurons, but no significant reduction in the number of neurons in the PVCN of gerbils between the age of 1 and 3 years. Ostapoff & Morrest (1989) argued that at most 5-6% of the PVCN neurons may be lost due to microcysts. Thus, these studies suggest that age is not associated with a prominent loss of neurons in PVCN.

The cross sectional area of DCN, PVCN and AVCN was determined for 11 young and 18 old gerbils in sections at defined positions along the rostro-caudal extension of the CN (Stehle, 2010; Gleich et al., 2007c). Comparing the group means of young and old gerbils revealed a significant reduction of the cross-sectional area by 12% in old as compared to young gerbils only for AVCN. The data showed a much higher inter-animal variability of AVCN cross-sectional area in old as compared to young gerbils. A subgroup of 8 old gerbils had cross-sectional areas below those from young gerbils (representing an average reduction of almost 25%) while cross-sectional area of the other 10 old gerbils varied within the range observed for young gerbils. Counts of the GABA- and glycine-immunoreactive neurons in the CN subdivisions (Stangl et al., 2009) revealed only for the GABAergic neurons in the AVCN a significant reduction (mean 35%) in old as compared to young gerbils. The analysis of the size (cross sectional area) of inhibitory neurons as a function of age showed only for GABAergic cells of the PVCN a significant reduction (mean 16%) in old gerbils. These data demonstrate distinct and specific age-dependent changes in the CN subdivisions of the gerbil. The shrinkage of AVCN (presumably due to a loss of neuropil) in approximately half of the old gerbils was not associated with a comparable shrinkage in DCN and PVCN. A loss of GABAergic cells was only observed for AVCN, while the size of GABAergic cells was only reduced in the PVCN of old gerbils. Presently, the functional consequences of these structural age-dependent changes in the CN of old gerbils are unknown.

4.2.2 The medial nucleus of the trapezoid body (MNTB)

The neurons of the MNTB are glycinergic. They convert the excitatory input from the contra-lateral VCN to inhibitory glycinergic projections predominantly to MSO and LSO. A light microscopic analysis of glycine immunoreacted sections showed that spongiform lesions, like those previously described for the CN, were very prominent in the MNTB of 3 year old gerbils, but were almost absent in 1 year old gerbils (Gleich & Strutz, 2002). Thus, spongiform lesions in MNTB develop with a delay of approximately 1-2 years compared to the CN. Spongiform lesions in old gerbils showed a gradient along the MNTB, decreasing from caudal towards rostral. The volume of MNTB was independent of age, as there was no shrinkage of the MNTB in old gerbils. In addition, there was no significant loss of glycinergic neurons in old as compared to young gerbils. In young and old gerbils, there was a systematic gradient of MNTB neuron size: MNTB neurons were largest in the ventro-lateral and smallest in the dorso-medial part of MNTB. According to the tonotopic organisation of MNTB, low-frequency neurons appeared larger on average than high-frequency neurons. Comparing soma size of young and old gerbils revealed a homogenous reduction of cross-sectional area by approximately 20% throughout the MNTB in old gerbils, without any indication that the shrinkage of neurons varied with the tonotopic organisation of MNTB. The reduced size of MNTB neurons in old gerbils may lead to a reduced glycinergic input into MSO and LSO (and other nuclei receiving input from MNTB) and consequently affect processing of binaural stimuli.

4.2.3 The lateral superior olive (LSO)

The light microscopic analysis of GABA and glycine immunostained sections through the LSO in gerbils revealed that this nucleus was rather resistant to age-dependent changes (Gleich et al., 2004). Although Ostapoff & Morest (1989) had reported the presence of microcysts in the LSO of 1-2 year old gerbils, we found no or only small lesions in the LSO of 7 gerbils over 3 years of age. Only 4 old gerbils showed more-prominent lesions that were mainly restricted to the medial (high frequency) limb of LSO, although all 11 old gerbils in this sample had prominent lesions in the MNTB. Thus, LSO appeared more resistant to the formation of spongiform lesions than the MNTB. Neither the rostro-caudal extension, nor the cross-sectional area of LSO varied with age, demonstrating that the LSO did not shrink in old gerbils. In addition, the number of neurons in Nissl stained sections, as well as the number of GABA- and glycine-immunoreactive neurons did not change with age: there was no loss of neurons in the LSO of old gerbils. The density of inhibitory neurons showed the same gradient along the tonotopic representation of the LSO in young and old gerbils: GABAergic and glycinergic neurons were more prominent in the low as compared to the high-frequency limb. The comparison of the size of inhibitory neurons revealed that the cross sectional area of GABAergic and glycinergic LSO neurons was not affected by age in the lateral low-frequency limb, while there was a significant reduction (≈ 30%) in the medial high-frequency limb. Overall, the LSO showed only limited age-related changes that were restricted to the high-frequency limb.

4.2.4 The medial superior olive (MSO)

The neurons of the MSO do not express GABA or glycine, but MSO was well recognised in sections through the gerbil brainstem that were immunostained with antibodies against

GABA and glycine (Dalles, 2009, Gleich, 2006; 2007). The number of MSO neurons was independent of age: there was no loss of MSO neurons in old gerbils. However, the cross sectional area of MSO neurons and the cross sectional area of MSO both decreased by 10% and 20% respectively in old as compared to young gerbils. The shrinkage of MSO in old gerbils is a combination of the shrinkage of MSO neurons and a reduction in the innervation density of MSO (loss of neuropil). Age-dependent structural changes in the gerbil MSO were quite pronounced.

4.2.5 The inferior colliculus (IC)

The analysis of age-dependent changes of the gerbil IC (Gleich et al., 2011) revealed a significant shrinkage of the IC cross-sectional area (13%) in old as compared to young gerbils. Although the mean number and cross-sectional areas of GABAergic cells in the IC were slightly smaller in old as compared to young gerbils, the difference between both groups was not significant in the sample of 7 young and 18 old gerbils analysed. The age-dependent changes in the GABAergic system of the gerbil IC appeared less pronounced than those previously described in rat (Caspary et al., 1995). This might be explained by differences in the degree of peripheral hearing loss of old rats and gerbils.

4.2.6 Variation of age-dependent structural changes between auditory nuclei and potential functional consequences

The structural changes in the different auditory nuclei discussed above (loss of neurons, shrinkage of neurons and shrinkage of the whole nucleus due to loss of innervation) vary considerably. The effect of age appeared least in DCN and LSO and most for AVCN and MSO. Unfortunately, the functional consequences of the age-dependent structural changes in a specific nucleus on auditory processing are typically not well understood except for MSO and LSO, where it has been shown that they process two distinct aspects of binaural sound analysis: MSO analyses inter-aural time differences while LSO analyses inter-aural level differences (see review in Irvine, 1992), two separate cues that can be used for localisation or lateralisation of a sound source. The limited age-dependent pathology in LSO and the more pronounced pathology of MSO suggest that lateralisation of a sound source in old gerbils should be less affected when based on inter-aural level difference and more affected when based on inter-aural time difference. Unfortunately, behavioural data in gerbils addressing this question are not available. However, Babkoff et al. (2002) showed that for a sample of 78 human subjects aged 21-88 years, tested by the presentation of click trains via head phones, lateralisation based on inter-aural level difference did not change with age while the inter-aural time difference for correct lateralisation increased with age. The correlation of the degree of age-dependent structural changes in LSO and MSO of the gerbil and the effect of age on lateralisation based on inter aural level- and inter aural time-difference in humans is an example for a potential causal relationship of structural and functional age-dependent pathology.

5. Psychoacoustic / behavioural measurements

The first behavioural audiogram of the gerbil was determined by Ryan (1976) using a shock avoidance procedure. Subsequently, Sinnott et al. (1997) developed a go-nogo procedure where gerbils initiate a test trial by jumping onto an observation platform and indicate the perception of the test stimulus by jumping off the platform. In this procedure, correct responses are rewarded by a small food pellet. By repeated presentation of a fixed set of test stimuli, where the parameter under investigation varies over a given range (e.g. sound pressure level), a psychometric function is constructed by plotting the correct response probability as a function of the stimulus parameter. The derivation of threshold and other parameters from psychometric functions of gerbils are described in detail in Gleich et al. (2006). In addition to measuring threshold for the detection of signals in quiet, more complex tasks require the detection of a stimulus that deviates form a constantly and repeatedly presented background stimulus. This approach has been used to characterise the ability to discriminate between synthetic speech-like stimuli (Sinnott & Mosqueda, 2003), determine the minimum audible gap duration in a broadband noise pulse (Hamann et al., 2004) and characterise forward masking (Gleich et al., 2007a) in gerbils.

5.1 The audiogram and age-dependent threshold elevation

Behaviourally-determined thresholds in up to 3-year-old gerbils using positive reinforcement (food reward; Hamann et al., 2002) resembled those previously reported by Ryan (1976) using shock avoidance. Behavioural thresholds of 30-36 month-old gerbils showed no significant elevation for broadband noise and 10 kHz and only a small degree of hearing loss at 2 kHz (mean 7.2 dB) compared to gerbils up to 1 year of age. Inter-animal variability of behavioural thresholds in gerbils older than 3 years increased and showed a higher mean loss. However, in clinical terms, the losses were only mild, typically less than 40 dB (Hamann et al., 2002). This pattern differed considerably from the description of hearing loss based on previous CAP and ABR measurements where the mean hearing loss was 10-20 dB at 2 years of age and increased to 25-30 dB for frequencies above 4 kHz in 3 year old gerbils (Hellstrom & Schmiedt, 1990; Mills et al., 1990). To address the question whether the different patterns of hearing loss observed by ABR and behavioural testing were due to methodology or the breeding line, Hamann et al. (2002) determined ABR thresholds in a group of 5 gerbils at the age of 28-29 months. On average, these gerbils showed a 14 dB hearing loss, whereas thresholds in 4 of these gerbils determined at 18 months of age were not elevated. Based on the ABR, these 5 gerbils developed more than 10 dB hearing loss between 18 and 28-29 months of age. Behavioural thresholds of these same gerbils were obtained a few months following ABR testing at an age of 31-33 months and were not found to be elevated compared to the behavioural thresholds of young gerbils. Thus, although ABR thresholds were clearly elevated in these gerbils at 28-29 months of age, the behavioural thresholds determined a few months later showed no hearing loss, the elevation of ABR thresholds in these old gerbils was not reflected in the behavioural thresholds. The difference between behavioural thresholds and thresholds determined by ABR in the frequency range of 1-8 kHz increased from 13-14 dB in young (< 12 months) to 25-30 dB in approximately 2 year old gerbils. A similar observation was described in Boettcher (2002a) for humans. The difference between ABR and behavioural thresholds was around 8 dB at 2 and 4 kHz in a group of young human subjects and increased to around 20 dB in a group of old human subjects. Thus, ABR based thresholds in old humans and gerbils may lead to an over-estimation of threshold loss compared to pure tone audiometry.

There is not a simple, straight-forward explanation for the age–dependent, increasing discrepancy between behavioural and ABR thresholds (Hamann et al., 2002). One factor is a decreased synchronisation of the neural responses that will lead to reduced amplitudes of evoked potentials and reduced slopes of the CAP and ABR growth functions. In addition, a specific loss of auditory nerve fibres with low spontaneous activity, that typically have higher thresholds than those with high spontaneous activity could contribute to reduced amplitudes of CAP and ABR without associated elevation of threshold (Schmiedt et al., 1996; Lin et al., 2011). The advanced age-dependent cochlear pathologies discussed above (see heading 3) will eventually lead to behavioural manifestation of hearing loss.

5.2 Temporal integration

Thresholds for tones increased by more than 10 dB in both normal hearing, young gerbils and old gerbils, as signal duration was reduced from 300 to 10 ms (Gleich et al., 2007b). Like in humans and other species, temporal integration was reduced in gerbils with hearing loss and varied as a function of threshold elevation.

In the presence of fixed-level modulated and un-modulated speech like maskers, threshold shift due to the masker was inversely related to threshold in quiet: sensitive gerbils showed more masking compared to gerbils with slightly elevated thresholds. Consequently, the temporal integration functions (plots of the masked threshold as a function of duration) became very similar for all 13 gerbils with an age varying between 7 and 43 months and the functions were independent of peripheral hearing. Compared to the unmodulated masker, thresholds for short signals (10 and 30 ms) showed slightly more masking , while those for long signals (300 and 1000 ms) showed slightly less masking in the presence of the modulated masker, suggesting that long signals can be detected in the troughs while detection of short signals interferes with the peaks of the modulated masker. These data suggest that temporal integration in normal hearing gerbils is not affected by age.

5.3 Gap detection

The gap detection paradigm determines the minimum duration for the detection of a short period of silence (gap) embedded in a broadband noise pulse. It has been widely used to characterise the temporal resolution of the auditory system. By selecting old human subjects with no or minimal peripheral hearing loss (determined by pure tone audiometry), Snell (1997) demonstrated that mean gap detection thresholds increased with age even in the absence of peripheral hearing loss: some old subjects showed impaired performance, while others retained good temporal resolution, resulting in an increased inter-individual variability of gap detection thresholds in old human subjects. Very similar results were obtained in gerbils (Hamann et al., 2004). When tested with a noise carrier presented 30 dB above the threshold for the carrier, the minimum audible gap in young gerbils was below 4 ms, while approximately 50% of the old gerbils had gap detection thresholds above 4 ms. The variation of the threshold for the noise carrier explained less than 20% of the variation of the gap detection threshold in gerbils. This suggests that peripheral hearing loss was not the dominant cause of impaired temporal resolution. These data point to central auditory processing deficits that result in increased gap detection thresholds in normal hearing old humans and gerbils and are consistent with results obtained by ABR in gerbils (Boettcher et al., 1996). The similarity of age-dependent changes in gap detection by humans and gerbils emphasises the usefulness of the gerbil model for the analysis of impaired auditory temporal processing.

5.4 Forward masking

Forward masking is a phenomenon through which threshold for a probe that follows a signal (masker) is elevated (masked) and recovers with time (≈ 100 ms) following the end of the masker. Increased masking and delayed recovery from preceding acoustic stimulation interferes with the detection of fluctuations and transients in sound signals and might contribute to age-dependent impairment of speech perception. In the analysis of the effect of age on forward masking in gerbils (Gleich et al., 2007a) a 2.85 kHz masker presented at 40 dBSPL and repeated continuously every 1.6 seconds served as a constant background signal. Animals had to detect trials where a short 2.85 kHz probe signal (20 ms) was presented 2.5 ms after the end of the masker. In addition to the masked threshold, the threshold for the probe signal without a masker was determined to characterise peripheral hearing. In a sample of 15 gerbils between 5 and 36 months of age, threshold for the probe in quiet was independent of age (mean 12 dBSPL). These animals showed no sign of peripheral hearing loss. In contrast, the masked thresholds of these gerbils increased from around 33 dB SPL at 1 year of age to 48 dBSPL at an age of 3 years. The efficacy of the masker increased by 15 dB between 1 and 3 years of age. The increased degree of forward masking in old gerbils in the absence of elevated thresholds in the condition without a masker suggests a deficit in central, rather than peripheral, auditory processing. An analysis of forward masking using ABR in humans also demonstrated increased forward masking in old subjects with normal audiometric thresholds and led to the conclusion that this was likely due to changes in central auditory processing (Walton et al., 1999). Thus, gerbils appear to be a useful model for the analysis of the interaction of age and forward masking.

5.5 Auditory spatial resolution

Age-dependent structural changes in auditory nuclei involved in binaural processing have been discussed above (see headings 4.2.3-4.2.5). Consistent with the pathology in MNTB, MSO and LSO, auditory spatial resolution was impaired in old gerbils (Maier et al., 2008). The minimum resolvable angle in a sound lateralisation task showed a higher degree of inter-animal variability in old (32 to 51 months), as compared to young (3-8 months), gerbils. The angle for pure tones (0.5 and 8 kHz) and narrowband noise centred at 0.5 and 2 kHz was ≈ 50-60° in old gerbils, approximately twice the angle found in young gerbils. Maier et al. (2008) suggest that spongiform lesions in the VCN compromise the excitatory input, while pathology of the MNTB affects the inhibitory input to LSO and MSO and contribute to impaired auditory spatial resolution in old gerbils.

5.6 Pharmacotherapy

The available data indicate that ageing is associated with a loss of inhibition in the central auditory pathway, which could contribute to impaired auditory temporal processing (Caspary et al., 2008). Age-dependent changes in neurotransmitter systems might be influenced by pharmacotherapy and the similarity of age-dependent deficits between humans and gerbils with respect to gap detection and forward masking makes the gerbil an ideal model to test the effect of candidate substances on performance. Some anti-convulsive drugs in the context of epilepsy were designed to interact with the GABA system.

For our first study, we chose to analyse the effect of Sabril® (vigabatrin) on gap detection (Gleich et al., 2003). Vigabatrin blocks the GABA converting enzyme GABA transaminase and consequently leads to elevated levels of GABA in the brain. The effect of vigabatrin at a dose of 50 mg/kg/day was dependent on the initial gap detection threshold. Performance in gerbils with initially low gap detection thresholds were not systematically affected by the drug, while those with initially elevated gap detection thresholds improved and normalised to a level comparable to sensitive animals. The beneficial effect of vigabatrin on impaired gap detection was reversible, with gap detection thresholds increasing after the end of the treatment. These data clearly demonstrate the potential use of pharmacotherapy for the treatment of impaired auditory temporal resolution. Unfortunately, severe side effects on the visual system prevent the therapeutic use of vigabatrin for the treatment of hearing loss.

In a subsequent study, we evaluated the effect of gabapentin on gap detection and forward masking in gerbils, since other studies suggested beneficial effects of gabapentin for certain forms of tinnitus (Gleich & Strutz, 2011). Gabapentin was initially designed as a GABA analogue for the treatment of epilepsy and is also used for the treatment of neuropathic pain. In gerbils, gabapentin had no beneficial effect on impaired gap detection or on elevated masked thresholds. Unexpectedly, the data showed that gapapentin at a dose of 350 mg/kg/day increased masked thresholds in young gerbils, while it had no significant effect in old gerbils that had elevated masked thresholds before gabapentin treatment. The lack of a beneficial effect on impaired gap detection and increased forward masking in old gerbils could be due to an insufficient effect of gabapentin on the GABA system, while the increased masked thresholds of young gerbils during gabapentin treatment might be related to its interaction with voltage-gated calcium channels.

6. Conclusion

At the level of the cochlea, pathology begins to affect the marginal cells of the stria vascularis and eventually leads to a reduction of the endocochlear potential in old gerbils. Loss of hair cells and loss of auditory nerve fibres and spiral ganglion cells are not major contributors to age-dependent peripheral hearing loss. Consequently, gerbils can be regarded as a good model for strial or metabolic presbyacusis.

Behavioural and evoked potential (CAP, ABR) measures of auditory sensitivity are useful to characterise hearing status; however, the degree of age-dependent threshold elevation depends on the method used: the discrepancy between thresholds determined psychoacoustically and by evoked potentials increases with age; evoked potentials indicate more threshold loss than behavioural methods in old gerbils and old humans.

Auditory nuclei in the ascending auditory pathway of gerbils show specific and distinct age-dependent structural changes, where some nuclei appear more affected than others. Structural changes in nuclei involved in binaural processing are associated with impaired auditory spatial resolution in old gerbils. For LSO and MSO, the degree of age-dependent pathology in gerbils can be correlated with age-dependent changes in human performance in sound lateralisation tasks, which are based on inter-aural level and inter-aural time difference cues. This suggests a causal relationship between structural and functional age-dependent changes.

The age-dependent decline of auditory temporal resolution determined by gap detection and forward masking in gerbils and humans is very similar and probably due to loss of inhibition or age-dependent disturbance of neurotransmitter balance in the auditory pathway. Augmentation of the GABA system by vigabatrin was effective in the treatment of impaired gap detection in gerbils and demonstrates that pharmacotherapy of central auditory processing deficits appears feasible, in principle. The challenge is to identify appropriate substances that act on the disturbed neurotransmitter balance in advanced age. The available data show that the gerbil is a suitable model to evaluate the efficacy of potential therapies for the treatment of impaired central auditory processing.

7. Acknowledgements

We thank Steven Marcrum for thorough proofreading and suggestions for improving the manuscript.

8. References

Adams, J.C. & Schulte, B.A. (1997). Histopathologic observations of the aging gerbil cochlea. *Hearing Research* Vol. 104, No. 1-2, (Feb. 1997), pp. 101-111, ISSN: 0378-5955

Babkoff, H.; Muchnik, C.; Ben-David, N.; Furst, M.; Even-Zohar, S. & Hildesheimer, M. (2002). Mapping lateralization of click trains in younger and older populations. *Hearing Research* Vol. 165, No. 1-2, (Mar. 2002), pp. 117-127, ISSN: 0378-5955

Boettcher, F.A. (2002a). Presbyacusis and the auditory brainstem response. *Journal of Speech,Language and Hearing Research* Vol. 45, No. 6, (Dec. 2002), pp. 1249-1261, ISSN: 1092-4388

Boettcher, F.A. (2002b). Susceptibility to acoustic trauma in young and aged gerbils. *Journal of the Acoustical Society of America* Vol. 112, No. 6, (Dec. 2002), pp. 2948-2955, ISSN: 0001-4966

Boettcher, F.A.; Mills, J.H. & Norton, B.L. (1993a). Age-related changes in auditory evoked potentials of gerbils. I. Response amplitudes. *Hearing Research* Vol. 71, No. 1-2, (Dec. 1993), pp. 137-145, ISSN: 0378-5955

Boettcher, F.A.; Mills, J.H.; Norton, B.L. & Schmiedt, R.A. (1993b). Age-related changes in auditory evoked potentials of gerbils. II. Response latencies. *Hearing Research* Vol. 71, No. 1-2, (Dec. 1993), pp. 146-156, ISSN: 0378-5955

Boettcher, F.A.; Mills, J.H.; Dubno, J.R. & Schmiedt, R.A. (1995). Masking of auditory brainstem responses in young and aged gerbils. *Hearing Research* Vol. 89, No. 1-2, (Sept. 1995), pp. 1-13, ISSN: 0378-5955

Boettcher, F.A.; Mills, J.H.; Swerdloff, J.L. & Holley, B.L. (1996). Auditory evoked potentials in aged gerbils: responses elicited by noises separated by a silent gap. *Hearing Research* Vol. 102, No. 1-2, (Dec. 1996), pp. 167-178, ISSN: 0378-5955

Caspary, D.M.; Milbrandt, J.C. & Helfert, R.H. (1995). Central auditory aging: GABA changes in the inferior colliculus. *Experimental Gerontology* Vol. 30, No. 3-4, (May-Aug. 1995) pp. 349-360. ISSN: 0531-5565

Caspary, D.M.; Ling, L.; Turner, J.G. & Hughes, L.F. (2008). Inhibitory neurotransmission, plasticity and aging in the mammalian central auditory system. *The Journal of Experimental Biology* Vol. 211, No. 11, (Jun. 2008), pp. 1781–1791. ISSN: 0022-0949

Cheal, M.L. (1986). The gerbil: a unique model for research on aging. *Experimental Aging Research* Vol. 12, No. 1, (Spring 1986) pp. 3-21. ISSN: 0361-073X

Czibulka, A. & Schwartz, I.R. (1991). Neuronal populations in the gerbil PVCN: Effects of age, hearing status and microcysts. *Hearing Research* Vol. 52, No. 1, (Mar. 1991), pp. 43-58, ISSN: 0378-5955

Czibulka, A. & Schwartz, I.R. (1993). Glial or neuronal origin of microcysts in the gerbil PVCN? *Hearing Research* Vol. 67, No. 1-2, (May 1993), pp. 1-12, ISSN: 0378-5955

Dalles, C. (2009). Der laterale Kern des Trapezkörpers (LNTB) und die mediale obere Olive (MSO): altersbedingte Veränderungen bei der Wüstenrennmaus (Meriones unguiculatus). *Dissertation* at the Medical Faculty of the University of Regensburg.

Eckrich, T.; Foeller, E.; Stuermer, I.W.; Gaese, B.H. & Kössl, M. (2008). Strain-dependence of age-related cochlear hearing loss in wild and domesticated Mongolian gerbils. *Hearing Research* Vol. 235, No. 1-2, (Jan. 2008), pp. 72-79, ISSN: 0378-5955

Faddis, B.T. & McGinn, M.D. (1997). Spongiform degeneration of the gerbil cochlear nucleus: an ultrastructural and immunohistochemical evaluation. *Journal of Neurocytology* Vol. 26, No. 9, (Sept. 1997) pp. 625-635. ISSN: 0300-4864

Fjell, A.M. & Walhovd, K.B. (2010). Structural brain changes in aging: courses, causes and cognitive consequences. *Reviews in the Neurosciences* Vol. 21, No. 3, (Jun. 2010), pp. 187-221 ISSN: 0334-1763.

Gleich, O. (2006). Altersbedingte Veränderungen auditorischer Hirnstammkerne (bei Nagetieren): Beeinträchtigen Defizite des inhibitorischen Systems die Verarbeitung komplexer Schallsignale? *Tagungs-CD der 9. Jahrestagung der Deutschen Gesellschaft für Audiologie*, ISBN 3-9809869-5-0, Köln, Feb. 2006

Gleich, O. (2007). Altersbedingte zentrale Hörstörungen und funktionelle Veränderungen der aufsteigenden Hörbahn. In: *Hören im Alter, Materialsammlung vom 13. Multidisziplinären Kolloquium der GEERS-STIFTUNG am 20. und 21. Februar 2006 im Wissenschaftszentrum Bonn, Band 16*, Specht, H. v., pp 57-76, Gustav Kleff GmbH & Co. KG, ISSN 0935-1213, Dortmund

Gleich, O. & Strutz, J. (2002). Age dependent changes in the medial nucleus of the trapezoid body in gerbils. *Hearing Research* Vol. 164, No. 1-2, (Feb. 2002), pp. 166-178, ISSN: 0378-5955

Gleich, O. & Strutz, J. (2011). The effect of gabapentin on forward masking and gap detection in gerbils. *Ear and Hearing* Vol. 32, No. 3 (Nov. - Dec. 2011), pp 741-749 ISSN: 0196-0202

Gleich, O.; Hamann, I.; Klump, G.M.; Kittel, M.C. & Strutz, J. (2003). Boosting GABA improves impaired auditory temporal resolution in the gerbil. *Neuroreport* Vol. 14, No. 14, (Oct. 2003), pp. 1877-1880, ISSN: 0959-4965

Gleich, O.; Weiss, M. & Strutz, J. (2004). Age-dependent changes in the lateral superior olive (LSO) of the gerbil (Meriones unguiculatus). *Hearing Research* Vol. 194, No. 1-2, (Aug. 2004), pp. 47-59, ISSN: 0378-5955

Gleich, O.; Hamann, I.; Kittel, M.C.; Klump, G.M. & Strutz, J. (2006). A quantitative analysis of psychometric functions for different auditory tasks in gerbils. *Hearing Research* Vol. 220, No. 1-2, (Oct. 2006), pp. 27-37, ISSN: 0378-5955

Gleich, O.; Hamann, I.; Kittel, M.C.; Klump, G.M. & Strutz, J. (2007a). Forward masking in gerbils: the effect of age. *Hearing Research* Vol. 223, No. 1-2, (Jan. 2007), pp. 122-128, ISSN: 0378-5955

Gleich, O.; Kittel, M.C.; Klump, G.M. & Strutz, J. (2007b). Temporal integration in the gerbil: The effect of age, hearing loss and temporally unmodulated and modulated speech-like ICRA noise maskers. *Hearing Research* Vol. 224, No. 1-2, (Feb. 2007), pp. 101-114, ISSN: 0378-5955

Gleich, O.; Thurnbauer, K. & Strutz, J. (2007c). Differentielle altersbedingte Veränderungen in den Unterkernen des Nucleus cochlearis der Wüstenrennmaus. In: *78th Annual Meeting of the German Society of Oto-Rhino-Laryngology, Head and Neck Surgery, German Society of Oto-Rhino-Laryngology, Head and Neck Surgery, 16.05. - 20.05.2007, Munich*, 19. 8. 2011, Available from: http://www.egms.de/en/meetings/hnod2007/07hnod035.shtml

Gleich, O.; Netz, J. & Strutz, J. (2011). Altersbedingte Veränderungen im Colliculus inferior der Wüstenrennmaus. In: *82. Jahresversammlung der Deutschen Gesellschaft für Hals-Nasen-Ohren-Heilkunde, Kopf- und Hals-Chirurgie e. V., 01.06. - 05.06.2011, Freiburg.*, 19. 8. 2011, Available from: http://www.egms.de/static/de/meetings/hnod2011/11hnod340.shtml

Gratton, M.A. & Schulte, B.A. (1995). Alterations in microvasculature are associated with atrophy of the stria vascularis in quiet-aged gerbils. *Hearing Research* Vol. 82, No. 1, (Jan. 1995), pp. 44-52, ISSN: 0378-5955

Gratton, M.A.; Smyth, B.J.; Schulte, B.A. & Vincent, D.A. Jr. (1995). Na,K-ATPase activity decreases in the cochlear lateral wall of quiet-aged gerbils. *Hearing Research* Vol. 83, No. 1-2, (Mar. 1995), pp. 43-50, ISSN: 0378-5955

Gratton, M.A.; Schmiedt, R.A. & Schulte, B.A. (1996). Age-related decreases in endocochlear potential are associated with vascular abnormalities in the stria vascularis. *Hearing Research* Vol. 102, No. 1-2, (Dec. 1996), pp. 181-190, ISSN: 0378-5955

Gratton, M.A.; Smyth, B.J.; Lam, C.F.; Boettcher, F.A. & Schmiedt, R.A. (1997a). Decline in the endocochlear potential corresponds to decreased Na,K-ATPase activity in the lateral wall of quiet-aged gerbils. *Hearing Research* Vol. 108, No. 1-2, (Jun. 1997), pp. 9-16, ISSN: 0378-5955

Gratton, M.A.; Schulte, B.A. & Smythe, N.M. (1997b). Quantification of the stria vascularis and strial capillary areas in quiet-reared young and aged gerbils. *Hearing Research* Vol. 114, No. 1-2, (Dec. 1997), pp. 1-9, ISSN: 0378-5955

Hamann, I.; Gleich, O.; Klump, G.M.; Kittel, M.; Boettcher, F.A.; Schmiedt, R.A. & Strutz, J. (2002). Behavioral and evoked-potential thresholds in young and old Mongolian gerbils (Meriones unguiculatus). *Hearing Research* Vol. 171, No. 1-2, (Sept. 2002), pp. 82-95, ISSN: 0378-5955

Hamann, I.; Gleich, O.; Klump, G.M.; Kittel, M. & Strutz, J. (2004). Age-dependent changes of gap detection in the Mongolian gerbil (Meriones unguiculatus). *Journal of the Association for Research in Otolaryngology* Vol. 5, No. 1 (Mar. 2004), pp. 49-57, ISSN: 1525-3961

Hellstrom, L.I. & Schmiedt, R.A. (1990). Compound action potential input/output functions in young and quiet-aged gerbils. *Hearing Research* Vol. 50, No. 1-2, (Dec. 1990), pp. 163-174, ISSN: 0378-5955

Hellstrom, L.I. & Schmiedt, R.A. (1991). Rate/level functions of auditory-nerve fibers in young and quiet-aged gerbils. *Hearing Research* Vol. 53, No. 2, (Jun. 1991), pp. 217-222, ISSN: 0378-5955

Hellstrom, L.I. & Schmiedt, R.A. (1996). Measures of tuning and suppression in single-fiber and whole-nerve responses in young and quiet-aged gerbils. *Journal of the Acoustical Society of America* Vol. 100, No. 5, (Nov. 1996), pp. 3275-3285, ISSN: 0001-4966

Henry, K.R; McGinn, M.D. & Chole, R.A. (1980). Age-related auditory loss in the Mongolian gerbil. *Archives of oto- rhino- laryngology* Vol. 228, No. 4., (Dec. 1980), pp. 233-238, ISSN: 0937-4477

Irvine, D.R.F. (1992). Physiology of the auditory brainstem. In: *Springer Handbook of Auditory Research Vol. 2: The mammalian auditory pathway: Neurophysiology*, Popper, A.N., Fay, R.R., pp. 153-231, Springer-Verlag, ISBN 0-387-97690-6, New York

Janssen, T.; Niedermeyer, H.P. & Arnold, W. (2006). Diagnostics of the cochlear amplifier by means of distortion product otoacoustic emissions. *ORL Journal for Oto- Rhino-Laryngology, Head and Neck Surgery* Vol. 68, No. 6 (Oct. 2006), pp. 334-339, ISBN: 978-3-8055-8204-9

Keithley, E.M.; Ryan, A.F. & Woolf, N.K. (1989). Spiral ganglion cell density in young and old gerbils. *Hearing Research* Vol. 38, No. 1-2, (Mar. 1989), pp. 125-133, ISSN: 0378-5955

Kelly, J.B. & Masterton, B. (1977). Auditory sensitivity of the albino rat. *Journal of Comparative and Physiological Psychology* Vol. 91, No. 4, (Aug. 1977), pp. 930-936, ISSN: 0021-9940

Kiang, N.Y.S. (1965) *Discharge Patterns of Single Fibers in the Cat's Auditory Nerve.* MIT Press, ISBN-10: 0-262-11016-4, Cambridge MA.

Lang, H.; Jyothi, V.; Smythe, N.M.; Dubno, J.R.; Schulte, B.A. & Schmiedt, R.A. (2010). Chronic reduction of endocochlear potential reduces auditory nerve activity: further confirmation of an animal model of metabolic presbyacusis. *Journal of the Association for Research in Otolaryngology* Vol. 11, No. 3 (Sept. 2010), pp. 419-434, ISSN: 1525-3961

Lin, H.W., Furman, A.C., Kujawa, S.G. & Liberman, M.C. (2011). Primary Neural Degeneration in the Guinea Pig Cochlea After Reversible Noise-Induced Threshold Shift. *Journal of the Association for Research in Otolaryngology* Vol. 12, No. 5 (Oct. 2011), pp 605-616 ISSN: 1525-3961

Maier, J.K.; Kindermann, T.; Grothe, B. & Klump, G.M. (2008). Effects of omni-directional noise-exposure during hearing onset and age on auditory spatial resolution in the Mongolian gerbil (Meriones unguiculatus) -- a behavioral approach. *Brain Research* Vol. 1220, (Jul. 2008), pp. 47-57, ISSN: 00068993

McGinn, M.D. & Faddis, B.T. (1987). Auditory experience affects degeneration of the ventral cochlear nucleus in mongolian gerbils. *Hearing Research* Vol. 31, No. 1-2, (Dec. 1987), pp. 235-244, ISSN: 0378-5955

McGinn, M.D.; Faddis, B.T. & Moore, H.C. (1990). Acoustic isolation reduces degeneration of the ventral cochlear nuclei in Mongolian gerbils. *Hearing Research* Vol. 48, No. 3, (Oct. 1990), pp. 265-274, ISSN: 0378-5955

McGinn, M.D. & Faddis, B.T. (1998). Neuronal degeneration in the gerbil brainstem is associated with spongiform lesions. *Microscopy Research and Technique* Vol. 41, No. 3, (May 1998), pp. 187-204, ISSN: 1059-910X

Mills, J.H.; Schmiedt, R.A. & Kulish, L.F. (1990). Age-related changes in auditory potentials of Mongolian gerbil. *Hearing Research* Vol. 46, No. 3, (Jul. 1990), pp. 201-210, ISSN: 0378-5955

Mills, J.H.; Boettcher, F.A. & Dubno, J.R. (1997). Interaction of noise-induced permanent threshold shift and age-related threshold shift. *Journal of the Acoustical Society of America* Vol. 101, No. 3, (Mar. 1997), pp. 1681-1686, ISSN: 0001-4966

Milne-Edwards, M. (1867). Observations sur quelques mammifères du nord de chine. *Annales des Sciences Naturelles* Vol. 5, No. 7, pp. 375-377. ISSN: 0150-9330

Ostapoff, E.-M. & Morest, D.K. (1989). A degenerative disorder of the central auditory system of the gerbil. *Hearing Research* Vol. 37, No. 2, (Jan. 1989), pp. 141-162, ISSN: 0378-5955

Radziwon, K.E.; June, K.M.; Stolzberg, D.J.; Xu-Friedman, M.A.; Salvi, R.J. & Dent, M.L. (2009). Behaviorally measured audiograms and gap detection thresholds in CBA/CaJ mice. *Journal of Comparative Physiology A, Neuroethology, Sensory, Neural, and Behavioral Physiology* Vol. 195, No. 10, (Oct. 2009), pp. 961-9. ISSN: 0340-7594

Rüttiger, L., Panford-Walsh, R., Schimmang, T., Tan, J., Zimmermann, U., Rohbock, K., Köpschall, I., Limberger, A., Müller, M., Fraenzer, J.T., Cimerman, J. & Knipper, M. (2007). BDNF mRNA expression and protein localization are changed in age-related hearing loss. *Neurobiology of Aging* Vol. 28, No. 4, (Apr. 2007), pp 586-601. ISSN: 0197-4580

Ryan, A. (1976). Hearing sensitivity of the mongolian gerbil, Meriones unguiculatis. *Journal of the Acoustical Society of America* Vol. 59, No. 5, (May 1976), pp. 1222-1226, ISSN: 0001-4966

Sakaguchi, N.; Spicer, S.S.; Thomopoulos, G.N. & Schulte, B.A. (1997a). Increased laminin deposition in capillaries of the stria vascularis of quiet-aged gerbils. *Hearing Research* Vol. 105, No. 1-2, (Mar. 1997), pp. 44-56, ISSN: 0378-5955

Sakaguchi, N.; Spicer, S.S.; Thomopoulos, G.N. & Schulte, B.A. (1997b). Immunoglobulin deposition in thickened basement membranes of aging strial capillaries. *Hearing Research* Vol. 109, No. 1-2, (Jul. 1997), pp. 83-91, ISSN: 0378-5955

Sakaguchi ,N.; Crouch, J.J.; Lytle, C. & Schulte, B.A. (1998). Na-K-Cl cotransporter expression in the developing and senescent gerbil cochlea. *Hearing Research* Vol. 118, No. 1-2, (Apr. 1998), pp. 114-122, ISSN: 0378-5955

Schmiedt, R.A. (1983). Cochlear potentials in quiet-aged gerbils: does the aging cochlea need a jump start? In: *Sensory Research: Multimodal Perspectives.* Verillo, R.T., pp. 91-103, Lawrence Erlbaum Assoc., ISBN: 0-8058-1342-X, Hillsdale NJ

Schmiedt, R.A. (1989). Spontaneous rates, thresholds and tuning of auditory-nerve fibers in the gerbil: comparisons to cat data. *Hearing Research* Vol. 42, No. 1, (Oct. 1989), pp. 23-35, ISSN: 0378-5955

Schmiedt, R.A. (1996). Effects of aging on potassium homeostasis and the endocochlear potential in the gerbil cochlea. *Hearing Research* Vol. 102, No. 1-2, (Dec. 1996), pp. 125-132, ISSN: 0378-5955

Schmiedt, R.A.; Mills, J.H. & Adams, J.C. (1990). Tuning and suppression in auditory nerve fibers of aged gerbils raised in quiet or noise. *Hearing Research* Vol. 45, No. 3, (May 1990), pp. 221-236, ISSN: 0378-5955

Schmiedt, R.A.; Mills, J.H. & Boettcher, F.A. (1996). Age-related loss of activity of auditory-nerve fibers. *Journal of Neurophysiology* Vol. 76, No. 4, (Oct. 1996), pp. 2799-2803, ISSN: 0022-3077

Schuknecht, H.F. & Gacek, M.R. (1993). Cochlear pathology in presbycusis. *Annals of Otology, Rhinology & Laryngology* Vol. 102, No. 1, Pt. 2, (Jan. 1993), pp. 1-16.

Schulte, B.A. & Schmiedt, R,A. (1992). Lateral wall Na,K-ATPase and endocochlear potentials decline with age in quiet-reared gerbils. *Hearing Research* Vol. 61, No. 1-2, (Aug. 1992), pp. 35-46, ISSN: 0378-5955

Schwartz, I. (1991). The superior olivary complex and lateral lemniscal nuclei. In: *Springer Handbook of Auditory Research Vol. 1: The mammalian auditory pathway: Neuroanatomy.* Webster, D.B., Popper, A.N., Fay, R.R., pp 117-167, Springer Verlag, ISBN 0-387-97678-7, New York

Sewell, W.F. (1984). The effects of furosemide on the endocochlear potential and auditory-nerve fiber tuning curves in cats. *Hearing Research* Vol. 14, No. 3, (Jun. 1984), pp. 305-314, ISSN: 0378-5955

Sinnot, J.M.; Street, S.L.; Mosteller, K.W. & Williamson, T.L. (1997). Behavioral measures of vowel sensitivity in Mongolian gerbils (Meriones unguiculatus): Effects of age and genetic origin. *Hearing Research* Vol. 112, No. 1-2, (Oct. 1997), pp. 235-246, ISSN: 0378-5955

Sinnott, J.M. & Mosqueda, S.B. (2003). Effects of aging on speech sound discrimination in the Mongolian gerbil. *Ear and Hearing* Vol. 24, No. 1, (Feb. 2003), pp. 30-37 ISSN: 0196-0202

Snell, K.B. (1997). Age-related changes in temporal gap detection. *Journal of the Acoustical Society of America* Vol. 101, No. 4, (Apr. 1997), pp. 2214-2220, ISSN: 0001-4966

Spicer, S.S.; Gratton, M.A. & Schulte, B.A. (1997). Expression patterns of ion transport enzymes in spiral ligament fibrocytes change in relation to strial atrophy in the aged gerbil cochlea. *Hearing Research* Vol. 111, No. 1-2, (Sept. 1997), pp. 93-102, ISSN: 0378-5955

Spicer, S.S. & Schulte, B.A. (1998). Evidence for a medial K+ recycling pathway from inner hair cells. *Hearing Research* Vol. 118, No. 1-2, (Apr. 1998), pp. 1-12, ISSN: 0378-5955

Spicer, S.S. & Schulte, B.A. (2002). Spiral ligament pathology in quiet-aged gerbils. *Hearing Research* Vol. 172, No. 1-2, (Oct. 2002), pp. 172-185, ISSN: 0378-5955

Stangl, P.; Gleich, O. & Strutz, J. (2009). Altersbedingte Veränderungen inhibitorischer Neurone im Nucleus cochlearis der Mongolischen Wüstenrennmaus (Meriones unguiculatus). In: *93. Jahrestagung der Vereinigung Südwestdeutscher Hals-Nasen-Ohrenärzte 17. - 19.09.2009, Neu-Ulm,* 19. 8. 2011, Available from: http://www.egms.de/static/de/meetings/hnosw2009/09hnosw31.shtml

Statler, K.D.; Chamberlain, S.C.; Slepecky, N.B. & Smith, R.L. (1990). Development of mature microcystic lesions in the cochlear nuclei of the Mongolian gerbil, Meriones unguiculatus. *Hearing Research* Vol. 50, No. 1-2, (Dec. 1990), pp. 275-288, ISSN: 0378-5955

Stehle, K. (2010). Altersbedingte Veränderungen des inhibitorischen Systems im Nucleus cochlearis der Mongolischen Wüstenrennmaus (Meriones unguiculatus). *Dissertation* at the Medical Faculty of the University of Regensburg.

Strutz, J. (1991). Die nichttumorbedingten zentralen Hörstörungen - Eine Übersicht. *HNO* Vol. 39, No. 9, (Sept. 1991), pp. 332-338 ISSN: 0017-6192

Stuermer, I.W.; Plotz, K.; Leybold, A.; Zinke, O.; Kalberlah, O.; Samjaa, R. & Scheich, H. (2003). Intraspecific allometric comparison of laboratory gerbils with Mongolian gerbils trapped in the wild indicates domestication in Meriones unguiculatus (Milne-Edwards, 1867) (Rodentia : Gerbillinae). *Zoologischer Anzeiger – A Journal of Comparative Zoology* Vol. 242, No. 3, pp. 249-266 ISSN: 0044-5231

Suryadevara, A.C.; Schulte, B.A.; Schmiedt, R.A. & Slepecky, N.B. (2001). Auditory nerve fibers in young and quiet-aged gerbils: morphometric correlations with endocochlear potential. *Hearing Research* Vol. 161, No. 1-2, (Nov. 2001), pp. 45-53, ISSN: 0378-5955

Tarnowski, B.I.; Schmiedt, R.A.; Hellstrom, L.I.; Lee, F.S. & Adams, J.C. (1991). Age-related changes in cochleas of mongolian gerbils. *Hearing Research* Vol. 54, No. 1, (Jul. 1991), pp. 123-134, ISSN: 0378-5955

Thomopoulos, G.N.; Spicer, S.S.; Gratton, M.A. & Schulte, B,A. (1997). Age-related thickening of basement membrane in stria vascularis capillaries. *Hearing Research* Vol. 111, No. 1-2 (Sept. 1997), pp. 31-41, ISSN: 0378-5955

Walton, J.; Orlando, M. & Burkard, R. (1999). Auditory brainstem response forward-masking recovery functions in older humans with normal hearing. *Hearing Research* Vol. 127, No. 1-2 (Jan. 1999), pp. 86-94, ISSN: 0378-5955

Wangemann, P. (2006). Supporting sensory transduction: cochlear fluid homeostasis and the endocochlear potential. *The Journal of Physiology* Vol. 576, No. 1, (Oct. 2006), pp. 11-21 ISSN: 0022-3751

Webster, D.B. & Plassmann, W. (1992). Parallel evolution of low-frequency sensitivity in old world and new world desert rodents. In: *The evolutionary biology of hearing.* Webster, D.B., Fay, R.R. & Popper, A.N., pp 633-636, Springer, ISBN 0-387-97588-8, New York

Winter, I.M.; Robertson, D. & Yates, G.K. (1990). Diversity of characteristic frequency rate-intensity functions in guinea pig auditory nerve fibres. *Hearing Research* Vol. 45, No. 3 (May 1990), pp. 191-202, ISSN: 0378-5955

Zwicker, E. & Fastl, H. (1990). *Psychoacoustics Facts and Models.* Springer, ISBN 3-540-52600-5, Berlin Heidelberg New York

Part 2

Childhood Hearing Loss

5

Families of Children with Hearing Loss and Parental Educational Practices

Bolsoni-Silva Alessandra Turini and Rodrigues Olga Maria Piazentin Rolim
Universidade Estadual Paulista – UNESP
Brazil

1. Introduction

The present chapter presents an empirical study of parental practices and behaviors related to children with and without hearing loss. Studies of families of children with hearing loss, as well as aspects related to the influence of parental practices upon the behavior of children give support to the present research.

1.1 Families of children with hearing loss

People with communication disorders caused by hearing loss may present complex manifestations involving linguistic, cognitive, behavioral, psychological and social alterations. The causes can be isolated or associated to clinical aspects of different neurological or genetic problems. Children with hearing loss (HL) may be considered as a high risk population due to the presence of indicators such as: language delay, which involve communication skills, low academic progress and social emotional level (Calderon, 2000). The presence of such impairments may cause some difficulties concerning the development of the children and the relationship with their parents.

Some preventive measures should be taken more actively including the primary ones which reduce the birth incidence of children with hearing loss and secondary ones that help in its early detection. (Gatto & Tochetto, 2007).

In addition to hearing screening programs researchers emphasize the importance of training health professionals to guide parents on how to communicate with their children. The need to decide beforehand (without having enough knowledge of their benefits) the communication form that is to be used with their children possibly is a stress trigger which may influence the quality of the interaction between parents and children. (Gravel & O´Gara, 2003). Early identification of hearing loss and the consequent counseling services available in the community may help parents establish effective relationships with their children (Marchesi, 1996), and if followed by intervention allows fast access to available technologies (Smith, 2008). If this happens before six months of age, the life of the child will be positively affected, increasing the prognosis of better school performance (Smith, 2008; Marscharck, 2001; Yoshinaga-Itano & Sedey, 2000).

In the Brazilian culture parents emphatically employ verbal behavior to interact with the children from an early age. This type of behavior provides no positive effect for children with hearing loss. Parents tend to reduce this and other types of communicative behaviors towards their deaf children as soon as they find out their children cannot hear them. A study was conducted with 19 parents in order to check feelings and expectations towards children with hearing loss. The results showed communication problems because the parents took a long time to make use of other communication means to facilitate the relationship between them (Boscolo & Santos, 2005).

In a literature review about family relationships and presence of children with hearing loss, it was observed that mothers were less equalitarian and spontaneous with deaf children than with the other children. They were also more restricting and controlling (Brito & Dessen, 1999). The relationship of the fathers with the children with hearing loss tended to be somewhat absent. The mothers assumed the care of the children and, consequently, their education (Brito, 1997). Fathers participated less intensively on the development of the children using more rational justifications, culturally more accepted, as the necessity of being absent due to work. However, fathers tend to present the same anguish and anxiety feelings reported by mothers (Canho, Neme & Yamada, 2006). The authors suggest intervention procedures geared towards the fathers in order to make them active participants in the upbringing of the children. In the Brazilian culture, the mother is responsible for taking care of the house, raising the children, including the ones with no disorder (Oliveira, Simionato, Negrelli & Marcon, 2004; Guarinello, 2004; Dias, Rocha, Pedroso & Caporali, 2005).

The authors above focus on the important role familiar interactions have for the development of deaf children. They represent opportunities for both of them to learn how to communicate with each other.

The early use of bimodal communication (oral and gestures), may prevent problems and promote mutually satisfactory interactions between parents and deaf children (Oliveira, Simionato, Negrelli & Marcon, 2004; Guarinello, 2004; Dias, Rocha, Pedroso & Caporali, 2005). Thus, interventions with children with hearing loss must also focus on their families. The use of sign language by the family helps these children to interact with the surrounding world, favoring satisfactory and appropriate relationships (Negrelli & Marcon, 2006; Lacerda, 2003).

Deaf children with deaf parents who learned the sign language during childhood had better school performance than deaf children with hearing parents. Deaf children learned to read and write two years before those with hearing parents (Marscharck, 1993). Nevertheless, 90% of the children with hearing loss have hearing parents. This fact may lead to super protective practices due to communication problems (Gargiulo, 2003).

Hearing parents expect their children to speak. They take longer to understand that other forms of communication are possible. Such communication difficulties between them may cause social skills deficits in the children (Boscolo & Santos, 2005).

Social skill may lead to a better development and help preventing behavioral problems. They may also aid the children to interact positively with people, increasing the possibility of social support as well as being able to solve problems.

Apart from hearing loss, studies have reported an inverse relation between social skills repertoire and behavior problems (Cia & Barham, 2009). Nevertheless, there is an assumption that children with hearing loss have a lack of social skills and more behavior problems, as compared to hearing children.

A review of Brazilian papers published between 1995 and 2005 has identified the relationship between parents and children with hearing loss (Bisol, Simioni & Sperb, 2008). However there are no reports comparing positive and negative practices of parents. There are no studies comparing those conducted in clinical and nonclinical groups.

One study compared parental educational practices of hearing families with deaf children, and hearing families with hearing children. The results obtained showed that parents of children with hearing loss (HL) expressed less feelings and opinions, and did not play very much with their children. The positive practices were most frequent among parents of hearing children. Nonetheless, the study did not control other important variables as the presence or absence of behavior problems in the children (Rodrigues et al. 2010).

1.2 Parental educational practices of mothers of children with hearing loss

Behavioral evaluation of children and parental educational practices are important and necessary to identify the difficulties and the resources they present. It permits the elaboration of behavioral diagnosis and effective interventions with the children or with their parents/caretakers. Evaluation procedures include: spontaneous report during the interview, oriented instruments (scales, inventory) and direct observation in a natural or structured environment. However, it is important to investigate parental practices and behavior of children through validated instruments. In this study a validated inventory Roteiro de Entrevista de Habilidades Sociais Educativas Parentais (RE-HSE-P) (Interview Guide of Parental Educational Social Skills - Bolsoni-Silva, Loureiro & Marturano, 2011)[1] was used. It evaluates positive and negative parental educational practices, as well as behavior problems and social skills of children reported by the mothers.

Behavior problems are classified as internalizing (isolation, depression, anxiety and somatic complaints) and externalizing behaviors (impulsiveness, aggression, agitation, challenging and anti-social characteristics) (Achenbach & Edelbrock, 1979). In any of the situations if they occur for at least six months they can be considered as emotional disorders (internalizing) or as disruptive behavior (externalizing) according to DSM-IV (APA, 2006). The externalizing behaviors are characterized by improper expression usually towards other people, with a tendency to harm them (Kazdin & Weisz, 2003). On the other hand, internalizing behaviors refer to harmful actions towards the person himself. However, in both cases they are considered inadequate for infantile social skills.

Infantile social skills have been reviewed by Calderella (Caldarella & Merrell, 1997). They identified a diversity of infantile social skills, as follows: 1) *peers relationship skills* (greeting, praising, helping, negotiating, inviting friends to play); 2) *self-control skills* (controlling humor, dealing with criticism); 3) *academic skills* (removing doubts, following teacher's instructions, working independently); 4) *adaptability skills* (following rules and instructions,

---

[1] This study kept the original denomination for RE-HSE-P. The corresponding name in English is Interview Guide of Parental Educational Social Skills.

using free time properly, answering requests); 5) *assertive skills* (starting conversation, accepting invitations, replying greetings). Nonetheless, other components of the children social skills may be present, such as: emotional expressiveness, civility, empathy, interpersonal problems solution, ability to make friends and social academic skills (Del Prette & Del Prette, 2006).

In a study with 48 preschoolers (24 with behavioral problem and 24 without), behavioral categories for the infantile social skills were suggested from evaluations of mothers and teachers. They were classified as: (a) **Social availability and cooperation**: Child makes requests, tries to help, asks questions, greets people, praises people, takes initiatives; (b) **Expression of feelings and coping**: expresses properly: thoughts, concerns and needs, shows distress, gives opinions, claims personal rights, is usually in a good mood and negotiates; (c) **Positive social interaction**: communicates in a positive manner, makes friends, plays with them, has nonverbal interaction (Bolsoni-Silva, Marturano, Pereira & Manfrinato, 2006).

Positive parental practices may avoid the appearance and/or the maintenance of difficulties in interactions established between parents and children. On the other hand, negative practices may increase the probability of their occurrences (Patterson, Reid & Dishion, 2002).

Positive educational practices include positive monitoring and moral behavior. Positive monitoring comprises the appropriate employment of attention and to grant privileges. Moral behavior implies promoting favorable conditions to the development of virtues and cultural values (empathy, notion of justice, responsibility, and work). Negative educational practices comprise negligence, permissiveness, negative monitoring, inconsistent punishment and physical abuse (Gomide, 2006).

Parental social educational skills constitute important behaviors to guarantee a positive parental practice. In order to study the parents-children interaction as parental educational social skills (ESS-P); such skills were classified as: communication (talking, asking) expression of feelings and coping (expressing positive and negative feelings, opinions, demonstrating concern, playing) and establishing limits (identifying and reinforcing socially skilful and nonskilful behaviors, setting rules, being consistent, agreeing with the spouse, fulfilling promises, identifying mistakes and apologizing) (Bolsoni-Silva, Loureiro & Marturano, 2011).

The interview guide (RE-HSE-P) was elaborated based on the propositions of authors involved in the social skills field (Del Prette & Del Prette, 1999; Caballo, 1991) and researchers involved in the study of parental practices (Patterson, Reid & Dishion, 2002; Reid, Webster-Stratton & Hammond, 2003). Authors of the Behavior Analysis field were consulted especially concerning the application of functional analyses in clinical practice (Goldiamond, 1974/2002; Meyer, Oshiro, Mayer, & Starling, 2008). The RE-HSE-P was validated and it has been employed in characterization studies (Bolsoni-Silva & Marturano, 2008) and as a pre and post-test measure at interventions (Bolsoni-Silva & Marturano, 2010) being effective in differentiating groups with and without problems. It has also being used in the identification of behavioral patterns of parents and children after intervention, by functional analysis.

The term functional analysis contains different definitions (Meyer, Oshiro, Mayer, & Starling, 2008) and it was elaborated from the Experimental Analysis of Behavior. For the clinical context it reinforces the relevance of evaluating several behaviors and multiple causes, considering antecedent variables (environment), response (reported or observed behavior) and consequent (events which occur after the answers). Considering parents-children interactions the consequent variables constitute the children's behaviors towards the parents' behavior and vice-versa (Goldiamond, 1974/2002).

In order to compare the parental educational social skills of two groups of mothers (one of children with hearing loss, and the other with hearing children without any behavior problems or other disorder) the RE-HSE-P was employed.

Differences were found between the clinical and nonclinical population, in relation to parental educational social skills (ESS-P), the infantile social skills, and the contextual variables. There were no differences between the groups in relation to negative practices and behavior problems. However, there were no evaluations for the sub-categories of the following behaviors: communication, expressiveness and the establishment of limits (Bolsoni-Silva, Loureiro & Marturano, 2011). Describing them may help in the identification of behavior which can be focus of rapid interventions without neglecting other needs of the studied population. Therefore, additional analyses must be performed comparing the interactions established between parents and children from the hearing loss (HL) group and from the nonclinical group.

The present study aims at comparing the quality of interactions established between parents and children, considering two groups: Clinical Group x Nonclinical Group (normative). Specific objectives were to describe and compare behaviors denominated as positive parental practices (Parental Educational Social Skills - ESS-P), negative parental practices (aggressiveness and no assertiveness), infantile social skills, and behavior problems.

2. Method

2.1 Participants

A total of 52 mothers took part in this study whose children presented hearing loss (n = 27) (HL Group) or children who were part of a normative/nonclinical sample (n = 26) (Normative Group). The children with hearing loss (HL) used Hearing Aids (HA - AASI Aparelho de Amplificação Sonora Individual) and had hearing parents. They were identified at CEDALVI/HRAC/USP (Center of Hearing, Language and Vision Disorders, in the Hospital for the Rehabilitation of Craniofacial Anomalies, at University of São Paulo, Bauru, São Paulo, Brazil). The normative/nonclinical sample (n = 26) comprised two studies: the first evaluated the effectiveness of an intervention procedure (Bolsoni-Silva, Salina, Versuti & Rosin-Pinola, 2008) and the other evaluated the parental practices of separated/divorced mothers (Boas & Bolsoni-Silva, 2010).

2.2 Inventory

The Roteiro de Entrevista de Habilidades Sociais Educativas Parentais (Interview Guide of Parental Educational Social Skills) - (RE-HSE-P - Bolsoni-Silva, Loureiro & Marturano, 2011) was used. It evaluates the occurrence and the quality of social skills applicable to educational practices and behavior of children, contingent to: starting conversation, asking questions in general (*Communication*), expressing positive and negative feelings and opinions (*Expressiveness*), affection, situations and strategies used to establish limits, identify children's behavior, what he/she likes and dislikes, accomplish promises (*Limits Establishment*). In total the inventory comprises 70 items and comprehends alpha of 0.846. They are organized into two factors: positive and negative interaction characteristics. The positive interactions are: educational social skills and infantile social skills. The negative ones are: negative practices and behavior problems.

2.3 Data collection procedures

Data from HL and normative groups were collected in the clinics. For the normative group the data were collected in their houses and/or at the children's schools. After the consent of the respondent the mothers signed an Informed Consent. The interviews were conducted according to a specific set of procedures. The answers were recorded for further categorization.

2.4 Treatment procedures and data analysis

Data were computed according to the given information and organized into previously reported categories. Comparisons were made between hearing loss and normative groups (*t Student Test*).

3. Results

The results were synthesized according to three broad categories of RE-HSE-P: *Communication, Expressiveness and Limits Establishment.*

Figures 1 and 2 present, respectively, the results of the participant's mothers behavior of "talking" and "asking" which are part of the *communication* category. Asterisks in the figures correspond to the items with *statistically significant differences.* The bars identify the clinical group and the lines the nonclinical group.

Analyzing the answers to the question *"Do you talk to your child?", "What subjects do you discuss?"* (Figures 1 and 2*)*, it was observed that both groups talked to their children in order to teach them what is correct or incorrect, mainly concerning externalizing behaviors (especially disobedience and aggressiveness). Notwithstanding, the nonclinical group more frequently than the clinical group talked about different subjects (clinical average 0.63, SD = 0.88; nonclinical average= 1.42, SD = 1,.5; p = 0.029), and in different periods of the day (clinical average = 0.26, SD = 0.45; nonclinical average = 0.70, SD = 2.11; p = 0.002). The children without hearing loss acted positively during these periods. They demonstrated socially skilful behaviors, such as: talking, keeping eye contact, giving attention to the mothers (nonclinical average = 1.81, SD = 1.09). The clinical group also demonstrated social skills (clinical average = 0.89, SD = 0.95), but with a statistically significant difference in inferiority (p = 0.001). Both groups sometimes answered with nonskilful behaviors (problems concerning externalizing or internalizing behaviors) during conversations,, with no statistical difference between the groups.

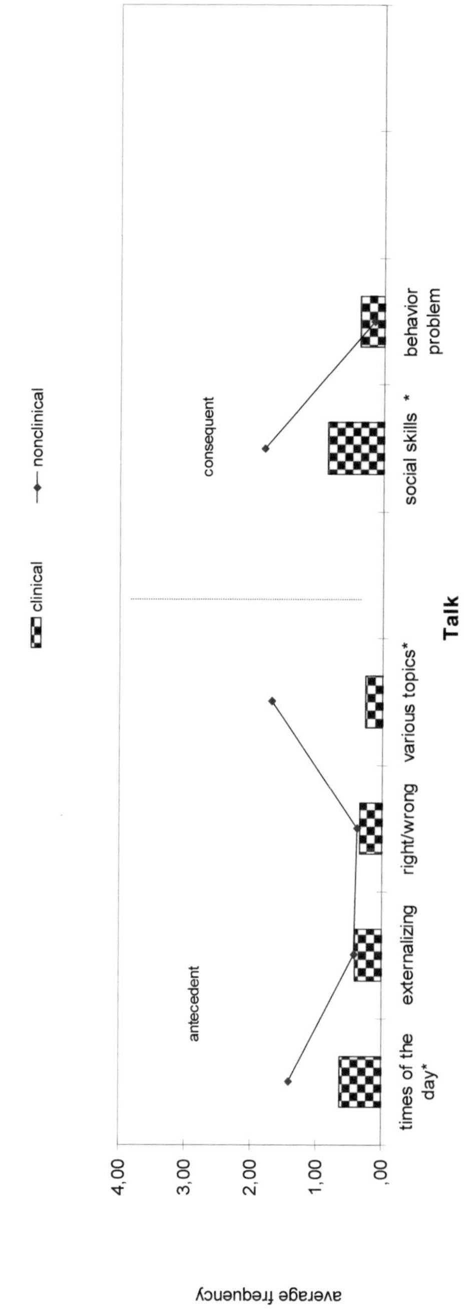

Fig. 1. Average frequency of antecedent variables and behavior of children when the mother talks to them.[2]

[2] The legends for every figure correspond to the ones from Figure 1.

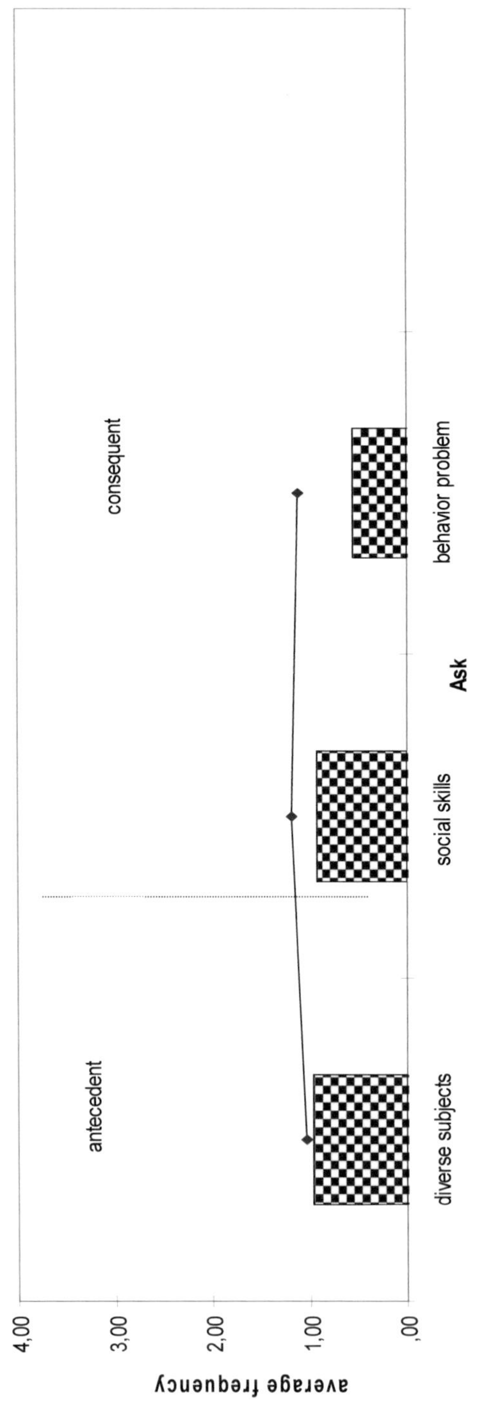

Fig. 2. Average frequency of antecedent variables and behavior of children when a mother questions them.

When the answer included "different periods of the day" to the question "When", the mothers reported the following: on the way to school, at night, after arriving from school, during the day, during hygiene care, in all the situations, on vacation, on weekends, late afternoon, at time to get up, during meal times, during homework time, on the traffic, arriving from a trip, arriving from work, when they were together, when going to bed.

As an answer to the question "Which subject?" mothers reported "different subjects" as follows: everyday life, leisure time, usefulness of objects (for instance: pans, brooms), meaning of concepts and objects, something that the child saw, a party, food, animals, plays, cars, father-mother relationship (marriage and separation), drugs, private events involving the mother and the child, personal hygiene, their own body, infantile books, soap operas/ cartoons/television programs, the mother's job, wishes and interest of the child, the future of the family and/or the child, offer help to the child, dangers facing the world, members of the family, which clothes to wear, religion, health, violence and other questions asked by the child.

About the interactions established for the mothers' questions the groups did not present differences. Both talked during different situations and sometimes the children answered in a socially skilful manner, and sometimes not.

Expressiveness corresponds to a category of parental educational practice and behavior of the children corresponding to four questions of the RE-HSE-P: "Do you express positive feelings towards your child?", "Do you express negative feelings towards your child?", Do you express your opinions to your child?", "Do you caress your child?". After each of these questions the respondent was required to talk about the quality of the interventions established between parents and children. The answers to these questions were analyzed and according to the occasions in which they occurred, were denominated as *context variables.* The obtained categories were as follows: in several situations, the mother's personal problems, treating the environment carelessly, after calling the attention of the child, due to his/her behavior, before something interesting that the child has done, during leisure time and when the child was not feeling well. Another set of categories refers to *features of mothers' behavior,* present in two classifications of ESSP-P: 1. Communicates and expresses feelings and coping and, 2. Negative educational practice (beating, shouting). The last set of categories refers to *features of the children's behavior* contingent to the mother's, described as skilful behavior and behavior problem (internalizing and externalizing). The results of the questions about "positive feelings" are demonstrated in Figure 3.

The ESS-P "Communication to express positive feelings" refers to the parents' behavior of expressing tenderness in relation to the child or the child's appropriate behavior. The ESS-P "Expresses feelings and coping" refers to: touches the child, plays, hugs and kisses. The comparison between groups shows that the clinical group expresses feelings less in a "communicating" way than the nonclinical group (clinical = 1.15, SD = 0.71; nonclinical average = 2.31, SD = 1.59; $p = 0.002$). The groups equally "express feelings and coping".

Figure 4 presents "Tenderness expression" for each group. It can be observed that the groups express tenderness towards good behaviors equally in leisure situations and when the child is not feeling well, specially the nonclinical group (clinical average = 0.04, SD =

0.19; nonclinical average = 0.35, SD = 0.63; p = 0.023). In these situations, the mothers of children without any deficiency are significantly more dedicated (clinical average = 0.04, SD = 0.19; nonclinical average = 0.35, SD = 0.63; p = 0.023) and as consequence, their children correspond more intensely to the expression of tenderness (clinical average = 0.04, SD = 0.19; nonclinical average = 0.35, SD = 0.63; p = 0.003).

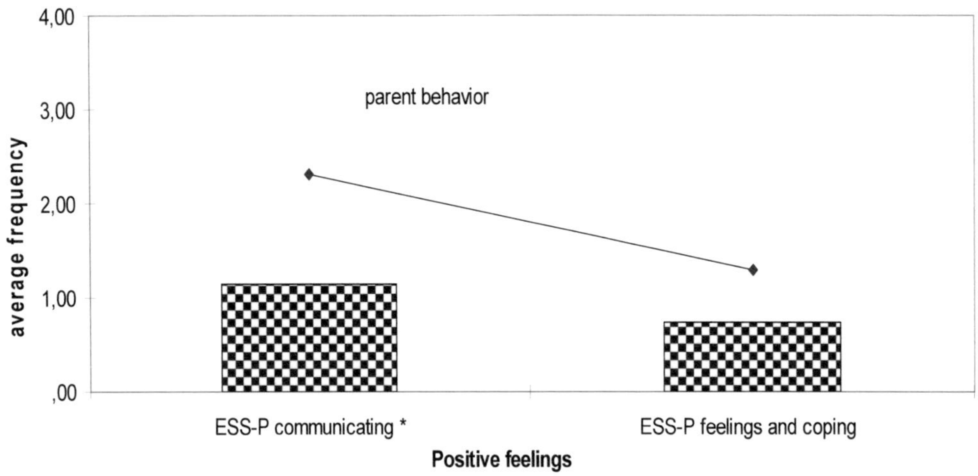

Fig. 3. Average frequency of how mothers express positive feelings to the children.

Figure 5 shows that both groups express opinions about different subjects. Nonetheless, the children from the nonclinical group behaved more frequently according to the category "Expression of feelings and coping" (clinical average = 0.48, SD = 0.51; nonclinical average = 1.15, SD = 1.00; p = 0.004). Some examples of how the child behaves are: hugs, accept the adults' opinion, thanks, gives support to parents when they are sad, gives his/her opinion, and explain his/herself.

Figure 6 presents the context and the mothers' and children's behaviors when mothers expressed negative feelings. Both groups expressed these feelings when they had personal problems, when were in dangerous environments, faced optimal behaviors of children, discussed several subjects and also after reprimands. Nonetheless, the nonclinical group used more negative educational practices (clinical average = 0.30, SD = 0.54; nonclinical average = 1.50, SD = 1.53; p = 0.004) in addition, these children expressed affection in these moments more frequently (clinical average = 1.11, SD = 0.89; nonclinical average = 2.08, SD = 1.62; p = 0.004).

The following examples can be considered as negative practices: verbal and/or non verbal threatening (deprive of privileges, beating), punishment (grounding), tightening the arm of the child, beating, shouting, fighting, getting nervous, calling names, talking a lot, saying "no" without explaining the reason, saying that will exchange the children for other ones, accusing/criticizing the spouse's behavior, cheating, imitating the incorrect behavior of the child and depriving the child from something he/she likes.

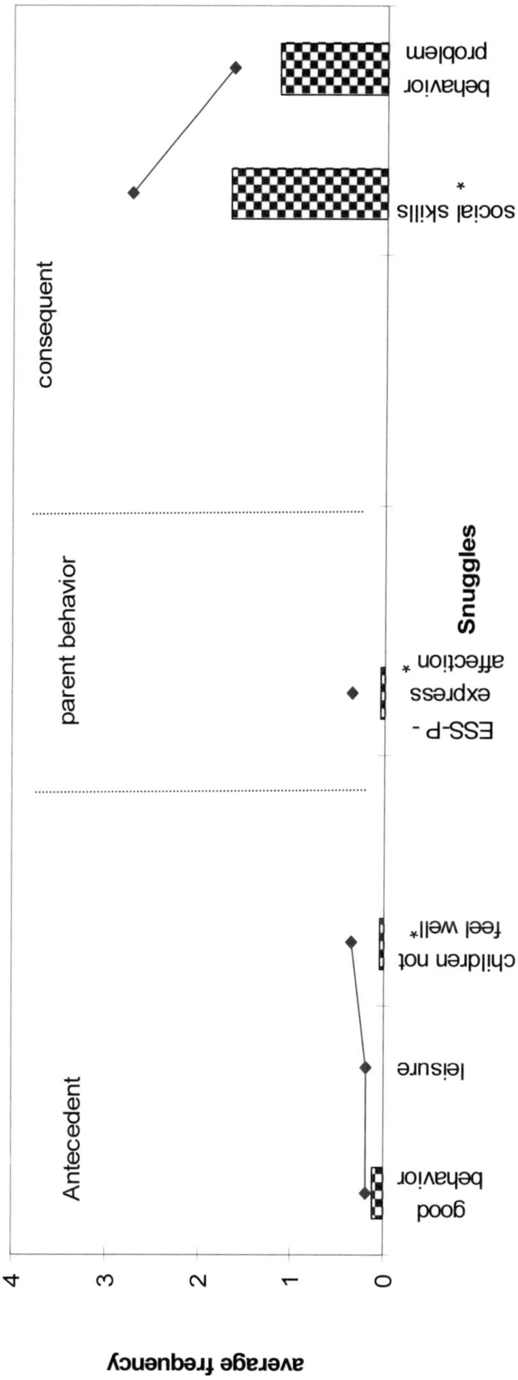

Fig. 4. Mean frequency of antecedent variables when mothers cuddled and behaviors of children in these interactions.

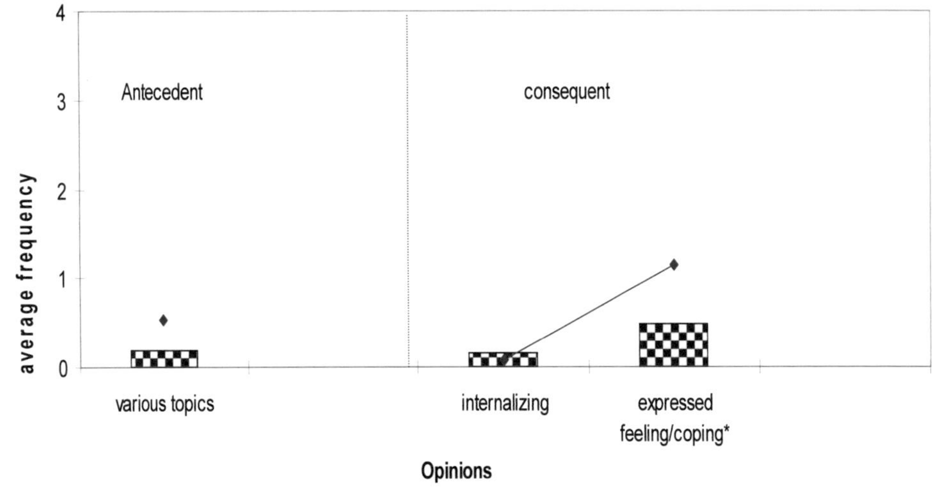

Fig. 5. Mean frequency of antecedent variables when mothers expressed opinions and behaviors of children in these interactions.

Establishment of limits consisted in another category of educational practices and children's behaviors corresponding to four questions of the RE-HSE-P: *"Why does it become important to establish limits?", "What do you do to establish them?", "Does your child do things that you like?", "Does your child do things that you do not like?"* After each of these questions the respondent is required to talk about the quality of the interactions established regarding the occasions in which they occurred, the type of the mother's behavior, and the child's behavior in relation to the mother's. The answers from the analyses of content according to RE-HSE-P, were classified into three subcategories: (a) context variables: facing the obedience of the child, teaching what is correct and incorrect, having control of the behavior of the child, protecting the health of the child, and in leisure environment; (b) mother's behaviors: b1) communicates and expresses feelings and coping and, b2) makes uses of negative practices (beating, shouting, being quiet/not doing anything) and, (c) children's behavior: skilful and behavior problems (internalizing and externalizing).

Figure 7 describes the results of the identification of appropriate behaviors and mothers-children interactions in these situations. Both groups consider as appropriate the obedience of the children, but the nonclinical group statistically highlights the expression of affection of the children (clinical average = 0.41, SD = 0.50; nonclinical average = 0.88, SD = 0.86; $p = 0.019$). Both groups use few negative practices, but do not report positive practices. Possibly in these situations even if the mothers identify the proper behavior they do not reinforce it. The children from both groups demonstrate behaviors corresponding to "expressing feelings and coping".

Figure 8 presents the interactions involved when the child demonstrates behaviors that mothers disapprove. Both groups do not like it when children are disobedient or when they are aggressive. Equally, in these occasions, the groups show behaviors considered as negative practices and, mothers also report that they are feeling bad (sad, angry,

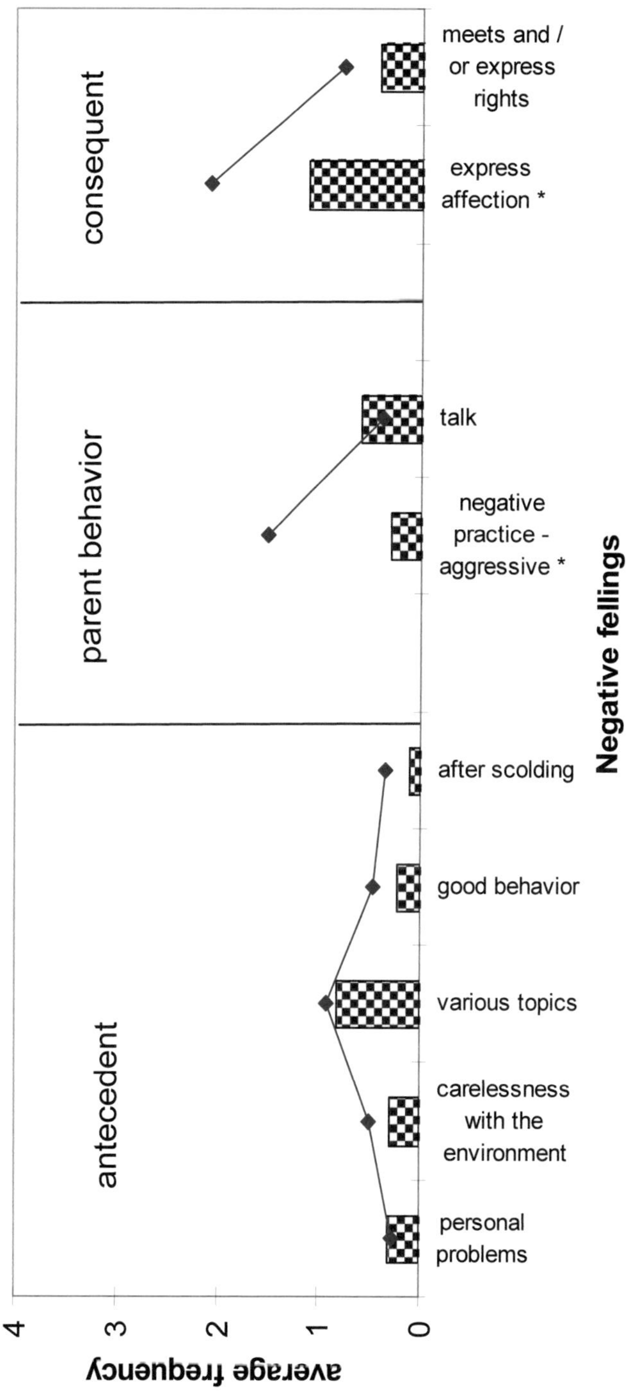

Fig. 6. Mean frequency of antecedent variables when mothers expressed negative feelings and children behaviors in these interactions.

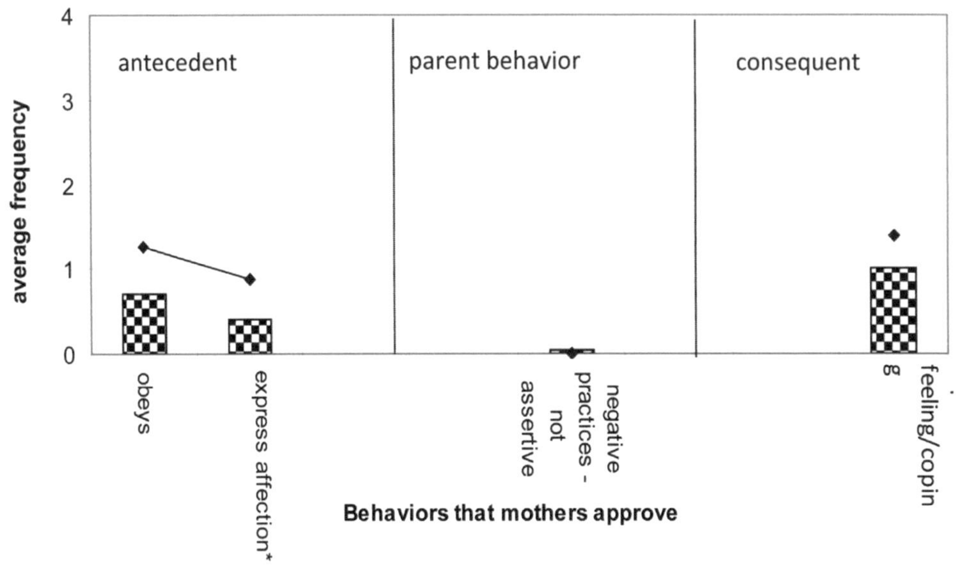

Fig. 7. Behaviors that mothers approve, maternal behaviors, and children's reactions.

disappointed), especially the clinical group (clinical average = 2.04, SD = 0.59; nonclinical average = 1.38, SD = 1.10; p = 0.011). Children from both groups obey in the same degree , present internalizing or externalizing behaviors, though, the children with deficiency apologize or give explanations more frequently (clinical average = 0.15, SD = 0.36; nonclinical average = 0.81, SD = 1.02; p = 0.004).

Figure 9 describes the reasons given by the mothers to establish limits, their behaviors and the behaviors of their children. It can be observed that mothers from both groups consider important the use of limits establishment to teach children how to behave correctly and safely according to social standards during meals and plays.

However, the nonclinical group, more than the hearing loss group, emphasizes intensely that it is important to establish limits in order to have control over the child's behavior (clinical average = 0.22, SD = 0.42; nonclinical average = 1.35, SD = 1.32; p = 0.000), to teach social relationship rules (clinical average = 0.07, SD = 0.27; nonclinical average = 0.46, SD = 0.86; p = 0.036) and when the child treats their belongings and the environment carelessly (clinical average = 0.37, SD = 0.63; nonclinical average = 0.92, SD = 1.16; p = 0.039).

Mothers of both groups reported that they demonstrated behaviors denominated as positive and negative educational practices, and informed that they felt fine behaving this way. Likewise, in these situations, the children demonstrated behaviors considered as problems, such as disobedience and aggressiveness.

Figure 10 shows global results comparing both groups. In Figure 10 it can be observed that mothers of the nonclinical group reported that they behaved in a social skilful way (clinical average = 6.07, SD = 2.05; nonclinical average = 10.31, SD = 3.78; p = 0.000) as did their children (clinical average = 5.70, SD = 2.30; nonclinical average = 11.00, SD = 4.72; p = 0.000).

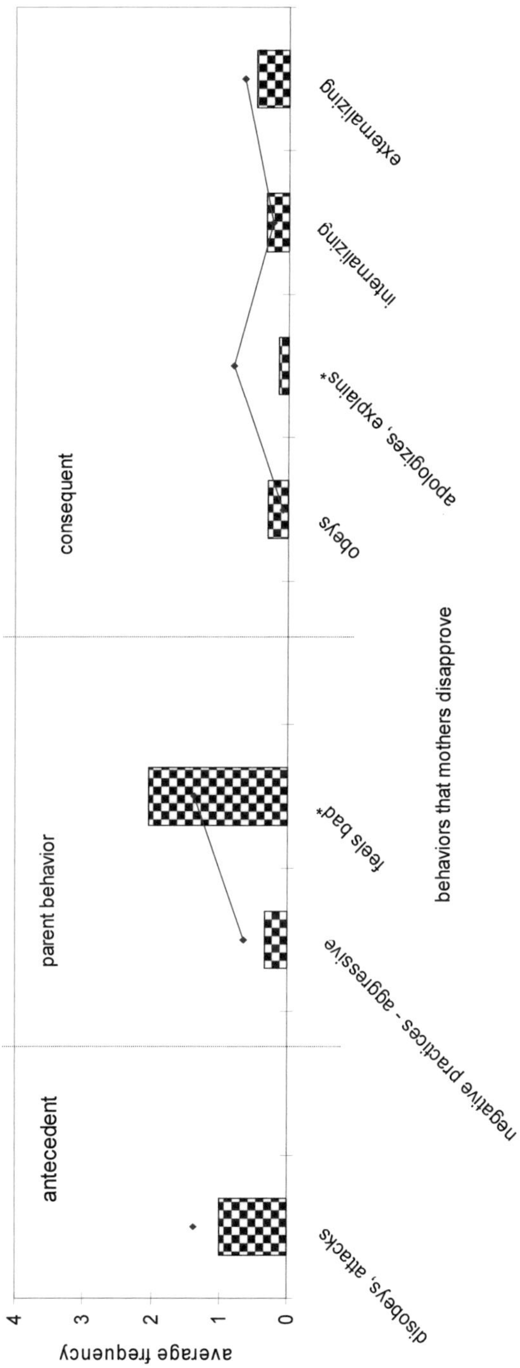

Fig. 8. Children's behaviors that mothers disapprove, maternal behaviors, and children's reactions

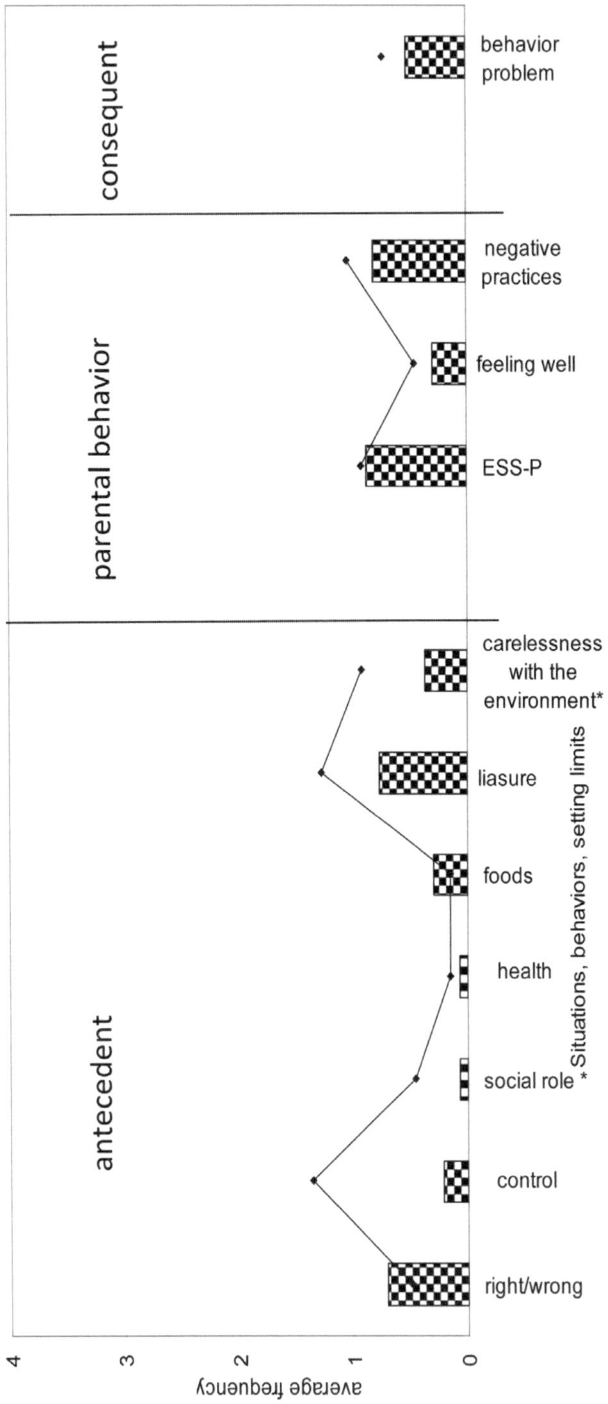

Fig. 9. Frequency of previous situations, maternal behaviors, and reactions of children before setting limits.

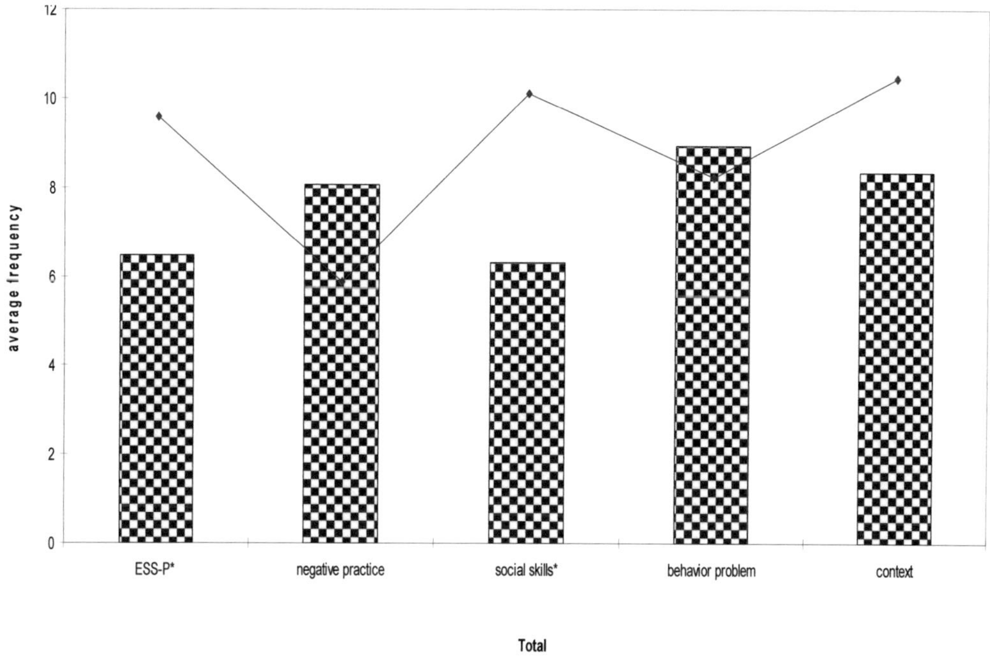

Fig. 10. Categories totals of RE-HSE-P.

4. Conclusion

The quality of interactions established between mothers and children with hearing loss were positively correlated with the social skills of the children and with the context variables. The results indicated that the interactions established between mothers and children favor the acquisition and maintenance of the social skills repertoire. For the hearing loss group both mothers and children presented a poor social skills repertoire in comparison to the normative group.

As for *Communication*, the HL group, when compared to the normative group reported talking to their children less frequently about subjects of their interests and in fewer social contexts. In these occasions the HL children presented poor social skills behavior.

Regarding *Expressiveness*, it was observed that the mothers of the normative group expressed affection and praised more frequently than those from the HL group. The children who belonged to the normative group again presented more social skills than HL group. On the other hand, mothers from the HL group used less punishing strategies for education when compared to the normative group.

For *Limits Establishment*, it was observed that mothers of children with hearing loss identified fewer approved behaviors when compared to the normative group, and children were less obedient.

When parents establish limits children of the normative group apologize and/or offer explanations (social skills) more frequently than children with HL.

Parents establish limits in order to teach their children society rules, and also to deal with children carelessness behaviors towards their own belongings and those at home. The mothers of the normative group recognized mostly that they acted incorrectly concerning the children education, qualifying "incorrect behavior" as beating and shouting (negative practices).

A hypothesis for the differences between the clinical and nonclinical groups could be related to the absence of oral expression of children with hearing loss. The mothers can communicate with their children, but, as the children do not have access to the spoken content it impairs the acquisition and maintenance of the social skills repertoire. The intervention programs which advise families on how to interact with their children must consider this aspect and propose an additional training, in order to guarantee more communication between parents and children. The results seem to suggest super protection (Gargiulo, 2003) from the mothers of children with hearing loss, considering that they establish few limits for the behavior of their children. The hypothesis of the study was partially confirmed. Children with hearing loss and their mothers reported fewer social skills. However, they did not present more behavioral problems than the normative population.

The results also showed a connection between positive parental practices and infantile social skills. It was observed the reduced use of negative practices and absence of behavior problems (Patterson, Reid & Dishion, 2001). The nonclinical group reported statistically lower incidence of negative practices. In both groups there was low occurrence of negative practices and behavior problems.

The RE-HSE-P (Bolsoni-Silva, Loureiro & Marturano, 2011) was useful to add some knowledge about interactions between mothers and children with hearing loss. In regard to social skills it has also favored the identification of behavioral patterns, specific for this population that indicated more behavioral deficits.

The results also emphasized the fact that many times mothers of children with hearing loss behaved just like the mothers in the nonclinical population. Some of the similar practices were: talking about several subjects, expressing affection, establishing limits, and facing behaviors that they did not approve. Children from the HL group also demonstrated social skills. Both parents and children need to have their social skills repertoire improved , but it becomes necessary to consider behaviors which are already present on their repertoires (Goldiamond, 1974/2002).

The externalizing and internalizing behaviors which were reported by the hearing loss group are insufficient to consider that the children have disruptive problems (APA, 2006). In addition, both groups present interactions which are classified as behavior problems. They could be avoided if the mothers learned how to reinforce (praise, thank) the good behaviors.

Studies about social educational skills show that talking to the children about several subjects, especially the ones of their interest in different situations promoted social skills and reduced the probability of behavior problems (Bolsoni-Silva, Loureiro, & Marturano, 2011). In the present research such behaviors were less frequently observed during interactions with hearing loss children, which possibly favors the children's poor repertoire of social skills.

These results are in accordance to the field literature which affirms that for this population there is a great difficulty in communicating (Boscolo & Santos, 2005). Other authors have also found out that mothers of children with hearing loss are less spontaneous than with normative children (Brito & Dessen, 1999). Additionally, mothers of children with hearing loss are less involved in their development, being more concerned in taking basic care rather than talking to them (Canho, Neme & Yamada, 2006). However, the results of the present research do not prove that low repertoire of social skills is associated to behavior problems, a finding in agreement with some other studies (Cia & Barham, 2009; Gargiulo, 2003).

For efficiently talking to children with hearing loss mothers are required to know sign language. Due to its additional cost they avoid learning it, impairing the promotion of better interactions and consequently the development of children's social skills (Lacerda, 2003; Negrelli & Marcon, 2006). Affection expressing behaviors are also less frequent in the clinical group. Children tend to see their mothers as models. When they are not affectionate they favor this deficit in their children.

In relation to limits establishments it can be observed that mothers of children with hearing loss used fewer negative practices than the normative population. Considering the results expressed in Figure 8 it can be observed that children from both groups disobey; that is a reason for mothers to establish limits. It can also be noticed that the mothers talk to their children with hearing loss who on their turn obey and justify themselves when behaving improperly.

Overall, the results of the present research confirm the findings of previous studies, concerning educational practices (little communication and little affection expressions) with children social skills deficits (Rodrigues, Carrara, Palamin & Bolsoni-Silva, 2010; Bolsoni-Silva, Rodrigues, Abramides, Souza & Loureiro, 2010).

Mothers of children with hearing loss are less equalitarian and spontaneous than with other children, besides being more restricting and controlling (Brito & Dessen, 1999). Data from the present research do not allow affirming about different practices, considering siblings with or without hearing loss. The results show that the mothers of children with hearing loss seem to establish limits in a skilful manner (talking) and that their children obey and express themselves similarly to the normative population.

Intervention procedures with this population should teach the importance of affection and communication, not only for the care, or to determine limits, but also in other situations of interest for the child. It is important to teach the social skills repertoires. The more skilful the mothers, the more skilful the children will be (Bolsoni-Silva, Loureiro & Marturano, 2011).

Skilful behavior is not always easy to achieve considering that mothers are frequently overloaded with chores. The Brazilian literature has pointed to the cultural aspect present on interactions between parents and children, in which the interaction of mother-children are the most studied, indicating aspects in their practices as more restricting and controlling, associated to anxiety and anguish patterns (Brito & Dessen, 1999; Oliveira, Simionato, Negrelli & Marcon, 2004; Guarinello, 2004; Dias, Rocha, Pedroso & Caporali, 2005). Nevertheless, studies with fathers have not been frequently developed (Brito, 1997; Canho, Neme e Yamada, 2006), taking into consideration its important role on the children's development. An early counseling and follow-up are extremely important as a mean of improving the interaction between father and child (Marchesi, 1996; Bisol, Simioni, and Sperb, 2008; Smith, 2008).

In conclusion, studies comprising children with hearing loss and their families have shown the necessity of preventive actions and early identification of the child's condition. This permits parents orientation, the involvement into alternative forms of communication with their children insuring their development, and reducing the possibility of behavior problems. However, it is mandatory for the parents to develop educational practices such as: expression of feelings, establishment of limits, in addition to praising and reinforcing their children's appropriate behaviors.

Studies concerning the interaction between the dyads father-child and mother-child specially with hearing loss are necessary and urgent. It's important to give special attention to children since preschool up to school age creating a fertile and promising situation for optimal parents-children interactions and thus promoting the development of the child with hearing loss.

5. References

American Psychiatric Association (2000). *Diagnostic and statistics manual of mental disorders* (6a. Ed.). The Association, ISBN: 10: 1433805618, Washington.

Bisol, C. A.; Simioni, J. & Sperb, T. (2008). Contribuições da Psicologia brasileira para o estudo da surdez. *Revista Psicologia Reflexão e Crítica*; Vol. 21, No. 3, (December 2007), pp. (392-400), ISSN: 0102-7972.

Boas, A. C. V. B. V. & Bolsoni-Silva, A. T. (2010). Habilidades sociais educativas de mães separadas e sua relação com o comportamento de pré-escolares. *Psico-USF;* Vol. 15, No. 3, (June 2010), pp. (301-310), ISSN: 1413-8271.

Bolsoni-Silva, A. T. & Marturano, E. M. (2010). Evaluation of group intervention for mothers/caretakers of kindergarten children with externalizing behavioral problems. *Revista Interamericana de Psicología/Interamerican Journal of Psychology*; Vol. 44, No. 3, (May 2009), pp. (411-417), ISSN: 0034-9690.

Bolsoni-Silva, A. T.; Loureiro, S. R. & Marturano, E. M. (2011). *Roteiro de Entrevista de Habilidades Sociais Educativas Parentais (RE-HSE-P). Manual Técnico*. Editora Vetor, ISBN: 978-85-7585-438-9, São Paulo.

Bolsoni-Silva, A.T.; Salina, A.; Versuti, F.M. & Rosin-Pinola, A. R. (2008). Avaliação de um programa de intervenção de habilidades sociais educativas parentais. *Psicologia Ciência e Profissão;* Vol. 28, No. 1, (February 2007), pp. (18–33), ISSN: 1414-9893.

Bolsoni-Silva, A. T. & Marturano, E. M. (2008). Habilidades sociais educativas parentais e problemas de comportamento: comparando pais e mães de pré-escolares. *Aletheia (ULBRA);* Vol. 27, No. 1, (January 2008), pp. (126-138), ISSN: 1413-0394.

Bolsoni-Silva, A. T.; Marturano, E. M.; Pereira, V. A. & Manfrinato, J. W. S. (2006). Habilidades sociais e problemas de comportamento de pré-escolares: comparando avaliações de mães e de professoras. *Psicologia: Reflexão e Crítica*; Vol. 19, No. 3, (March 2006), pp. (460-469), ISSN: 0102-7972.

Bolsoni-Silva, A. T.; Rodrigues, O. M. P. R.; Abramides, D. V. M.; Souza, L. S. & Loureiro, S. R. (2010). Práticas educativas parentais de crianças com deficiência auditiva e de linguagem. *Revista Brasileira de Educação Especial*; Vol. 16, No. 2, (August 2010), pp. (265-282), ISSN: 1413-6538.

Bolsoni-Silva, A. T. & Loureiro, S. (2010). Validação do Roteiro de Habilidades Sociais Educativas Parentais - RE-HSE-P. *Avaliação Psicológica*; Vol. 9, No. 1, (February 2010), pp. (63-75), ISSN: 1677-0471.

Boscolo, C. C. & Santos, T. M. M. (2005). A deficiência auditiva e a família: sentimentos e expectativas de um grupo de pais de crianças com deficiência da audição. *Distúrbios da Comunicação*; Vol. 17, No. 1, (February 2005), pp. (69-75), ISSN: 2176-2724.

Brito, A. M. W. & Dessen, M. A. (1999). Crianças surdas e suas famílias: um panorama geral. *Psicologia: Reflexão e Crítica*; Vol. 12, No. 2, (March 1999), pp. (429-445), ISSN: 0102-7972.

Caballo, V. E. (1991). El entrenamiento en habilidades sociales. In *Terapia y modificacion de conducta* V. E. Caballo (Org.), pp. (403-443), Siglo Veintiuno, ISBN: 84-323-0808-0, Madri, Spain.

Caldarella, P. & Merrell, K. W. (1997). Common dimensions of social skills of children and adolescents: a taxonomy of positive behaviors. *School Psychology Review*; Vol. 26, No. 2, (March 1997), pp. (264-278), ISSN: 0279-6015.

Calderon, R. & Greenberg, M.T. (1999). Stress e coping in hearing mothers of children with hearing loss: factors affectting mother and child adjustment. *American Anals of the Deaf*; Vol. 144, No. 1, (March 1999), pp. (7-18), ISSN: 0002-726X.

Calderon, R. (2000). Parental involvement in deaf children's education programs as a predictor of child's language, early reading, and social-emotional development. *Journal Deaf Studie Deaf Education*; Vol. 5, No. 2, (October 1999), pp. (140-155), ISSN: 1081-4159.

Canho, P. G. M., Neme, C. M. B., & Yamada, M. O. (2006). A vivência do pai no processo de reabilitação da criança com deficiência auditiva. *Estudos de Psicologia*; Vol. 23, No. 3, (February 2006), pp. (226-269),ISSN: 0103-166X.

Cia, F. & Barham, E. J. (2009). Repertório de habilidades sociais, problemas de comportamento, autoconceito e desempenho acadêmico de crianças no início da escolarização. *Estudos de Psicologia*; Vol. 26, No. 1, (September 2007), pp. (45-55), ISSN: 0103-166X.

Del Prette, Z. A. P. & Del Prette, A. (2006). *Psicologia das habilidades sociais na infância*, Editora Vozes, ISBN: 853263144 - 4, Petrópolis, Brazil.

Del Prette, Z. A. P. & Del Prette, A. (1999). *Psicologia das Habilidades Sociais: Terapia e educação*, Editora Vozes, ISBN: 85.326.2142-2, Petrópolis, Brazil.

Dias, T. R. S.; Rocha, J. C. M.; Pedroso, C. C. A. & Caporali, S. A. (2005). Educação bilíngüe de surdos: grupos familiares. Retrieved from <HTTP://www.educacaoonline.pro.br/ educacao_bilingue.asp.>

Gargiulo, R. M. (2003). *Special Education in contemporary society: an introduction to excepcionality*, Thomson Learning, ISBN: 13: 978-0534626419, Wadsworth, United States of America.

Gatto, C. I. & Tochetto, T.M. (2007). Deficiência auditiva infantil: implicações e soluções. *Revista CEFAC*; Vol. 9, No. 1, (December 2006), 110-15, ISSN: 1516-1846.

Goldiamond, I. (2002/1974). Toward a constructional approach to social problems: ethical and constitutional issues raised by applied behavioral analysis. *Behavior and Social Issues*; Vol 2, (March 2002) pp.108-197, ISSN: 1064-9506.

Gomide, P. I. C. (2006). *Inventário de Estilos Parentais. Modelo teórico: Manual de aplicação, apuração e interpretação*, Editora Vozes, ISBN: 8532632483, Petrópolis, Brazil.

Gravel, J. S. & O'Gara, J. (2003). Communication options for children with hearing loss. *Mental Retardation and Developmental Disabilities Research Reviews*; Vol. 9, (November 2003), pp. (243-251), ISSN: 1940-5529.

Guarinello, A. C. (2000). A influência da família no contexto de filhos surdos. *Jornal Brasileiro de Fonoaudiologia*; Vol. 3, (March 2000), pp. (28-33), ISSN: 1517:5308.

Lacerda, C. B. F. (2003). A família ouvinte de sujeitos surdos: reflexões a partir do contato com a língua de sinais. *Temas em Desenvolvimento*; Vol. 67, No. 12, (March 2003), pp. (34-41), ISSN: 0103-7749.

Kazdin, A. E. & Weisz, J. R. (Orgs.) (2003). *Evidence-based psychotherapies for children and adolescent*, Guilford, ISBN: 10: 1593859740, New York, United States of America.

Marschark, M. (2001). Language development in children who are deaf: a research synthesis. *Alexandria, V.A. National Association of State Directors of Special Education*, ISSN: 1183-322X.

Marschark, M. (1993). *Psychological development of deaf children*, Oxford University, ISBN: 13: 9780195115758, New York, United States of America.

Meyer, S. B.; Oshiro, C.; Mayer, R. C. F. & Starling, R. (2008). Subsídios da obra "Comportamento Verbal" de B. F. Skinner para a terapia analítico-comportamental. *Revista Brasileira de Terapia Comportamental e Cognitiva*; Vol. 10, No. 1, (January 2008), pp. (105-118), ISSN: 1981-9145.

Negrelli, M. E. D. & Marcon, S. S. (2006). Família e a criança surda. *Ciência, Cuidado e Saúde*; Vol. 5, No. 1, (December 2005), 98-107, ISSN: 1677-3861.

Oliveira, R. G.; Simionato, M. A. W.; Negrelli, M. E. D. & Marcon, S. S. (2004). A experiência de famílias no convívio com a criança surda. *Revista Acta Scientiarum*. Health Sciences; Vol. 6, No. 1, (November 2003), pp. (183-191), ISSN: 1679-9291.

Patterson, G.; Reid, J. & Dishion, T. (2002). *Antisocial boys. Comportamento anti-social*, ESETec Editores Associados, ISBN: 10: 091615405X, Santo André, Brazil.

Reid, J.; Webster-Stratton, C. & Hammond, M. M. (2003). Follow-up of children who received the incredible years intervention for oppositional defiant disorder: maintenance and prediction of 2-year outcome. *Behavior Therapy*; Vol. 34, (March 2003), pp. (471-491), ISSN: 0731-7107.

Rodrigues, O. M. P. R.; Carrara, M. P.; Palamin, M. E. G. & Bolsoni-Silva, A. T. (2010). Práticas educativas parentais: a deficiência auditiva pode fazer a diferença? *Revista Pensando Famílias*; Vol. 14, No. 1, (March 2010), pp. (141-162), ISSN: 1679-4947.

Smith, D. D. (2008). *Introdução à Educação Especial: ensinar em tempos de inclusão*, Editora Artmed, ISBN: 13: 9788536311135, Porto Alegre, Brazil.

Yoshinaga-Itano, C. & Sedey, A. (2000). Early speech development in children who are deaf of hearing: interrelationships with language and hearing. *Volta Review*; Vol. 1000, pp. (181-211), ISSN: 0042-8639.

6

Early Intervention with Children Who Have a Hearing Loss: Role of the Professional and Parent Participation

Zerrin Turan
Anadolu University
Turkey

1. Introduction

Early intervention is defined as "a set of services for children six years of age or younger who are at risk of or who currently have developmental delays or social emotional problems" (Guralnick, 2005, as cited in Mahoney & Wiggers, 2007). The underlying premise for early intervention is that children's developmental or social-emotional problems can be either prevented or remediated through specialized services and activities designed to maximize their developmental learning (Bailey, et. al., 1998; Baguley, et al., 2000; Bluebanning , et. al., 2004). Early intervention is grounded in the conviction that the first five years of life are a span during which there is unique opportunity to prevent or reverse children's developmental problems. The rapid brain growth that occurs at this time of children's lives is believed to be associated with critical periods during which children are uniquely prepared to benefit from developmental stimulation that is matched to their individualized needs and abilities (Mahoney & Wiggers, 2007; Ryugo, Limb & Redd, 2000). In other words there are clearly defined times when the physiological readiness of the organism must coincide with the occurrence of specific externally derived experiences (Ryugo, Limb & Redd, 2000).

Many early intervention programs, particularly programs for children up to age three, provide comprehensive services to families, including social support, service coordination as well as information about child's development (Brown & Arehart, 2000; Brown & Nott, 2005; Mahoney & Wiggers, 2007). Generally it is believed that services that reduce the burdens and stressors families experience can make it easier for parents to focus on the needs and care of their children (Bailey, et. al., 1998; Childress, 2004; Dunst, 2002; Kratochwill, et. al., 2007; Odom & Wolery, 2003). It is also argued that parents must play an active role in their children's development. The argument rests on research results which indicate effectiveness of early intervention services is related to the effect they have on the way parents care for or interact with their children (Bailey, et. al., 1998; Clark, 2007; Kaiser & Hancock, 2003; Mahoney, 2009; Rice & Lenihan, 2005). Therefore it is suggested that professionals who work in early intervention services should collaborate with parents instead of directly shaping children's developmental skills.

Like other areas of special education the necessity for early identification and intervention for language development of children with a hearing loss has long been realized and auditory oral/verbal programs have offered intervention for parents to development of spoken language of their children. However progress in universal newborn hearing screening has altered the age range that professionals used to work with. They have to deal much younger children than the past. The advancement in hearing technology has increased the hearing capacity of these young children. Digital hearing aids and cochlear implants provide richer stimuli than ever. Therefore it seems necessary to reconsider the intervention approaches regarding the age of these children and the new role of the professional.

In this chapter the basic issues on the early management of a hearing loss and the rationale of family based services will be described, the professional's role as a partner with parents in early intervention for babies with a hearing loss will be discussed and the factors which facilitate language development and their use in intervention process will be summarized.

2. Early identification of a hearing loss

Hearing loss which occurs congenitally or early in life prevents language development in its normal discourse since hearing is our primary sense to acquire spoken language. Therefore some steps should be taken to help babies with hearing loss to achieve speech and language skills.

It has been widely acknowledged that children born with a hearing loss can acquire and develop spoken language if they are identified and fitted with appropriate hearing technology early in their lives and receive quality intervention services (Clark, 2007; Cole & Flexer, 2007; DesJardin, et. al., 2006; Estabrooks, 2006). Younger the age of diagnosis and intervention, better the development of spoken language (White, 2006; Yosinago-Itano & Apuzzo, 1998; Yosinago-Itano & Sedey, 2000). For this reason, it is aimed to identify and fit the hearing aids within the first 3 months of life and to start the intervention program no later than 6 months of age.

Technology for automated hearing screening with otoacoustic emissions (OAE) and with auditory brainstem responses (ABR) permits fast, accurate and cost-effective identification of hearing loss in infants within hours after their birth. During the last two decades universal newborn hearing screening (UNHS) were supported as official policy in most developed countries (Department of Public Health, 2009; NDCS; 2004). It is also steadily expanding in developing countries; giving way to early identification and management of any kind of a hearing loss in infants and young children throughout the world.

Early identification and fitting of hearing aids/cochlear implant provide opportunities to stimulate auditory pathways during the critical periods of language acquisition and enables normal development of language. Although it is flawed, sensory stimulation which is provided through the hearing aids or cochlear implants supports the development of the neural network within the auditory system (Ryugo, et.al., 2000). On the other hand, a language enhancing environment should also be created to make maximum use of the sensory stimulation since learning is required for language acquisition (Clark, 2007; Cole & Flexer, 2007; Lieven, 1994; Otto, 2006 ; Sokolov & Snow, 1994).

In course of language development the first two years of life are seen to be critical.

3. Language development in infancy

Language development is one of the most remarkable achievements in childhood. Sometime during their second year most children begin to talk and apparently little time is required in using language to address their needs and carry on social interactions. During the last 50 years language acquisition has been studied with respect to what is learned, when it is learned and what factors or variables seem to explain the process of acquisition. While no single theory provides complete and irrefutable explanation of language acquisition, each theory contributes significant ideas and concepts which over time has clarified the awareness of the ways language is acquired (Bloom, 1993; Otto, 2006; Pine, 1994; Rice, 1996).

Theories which try to explain the language acquisition can be summarized under four broad categories. The nativist and the cognitive developmentalist perspectives emphasize the contributions of "nature" whereas the behaviourist and interactionist perspectives focus more on "nurture".

Nativist perspective emphasizes inborn or innate human capabilities as being responsible for language acquisition. Linguist Noam Chomsky is the major theorist associated with the nativist perspective. He contends that all people inherently have the capacity to acquire language due to cognitive structures that process language differently from other stimuli (Otto, 2006). A major focus of the nativist perspective is on the acquisition of syntactic knowledge. Semantic knowledge is also considered with respect to its relation to syntax (Pool, 2005). Chomsky proposes that universal grammar which is "the system of principles, conditions and rules that are elements or properties of all human languages" (Chomsky, 1975, as cited in Otto, 2006). As evidence of the universality and instinctive nature of language it is argued that no mute civilizations have ever been discovered throughout history. Since language exists in every culture it is concluded that it must arise from human biological instinct rather than from the existence of the culture (Otto, 2006).

Cognitive developmental perspective is based on the work of Jean Piaget (Baldwin, 2005). The emphasis of this perspective is that language is acquired as maturation occurs and cognitive competencies develop. While the nativist perspective emphasizes the inborn language mechanism, the cognitive developmental perspective assumes that cognitive development is a prerequisite and foundation for language learning. This perspective proposes that language is learned using the same learning mechanisms that the child uses for other learning. Thus there is no unique language mechanism. The close relation between the cognitive development and language is based on the belief that, for language to develop, specific cognitive growth must occur first (Baldwin, 2005; Bloom, 1995).

Behaviourist perspective states that learning occurs due to associations established among stimuli, responses and events that occur after the response behaviour. Language is learned as a result of these associations. The child is considered to be a "blank slate" and reinforcement of a child's verbal and nonverbal responses to language directed at him is responsible for language learning. Thus language is "taught" through situations in which children are encouraged to imitate other's speech and to develop associations between verbal stimuli and objects. Reinforcement often takes the form of attention, repetition and approval. This kind of learning is called operant conditioning. The use of the word "operant" acknowledges the child's active role in the learning process. It occurs when environmental consequences occur that are contingent on the specific behaviour. For example when an infant is producing sound and says "ma-ma" the parent may rush to the infant, show signs of delight and say "Oh, you said ma-ma". This positive response from the parent increases the chances the infant will repeat these sounds. Likewise, speech that elicits no response or ignored is less likely to be repeated (Otto, 2006).

Interactionist approach contends that children acquire language through their attempts to communicate with the world around them. Sociocultural interaction has the primary role and therefore is the main focus of this perspective. Language is acquired by individuals out of a need to function in society and an accompanying need for knowledge of how language functions in that society (Halliday, 1996). The primary role of social interaction in language acquisition is based on the observation that children acquire an awareness of specific communicative functions or intentions (such as indicating, requesting and labelling) before they are able to express themselves linguistically. This can be seen in the joint attention and verbal turn taking that often occurs between prelinguistic infants and their parents or caregivers (Bruner, 1983; 1990). These early understandings of how language functions provide a foundation on which the linguistic competencies are acquired. Environmental supports for language acquisition can be observed in the interaction patterns found in conversations such as listening, responding to what was said, repeating for clarification and asking questions (Cole & Flexer, 2007). Another important aspect of this approach is its focus on the language as *process* of acquisition rather than the language as *product* (Otto, 2006).

Overall the outcomes of research which has different theoretical backgrounds indicates that there is remarkable similarity in the general acquisition sequence for language skills across language and cultures although there is considerable individual variability in language learning strategies and rate of acquisition (Lieven, 1994; Pine, 1994). It is clear that children learn language as a means of talking about what they know so they can accomplish social goals important to them (Halliday, 1996; Thompson, 2005; Vygotsky, 1996) and it is agreed that language emerges from the child's explorations of the world in a rich social setting (Baldwin, 2005; Bloom, 1993; Rice, 1996).

Current thinking behind the language intervention for babies and young children with a hearing loss is more closer to interactionist view suggests that children with a hearing loss have the same innate capacity to develop fluent spoken language as do children with normal hearing provided that they are given the same opportunities (Childress, 2004; Clark, 2007; Cole & Flexer, 2007;). Clark (2007) states that "same opportunity"is sometimes difficult to create. Because knowledge of the presence of a hearing loss in a child often puts pressure on the significant adults in the child's environment. The pressure that parents experience usually lead them to alter their natural interaction with their baby. The purpose of early intervention was therefore defined as to support and assist families in providing language learning opportunities for their infant within the activities, routines and events of everyday life in an interactional natural way rather than "teaching language". The professionals who work in early intervention should be guiding and coaching parents to establish an appropriate quality interaction with their babies (Bailey et. al., 1991; Baguley & Bamford, 2000; Clark, 2007; DesJardin, et.al, 2006; Mahoney & Perales, 2003; Mahoney 2009; White, 2006).

4. Parent-child interaction in language development and early intervention

Studies concentrated on parent-child interaction in language development indicate that there are some speech adjustments which adults make when they interact with young language learners. The speech addressed to children consists of short, well-formed utterances and simple sentences. It is characteristically higher in pitch, more exaggerated in intonation and slower in tempo than speech among adults. It is highly redundant with lots of repetitions and closely tied to the immediate context (Bornstein & Tamis-LeMonda, 1997; Bornstein, et.al., 1999; Pine, 1994). This kind of speech is called "motherese" or child directed speech by several reserchers (Cole &Flexer, 2007, Eastabrooks, 2006; Otto, 2006; Pine, 1994).

To answer the reasons for using speech adjustments several explanations were suggested and a general consensus is reached arguing that speech adjustment to young children are motivated by a desire to communicate rather than to teach the language (Bruner, 1990; Cole & Flexer, 2007; Lieven, 1994; Pine, 1994; Sokolov & Snow, 1994). It is suggested that these adjustments have two main functions: the facilitation of understanding and sustaining of attention (Cole & Flexer, 2007; Pine, 1994). It has a conversational nature but at the same time it helps to direct and control child's behaviour (Bornstein & Tamis-LeMonda, 1997; Bornstein, et.al., 1999). The speech adjustment can be properly understood by putting it back to the context in which it occurs but the context is itself multifaceted and extends far beyond the dyad itself, not only to the family in which child is growing up, but also to the culture or subculture of which it forms a part (Lieven, 1994).

Young children's social and communicative skills were also found to be more precocious than their language skills during their interactions with adults and argued that it could serve as a facilitative source for language development (Bruner, 1983; 1990). Children were seen as active learners in interaction process rather than passive learners. The term "cognitive apprenticeship" is used to explain the child's learning and problem solving from "*actively* observing and participating in culturally defined problems with more skilled members in their society" (Sokolov & Snow, 1994, p. 44). Based on these observations, the connection between prelinguistic communicative intents in children and adults were studied widely in early language development and it was suggested that what children acquire and encounter is "language in use" during the language development process (Halliday, 1996). Language is a resource for making meaning and meaning is reflexive of the context. It is social, semantic and holistic (Thompson, 2005). Therefore communication and context of conversational interaction is central in the acquisition of language and the data from controlled experiments must be completed by observational studies of children in their natural environments as well (Halliday, 1996). Bruner (1983) supported this view and argued that the study of communicative precursors to formal language was important and quite independent of the nature-nurture controversy suggesting to concentrate more on intention between the adult and the child.

These summarized concepts are also relevant to intervention practices for children with a hearing loss (Brown & Nott, 2005; Clark, 2007; Estabrooks, 2006; Sokolov & Snow, 1994) especially for the ones before 3 years of age. Basic assumption is that if adequate auditory and linguistic experience is provided to most children who have hearing loss from an early age; cognitive and linguistic functioning can be expected to follow the normal course of development (Clark, 2007; Geers, 2004, as cited in Cole and Flexer, 2007; Houston, et.al., 2003; Moller, 2000; Rice & Lenihan, 2005; Spencer, 2004; Wallace, et.al., 2000; Warren, 2000).

The most reasonable course to follow in carrying out intervention is, establishing a normal language learning environment (Brown & Nott, 2005; Clark, 2007; Cole & Flexer, 2007; Hogan. et.al., 2008). The sequence of language learning is expected to include normal processes such as the intertwining of linguistic and cognitive activity. Parents are the social agents that best understand child's intentions and thus can best provide the scaffolding that they needed during the early development (Brown & Nott, 2005; Bloom, 1993; Bruner,1983; Wilson, 1998; Mahoney & Wiggers, 2007; Mahoney, 2009).

5. Effects of a hearing loss in interaction

Studies in the past conducted with children older than 18 months of age showed that parents of children who have hearing loss undergo controlling, discouraging and negative interactions with their children which provide a less facilitative environment for language acquisition and for social and cognitive development (Schlesinger & Meadow, 1972). Some studies argued that linguistic competence of the child would determine the parent's interaction with the child. If the child's language level is behind their chronological age parental control, simplicity and directivenes in language are increased and becomes different than the language used while addressing normal hearing children at the same age. (Gregory, et. al., 1979). Even in the earliest stages, differences in interactive behaviour were reported. Meadow, et. al. (1981) indicated that deaf infants of three, five and eight months had more physical contact with their mothers than hearing infants, suggesting that mothers of deaf children exploit the tactile kinaesthetic channel for gaining and holding attention rather than well known child directed speech features such as shorter utterances. Hughes and Huntington (1986) reported distorted speech and phonologic/prosodic characteristics in some mothers' of deaf children. They were easily recognized by listening to audiotaped voices during their interaction with the child. It is argued that distorted speech and altered intonation make the speech even more difficult to understand since they effect the second formant information. These kind of interactive differences possibly had negative effects on language development of children with hearing loss in later ages.

Early identification, amplification and intervention provide a chance to prevent deviances from normal interaction by providing auditory information to the child and supporting parents in their interactive skills immediately. Indeed it becomes possible to follow normal developmental patterns in language development without considerable delay and in most cases with no delay at all (Brown & Arehart, 2000; DesJardin, et.al., 2006; Moller, 2000; Hoberg-Arehart & Yoshinago-Itano, 1999; Houston, et.al., 2003; Robinshaw, 1995; Spencer, 2004; Wallace, et.al., 2000; White, 2006, Yoshinago-Itano & Apuzzo, 1998). Starting with the diagnosis of the hearing loss, parents should be encouraged to follow normal interaction patterns during their daily life.

Daily activities such as feeding, cleaning, dressing and simple play routines provide excellent opportunities of language learning for babies younger than one year old. The repetitive nature of the daily routines consolidates the experience and the language that accompanies them. By talking about the things they do during these activities parents are most likely to provide meaningful language input to the child. Following the baby's gaze and responding to his/her vocalizations help parents to regulate turn taking and to understand his/her intentions. (Brown & Nott, 2005; Clark, 2007).

The professional should guide and coach the parents in such a way that they come to realize that listening and speaking are a way of life for development of language in babies with a hearing loss. The parents' awareness should be heightened on how much they are already doing naturally and to encourage them to do more of it. The idea is not to intrude into the child's self-absorbed exploratory play in order to engage him/her in talk every waking minute, but to select or create opportunities for verbal interaction (Cole & Flexer, 2007). Auditory stimulation is the base of these kind of intervention and if language acquisition through audition is attempted, correct use of hearing aids or cochlear implants throughout the day has the utmost importance.

6. Management and practical aspects in intervention

6.1 Amplification and listening environment

Hearing aids and cochlear implants properly adjusted are the core of auditory oral or verbal intervention programmes. It is possible to fit and adjust internal settings of the hearing aids or cochlear implants with objective techniques in today's technology. Digital hearing aids are so flexible that they can be easily set for very young ones and it is possible to programme cochlear implants using NRT (Hughes, et.al., 2000), eSRT (Kosaner, et. al., 2009) and cortical responses (Sharma, et. al., 2005) even for babies younger than one year old. Combined with careful behavioural observations at home and clinics it does not take long to achieve optimum adjustment of the hearing aids or cochlear implants. However, the main issue is the effective use of hearing devices after fitting (Brown & Nott, 2005; Clark, 2007; Cole & Flexer, 2007).

Particular attention should be paid to train parents in effective use of hearing aids/cochlear implants during all waking hours of the baby. The parents must accept their responsibility in constant and efficient use of hearing aids or cochlear implants since babies spend all of their time with the family. When parents purchase the hearing aids it is the professional's role to help and supervise parents until they feel comfortable enough to check and fit the devices onto the baby properly (Clark, 2007). Guiding parents in hearing aid use and solving the problems related to hearing aids improves parents confidence in dealing with the devices and motivates them in efficient use. They should be advised about the frequently checking the external controls of the devices and batteries during the day because babies and young children are not capable of signalling the problems of the incoming sound. Adults must detect and solve the problems in the hearing aids/cochlear implants to provide constant flow of the auditory information. It is possible to lock external control settings of the digital hearing aids/cochlear implants during programming of the device which provides confidence about the exact settings in daily use. Batteries should be checked if they keep supplying the power during the day.

Feedback is the major problem while using hearing aids with the very young ones since the pinna is too small and soft to support the weight of the hearing aid and the neck support at this age is weak. It is possible to prevent feedback problem by using soft ear moulds and specially designed long spiral shaped tubing which allows attaching the hearing aids over shoulders until the baby start to hold his/her neck securely and sit up with no support.

Parents also need to know that hearing aids/cochlear implants does not restore the hearing to the normal. It is necessary to inform parents on deteriorative effect of the background noise over speech sounds and the negative effect of the microphone distance on speech perception. It is easier to accomplish optimum microphone distance with babies during their first year in life since we talk to them literally in an "ear shot" while holding them in arms or in their cribs. It is also advised to use a FM system in noisy conditions.

Parents should also be warned to be sensitive about voice clashes. It occurs while more than one person is talking at the same time during their interaction with the baby. As an inexperienced listener it is very difficult for a young child to know whom to attend to and it would deteriorate the intelligibility of the speech signals via hearing aids.

It helps in constant and efficient use of the hearing aids if parents are convinced that their baby can hear with the amplification (Clark, 2007; Cole & Flexer, 2007, Estabrooks, 2006). Often, early indications or clues of the child progressing are the most effective and immediate encouragement for the parents. This can be achieved by demonstrating the child's responses to the sound during the intervention and leading parents to observe their child's responses to the sound at home. The professional can guide the parents about early indicators of the child's hearing. These indicators include alertness to sound, turning to sound, quieting to sound, increased vocalizing, decreased vocalizing while listening and/or increased variety in vocalized sounds. The questions about child's responses to the sound help parents to observe more closely their child. Seeing the responses to the sound motivates parents in efficient use of hearing aids, they become sensitive for monitoring progress in the child.

6.2 Intervention sessions

Frequency, duration and place of an intervention session varies depending on the state policies in a given country and theoretical base and facilities of the intervention centres. Intervention could be home-based or centre-based, it could be once or twice in a week or a month (Department of Public Health, 2009; NDCS, 2004; Hogan, 2008).

Home based intervention has the advantage of knowing families' real life and planning the intervention accordingly. It is also possible to create close to natural environments at centre based programs. Duration of a session is usually reported 45 minutes to 1.5 hours (Brown & Nott, 2005; Clark, 2007, Estabrooks, 2006; Hogan, 2008).

In each session observing parents while interacting with the child is suggested (Brown & Nott, 2005; Clark, 2007; Estabrooks, 2007). Observing parents in interacting with the child serves several purposes. Firstly, the professional can evaluate the parents' strengths and weaknesses during their interaction with the child and guide the parents accordingly. Second, they have an opportunity to practice the new skills they acquired. Third it provides a chance to observe and monitor the progress in the child. It must be remembered that the main aim is to lead the parents toward confidence, competence and independence in handling their child with hearing loss (Bailey, 1998; Childress, 2004; DesJardin, et.al., Estabrooks, 2007; Kaiser & Hancock, 2005). Therefore all the positive aspects of the interaction should be mentioned and explained to the parents. The parents become more receptive to the suggestions given by the professional when they realize their strengths. In every session only one feature of what has been observed should be discussed for improvement (Clark, 2007).

The educational materials used in the sessions should be familiar and available at home. Using materials which are developmentally not appropriate to the child or are not available at home might be discouraging for the parents (Childress, 2004; Dunst, 2002; Mahoney, 2009; Odom& Wolery, 2003). Parents also may bring the toys, books or other materials to the session. For the babies younger than 6 months of age simple turn taking games, hiding and finding toys, popping up games and daily care routines of the infant can be used to interact in a language enabling way. When they grow a little older, simple household routines like sorting clothes to be washed, making fruit juice and tidying up can be performed. Parents must understand to recognize opportunities to facilitate language learning during the daily activities through following child's interest and being sensitive to communicative intentions of the child. Once parents understand to use language facilitating strategies in daily routines, they become active partners in creating these opportunities (Brown & Nott, 2005; Clark, 2007; Kaiser & Hester, 1995; Kaiser & Hancock, 2003; Wilson, 1998).

Some time during the session must be spent in discussing the things parents have done with the child since the last time they have been to the session. Also parents must be asked if they want to discuss any thing related to the child's development or progress. The parents should feel free to share their concerns or questions with the professional as well as positive signs of the progress. The professional should be able to refer parents to related professionals if their concerns are beyond the scope of the intervention process such as suspicion of a second handicap, neurological problems or necessity of psychiatric evaluation (Estabrooks, 2007; Clark, 2007; Lutherman, 2004).

Each session should include a musical activity or a listening game to improve listening skills of the child. Parents often need help to create suitable activities during the first few sessions. Therefore it is advised to dedicate time for age appropriate and enjoyable listening activities in each session. Parents must understand that these activities improve listening skills and are also enjoyable. Singing lullabies, rhymes and simple repetitive songs are highly recommended to widen the child's listening experience and to develop a sense of rhythm (Clark, 2007; Cole & Flexer, 2007; Estabrooks, 2007). Naturally occurring sounds at home such as door bell, telephone ring, and sounds from outside can also be used to develop listening skills. Parents are advised to listen to the sounds at home themselves first, then draw the attention of the child to the sound and to show them the source.

At the end of the session it is better to discuss language enabling activities and areas of language that might be focused at home. Caution should be taken that parents provide a language enhancing environment to the child. It must be remembered that language is a complex, specialized skill that develops in a child spontaneously and it is not something that parents teach their children (Pinker, 1994, as cited in Clark, 2007).

Sometimes it is better for the parents to see the professional interacting and talking with their child in a natural way. Professional's attitude towards the child encourages parent to expect age appropriate development. It is highly motivating especially after the diagnosis for some parents to see someone treating their child in a normal way who is not solely focusing on the hearing loss.

7. Role of the professional

Advice given in the early years to the parents of children who have a hearing loss has long lasting effects on the children's development and future lives. The professionals who first come into contact with families seeking advice on how best to manage a young child who has a hearing loss bear tremendous responsibility for their futures (Clark, 2007). Their role is complex and challenging. It is different from other professional roles such as teachers or case managers, although it may include some aspects of these roles (Bailey, et.al., 1991; Hoberg-Arehart & Yoshinago-Itano, 1999; Kaiser & Hancock, 2003). Professionals who work with young children with disabilities must know how to partner with families, including working together to address child and family needs. Studies on parent participation indicate that intervention efforts are enhanced when families participate in early childhood programs (Bailey et al., 1998; Baguley, 2000; Bluebanning, 2004; Mahoney & Wiggers, 2007; Mahoney, 2009; White, 2006; Wilson, 1998).

If a family centred and participation-based philosophy is adopted, roles of parents and professionals become different from traditional practice on the basis of four primary features: (a) activity leader, (b) use of natural materials, (c) role of the parent, and (d) role of the provider. (Brown & Nott, 2005; Campbell & Sawyer, 2009; Dunst, 2002) In traditional practice, the professional is generally the activity leader, materials that are not likely to be natural to the home setting are used in intervention, the parent most frequently plays a passive role such as an observer, and the professional is the primary person interacting with the child. This type of intervention approach has been identified by a number of labels including one-on-one intervention or direct intervention (Dunst, 2002). In a participation-based approach, the focus is on promoting a child's participation within typical family activities and routines. The activity leader is the parent or child, materials natural to the activity or routine are used, the parent actively interacts with the child, and the professional plays a role of facilitator (Campbell & Sawyer, 2009; Childress, 2004; Dunst, 2002; Macy, et. al., 2009; Mahoney, 2009;) suggesting appropriate techniques and strategies to facilitate language development and sometimes interacting with the child to model the parents at certain techniques (Clark, 2007; Estabrooks, 2006).

In order to work effectively in the field, the professional must be fluent in specific intervention they will teach parents (Kaiser & Hancock, 2003). Fluency requires mastery of specific intervention procedures, understanding of the conceptual basis of the intervention and its main assumptions. The conceptual knowledge is required in order to explain the rational behind the each aspect of the procedure to parents, to place the intervention in the framework of the child's developmental characteristics, to relate the parents' behavior to the goals of the intervention and the family's goals for the child and themselves and to answer parents' questions (Brown & Nott, 2005; Estabrooks, 2006; Hogan, 2008).That is consistent with the findings indicating technical knowledge and skills of the service providers, parent education and diagnostic evaluations/ assessment of the child as the most beneficial aspects of early intervention experiences among the other properties as well (Foran & Sweeney, 2010).

The ability to present the intervention in a way that is understood by the parents is another aspect which is crucially important (Kaiser & Hancock, 2003). The professional must be able to instruct parents on interacting in a language enabling way with their child and to troubleshoot with parents in their use of it in order to provide specific feedback, guidance and coaching toward effective implementation (Brown & Nott, 2005; Estabrooks, 2006; Kaiser & Hester, 1995; Kaiser & Hancock, 2003). This can be achieved by observing parents while they are interacting with their baby during play or daily activities. Depending on these observations, the needs of a specific parent child relationship at a specific language learning stage can be decided (Brown & Nott, 2005; Clark, 2007; Estabrooks, 2006). From the start parents must understand that the professional's task is to observe and to offer advice on the type of interaction that the professional sees them enjoy with the child. Initially some parents are resistant to this approach because they want to the child to receive therapy from the professional (Clark, 2007).

Observing parent child-interaction either in daily activities or at play the professional gathers information on contingent responsiveness between the parent and the child, amount of joint attention, and how it is created and maintained by both parties, parent's awareness on language facilitative opportunities. These are all critical for planning the intervention sessions. Parents are a valuable source of information about their child and their observations and judgements should be included while planning the intervention (Campbell & Sawyer, 2009; Eriks-Brophy, et.al., 2006; Knopf & Swick, 2008).

It is seen as a professional's responsibility to encourage parents to involve actively in the intervention sessions in a way that is most suitable for the family. The professionals must realize uniqueness of each family to achieve this. It must also be kept in mind that relationships and interaction patterns within a family system are more complex than formerly believed. Family members assume familial roles and functions with proximal and distal features (Campbell & Sawyer 2009). Therefore, the needs, priorities, resources, desires, and wisdom of a child's family should be taken into account. The presence of hearing loss in the child does not mean that the family has to alter what would have been its natural child rearing practice to fit the professional's concept of child rearing. The only time professional alters the way a child is managed is when there is behaviour that is inhibiting the development of listening and of spoken language (Clark, 2007).

In recent years interpersonal relationship between parents and the professionals has gained considerable attention as another important aspect of successful intervention process. Research on the subject indicates its role in the development of family centred practices aiming to empower parents in special education (Knight & Woodsworth, 1999; Kratchowill, et. al., 2007; Lutherman, 2004; Macy, et. al., 2009).

Park and Turnbull (2003) created a framework distinguishing interpersonal and structural components of effective partnership. They identified from the literature a series of interpersonal relationship attitudes, skills and beliefs that appear to contribute to effective partnership among families, professionals and agencies. Collaborative partnership characterized by factors such as trust, respect, communication, shared vision and cultural sensitivity were identified as critical for effective partnership. However these are subjective terms and their meaning can be different from one person to another.

Bluebanning et al. (2004) emphasized the need for the operational definition of these terms. They argued that the clear operational definition of these terms may help professionals to develop a better understanding of the family perspectives leading to establish good quality early intervention services. Their study focused on parents' and professionals' descriptions of the terminology which are widely used in family centered, collaborative intervention programs. They described six collaborative themes and their behavioural indicators is stressed by parents and professionals. Themes are defined as communication, commitment, equality, skills, trust and respect. Parents and professionals described behaviours related to each of these themes in substantial good agreement except commitment and equality. Parents talked of wanting professionals to "go the extra mile" and to be like one in the family in their involvement with them. Professionals expressed the same sentiments but they also expressed reservations about taking these concepts too far. These reservations centred on the perceived need to "empower" families to take charge of advocating for their child and themselves, and the concern that doing "too much" might foster co-dependency and actually harm the family. The questions of when being "like family" gets in the way of doing one's job and when "empowering" becomes disenfranchising are issues referring to the boundaries between families and professionals. It is argued that the subject needs further research for effective guidelines on creating appropriate boundaries between families and professionals that preserve warm and committed relationships without disempowering families.

8. Conclusion

The children who are born with a hearing loss or acquired it early in life have never before had such a potential to hear, listen and talk. Advances in technology such as digital hearing aids and cochlear implants make language development through audition possible. This particular group of children can hear the sounds around them with greater ease than in the past. By early detection of the hearing loss and early intervention, these children have a chance to develop spoken language comparable to those of their hearing counterparts since they catch up the critical periods for language learning.

Intervention programmes aim to establish normal interaction patterns which facilitate language development in infants and children with a hearing loss. These programs assume that children with a hearing loss have the same innate capacity with normal hearing children for language acquisition. By providing the same opportunities they can develop spoken language which is comparable to normal development.

Parents are seen as partners in this approach and have the responsibility to ensure use of hearing aids/cochlear implants within all waking hours of the child. Professionals work with parents to elaborate their communicative strategies with the young child in their daily lives. They were encouraged to independently handle their child with a hearing loss.

Professionals who work in the field are expected to give information that is timely, accurate and at the appropriate level of the individual parent. They need to possess active listening skills to define and address identified problems or needs. They should be foster confidence, competence and independence in parents. They must have strength in providing strategic guidance to parents by adopting the role of a mentor or coach.

9. References

Bailey, B. D. Jr., Palsha, S. A. & Simeonsson, R. J. (1991). Professional Skills, Concerns and Perceived Importance of Work With Families in Early Intervention. *Exceptional Children,* Vol. 58, Available from http://www. questia.trustedonlineresearch/

Bailey, B. D. Jr., McWilliam, R.A., Darkes, L. A., Hebbeler, K., Simeonsson, R. J., piker, D., & Wagner, M. (1998). Family Outcomes in Early Intervention: A F ramework for Programme Evaluation and Efficacy Research. *Exceptional Children,* Vol. 64, Available from http://www. questia.trustedonlineresearch/

Baguley, D.; Davis, A. & Bamford, J. (2000) The Principles of Family-Friendly Hearing Services for Children. *British Society of Audiology News,* Vol. 29, pp. 35-39, Available from http://www.deafnessatbirth.org.uk/content2/support/services

Baldwin, J.A. (2005). Jean Piaget. In: *Key Thinkers in Linguistics and The Philosophy of Language,* 205-207, S. Chapman & C. Routledge (Eds.), Oxford University Press, ISBN 0-19-518768-8, Oxford, New York

Bloom, L. (1993). *The Transition from Infancy to Language,* Cambridge University Press, ISBN0-521-48379-4, Cambridge, Melbourne

Bluebanning, M., Summers, J. A., Frankland, H. C. Nelson, L. L. & Beegle, G. (2004) Dimensions of Family and Professional Partnerships: Constructive Guidelines for Collaboration. *Exceptional Children,* Vol. 70, No. 2, pp. 167-184

Brown, A. S. & Arehart, K. H. (2000) Universal Newborn Hearing Screening: Impact on Early Intervention Services. *The Volta Review,* Vol. 100, No. 5, pp. 85-117

Brown, P.M. & Nott, P. (2005). Family-Centred Practice in Early Intervention for Oral Language Development: Philosophy, Methods and Results. In: *Spoken Language Development of Deaf or Hard of Hearing Children,* 136-165, P. E. Spencer (Ed), Available from http://site.ebrary.com/lib/anadolu/Doc?id=10091866

Bornstein, M.H. & Tamis-LeMonda, C.S.(1997) Maternal responsiveness and infant mental abilities: specific predictive relations. Infant Behaviour and Development, 20 (3), 283-296.

Bornstein, M.H., Tamis-LeMonda, C.S. & Haynes, O.M. (1999) First words in the second year: continuity, stability and models of concurrent and predictive correspondance in vocabulary and verbal responsiveness across age and context. Infant Behaviour and Development, 22(1), 65-85.

Bruner, J. (1983) *Child's Talk: Learning to Use Language.* W. W. Norton, ISBN 0-393-95345-9, New York

Bruner, J. (1990). *Acts of Meaning.* Harvard University Press, ISBN 0674-00361-6, Cambridge

Campbell, P. H. & Sawyer, L. B. (2009). Changing Early Intervention Providers' Home Visiting Skills Through Participation in Professional Development. *Topics in Early Childhood Special Education,* Vol.28, No. 4, pp. 219-234, Available at: http://online.sagepub.com

Clark, M (2007). *A Practical Guide to Quality Interaction With Children Who Have a Hearing Loss,* Plural Publishing, ISBN 1-597556-112-6, San Diego, Oxford, Brisbane

Childress, D.C. (2004). Special Instructions in Natural Environments: Best Practices in Early Intervention. *Infants and Young Children,* Vol. 17, No. 2, pp. 162-170

Cole, E.B. & Flexer, C. (2007). *Children With Hearing Loss: Developing Listening and Talking Bith to Six,* ISBN 978-1-59756-158-7, Plural Publishing, San Diego, Oxford, Brisbane.

Department of Public Health Interagency Coordinating Council (2009). Partnering for the Success of Children With Hearing Loss Task Force Report. Available from www.mass.gov/dph/earlyintervention

DesJardin, J. L., Eisenberg, L. S., & Hodapp, R. M. (2006) Sound beginnings: Supporting Families of Young Deaf Children With Cochlear Implants. *Infants & Young Children,* Vol. 19, No. 3, pp. 179-189

Dunst, C. J. (2002). Family Centred Practices: Birth Through High School. *The Journal of Special Education,* Vol. 36, No. 3., pp. 139-147

Eriks-Brophy, A., Durieux-Smith, A., Olds, J., Fitzpatrick, E., Duquette, C., & Whittingham, J. A. (2006) Facilitators and Barriers to the Inclusion of Orally Educated Children and Youth with Hearing Loss in Schools: Promoting Partnerships to Support Inclusion. *The Volta Review,* Vol. 106, No. 1, pp. 53-88

Estabrooks, W. (2006). *Auditory Verbal: Therapy and Practice.* AG Bell, ISBN 978-0-88200-223-1, Washington, DC

Foran, S., & Sweeney, J. (2010) Accessing Specialist Early Intervention Services for Pre-School Children: A Lack of Co-ordination in the Delivery of Early Intervention to Children with an Intellectual Disability in Ireland Led to Examine the Lived Experiences of Families Accessing Services. *Learnıng Disability Practice,* Vol.13 No.2

Gregory, S., Mogford, K., & Bishop, J. (1979). Mothers' Speech to Young Hearing Impaired Children. *Journal of the British Association of the Teachers of the Deaf,* Vol. 3, pp. 42-5

Halliday, M. A. K. (1996). Relevant Models of Language. In: *Language Development: A Reader for Teachers,* 36-41, B.M. Power & R.S. Hubbard (Eds.), Pearson-Merril Prentice Hall, ISBN 0-13-191032-9 New Jersey, Ohio. (Original Source: Relevant Models of Language, 1969, *Educational Rewiev,* Vol. 22, pp. 26-37)

Hoberg-Arehart, K., & Yoshinago-Itano, C. (1999). The Role of Educators of the Deaf in The Early Identification of Hearing Loss. *American Annals of the Deaf,* Vol. 144, no. 1, pp. 19-23

Hogan, S., Stokes,J., White, C., Tyszkiewicz, E., & Woolgar, A. (2008). An Evaluation of Auditory Verbal Therapy Using the Rate of Early Language Development as an Outcome Measure. *Deafness Educ. Int.* Vol. 10, pp. 143–167

Houston, D. M., Ying, E.A., Pisoni, D. B. & Kirk, I.K. (2003) Development of Pre-Word Learning Skills in Infants with Cochlear Implants. *The Volta Review,* Vol. 103, No. 4, pp. 303-326

Hughes, M. L., Brown, C., Abbas, P., et.al. (2000) Comparison of EAP Threshold Measures with MAP Levels in the Nucleus 24 Cochlear Implants: Data from Children. *Ear & Hearing,* Vol. 21, No: 2, pp. 164-174

Hughes, M. E., & Huntington, J. N. (1983). Subjective Listener Judgements of Mothers' Speech to Normally Hearing and Hearing Impaired Children. *Journal of the British Association of the Teachers of the Deaf,* Vol. 7, pp. 18-23

Kaiser, A.P. & Hester, P.P. (1995). Preparing Parent Trainers: An Experimental Analysis of Effects on Trainers, Parents and Children. *Topics in Early Childhood Special Education,* Vol. 15, No. 4, ISSN 0271-1214

Kaiser, A. P., & Hancock, T. B. (2003). Teaching Parents New Skills to Support Their Young Children's Development. *Infants & Young Children,* Vol. 16, No. 1, pp. 9-21

Knight, D. & Wadsworth, D. (1999) Is the Development of Family/School Partnership Promoted in the Nation's Special Education Teacher Preparation Programmes? *Contemporary Education,* Vol. 70, No. 3, pp. 22-29

Knopf, H. E., & Swick K. J. (2008). Using Our Understanding of Families to Strengthen Family Involvement. *Early Childhood Educ J,* Vol. 35, pp. 419–427, ISSN 10643-007-0198

Koşaner, J., Anderson, I., Turan, Z., Diebl, M. (2009). The Use of eSRT in Fitting Children With Cochlear Implants. *Journal of International Advanced Otology,* Vol.5, No. 1, pp. 70-79

Kratochwill, T. R., Volpianski, P., Clements, M. & Ball, C. (2007). Professional Development in Implementing and Sustaining Multitier Prevention Models: Implications for Response to Intervention. *School Psychology Review,* Vol.36, No.4, pp. 618-631, ISSN 0279-6015

Lieven, E.V.M. (1994). Crosslinguistic and Crosscultural Aspects of Language Addressed to Children. In: *Input and Interaction in Language Acquisition,* 56-73, C. Gallaway & B.J. Richards (Eds.), Cambridge University Press, ISBN 0-521-43725-3, Cambridge, Melbourne

Luterman, D. (2004) Counselling Families of Children with Hearing Loss and Special Needs. *Volta review,* Vol. 104, No. 4 (monograph), pp.215-220

Macy, M., Squires, J.K., & Barton, E. E. (2009) Providing Optimal Opportunities Structuring Practicum Experiences in Early Intervention and Early Childhood Special Education Preservice Programs. *Topics in Early Childhood Special Education,* Vol. 28, No. 4, pp. 209-218, Available at http://tecse.sagepub.com

Mahoney, G. & Perales, F. (2003). Using Relationship-Focused Intervention to Enhance The Social-Emotional Functioning of Young Children with Autism Spectrum Disorders. *TECSE,* Vol. 23, No. 2, pp. 77-89

Mahoney, G. & Wiggers, B. (2007). The Role of Parents in Early Intervention: Implication for Social Work. *Children and Schools,* Vol. 29 , No. 1, pp. 7-15

Mahoney, G. (2009) Relationship Focused Intervention (RFI): Enhancing the Role of Parents in Children's Developmental Intervention. *International Journal of Early Childhood Special Education (INT-JECSE),* Vol. 1, No. 1, pp. 79-94

Meadow, K. P., Greenberg, M. T., Erting, C., & Charmichael, H. (1981). Interactions of Deaf Mothers and Deaf Preschool Children: Comparisons with 3 Other Groups of Deaf and Hearing Dyads. *American Annals of the Deaf,*Vol. 126, pp. 454-68

Moller, M.P. (2000) Early Intervention and Language Development in Children Who are Deaf or Hard of Hearing. *Paediatrics,* Vol. 106, No. 3, e43 (electronic version).

NDCS, (2004) Communicating With Your Deaf Child. In: *Communicating With Your Deaf Child, NDCS,*19.03.2007, Available from http: // www. ndcs. org.uk /family _ support/ communication

Odom, S.L., & Wolery, M. (2003). A Unified Theory of Practice in Early Intervention/Early Childhood Special Education: Evidence Based Practices. *The Journal of Special Education,* Vol. 37, No. 3, pp. 161-173

Otto, B. (2006). *Language Development in Early Childhood,* Pearson-Merril Prentice Hall, ISBN 0-13-118771-6, New Jersey, Ohio

Pine, J.M. (1994). The Language of Primary Caregivers, In: *Input and Interaction in Language Acquisition,* 15-37, C. Gallaway & B.J. Richards (Eds.), Cambridge University Press, ISBN 0-521-43725-3, Cambridge, Melbourne

Pool, G. (2005). Noam Chomsky, In: *Key Thinkers in Linguistics and The Philosophy of Language,* 53-60, S. Chapman & C. Routledge (Eds.), Oxford University Press, ISBN 0-19-518768-8, Oxford, New York

Rice, M. (1996). Children's Language Acquisition. In: *Language Development: A Reader for Teachers,* 3-12, B.M. Power & R.S. Hubbard (Eds.), Pearson-Merril Prentice Hall, ISBN 0-13-191032-9, New Jersey, Ohio

Rice, G.B. & Lenihan, S. (2005) Early Intervention in Auditory/Oral Deaf Education: Parent and Professional Perspectives. *The Volta Review,* Vol. 105, No. 1, pp. 73-96.

Robinshaw, H.M. (1995) Early intervention for hearing impairment: differences in timing of communicative and linguistic development. British Journal of Audiology. 29, 315-334.

Ryugo, D. K., Limb, C.J. & Redd, E.E. (2000). Brain Plasticity: The Impact of the Environment on the Brain as It Relates to Hearing and Deafness. In: *Cochlear Implants: Principles and Practices,* pp. 33-57, J.K. Niparko (Ed.), Lippincott Williams & Wilkins, ISBN 0-7817-17-82-5, Philadelphia

Schlesinger, H. S., & Meadow, K. P. (1972). *Sound and Sign: Childhood Deafness and Mental Health.* UCLA Press, Berkeley (ISBN not available)

Sharma, A., Martin, K., Roland, P., Bauer, P., et. al., (2005). P1 Latency as a Biomarker for Central Auditory Development in Children with Hearing Impairment. *Journal of the American Academy of Audiology,* Vol. 16., pp. 564-573

Snow, C. E. (1972). Mothers' Speech to Children Learning Language. *Child Development,* Vol. 43, pp. 549-65.

Sokolov, J.F. & Snow, C. E. (1994). The Changing Role of Negative Evidence in Theories of Language Development, In: *Input and Interaction in Language Acquisition,* 38-55, C.

Gallaway & B.J. Richards (Eds), Cambridge University Press, ISBN 0-521-43725-3, Cambridge, Melbourne

Spencer, P.E. (2004). Individual Differences in Language Performance after Cochlear Implantation at One to Three Years of Age: Child, Family and Linguistic Factors, *Journal of Deaf Studies and Deaf Education,* Vol.9, No. 4, pp. 398-411

Thompson, G. (2005). Halliday, M.A.K . In: *Key Thinkers in Linguistics and The Philosophy of Language,* 116-122, S. Chapman & C. Routledge (Eds.), Oxford University Press, ISBN 0-19-518768-8, Oxford, New York

Tucker, I., Hughes, M. E., & Glover, M. (1983). Verbal Interaction with Preschool Hearing Impaired Children: A comparison of Maternal and Paternal Inputs. *Journal of the British Association of Teachers of the Deaf,* Vol. 7, pp. 90-8

Wallace, V., Menn, L. M. M. & Yoshinago-Itano, C. (2000). Is Babble the Gateway to Speech for All Children? A Longitudinal Study of Children Who Are Deaf or Hard of Hearing. *The Volta Review,* Vol. 100, No. 5, pp. 121-148

Warren, S. F. (2000) The future of early communication and language intervention. Topics in Early Childhood Special Education, Vol. 20, No.1,

White, K. R. (2006) Early Intervention for Children with Permanent Hearing Loss: Finishing the EHDI Revolution. *The Volta Review,* Vol. 106, No. 3, pp. 237-258, ISSN 0042-8639

Wilson, R.A. (1998). *Special Educational Needs in Early Years.* Falmer Press Limited, ISBN 0-10-095173-9, London

Vygotsky, L. S. (1996). On Inner Speech. In: *Language Development: A Reader for Teachers,* 13-17, B.M. Power & R.S. Hubbard (Eds.), Pearson-Merril Prentice Hall, ISBN 0-13-191032-9 New Jersey, Ohio. (Original Source: Thought and Language, 1962. MIT Press: Cambridge, MA)

Yoshinago-Itano, C. & Apuzzo, M. R. L. (1998) Identification of Hearing Loss After Age 18 Months Is Not Early Enough. *American Annals of the Deaf,* Vol. 143, No. 5, pp. 380-387

Yoshinago-Itano, C. & Sedey, A.L. (2000) Language, Speech and Social Emotional Development of Children Who are Deaf or Hard of Hearing: The Early Years (monograph). *The Volta Review,* Vol. 100, No.5, pp.

Part 3

Injuries & Traumas

7

Hearing Loss in Minor Head Injury

Lingamdenne Paul Emerson
Christian Medical College, Vellore
India

1. Introduction

Hearing loss is a common problem encountered in ENT practice. Recognition of hearing loss as a problem by the patient usually occurs when speech frequencies are affected or when there is a sudden hearing loss. Hearing loss following head trauma or head injury is a major medical problem in adults (Bergemalm P-O&Borg.E. 2001) as well as children (Hough JVD &Stuart WD, 1968). The loss may go unnoticed when the speech frequencies are not affected. Sensorineural hearing loss at high frequencies is a frequent finding associated with head injuries (H.Alexander Arts). Hearing impairment can be due to central or peripheral causes, middle ear or cochlea being the most common site of peripheral injury. The most pronounced injury is fracture of temporal bone (Dahiya.R &Keller J.D, 1999). In both clinical and animal experimental studies it has been shown that there are various sites of pathology ranging from hair cell damage and degeneration of the organ of corti, ischemia of the 8th nerve to damage of central auditory pathways (due to compromise of blood supply to the inner ear) either partly or totally. In most cases hearing impairment dissipates during subsequent post traumatic period, but some times it may persist or progress.

The causes of progression of hearing loss are not well known. Several explanations have been proposed such as development of perilymphatic fistula, secondary degenerative changes in cochlea following inner ear concussion possibly due to consequences of pre-existing autoimmune disease (or trauma itself may initiate such a reaction towards specific inner ear proteins). Progression of hearing loss can be attributed to the synergistic effects between trauma, noise exposure, medication and meningitis.

In developing countries roads are used not only by modern cars and buses, along with locally developed vehicles for public transport (three-wheeled scooter taxis, auto rickshaw's), scooters and motorcycles, bicycles, but also by rickshaws, and animal or human drawn carts that has resulted in disproportionate increase in road traffic accidents compared to developed countries. Minor head injuries (WHO 2004) constitute a major portion of all accidents. Evaluation of these patients revealed presence of hearing loss in the high frequency range. Hence auditory assessment is needed in this group of patients.

Evaluation of hearing loss in patients who sustain minor head injury has not been done in the Indian subcontinent. Therefore, this prospective study was done to evaluate the incidence of hearing loss and estimate its progression or regression by serial assessment over a period of six months

2. Classification of head injury

Hearing loss is a well known entity following head injury. The degree of hearing loss may vary depending on the severity of the head injury. The severity of Head injury is measured clinically using the Glasgow coma scale scoring system (G.C.S). The Glasgow Coma Scale was first published by Teasdale and Jennett in 1974. Several years later it was modified by Jennett and Teasdale and by Rimel et al (Rimel RW et al 1981, 1982) .This scoring system provides the best measure of severity of head injury. The score is the sum of the scale's three measures of eye opening, best motor and verbal responses. This ranges from a score of 3 for a patient with no motor, verbal response or eye opening to painful stimuli, to 15 for a patient who is oriented, follows commands, and has spontaneous eye opening. Patients, who do not follow commands, speak or open their eyes, with a score of 8 or less, are by definition in coma. Head injury is defined as mild when the GCS score is either 13 or 14–15, moderate by a score of 9–12 or 13, and severe by a score of 3–8. The GCS score on admission, and its prognostic usefulness, are easily confounded by other factors particularly substance misuse, but sequential monitoring after admission plays a crucial role in detecting early deterioration and in its management.

Culotta (Culotta VP et al, 1996) following a retrospective study found that patients with a GCS score of 13–15, represent a heterogeneous group with statistically significant different head tomography abnormalities. On the basis of findings they suggested separating patients with GCS score 13–14 into a different category from patients with a GCS score of 15, thus effectively redefining minor head injury. These findings were confirmed by a similar study by Gomez (Gomez PA,et al1996). Hsiang , on the basis of a cohort study of 1360 patients with GCS score of 13–15 suggested that this group of patients could also be divided into two subgroups, mild head injury and high risk mild head injury(Hsiang JNK et al,1997). Mild head injury is defined as GCS 15 without radiographic abnormalities, high risk mild head injury being defined as GCS 13–14, or a GCS 15 with acute radiographic abnormalities. More recently Swann and Teasdale recognizing the limitation of the GCS with regard to minor head injury have suggested another sub classification. Mild head injury is defined as GCS 13–14. Minor head injury is defined as GCS score of 15. The authors recognized in their monograph that this is a somewhat arbitrary definition. However in Clinical practice GCS is used in evaluation of Head injury (Swan IJ,Teasdale Gm 1999)

Glasgow coma scale and score (Table-1). Glasgow coma score: (E+M+V) = 3–15.

EYE OPENING	BEST MOTOR RESPONSE	VERBAL RESPONSE
Spontaneous - 4	Obeys commands - 6	Oriented - 5
To speech - 3	Localizes to pain - 5	Confused, Disoriented-4
To pain - 2	Withdraws (Flexion) - 4	Inappropriate words - 3
None - 1	Abnormal flexion -3	Incomprehensible sounds -2
	Abnormalextension - 2	No verbal response -1
	No motor response - 1	

Table 1. Glasgow coma score

In India, in the year 2000, official statistics revealed that 80,118 persons died and 3, 42,200 were injured in road traffic accidents . However this is an underestimate, as not all accidents are reported to the police. A study done in Haryana (India) recorded all traffic-related injuries and deaths through bi-weekly home visits to all households in 9 villages for a year. This study showed that the ratio between critical, serious and minor injuries was 1:29:69. (Varghese .M .Mohan.D 2003).

2.1 Definition of a mild head injury

A mild head injury can be defined as an injury caused by blunt trauma and/or sudden acceleration /deceleration which produces a period of unconsciousness for 20 minutes or less, a Glasgow coma scale score of 13-15, no focal neurological deficit, no intracranial complications and computed tomographic findings limited to a skull fracture without evidence of contusion or hematoma.Despite the dissemination of information that is available on diagnostic criteria, controversies still exist in defining mild head injury and collecting patients.

Estimating the duration of unconsciousness is difficult when witnesses are not available, second if the patient is intoxicated at the time of hospital admission it can obscure the assessment of severity of head injury.

3. Hearing loss in head injury

Deafness due to head injury is known since ancient times, the earliest account of which is the Edwin Smith papyrus, (Marc stiefel, 2006) the world's earliest known medical document, written around 1600 BC, but thought to be based on material from as early as 3000 BC. It is a textbook on trauma surgery, and describes anatomical observations physical examination, diagnosis, treatment, and prognosis of numerous injuries in exquisite detail. The symptoms and signs of head injury were given in considerable detail. It was noted that brain injuries were associated with changes in the function of other parts of the body. Feeble pulse and fever are associated with grievous injuries and deafness as well as aphasia are recognized in fractures of the temporal region.

Sushrutha who is known as "Father of Surgery" in India, even though he does not attach significance to the brain, however, considers head as the centre of all special senses and describes certain cranial nerves connected with specific sensory functions. He described two nerves lower down the back of the ear (vidhura), which, if cut, produce deafness; a pair of nerves (phana) situated inside the two nostrils, which if cut, cause anosmia. A pair of nerves below the outer end of the eye-brow, near the external corner of the eyeball (apanga) which if cut, cause total blindness.

Alexander and Scholl (Alexander AF and Scholl) as early as 1938 reported a 31% incidence of hearing loss in patients with head injury. In 1939 Grove (Grove W.E) reported an incidence of 32.6% of sensorineural hearing loss and suggested that bleeding in the inner ear was the cause whereas Uffenorde (Uffenorde W, 1924) stated that stretching of the fibers of the cochlear nerve in the internal auditory canal bought on the hearing loss after head injury. Similar results were reported by Gurdijan,(Gurdijan ES 1933) Fradis and Podoshin (Podoshin .L&,Fradis.M,1975) and M R Abd al Hady (M.R.Abd AL-HADY et al,1990). Griffiths (M.V.Griffiths)in 1979 reported an incidence of 56% of sensorineural deafness in cases of mild head injury . He stated that there may be difference in outcome depending on the type of violence. A blow to the head with a soft object seems to cause less damage to the hearing system than a blow to the head with a hard object with the same power at impact. The greater hearing loss according to him is due to an acoustic component.

The site of injury is important, frontal injuries resulting in a comparatively low incidence of hearing loss as compared to temporal blows. The type of audiogram recorded is an important indicator in assessing prognosis. Vertigo according to them has its own separate etiology and should be assessed and treated separately and not as a part of the post concussion syndrome.

In the immediate post injury period the incidence of hearing loss is 56% and vertigo is 24% which is very high when compared to controls (8%).Hearing loss recovered within three months. Accordingly, the mechanism of low frequency hearing loss is seen in patients with hydrops and suggests a similar peripheral mechanism. He stated that the lesions lie in the peripheral labyrinth due to edema or hydrops both of which subside with excellent prognosis. High frequency hearing loss may be caused by concussion and intense acoustic stimulation, concussion being reversible. Griffiths study showed a residual hearing loss in 14% of patients even after six months in cases of head injury with concussion without fracture.Vartiannenn (E.Vartianen et al, 1985) reported that in children who suffered blunt head trauma, 30% were found to have hearing loss of whom 16.3% had CHL and 13% had SNHL. One third of them recovered normal hearing with in six months. Similar results were reported by Zimmerman (William D.Zimmerman et al, 1993) Ludwig podoshin, (Podoshin .L. & Fradis.M, 1975) reported that conductive hearing loss due to head injury usually disappears in two months, if it persists ossicular discontinuity must be suspected.

According to Andrew T Lyos (Andrew.T.Lyos et al, 1995) in case of temporal bone fracture, immediate profound hearing loss may be caused by avulsion of the nerve or severe damage to the membranous labyrinth. Concussion directly to the otic capsule or acoustic trauma via the ossicular chain is well described. If it is not severe, it produces transient cochlear hyperemia resulting in temporary threshold shift. Feldman (Feldman H, 1987) stated that, sudden hearing loss with delayed onset can also occur following head trauma, thus it may be due to the sequelae consisting of perilymph fistula in one of the windows or a fracture of the labyrinthine capsule, which may manifest for the first time after a period of years or even decades.

Allison M Scott (Allison.M.Scot et al, 1999) found that in addition to low and high frequency hearing loss, audiograms with single and double sensorineural notches in mid frequency region may be related to head trauma.

The site of hearing impairment can be peripheral or central although the peripheral structures i.e., the middle ear and cochlea represent the most common site of injury. Nassulphis (Nassulphis P et al, 1964) found damage in the Reissner membrane and degeneration of the organ of corti in the spiral ganglion and cochlear nerve in several patients suffering from hearing loss following head injury. According to Schuknecht and Davison (Harold F.Schuknecht & Roderick C.Davison, 1956) auditory symptoms following head injury can be grouped according to the classification of labyrinthine damages which are:(a). Longitudinal fracture of temporal bone (b). Transverse fracture of temporal bone (c). Labyrinthine concussion. Labyrinthine concussion may be described as perceptive deafness and vertigo resulting from a blow to the head without fracture of bony labyrinth capsule. The nystagmus is positional and may persist for several months. The underlying pathology was thought to be due to injury to the utricle and saccule. Histopathological evidence showed rupture of the membranous walls of the utricle and saccule and degenerative changes in the macula of the saccule. This injury is commonest in ear with longitudinal fracture of the temporal bone, secondly in an ear opposite a temporal bone fracture and thirdly in a head injury with no evidence of skull fracture. According to them to produce labyrinthine concussion a head injury must be severe enough to cause loss of consciousness.

Hearing loss is worst in the high frequency range and the peak loss is usually at 4000 Hz. The vertigo attacks are of postural type as described for patients having longitudinal fracture.

Experiments on animals show that the deafness is due to injury of the organ of corti, identical with that which results from a shock pulse in the air as a bomb blast or a pistol shot. They found that it results in violent displacement of the basilar membrane and organ of corti, that both reversible and irreversible cellular injuries result. They estimated hearing loss in animals, cats subjected to head injury. The hearing loss was estimated by audiogram and compared with a cochlear chart and found that the primary effect of trauma is to the organ of corti and the nerve degeneration is secondary. It is in fact the presence of damage to the organ of corti which ruled out nerve injury as a primary effect. The slightest detectable histological changes consisted of anatomical derangement of outer hair cells and their supporting cells. In mild injuries the outer hair cells which are normally tall and rectangular appeared shorter and wider and the nuclei were smaller and the chromatin was condensed. In severe lesions there was a loss of external hair cells and the beginning of cytological changes in the Dieters cells and the supporting cells, further progressive stages of injury consisted of flattening of the organ of corti and finally its complete disappearance. In labyrinthine concussion histological examination of the auditory system revealed the significant pathological changes to lie in the cochlea, when there was damage to the organ of corti severest in the upper basal turn, the region serving 4000Hz frequency. Thus according to them partial permanent deafness occurs in about 50% of patients who sustain a blow to the head to produce unconsciousness. Even a mild head blow without loss of consciousness can occasionally result in deafness.

According to Makashima and Snow (Kazumi Makashima & James .B. snow, 1975) experimental findings by means of assessment of preyer reflex and cochlear potentials in guinea pigs after stimulating head injury by shaking them in a padded cage till they became unconscious showed that in animals which did not have fracture of the skull showed hemorrhage in and laceration of the 8th nerve where it exits from the medulla oblongata. Animals killed after 6 days and 30 days showed slight to moderate degeneration of outer hair cells and Hensens cells in the apical and middle turns of the cochlea, changes in the Stria vascularis were minimal.

The oto-neurological manifestations vary from patient to patient with head injury. Variability exists in type, severity and mode of onset of symptoms and signs. In some patients deterioration of hearing and vestibular functions occurs immediately after head injury and it may be transient or permanent. In other patients the symptoms may not manifest until later and deterioration of function may continue. According to them these facts suggest that there are various forms of trauma in the temporal bone and central pathways could be responsible for the deterioration of function.

In a study done by E B Dorman (E.B Dorman et al 1982) the hearing loss was noted to be due to cochlear dysfunction. No 8th nerve or central abnormalities were detected. Various hypotheses have been put forward to explain the hearing loss that appears after brain concussion.

According to Per-Olof Bergemalm (Per-olof Bergemalm, 2003) in cases of closed head injury 74% of patients showed progression of > 15dB HL which was significantly greater than the spontaneous progression in the control group. Age and temporal bone fractures were risk factors for progression but not brain contusion or Swedish Reaction Level Scale (RLS) They found an association between early PTA (Pure tone Audiometry) and progression as well as regression i.e. poorer the initial PTA the greater the progression indicating the increased instability of the auditory system. The cause of progression is usually unknown. One of the possibilities is the development of perilymphatic fistula, other reasons may be secondary degenerative changes in the cochlea following inner ear concussion and hypoxia following disturbance of micro-circulation. It has also been speculated whether progression is due to pre-existing autoimmune disease or whether the trauma itself may initiate such a reaction towards specific inner ear proteins. There may also be synergistic interaction between trauma and the effects of noise exposure (Neuberger M Korpert K et al 1992) and the use of oto-toxic agents and medication (Jacobson CA&.Jacobson JT, 1989)

According to Vernon and Press (Vernon JA, & Press LS, 1994) only 8% of the patients who sustained head injury complained of tinnitus.

Dizziness is a frequent complication of head injury. Numerous studies have attempted to quantify the incidence of neuro-otological abnormalities in patients with post traumatic dizziness. Toglia (Toglia J U et al, 1970) found out that 61% of patients had vestibular dysfunction. Gannon (Gannon RP et al, 1978) reported 32% and Wilson reported 57% neuro-otological test abnormalities in patients who sustained minor or moderate head injury. In case of recurring case of dizziness an organic etiology must be suspected. Hearing loss in the higher frequencies is sometimes seen as early as by age 20(Rakel R E, 2005) It increases systematically to age 60 (and beyond) and is largest at 4 kHz and 6 kHz and is much larger in males than in females.

A small Sensorineural hearing loss of 25dB at the age of 25 has little medical or social relevance, however by the age of 70 a hearing loss as a result of ageing is added to the pre-existing hearing loss. This results in a moderate to severe sensorineural hearing loss. In other words a seemingly minor hearing loss at a very young age may become severe when combined with other factors which affect hearing.

4. Anatomy of the ear and temporal bone

From the point of view of injury to the ear the anatomy can be divided into preauricular pinna, post auricular region, tympanic membrane, external auditory canal, middle ear and inner ear. Preauricular region is the region of the ear in front of the auricle. Post auricular region is the region behind the auricle. The temporal bone is a composite structure and cconsists of tympanic bone, mastoid process, squamous and petrous parts. The tympanic bone forms the anterior, inferior and parts of the posterior wall of the external auditory canal. Laterally the tympanic bone borders the cartilaginous external auditory canal. The sqamous portion of the temporal bone serves as the lateral wall of middle cranial fossa and interfaces with the parietal bone superiorly and with the zygomatic process and the sphenoid anteriorly.

The mastoid portion of temporal bone is the inferiorly extending projection seen on the lateral surface of the temporal bone. It is composed of a squamous portion laterally and petrous portion medially separated by korner's petro squamous septum. The petrous portion (Greek for 'rock like') guards the sensory organs of the inner ear.

The tegmen tympani is the bony roof of the tympanic cavity, and separates it from the dura of middle cranial fossa. It is formed in part by petrous and part by the squamous bone, and the petrosquamous suture line, unossified in the young does not close until adult life.

The floor consists of a thin plate of bone which separates the tympanic cavity from the dome of the jugular bulb, sometimes it is deficient. The anterior wall of tympanic cavity is narrow as the medial and lateral walls converge. The lower portion of the anterior wall is larger than the upper and consists of a thin plate of bone covering the carotid artery.

4.1 The cochlea

The bony cochlea lies in front of the vestibule and has an external appearance rather like the shell of a snail. The shell has approximately two and one half turns and its height is about 5mm while the greatest distance across the base is about 9 mm.

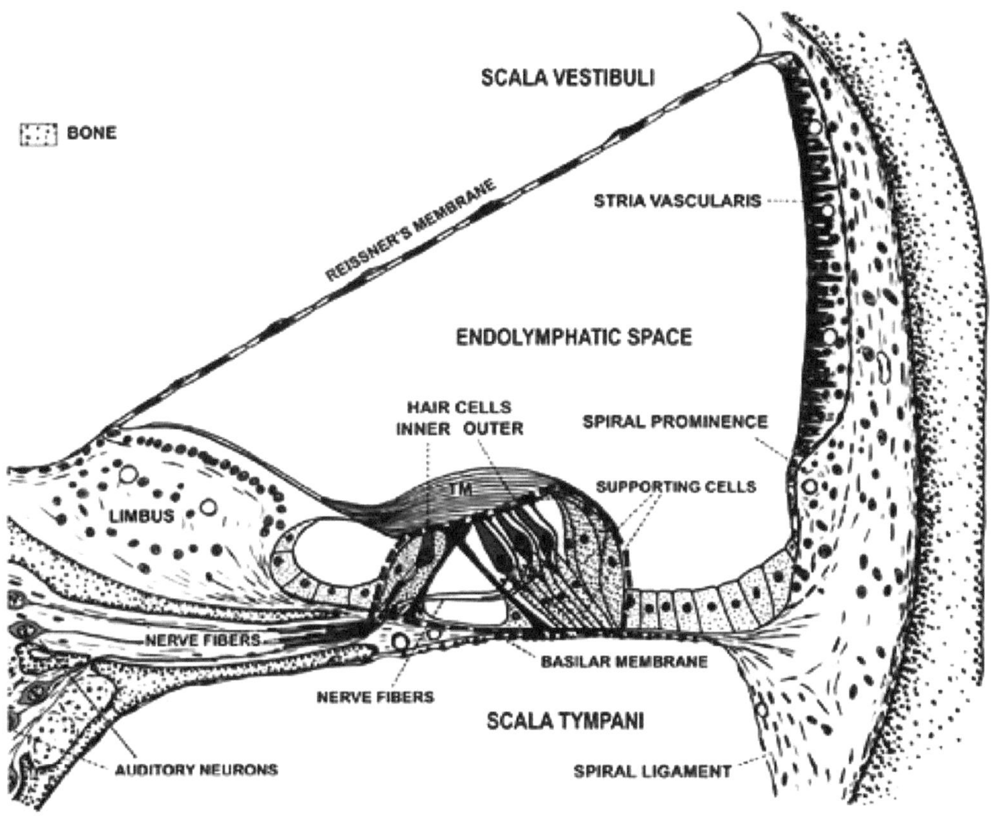

Fig. 1. Cross section of the cochlea
(SOURCE: www.nap.edu/openbook. page=35 Modified from Davis and Associates (1953)

The basilar membrane which separates the scala media from the scala tympani consists of connective tissue fibers embedded in an acellular matrix. The organ of corti, tectorial membrane along with the basilar membrane makes up the cochlear partition. (Fig-1).

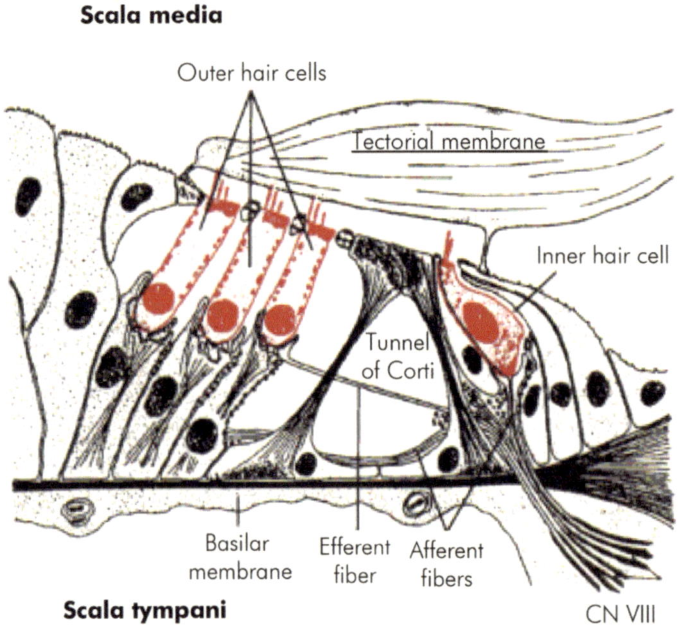

Fig. 2. Organ of corti (Nolte (1993) The Human Brain 3rd Ed. Fig. 9-34B, p. 213. Cross-section through the Organ of Corti)

The organ of corti (fig-2) is a ridge like structure containing the auditory sensory cells and a complex arrangement of supporting cells. The sensory cells are arranged in two distinct groups as inner and outer hair cells. There is a single row of inner hair cells, although occasionally extra hair cells may be apparent, and also three, four or five irregular rows of outer hair cells, with frequent gaps where individual hair cells are absent. Each hair cell consists of a body, which lies with in the organ of corti, and a thickened upper surface called the cuticular plate, from which projects a cluster of stereocilia or hairs. The stereocilia contains a core of actin molecules packed in a para crystalline array and covered with a cell membrane. The stereocilia are connected to each other along the sides by fine filaments called the side links. The tip of each stereocilium is connected to the sides of the next tallest stereocilium by a longer filament known as a tip link. The body of the inner hair cells is flask shaped, with a small apex and large cell body. The long axis of cell is inclined towards the tunnel of corti, and nerve fibers and nerve endings are located around the lower half of the body. The stereocilia projecting from the thickened cuticular plate are arranged in two or three rows parallel to the axis of the cochlear duct. The body of the outer hair cell is cylindrical with the nucleus lying close to the lower pole, where afferent and efferent nerve endings are attached. There are several rows of stereocilia but the configuration varies from a W shape at the base, through a V shape in the middle coil, to almost a linear array at the apex. The number of stereocilia also decreases in the passage from base to apex, where as the length increases, although not in a linear fashion. The hair cells are supported with in the organ of corti by several types of specialized, highly differentiated cells. These are the pillar cells, Dieters cells and Hensen's cells. In the fetus and the newborn there are about 3500 inner hair cells and 13000 outer hair cells.

5. Audiometric tests

5.1 Pure tone audiometry

It is the most commonly used method of measuring hearing acuity. It is a subjective test. The frequencies usually tested are at octave steps i.e., 125, 250, 500, 1000, 2000, 4000, 8000 Hz. A pure tone audiometer is an electronic instrument capable of producing pure tone sound of different frequencies at variable intensities. It helps in qualitative and quantitative diagnosis of hearing loss.

5.2 Tympanometry

It is the measurement of acoustic emissions in the external auditory meatus as a function of air pressure within the external auditory meatus. It provides a rapid atraumatic and objective technique for evaluating the integrity of (a) Middle ear transmission system, (b) Estimating middle ear pressure, (c) Estimating volume of ear canal or middle ear, (d) Evaluating Eustachian tube function.

Type A Tympanogram indicate normal middle ear pressure as indicated by tympanogram peak at 0 daPa. Normally middle ear pressure typically falls between +50 and -100 daPa.

Volume measurements more than 2 ml in children and 2.5ml in adults are usually indicative of tympanic membrane perforation or patent pressure equalization tube.

Mild cochlear hearing loss has little effect on acoustic reflex thresholds for tonal stimuli. for patients with hearing losses that exceed 70 dB reflexes are typically absent.

5.3 Oto-acoustic emissions

As early as 1948, Gold (Gold.T,1948) discovered that the outer hair cells of the cochlea could produce energy by an active mechanical process. However it was not until 1978 that Kemp (Kemp 1978) by a series of basic and clinical experiments demonstrated that the cochlea was capable of producing low intensity recordable sounds called oto-acoustic emissions (Fig-3). Oto-acoustic emissions (OAEs) can be defined as the audio frequency energy which originates in and is released from the cochlea, transmitted through the ossicular chain and tympanic membrane and measured in the external auditory meatus. They can occur either spontaneous or in response to acoustic stimulation. OAEs are believed to reflect the active biomechanical movement of the basilar membrane of the cochlea (Fig-4). This retrograde traveling wave is thought to be responsible for the sensitivity, frequency selectivity and wide dynamic range of the normal auditory system. Oto-acoustic emissions (OAEs) are believed to be the by product of pre-neural mechanisms of the cochlear amplifier and in particular, to be linked to the normal functioning of the outer hair cells. Oto-acoustic emissions are vulnerable to a variety of agents such as acoustic trauma (Hamernik RP, 1996) hypoxia, (Rebillard.G Lavigne& Rebillard.M) and oto-toxic medications (Ress .B D et al, 1999) that cause hearing loss by damaging outer hair cells.

Taking into account estimates of amplification provided by outer hair cells, complete destruction of OHC'S alone could result theoretically, in a hearing loss of 60 dB. Early investigations in to OAE'S proved that they are not present when the sensorineural hearing loss exceeds 40-50dB (Collet L, 1989), (Gorga, Michael P, 1997).

DPOAEs measures have shown excellent intra-subject test reliability which allows monitoring of dynamic changes of cochlear function (V.Rupa, 2001)

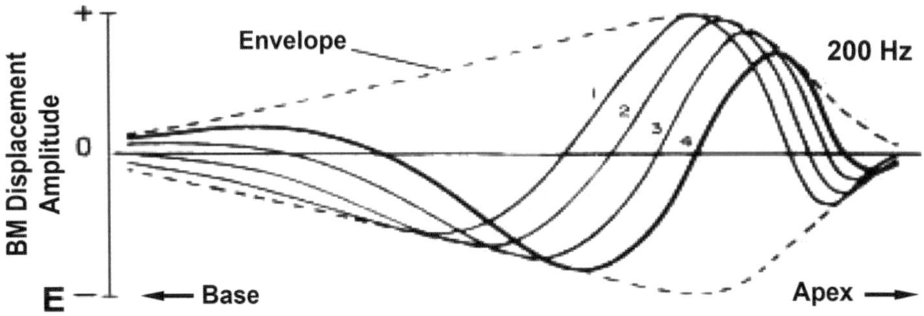

Fig. 3. Basilar membrane displacements produced in cadaveric human cochlea in response to 200Hz at 4 separate points of time. Envelope of travelling wave is also noted

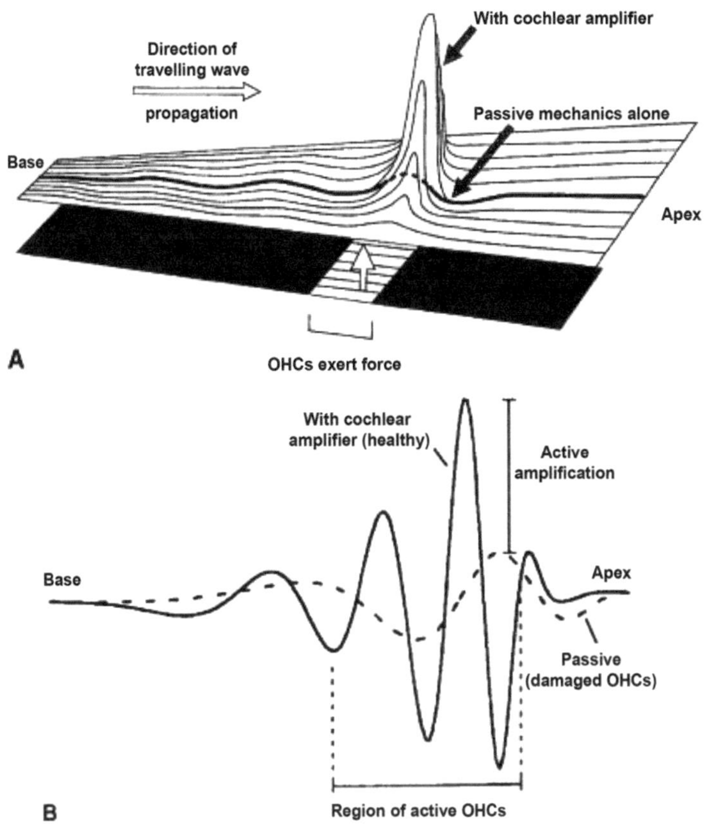

Fig. 4. Schematic representation of travelling wave along basement membrane

It has been established that DPOAEs are reduced or eliminated by compromise of middle ear conduction pathway. Normal middle ear functioning is pre-requisite for measuring DPOAE and it is therefore important to include immitance measurements while recording DPOAEs. This means is also used to confirm the presence of any middle ear pathology in MHI.

6. Study

In the study done in the ENT department of Christian Medical College India, 60 patients with history suggestive of mild head injury were evaluated over a period of six months.

INCLUSION CRITERIA: All patients with (a) history suggestive of Mild Head injury (MHI) Glasgow coma scale scoring system [GCS] 13 - 15 and improving (b) age between 6 - 60 years,(c) Patients discharged from casualty after observation period of 24 hours,(d) History of loss of consciousness of less than 20 minutes.

EXCLUSION CRITERIA: Patients with past history of ear disease, previous head injury or noise trauma. and patients having family history suggestive of autoimmune disease and hearing loss.

A detailed evaluation of the severity of injury using Glasgow coma scale scoring was done. Radiological investigations like X-Ray of skull (antero-posterior and lateral) and CT scan were used to detect skull fractures.

The external auditory canal and tympanic membrane were assessed to rule out any signs of temporal bone fracture like bleeding from external auditory canal, palpable step deformity, tympanic membrane perforation or haemotympanum. If the external auditory canal was filled with clotted blood patient was called for assessment after a period of one week. Eyes were checked for nystagmus and conjugate deviation. Facial nerve function tests were done and when the patient was cooperative facial nerve function was graded according to House Brackmann scale (House JW, &Brackmann DE 1985)

Pure tone audiometry was done and Hearing thresholds of 15-25 dB across the frequencies were considered to be as normal. Tympanometry was done using a probe tone frequency of 226Hz. An ipsilateral stapedial reflex at 1000 Hz was elicited. The ipsilateral acoustic reflex threshold was seen as normal if the level at which it is elicited falls between 70db and 100db.

DPOAE testing was done at 1000Hz, 2000Hz, 3000Hz, 4000Hz, and 6000Hz.

Repeat evaluation was done after a period of three and six months. A detailed oto-neurological evaluation was done in all three visits and patients were specifically asked for symptoms of hearing loss tinnitus and vertigo

6.1 Results and analysis

Road traffic accidents (RTA) were the most common cause of Minor head injury as seen in all studies. The incidence of road traffic accidents in age groups 20-50 years, in our study, (Fig-5) was similar to the study done by Ludwig podoshin and M R Abd AL-Hady. A vast majority (75%) of the RTA's (Road traffic accidents) (Fig-6) were two wheeler accidents and none wore helmets at the time of accident.

Majority (83%) were males and 66% were between ages of 20-50 years.

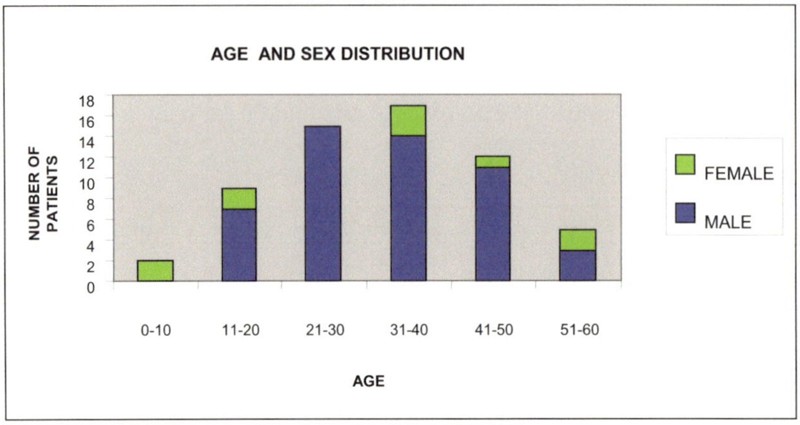

Fig. 5. Age amd sex distribution

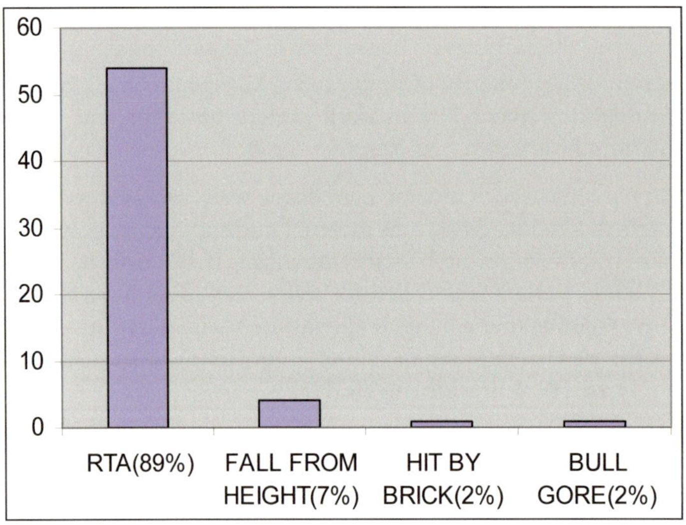

Fig. 6. Mode of injury

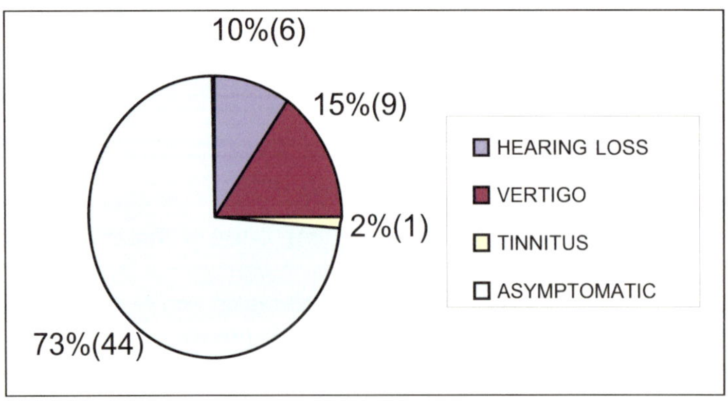

Fig. 7. Symptoms

Out of 60 patients 73% were asymptomatic, 15% complained of vertigo, 10% complained of hearing loss, and 2% complained of tinnitus (Fig-7).

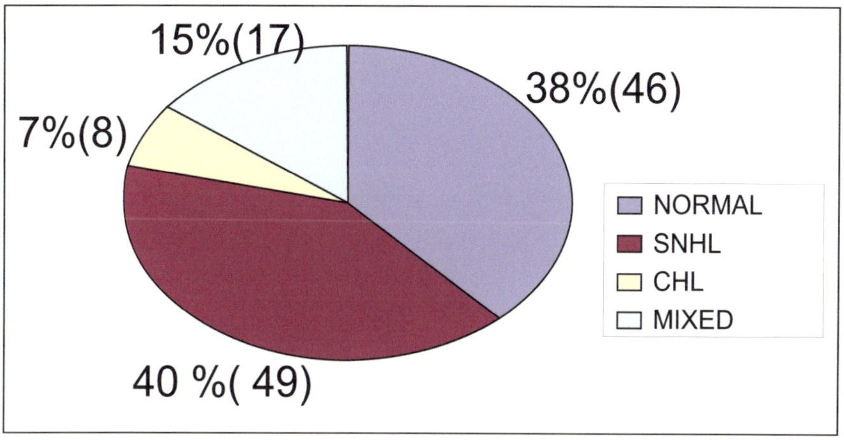

Fig. 8. Hearing loss in patients with MHI

Out of 60 patients (120 ears tested), 38 % had normal hearing, 40% had sensorineural hearing loss, 7% had conductive hearing loss, and 15 % had mixed hearing loss (fig -8).

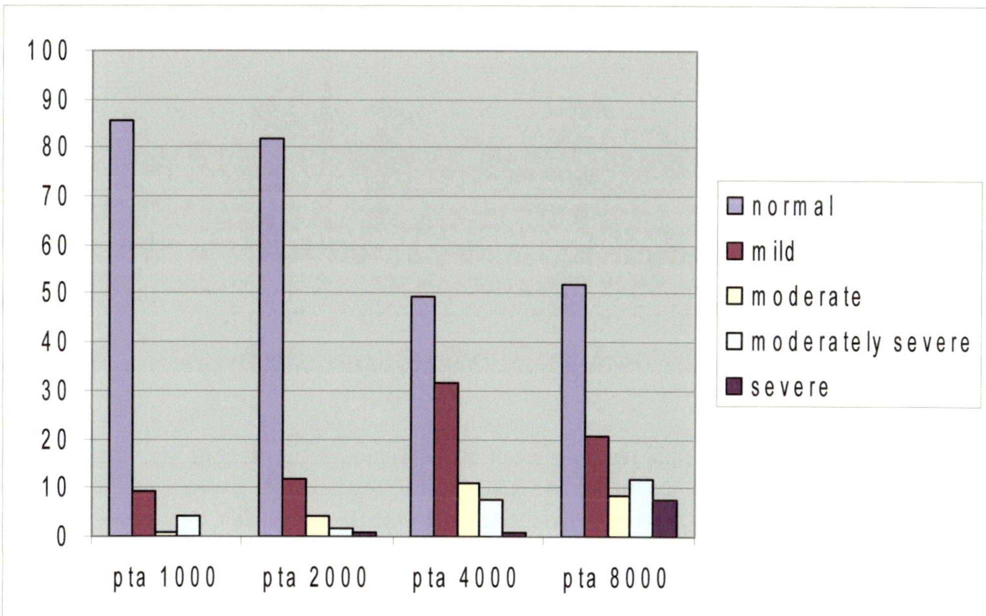

Fig. 9. Pure tone audiometry

Pure tone audiometry assessment of hearing immediately post trauma with respect to frequencies affected revealed that hearing loss was mainly in the high frequency region with greatest loss noticed at 4000 Hz and 8000 Hz (Fig-9). Significant hearing improvement on PTA was found at all the four frequencies with in three months after trauma , 1000Hz (p-value 0.014) , 2000Hz (p-value 0.006), 4000Hz (p-value<0.001), and 8000Hz (p-value 0.002)(Fig-10) ,(Fig-11),(Fig-12) .

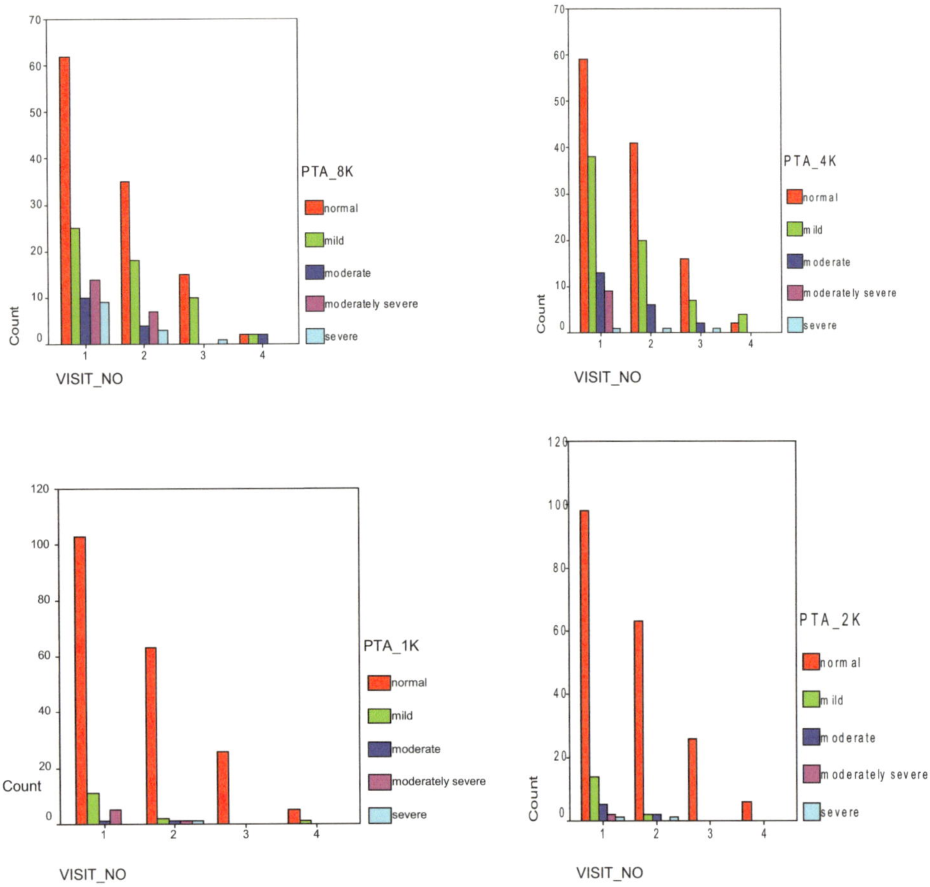

Fig. 10. Serial Pure Tone audiometry at 1000Hz,2000Hz,4000Hz,8000Hz over a period of six months

DPOAEs are present across most frequencies at and above 1000Hz in 99 to 100% of ears with normal hearing and they are absent when sensorineural hearing loss exceeds 40-50dB which was similar in our study. No studies were found in literature where DPOAE was assessed in minor head injury.

It was seen that DPOAE was absent in 38.6% at 1000Hz, 36% at 2000Hz, 29.8% at 4000Hz in patients even with normal PTA thresholds after mild head injury.

In case of Mild hearing loss on PTA, there was absence of emissions in 70% at 1000 Hz, 69% at 2000Hz, 83% at 4000Hz. This would suggest that damage to outer hair cells becomes more pronounced when there is manifest hearing loss on PTA. In few cases with normal hearing, DPOAEs were absent through out the evaluation time period suggesting irreversible damage to outer hair cells (Fig13, 14, 15).

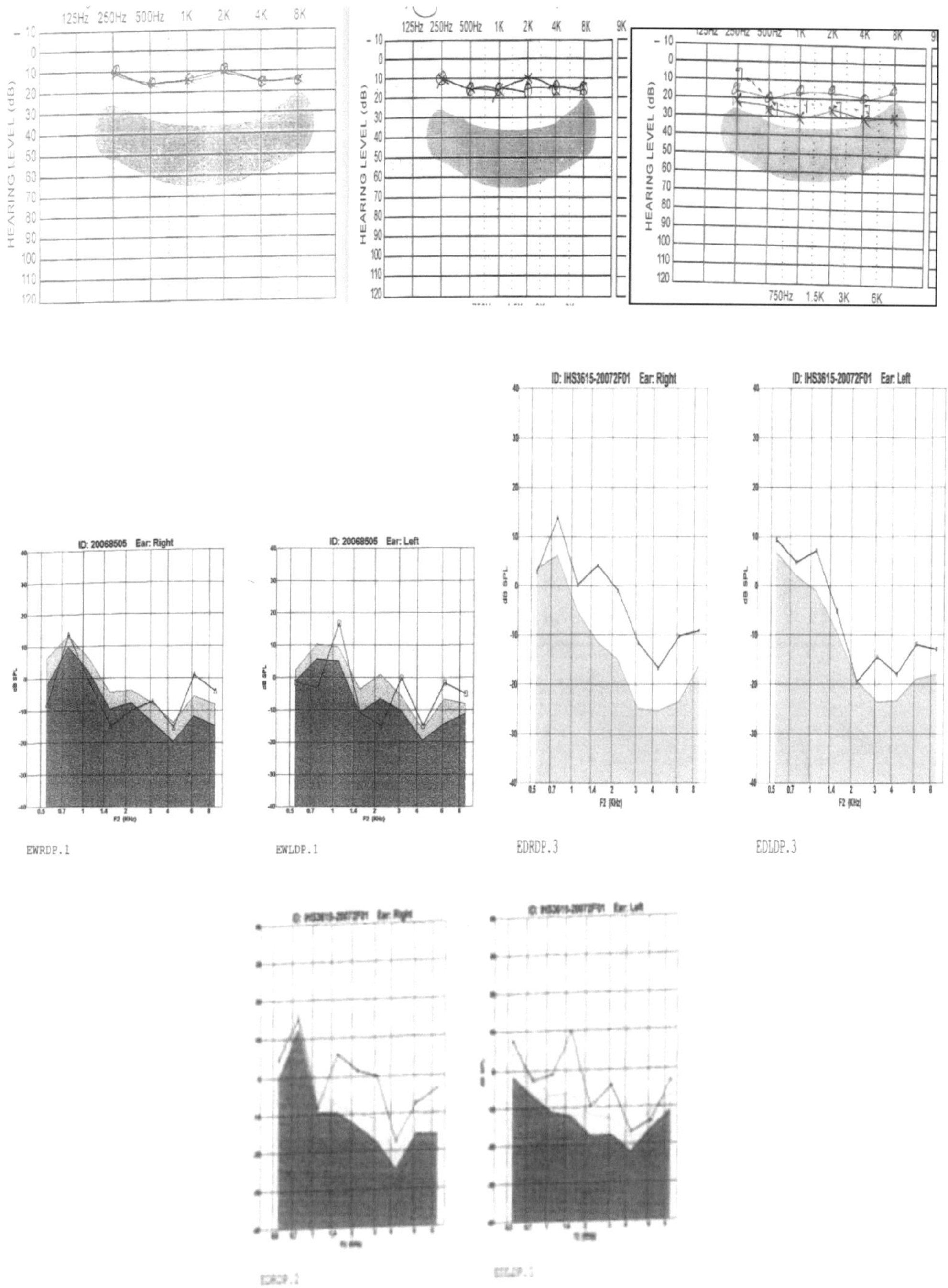

Fig. 11. Pure tone audiometry showing progression of hearing loss affecting frequency of 4000hz,8000hz in patient with left frontal bone fracture. Absence of DPOAEs at 4000hz from the time of trauma

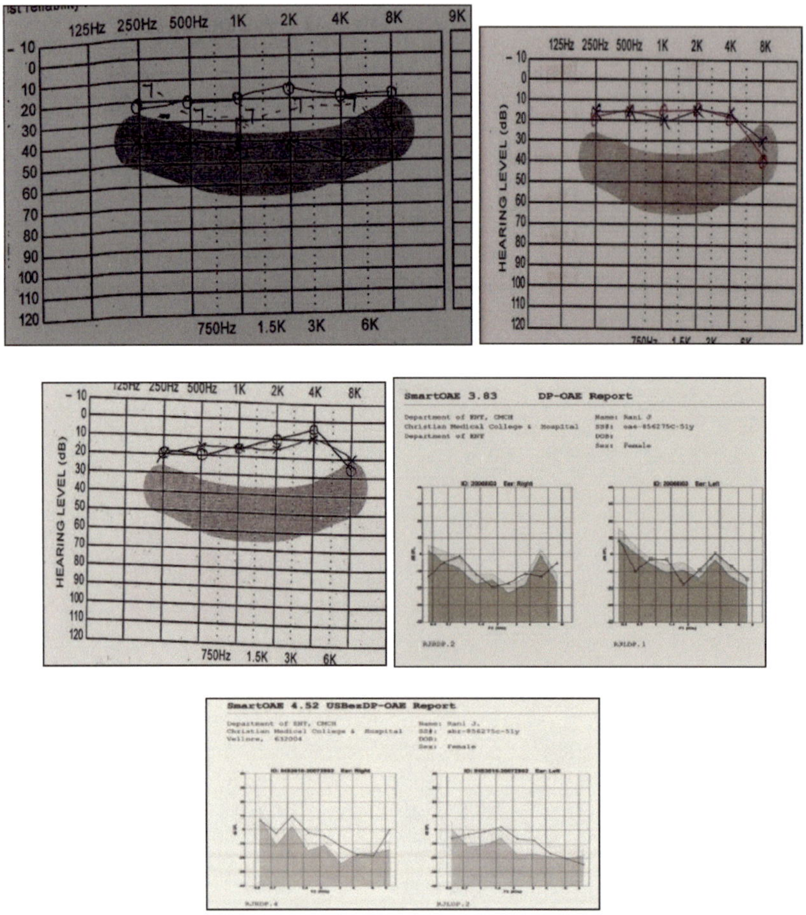

Fig. 12. Pure tone Audiometry and DPOAEs showing conductive hearing loss post trauma which returned to normal over a period of six months, but continues to have absent emissions at 4000 Hz, 6000 Hz

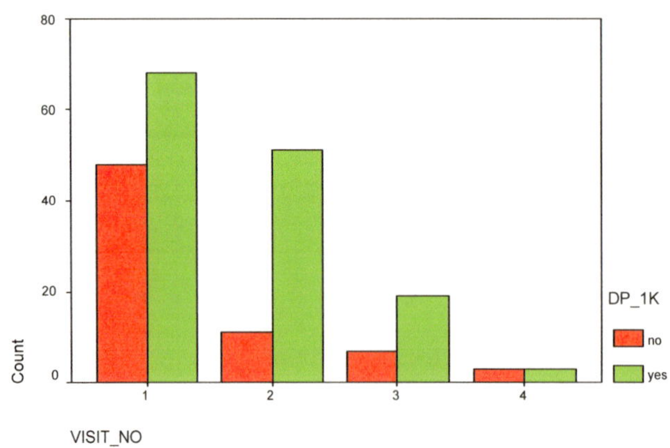

Fig. 13. DPOAE at 1000kz

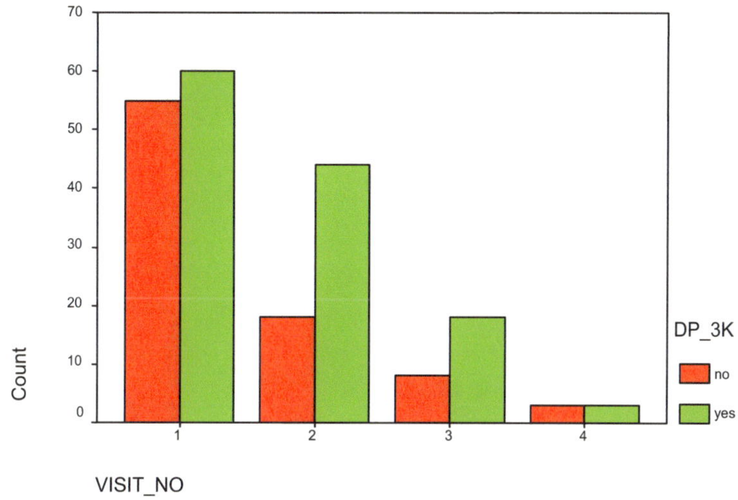

Fig. 14. DPOAE at 3000kz

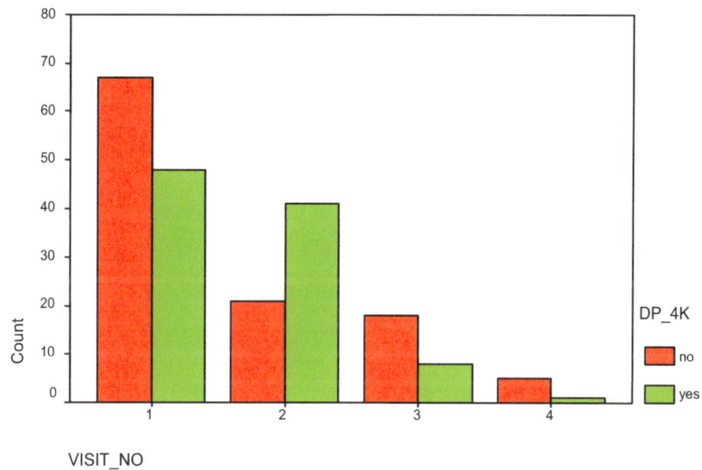

Fig. 15. DPOAE at 4000kz

As the hearing improved oto-acoustic emissions were detectable, however in cases where the hearing loss progressed, emissions could not be recorded. Changes in DPOAEs were found to be statistically significant only at 3000 Hz (p value-0.002) and 4000Hz (p value-0.003), in mild head injury.

Dix-Hallpike positional test was positive in three patients for whom Epley's repositioning maneuver was done and rests of the patients were treated with labyrinthine suppressants. One patient complained of tinnitus.

On examination hemotympanum was noticed in 2 patients which resolved over a period of three months. 1 patient presented with laryngeal trauma, rest of the patients had bleeding either from the nose or the ear.

Bleeding from the ear was noticed to be due to laceration in the external auditory canal. Patients having ear bleeding were called after a week for auditory assessment, no active intervention was needed. 1 patient had ottis externa which was treated conservatively.

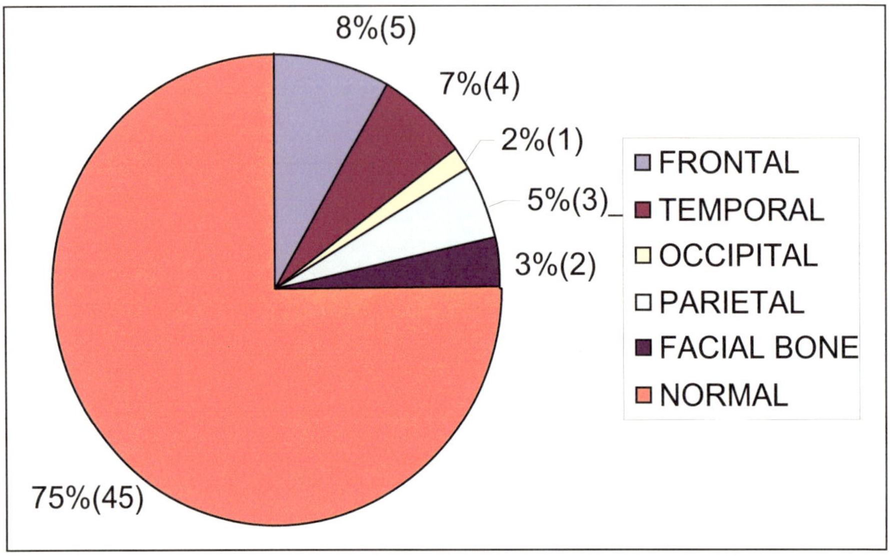

Fig. 16. Distribution of fractures

Out of 60 patients a total number of 15 patients were found to have skull fractures (fig-16).

Of 5 patients with frontal bone fractures bilateral hearing loss was noticed in all the patients, of which mixed hearing loss improved but did not become normal.

In patients who sustained temporal bone fractures, mixed fractures were seen in two patients, one patient had longitudinal fracture, and one had transverse fracture. Sensorineural hearing loss was found in four ears, mixed hearing loss was found in one ear, conductive hearing loss was noticed in one ear, and two ears were found to be normal.

Sensorineural hearing loss was noticed in the patient who sustained a fracture of the occipital bone.

Out of the three patients who sustained parietal bone fractures two patients were found to have normal hearing, the third patient had sensorineural hearing loss in one ear which became normal and mixed hearing loss in the other ear that improved.

Bilateral sensorineural hearing loss was detected in patients who sustained facial bone fractures.

Only one patient with parietal bone fracture with normal hearing complained of vertigo in which positional test was negative and was treated conservatively.

Out of the four patients who fell from a height three patients had normal hearing and one had conductive hearing loss. Parietal bone fracture was detected in one patient who had normal hearing. Hearing loss progressed in one patient.

Delayed facial nerve paresis was seen in one patient who presented with history of bull gore injury which recovered within 3 months.

7. Conclusion

This prospective study was done in a tertiary care teaching hospital to look at the incidence of hearing loss in patients who sustained minor head injury. The behavior of hearing loss was evaluated by serial assessment of hearing. Road traffic accidents (RTA) were the most common cause of Minor head injury as seen in all studies. The incidence of road traffic accidents in age groups 20-50 years, in our study, was similar to the study done by Ludwig podoshin and M R Abd AL-Hady. Whereas in the study done by Griffith, the majority were seen in late teens.

Two wheeler accidents were found to be the commonest cause of RTA causing minor head injury in our study, whereas another study (George .G.Browning at al 1982) reported that assault / fight was the major etiology causing minor head injury. 75% of the RTA's were two wheeler accidents and none of them were wearing helmets at the time of accident. In about 40% of our patient's consumption of alcohol would have contributed to the road traffic accident.

Symptoms of hearing loss were found in only 10% of patients which is in agreement with Harold F.Schuknecht (1956) and Kazumi Makashima et al (1975) due to the involvement in high frequency region. The symptoms of vertigo were found to be 15% which is low as compared with Toglia JU et al (1970) who reported an incidence of 61% and Rosalyn et al (1995) who reported 95% of patients with symptoms of vertigo . Additionally a low Incidence of tinnitus was observed which is in agreement with Griffith. The incidence of Hearing loss in our study is 62% which is in agreement with a previous study Griffith (56%) with males being most affected.

The commonest type of hearing loss was sensorineural loss confined to high frequencies. The degree of hearing loss determined the out come, and it was found in our study that patients who had moderate to severe hearing loss at the time of injury had a poorer prognosis as compared to those with normal hearing. Like the results of other studies temporal bone fractures had a higher incidence of hearing loss as compared to other facial bone fractures.

In our study in India, Road traffic accidents (RTA) were the most common cause of Minor head injury. 75% of the RTA's were two wheeler accidents and none of them were wearing helmets at the time of accident. In about 40% of our patient's consumption of alcohol might have contributed to the road traffic accidents.

Only 10% of patients complained of hearing loss ,however on evaluation 62% were found to have hearing loss. The commonest type of hearing loss was sensorineural loss confined to high frequencies. The prognosis was poor if the hearing loss was more severe. The degree of hearing loss determined the outcome, and it was found in our study that patients who had moderate to severe hearing loss at the time of injury had a poorer prognosis. Temporal bone fractures have a higher incidence of hearing loss, the symptoms of vertigo was found to be 15%. Incidence of tinnitus is low after minor head injury. DPOAE assessment at 3000 Hz and 4000 Hz is significant in assessing outer hair cell damage when compared to Pure Tone Audiometry in sub clinical hearing loss.

8. Acknowledgements

I wish to express my deep gratitude to Dr. John Mathew, Professor and Acting Head-unit-II, and Dr. Achamma Balraj, Professor Department of ENT, Christian Medical College Vellore, for their able guidance in conducting this study .

I wish to thank Dr. Anand Job, Medical superintendent, Professor and Head of unit-I, Department of ENT, and Dr. Pushparaj Singh, Head of Department of Accident and Emergency medicine for consent to use hospital facilities during the study period.

Last but not the least, I would like to thank my Parents, brother, wife, daughter, colleagues and staff of ENT for their help in making this study a reality.

I wish to thank Christoffel Blinden Mission SARO South for the financial support for Publication of this Chapter.

9. References

Andrew.T.Lyos.Michael A .Marsh et al .Progressive Hearing loss after Transverse Temporal Bone Fracture Arch Otolaryngol Head Neck Surg Vol 121 Jul 1995: pp 795-799

Allison.M.Scot..Christopher D.Bauch et al .Head Trauma and Mid-Frequency Hearing loss. American journal of Audiology Vol 8 December 1999: pp 101-105

Alexander AF,Scholl R:Beschwerden und stoerungen in Hoehr und gleichgewichtsogan bein Nachuntersuchung schaedelverlezter.Monatsschr Ohren 72 1938: pp 1021

Anthony Wright .Anatomy and ultrastructure of the human ear .In Scott-Browns's Otolaryngology, 6thedition volume 1 Alan.G Kerr .Butterworth-Heinemann, oxford ;1: 11-49

Bergemalm P-O.Borg.E., Long term objective and subjective audiologic consequences of closed head injury.Acta Otolaryngol 2001;121: pp 724-734

Collet L. Evoked Oto-Acoustic emissions and sensorineural hearing loss .Arch Otolaryngol Head and Neck surgery 115: pp 1060-1062

Culotta VP semementilli ME, Gerald. Ket al.clinico-pathological heterogenicity in the classification of mild head injury. Neurosurgery 1996; 38: pp 245-250

Dahiya.R, Keller J.D et al ,Temporal bone fractures :otic capsule sparing versus otic capsule violating clinical and radiographic considerations Trauma 1999:47:pp 1079-83

E.B Dorman,NZ Med Journal 1982;95: pp 454-455

E.Vartianen, S.Karjalainen et al, Auditory Disorders following Head Injury in children, Acta Otolaryngol[stockh]1985;99: pp 529-536

FELDMAN H., Sudden Hearing loss with Delayed onset following Head Trauma. Acta otolaryngol 1987; 103:pp 379-383.

Gannon RP.Wilson GN et al .Auditory and vestibular damage in head injuries at work. Arch otolaryngol, 1978 ,104: pp 404-408.

George .G.Browning .Iain R.C Swan et al. Hearing loss in Minor Head Injury. Arch Otolaryngol vol 108 1982: pp 474-477

Gold.T, The physical basis of the action of the cochlea. Proc R Soc Loud B Biol Sci 1948;135: pp 492-498

Grove W.E, Skull fractures involving the ear.Laryngoscope 1939; 69: pp 833-870

Gorga, Michael P; Neely, Stephen .T et al .From Laboratory to clinic: A large scale study of distortion product otoacoustic emissions in ears with normal hearing and ears with hearing loss. Ear Hear Vol 18(6) December 1997 : pp 440-455

Gomez PA,lobato RD,Ortega JM,et al.Mild head injury: Differences in prognosis among patients with a Glasgow coma scale score of 13-15 and analysis of factors associated with abnormal CT findings.Br J Neurosurgery 1996;10: pp 453-460

Gurdijan ES:Studies on Acute cranial and intracranial injuries.Ann Surg 1933 :pp 327-367.

H.Alexander Arts. Sensorineural Hearing loss:Evalaution and management in adults. In Charles.W.Cummings OTOLARYNGOLOGY AND HEAD AND NECK SURGERY 4TH Edition Elsevier Mosby` Part 14,Chapter 155- pp 3542

Harvey s.Levin, Outcome from mild head injury. In Raj .K.Narayanan .Jack .E.Wiberger NEUROTRAUMA Mc-Graw Hill: chap-50 pp 749-754

Harold F.Schuknecht and Roderick C.Davison,,Deafness and Vertigo from Head Injury,AMA Archives of Otolaryngology 1956: pp 513-528

Hamernik RP .The cubic distortion product oto-acoustic emissions from the normal and noise damaged chinchilla cochlea. J Acoust Soc Am 1996;100: pp 1003-1012

House JW, Brackmann DE. Facial Nerve Grading System.Otolaryngol Head and Neck surgery 1985; 93: pp 14

Hough JVD ,Stuart WD.Middle ear injuries in skull trauma. Laryngoscope 1968;78:899

Hsiang JNK,Yeung T,Yu ALM ,et al. High Risk mild head injury J Neurosurgery 1997:87 : pp 234-238

Jacobson CA.Jacobson JT et al.Hearing loss in prison inmates. Ear Hear 1989;10: pp178-183

Kazumi Makashima,James .B.snow. Pathogenesis of Hearing loss in Head Injury, Studies in Man and Experimental Animals. Arch Otolaryngol Vol 101 July 1975:pp 426-432

Kemp DT. Stimulated acoustic emission from with in the hearing system. J.Acoustic Soc Am 1978;64: pp 1386-1391

Marc stiefel.Arlene Shaner et al .The Edwin Smith Papyrus: The Birth of Analytical Thinking in Medicine and Otolaryngology,Laryngoscope116 Feb 2006:pp 182-188

M.R.Abd AL-HADY .O Shehata et al. The Journal of Laryngology and Otology Vol 104 December 1990: pp 927-936

M.V.Griffiths .The incidence of auditory and vestibular concussion following minor head injury. The Journal of laryngology and Otology 1979 March;Vol 93: pp 253-265

Nassulphis P:Die Schaedigung des innenohres und seines nerven nach Schaedeltrauma. Msch Ohr-Heilk,Jahg feb: 79-80, June,1964 :pp 222-252

Neuberger M Korpert K et al Hearing loss from industrial noise, head injury and ear disease. Audiology 1992 ;31: pp 45-57

Per-olof Bergemalm. Progressive Hearing loss after closed Head Injury: A Predictable Outcome?. Acta Otolaryngol 2003 ;123: pp 836-840

Podoshin .L., Fradis.M:Hearing loss after Head Injury.Arch otolaryngol 1975;101: pp 15-18

Rakel R E. Textbook of family practice. 6th Ed .Philadelphia PA .WB Saunders 2005 : pp 443-449

Rebillard.G Lavigne-Rebillard.M. Effect of reversible hypoxia on the compared time courses of endocochlear potential and 2f1-f2 distortion products. Hear Res 62:pp 142-148

Ress .B D, Sridhar K.S et al .Effects of Cis-platinum chemotherapy on Oto-Acoustic Emissions. The development of an objective screening protocol.Otolaryngol Head Neck Surg 1999; 121: pp 693-701.

Rimel RW, Giordani B,Barth JT et al. Disability caused by minor head injury. Neurosurgery 1981:9:pp 221-8

Rimel RW, Giordani B,Barth JT et al. Moderate head injury: Completing the clinical spectrum of brain trauma. Neurosurgery 1982;11: pp 344-51

Robert .J.Ruben .MD .Hearing loss and deafness. Ear Nose and Throat Disorders .Merck .Accessed at www .merck.com

Rosalyn A Davies. Linda M Luxon.Dizziness following head injury: A neuro-otological study. J Neurol 1995 ;242: pp 222-230

Starmark JE .Stalhammar D.et al .The Reaction Level Scale [RLS85].Manual and Guidelines Acta Neurochir 1988;:91:pp 12-20

Swan IJ, Teasdale Gm. Current concepts in the management of patients with so called' minor' or mild head injury, Trauma 1999;1: pp143-55

Teasdale G, Jennett B. Assessment of coma and impaired consciousness. A practical scale.Lancet1974;2:pp 81–4

Toglia JU .Rosenberg PE et al .Post traumatic dizziness: Vestibular, audiologic and medico-legal aspects. Arch of Otolaryngol ,1970,92: pp 485-492

Uffenorde W:Histologishe Befunde.Beiter Z Anat physiol Pathol Therap Ohrens 1924; 21:pp 282-285

Varghese. M. Mohan. D,Transportation Injuries in rural Haryana,North India. Proceedings International conference on Traffic safety, New Delhi. Macmilan India limited:2003: p 326-329

Vernon JA, Press LS. Characteristics of tinnitus induced by head injury. Arch Otolaryngol Head Neck Surg 1994;120:pp547–51

V.Rupa, Clinical utility of distortion product Oto-acoustic emissions. Indian journal of otolaryngology Head and neck surgery 2001;Vol 54: pp 88-90

World report on road traffic injury prevention,Peden marge,Scurfeild et al Editors, Edition 2004,GENEVA ,WHO .

William D. Zimmerman Toni. M Ganzel. et al .Peripheral Hearing Loss following Head Trauma in Children Laryngoscope 103 January 1993 : pp 87-91

Wilson GN .Gannon PR .Auditory and vestibular damage in 100 work -related head injuries .J Laryngol otol ;95: pp 1213-1219

8

Conductive Hearing Loss Due to Trauma

Olushola A. Afolabi, Biodun S. Alabi,
Segun Segun-Busari and Shuaib Kayode Aremu
University of Ilorin Teaching Hospital, Ilorin, Kwara State
Nigeria

1. Introduction

Hearing impairment is one of the most frequent sensory deficits in humans, affecting more than 250 million people in the world. Consequences of hearing loss include inability to interpret speech, often resulting in a reduced ability to communicate and delay in language acquisition. Untreated hearing loss may also cause economic and educational disadvantage, social isolation and cause stigmatization.

There are three basic types of hearing loss based on the part of auditory system with the damage: conductive hearing loss, sensorineural hearing loss, and mixed hearing loss.

Conductive hearing loss is the most common cause of hearing impairment both in children and in the adults and the incidence is significantly higher in children. In conductive hearing loss, the inner ear functions normally, but sound vibrations are blocked from passage through the ear canal, ear drum or across the tiny bones located in the middle ear. Patients with conductive hearing loss hear perceive bone-conducted sounds presented with a small vibrator to the skull with better thresholds than sounds presented through earphones. Conductive hearing loss is usually mild to moderate in degree and can be unilateral or bilateral and in most cases unilateral. Most type of conductive hearing loss is correctable by relatively minor medical or surgical treatments. More significant conductive hearing loss may be associated with skull and/or facial malformations which may require surgery for its correction.

Trauma generally is a major cause of morbidity and mortality in any society [Paul & Peter 2001]. Generally, trauma to the ear may result in fracture of the external auditory canal, tympanic membrane perforation, fracture to the ossicular chains, fracture of the temporal bone itself, damage to the cochlea or the facial nerve. Lesser bone trauma causes damage to the ossicular chains [Fradis & Podoshin 1975.] Hearing loss from trauma occurs in 22.5% of cases of temporal bone trauma and of these cases 16-30% have conductive hearing impairment [Fradis & Podoshin 1975, Ghoyareb B.Y et al 1987]. Hearing loss is defined as the averaged hearing loss at 1000, 2000 and 4000 Hz, measured by pure tone audiometry. This definition, although different from WHO/ISO definitions, is currently used in Nigeria because of its higher relevance to speech discrimination. It also corresponds to the standard proposed by the British Association of Otolaryngology and the British Society of Audiology (1983). Hearing is said to be impaired when the hearing level is above 25dB in the best ear. Hearing loss can have a profound impact on an individual's emotional, physical, and social well-being. People with hearing loss are more likely to report symptoms of depression, dissatisfaction with life, reduced functional health and withdrawal from social activities. This chapter aims to profile hearing loss due to trauma and its aetiology.

1.1 Anatomy and physiology of conductive hearing loss due to trauma

The ear consists of three parts namely external, middle and inner ear. Conductive hearing loss occurs due to damage to the external or middle ear (Figure 1).

The external ear consists of the pinna, and external auditory canal. The external auditory canal is about 2.5cm long. The external auditory canal extends from the concha to the tympanic membrane. The middle ear is made up of the Tympanic cavity, Aditus ad-antrum, mastoid air cells and Eustachian tube. It contains the ossicles, nerves and muscles and extends from the medial end of the tympanic membrane to the stapes footplate (figure 1.0).

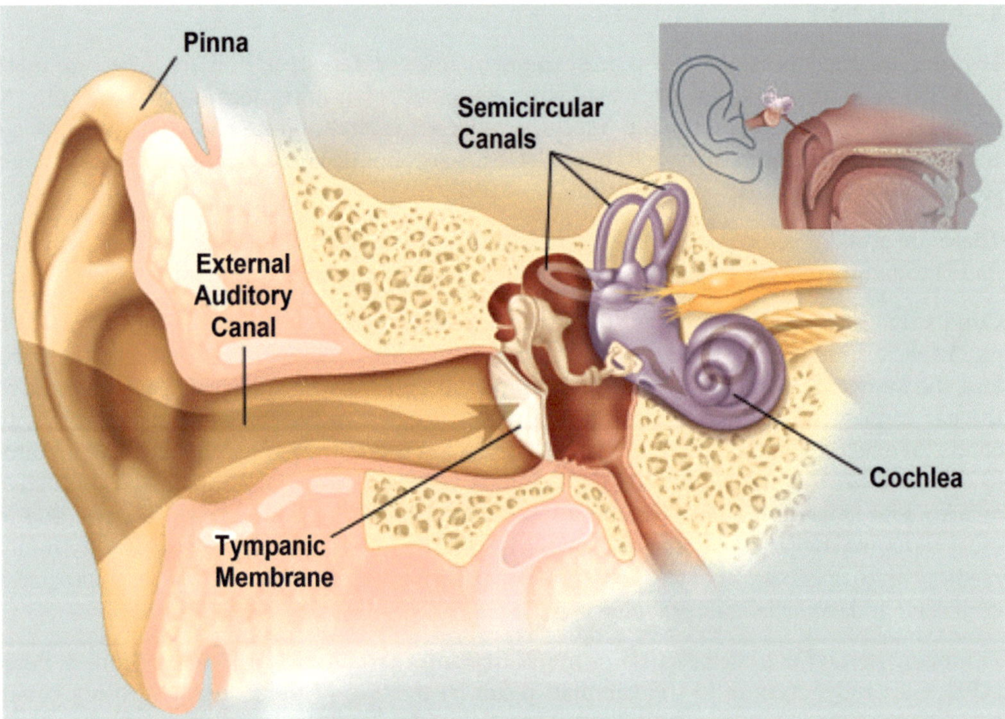

Fig. 1. Anatomical Diagram of the Ear

1.2 Physiology of hearing

Sound in the form of air waves arrives at the auricle and is transmitted through the external auditory canal. Sound then causes the tympanic membrane to vibrate. Vibration energy in the tympanic membrane is transmitted through the ossicles to the oval window into the cochlea. Pressure vibrations are transmitted into the scala vestibuli and into the cochlea. Vibrations of the scala vestibuli are greatest at the location where the resonance frequency of the cochlea corresponds to the frequency of the transmitted sound waves. In this way, a topographic representation of sound is possible. The basilar membrane vibrates which causes deflection of the stereocilia, and stimulation of the cochlear nerve. Injury to middle ear causes hearing loss. The is due to the problem of impedance: the resistance of transfer of energy between two media. This can be understood by analogy with transmission of light through water. When sun shines on water some of the light is reflected, while the remaining is transmitted through the water. This is manifested as a glare on top of the water and also visibility below the surface. Without the middle ear, most of the sound would bounce off of the surface of the oval window and less sound would be transmitted into the cochlea. This is because sound must pass from one medium (air) into another (liquid) in order to stimulate the cochlea.

The middle ear reduces the problem of impedance mismatch through several mechanisms. The effective ratio of these areas of the tympanic membrane to the oval window is about 14:1 (Roger and Maurice 1992). A second mechanism by which the middle ear overcomes impedance mismatch is through the ossicles. The malleus is 1.3 times longer than the incus. The ossicles also constitute a lever mechanism with a mechanical advantage of 1.3:1 (Roger and Maurice 1992, Lee KJ 1995). The product of these areas and lever ratios represent the transfer ratio of the whole mechanism. 14 x 1.3 = 18:1 (Roger and Maurice 1992). The vibration of cochlea fluids are processed and analyzed in such a way that data representing frequency, intensity and phase are transmitted as impulses along the auditory nerve via auditory pathway to brain for interpretation (Gibson 1978).

Thus injury to either the tympanic membrane or the middle ear ossicles from trauma will result in loss of this physiological function causing impedance mismatch ultimately resulting in impaired hearing (Roger 1992, Lee KJ1995).

The ear can be stimulated either with sound pressure waves or via vibrations applied directly to the skull. The latter is noted on audiograms as bone conduction and is used to distinguish the sensorineural component of hearing. There are three mechanisms in which vibratory energy placed directed onto the skull will cause stimulation of the cochlea:

This can be through

i. Distortional
ii. Inertia-Ossicular
iii. Osseo-tympanic mechanism

1. The distortional mechanisms is due to vibration directly distorting the skull. As the cochlea is part of the skull, it would be distorted as well. Because the round window yields more than the oval window, the scala vestubuli and scala tympani have different compliances. This results in the deflection of the basilar membrane and deflection of steriocillia with stimulation of the auditory nerve. However in fractured temporal bone (longtitudinal or transverse fracture) affecting either the oval window, cochlea or semicircular canal, this smooth mechanism is interrupted (Stanley 2009)
2. The inertial-ossicular mechanism of conductive hearing relates to the ability of vibration energy directed to the skull to cause motion of the ossicles. Vibration to the skull will cause the ossicles to move. Ossicular movement imparts its energy to the oval window which stimulates the cochlea. However, this is dependent on the direction of vibrations in the skull. If the direction of vibration is parallel to the axis of the movement of the ossicles, inertial-ossicular mechanism of conductive hearing takes place. If there is is

temporal bone injury resulting in fracture of the temporal bone or ossicular joint, fracture results in change or loss in the axis of ossicular movement and causes conductive hearing loss. If the vector of skull vibration is perpendicular to the axis of the movement of the ossicles, the effect is negligible. As a vibrating object, the ossicles have a resonance frequency. Therefore the inertial-loss mechanism of conductive hearing is more prominent about the resonance frequency of the ossicles.

3. The osseo-tympanic mechanism of bone conductive hearing is best illustrated by occlusion of the external auditory canal. Occlusion may be as a result of pathologic conditions such as fracture to the temporal bone with blood clots occluding the external auditory canal or cerumen impaction. Vibration energy is transmitted through the skull, causing a vibration of the soft tissues of the external auditory canal. This vibratory energy is transmitted into the air of the external auditory canal. Some energy escapes the external auditory canal while some reaches the tympanic membrane. The tympanic membrane is thus stimulated; energy is transferred to the ossicles and onwards to the cochlea. This explains why when the external ear canal is occluded, the bone-conduction threshold improves. Vibration energy into the external auditory canal bounces back from the object occluding the external auditory canal. Less sound energy is lost and more is reflected onto the tympanic membrane.

1.3 Aetiopathogenesis

Hearing loss due to trauma is a common phenomenon worldwide. This could arise from assaults, road traffic injury, domestic, industrial and sports injuries. These are relatively on the increase in our society. Trauma to the head causing conductive hearing loss commonly involves the external ear, middle ear and temporal bone in road traffic injuries. The sources of injury or accidents most frequently encountered are those involving motor vehicles; however, industrial and athletic injuries may also present potential lesions to the temporal bone and middle ear. Appropriate use of safety devices, both in automobiles and in industrial and athletic activities, to protect the skull and head from trauma may eliminate or reduce many of these problems. However, compliance with advised safety precautions is often not adequate.

1.4 External auditory canal injury

Two types of injury are likely to involve the external auditory canal: blunt and penetrating trauma, thermal and caustic burns. Isolated blunt trauma to the ear canal is most often caused by the insertion of a foreign object into the ear to scratch the skin or to remove wax. The skin of the ear canal, particularly the anterior and inferior part of the canal, is quite thin, with a minimal sub-epithelial layer. The tender skin of this portion of the canal is easily abraded and will bleed readily, particularly if the patient is on anticoagulant or anti-platelet therapy. In most instances, the pain and the sight of blood from the ear canal cause the patient to seek medical attention. In some cases, however, a secondary infection develops, and pain, hearing loss, or infected drainage causes the patient to seek help. The canal should be gently cleaned using microscopic technique, and blood clots, debris, and wax should be removed. When the bleeding site has been identified, placing a small pledget of Gelfoam coated with antibiotic ointment over it can readily control the bleeding. Alternatively, Gelfoam soaked with topical thrombin can be applied to the bleeding site. In rare cases, the site must be cauterized and then packed with a Merocel wick. In contrast, the skin of the posterosuperior part of the canal is much thicker and is more resistant to abrasions and injuries. Posterior lacerations usually stop bleeding because the subepithelial layer is more developed; therefore, vessels in this area readily contract and clot off.(Mitchell KS 2003)

After cleaning of the canal under good illumination, the tympanic membrane is inspected to determine the extent of injury. If an injury to the middle ear or temporal bone is discovered, a complete neurotologic examination is performed to evaluate the patient. Audiometric assessment can also be done to assess the degree of hearing loss. Blunt injuries to the temporal bone typically result from the head being forced against a stationary object in a deceleration injury or from an object being thrown directly at the head. Most injuries involving this region occur as a result of a glancing blow to the temporal region.

Although soft tissue injuries to the auricle and canal occur, they are often accompanied by fractures of the external auditory canal, middle ear structures, otic capsule, or surrounding structures. Mandibular injuries, particularly those that drive the mandible posteriorly into the jaw joint, will occasionally fracture the anterior wall of the ear canal, resulting in laceration of the skin and exposure of bone. Following blunt trauma to the ear and temporal bone, the external auditory canal should be carefully cleaned and bleeding controlled as described earlier. If exposed bone is found, it should not be debrided at this point but rather assessed later when the canal has healed. Radiographs, including facial bone computed tomographic (CT) scans and pantomographic mandibular views, should be obtained in these patients to define the injuries.

Occasionally, a direct blow to the auricle results in an isolated fracture of the external auditory canal and mastoid process. This is a fracture not involving the deeper parts of the temporal bone that are in contact with the dura matter. Regardless of where the fracture has occurred, the clinician should be aware that squamous cell epithelium can be entrapped by the fracture fragments, leading to the development of a canal cholesteatoma. Canal fractures can also lead to chronic infection, bone sequestration, and stenosis of the canal. The development of any of these sequelae may necessitate surgical débridement, grafting, reconstruction, or meatoplasty to ensure a healthy open ear canal. Penetrating injuries of the external auditory canal are usually caused by gunshot or stab wounds. This may be anteriorly through the parotid gland which often involves the external auditory canal or posteriorly through the mastoid bone also involving the external auditory canal. As a consequence, facial nerve injury, tympanic membrane perforation, and ossicular dislocation can result from gunshot wounds of the external auditory canal.

The facial nerve is most likely to be injured at the stylomastoid foramen apparently because it is relatively fixed at that point. In the absence of any of these additional injuries (mastoid or parotid) gunshot wounds of the ear canal require cleaning, a light dressing, and prophylactic antibiotics. Occasionally, the canal must be stented using Silastic with sofratulle protection with steroid based antibiotic drop impregnated in it or sofratulle with steroid based antibiotic impregnated rolled and stuck into the canal. Lacerations of the external auditory canal can occur either anteriorly or posteriorly and are often accompanied by partial avulsion of the auricle. These patients should be carefully evaluated for injury to the facial nerve and the great vessels; radiographic studies including arteriography may be indicated in these patients. Most external auditory canal lacerations require cleaning, gentle débridement, and suturing to realign the various parts of the ear canal and auricle. Surprisingly, stenosis does not usually occur in these patients.

Burns and caustic injuries to the ear canal often represent a potentially complicated situation in that severe burns can lead to circumferential scarring and stenosis of the canal. Most of these injuries are attributable to one of three mechanisms: a thermal burn, a caustic burn, or a welding injury. Thermal and caustic burns of the ear canal are usually associated with additional injury to the auricle, which may in itself lead to loss of cartilage, cicatrix formation, and stenosis of the canal. Most thermal burns of the ear canal are caused by flash injuries, fires, lightning strikes, or hot liquids such as oil. Similar to burns elsewhere on the body, the depth and extent of the burn should be determined and documented. Superficial thermal burns of the ear canal are usually treated with the application of antibiotic ointment. If more than half of the ear canal is involved or has third-degree burns, in addition to the application of antibiotic ointment, the canal is stented with soft Silastic tubing. Canal stenting is performed in an effort to prevent stenosis of the canal, which leads to the trapping of squamous debris and ultimately a destructive ear canal cholesteatoma. Stenosis of the canal is treated aggressively with corticosteroid injections, frequent dilations, and, in some cases, skin grafting or even meatoplasty. Caustic burns are usually caused by a chemical spill or a foreign object such as an alkaline battery. Thermal and acid burns cause coagulation necrosis, whereas alkaline burns cause liquefaction necrosis and leads to much more extensive injury over time (Mitchell KS 2003).

Kavanagh and Litovitz reported a series of battery-related injuries to the ear canal that were much more frequent and severe than expected, including tympanic membrane perforation, exposed bone of the ear canal, sensorineural hearing loss, ossicular destruction, and facial paralysis (Kavanagh KT and Litovitz T 1986). They also noted that otic drops must be withheld in these patients as they provide an external electrolyte bath for the battery, enhancing leakage and generation of an external current with subsequent tissue electrolysis and hydroxide formation. The foreign body should be removed as soon as possible, under general anesthesia if needed (Capo JM, Lucente FE 1986). Once the injury has been assessed, caustic burns are treated much like thermal burns described earlier, with microscopic cleaning, antibiotic eardrops, and stenting if indicated.

Welding injuries occur when hot slag or molten metal enters the meatus, usually resulting in either a small and localized burn of the ear canal or a tympanic membrane perforation. In most patients, microscopic cleaning, ciprofloxacin and hydrocortisone otic drops, and observation are the only measures indicated for welding injuries of the external auditory canal.

1.5 Middle ear and Tympanic membrane injury

The temporal bone and middle ear are composed of very dense bone. Relatively minor blows to the head would rarely cause a significant injury to the temporal bone and middle ear. The source of the injury that may involve the temporal bone must be of rather intense force.

The injury seen with trauma to the head may be either from two major categories: blunt trauma to the skull and penetrating trauma to the skull. The nature of the injury will vary considerably based on the type of trauma delivered directly to the head. The degree of hearing loss suffered by the patients also varies as discussed below. Trauma to the tympanic membrane and the middle ear can be caused by (1) overpressure, (2) thermal or caustic burns, (3) blunt or penetrating injuries, and (4) barotrauma. Of all these overpressure seems to be the most common. The major causes of overpressure include slap injuries and blast injuries. Slap injuries are extremely common and can be a result of either a hand or water slap. Slap injuries usually result in a triangular or linear tear of the tympanic membrane Most of these perforations cause mild hearing loss, aural fullness, and mild tinnitus. Blast injuries, although much less common in Nigeria, are potentially much more serious. Blast injuries may be caused by bomb explosions, gasoline explosions, rock blasting and air-bag deployment in automobile accidents. Blast injuries from bomb and gasoline explosions not only disrupt the tympanic membrane but also can cause temporal bone fracture, ossicular discontinuity, or high-frequency sensorineural hearing loss owing to cochlear injury. Following an overpressure injury, blood, purulent secretions, and debris should be carefully suctioned from the ear canal, and the perforation size and location should be recorded. Irrigation and pneumatic otoscopy should be specifically avoided in these patients. The ability to hear a whisper as well as tuning fork tests should be documented, and an audiogram should be obtained as soon as the patient's condition allows. A complete neurotologic examination should also be performed in these patients to document the status of the cranial nerves including the facial nerve and the vestibular nerve as well as the central nervous system. If the tympanic membrane perforation is dry, it should be observed and patient advised to keep the ear dry also ototopical ear drops are not indicated. If there is CSF leakage or mucopurulent discharge from the middle ear through the tympanic membrane perforation, the clinician should determine and note if this is consistent with cerebrospinal fluid (CSF). If a CSF leak is suspected, immediate CT scan of the temporal bone should be obtained to rule out a fracture. If the drainage is not consistent with CSF, oral antibiotics and ciprofloxacin with hydrocortisone otic drop should be applied in the form of wick dressing is done. A history of vertigo or nausea and vomiting and an audiogram showing a conductive hearing loss of more than 30 dB suggest disruption of the ossicular chain. Profound sensorineural loss also may signify oval window or cochlear damage.

Thermal injuries to the tympanic membrane include welding and lightning injuries. Welding injuries often result in non-healing perforations of the tympanic membrane, either as a result of infection or possibly because the slag acts to cauterize or devascularize the tympanic membrane as it passes through it. If infection occurs, the patient is treated with systemic antibiotics such as ciprofloxacin and steroid-based topical ear drops hydrocortisone otic drops. If the perforation is dry, it should be observed for a period of 12 weeks for spontaneous healing. If the drumhead does not heal, surgical closure in the form of tympanoplasty should be performed. Lightning and electrocution injuries are also a form of thermal injurie which are not rare, and the most frequent injury to the ear is perforation of the tympanic membrane ((Panosian MS, Dutcher 1994) The most common vestibular disturbance is transient vertigo. Other clinical findings include sensorineural hearing impairment, conductive hearing loss, tinnitus, temporal bone fracture, avulsion of the mastoid process, burns of the ear canal, and facial nerve paralysis (ogren and Edmund 1995). Management is similar to the welding injury as the tympanic membrane perforations caused by the lightning injury often do not heal, probably as a result of cauterization or devascularization of the tympanic membrane, much like welding injuries.

Caustic injuries to the tympanic membrane can cause its perforation. With alkaline agents, the tympanic membrane is damaged by liquefaction necrosis, that is, the alkaline caustic penetrates the tympanic membrane, causing occlusion of the vasculature that may extend farther than the visible perforation.

As a result, the size of the perforation may not be fully appreciated until all of the inflammation is resolved. Furthermore, after caustic injuries, other middle ear pathologies observed include an extensive granulation reaction with scarification, ossicular fixation, chronic infection of the middle ear mucosa, canal blunting where the raw surfaces that surround the canal form a cicatrix, leading to narrowing of the ear canal and loss of the vibratory surface of the tympanic membrane. Other complications are chronic myringitis on the surface of the tympanic membrane, creating a raw weeping surface with granulation on the surface of the drumhead. Treatment involved the use of systemic antibiotics, steroid-based topical ear drops for aural dressing, audiologic assessment and a complete neurotologic evaluation to determine the extent of injury. When the ear has stabilized, and preferably when drainage has diminished, the middle ear and tympanic membrane can be reconstructed surgically.

In Nigeria compared to the developed world it is difficult to know the economic impact of this injury both financially and otherwise. It is estimated that the annual cost of dealing with this tragedy is more than $100 billion in the USA. In a study done by the National Academy on Aging Society (NAAS) in 1999, it was found that the average value for time lost in a conductive injury due to trauma in the workplace costs more than US $8,000. [NAAS 1999]. However this data are not available for the developing countries. Trauma patients consume more health care resources than heart and cancer patients combined, and whereas mortality from heart disease and cancer is declining, the incidence from trauma is increasing [Boden&Galizzi 1999, Shires GT et al 1994].

Blunt trauma to the skull most frequently occurs as the result of the head being thrown against a solid or semisolid object, or an object being thrown directly at the head. Soft tissue injuries of the external auditory canal may occur with blunt trauma, particularly trauma that is glancing in nature, that is, delivered in a sharp angle to the side of the head as opposed to a 90-degree injury. Fractures of the middle ear structures, otic capsule, and structures surrounding the otic capsule may occur from blunt trauma. The most common form of temporal bone fracture, occurring from blunt trauma, is the longitudinal fracture of the temporal bone. It is estimated that 70% to 90% of temporal bone fractures are longitudinal (Cannon and Jahrsdoerfer, 1983; Dolan, 1989; Nelson, 1979). These fractures most commonly result from direct lateral blunt trauma to the skull in the parietal region of the head. In considering the effect of a fracture of the skull and its relationship to the temporal bone, it is helpful to think of the fracture occurring initially in a weaker portion of the calvarium, such as the squamous portion of the temporal bone, and the fracture line extending toward the temporal bone. Recognizing that the otic capsule is extremely dense bone, the fracture will occur around the otic capsule, taking the course of least resistance (Dahiya et al 1999. The course of least resistance usually involves major foramina in the skull base, the most common being that of the carotid artery and the jugular bulb. Fractures are frequently near the roof of the external auditory canal and run parallel along the petrous apex extending anteriorly to the foramen lacerum and the carotid artery. The line may also extend into the temporomandibular joint regions.

2. Methodology

This is a retrospective review of 64 patients seen at the Ear, Nose and Throat clinic and the accident and emergency unit of the University of Ilorin Teaching hospital, Ilorin, Nigeria over a ten year period between January 1998 to Dec 2007. The patients had history of bleeding from the ear due to trauma from various causes. Patients with multiple traumas were also included and these had traumatic tympanic membrane perforation as part of the presentation. The data retrieved included the bio-data, the clinical presentation, source of injury, the clinical findings and the outcome of the patients. These were entered into an SPSS version 11.0 computer soft ware and analyzed descriptively.

3. Results

Seventy patients were found to have traumatic tympanic membrane perforation. However 6 individuals were excluded because of incomplete data. Thus only 64 patients' records were analyzed and formed the basis for this study. Age range of the patients was between 6 months to 50 yrs with a mean age of 29.2yrs and modal age of 35 years. About 5 (7.9%) of them were ≤5years and majority of the patients were between 35 and 50years of age (Table 1).

There were 46 (71.9%) males and 18 (28.1%) females with a male to female ratio of 2.5:1. Males were affected in most of the aetiologies except in "fall" where no male patient was recorded (table 2).

The commonest aetiology for trauma was from slaps, followed by road traffic injury (RTI) in 35.9% and 23.5% patients, respectively (Table 3).

Majority of the slap injury were from fights, security agents, senior students and cultist synonymous with Gangsterism (group of criminals especially those who are armed and use guns or group of students acting as terrorists within the school system.)at schools in 30.5%, 17.4% and 17.4% respectively. (Table 4)

Traumatic tympanic membrane perforation affected 36 left ears and 28 right ears. Majority of the patients (95%) had associated sudden hearing loss. Tinnitus was present in 52% while 24 (37.5%) of the patients had progression to chronic suppurative otitis media (Table 5). It was observed that majority of the patients failed to follow up clinical visits once the symptoms of bleeding and pain had subsided. An average of three follow up visits per patient was recorded. Out of the few %that came for follow up check ups, only 7.8% had neo-membrane formation.

Age in years	**Number & Frequency (%)**
6months- 5yrs	5 (7.9%)
6years-10yrs	1 (1.6%)
11-20yrs	15 (23.5%)
21-34yrs	19 (29.7%)
35-64yrs	24 (37.7%)

Table 1. Age distribution of patients with traumatic TM perforations.

Predisposition	Number & Frequency Male	Female
Slap	15	08
Instrumentation	04	03
Self during ear cleaning	05	02
RTI	09	01
Foreign body	10	03
Explosion	03	
Fall		01
Total	46	18

Table 2. Predisposition and sex of patients.

Aetiology	Number &Frequency (%)
Slaps	23 (35.9%)
Instrumentations	7 (10.9%)
Self Ear cleaning	7 (10.9%)
Road Traffic Injury	15 (23.5%)
Foreign body	08 (12.5%)
Explosions	3 (4.7%)
Falls	1 (1.6%)

Table 3. Aetiological profile of TM perforations.

Sources of slap	Number & Frequency (%)
Security Agent	4 (17.4)
Assault from Fight	7 (30.5)
Spouse	2 (8.7)
Armed Robbery	3 (13.0)
Senior student/cultists	4 (17.4)
Sibling	3 (13.0)

Table 4. Sources of Slaps.

4. Discussion

Trauma to the ear can be classified on the basis onf the anatomical location or the type of injury. This could be a simple blunt trauma to the pinna; laceration of the pinna, avulsion of part or the whole of the pinna; tympanic membrane perforation; dislocation of the ossicles; longitudinal and transverse fractures of the petrous temporal bone with associated loss of inner ear and facial nerve function (Ologe FE 2002, Toner JG & Kerr AG 1997, Okafor BC 1983, Ijaduola GTA 1986, Bhattia PL 1987, Ladapo AA 1979, Ijaduola GTA and Okeowo PA 1986). Previous studies have shown that trauma to the tympanic membrane and the middle ear can be caused by overpressure (slap, fight, assault from security agents and road traffic injury (RTI)), thermal or caustic burns, blunt or penetrating injuries such as instruments and barotraumas (Mitchell K. S 2003, da Lilly-Tariah OB and Somefun OA 2007). Overpressure is by far the most common mechanism of trauma to the tympanic membrane (Mitchell K. S 2003) in our environment. Traumatic perforation of the tympanic membrane may be caused by direct impact of fluids and direct pressure from outside.

The tympanic membrane (TM) is an important component of sound conduction as its vibratory characteristic is necessary for sound transmission in human beings (Richard R. G and Mark R.G 2003)

Traumatic tympanic membrane perforation findings from our study are similar to findings elsewhere from the world (Ologe FE 2002, Mitchell K. S 2003, da Lilly-Tariah OB and Somefun OA 2007). Male to female ratio was found to be 2.5:1 with high predominance among males (72%). This is expected, as trauma is more common in this group of patients similar to other reported series (Ologe FE 2002, da Lilly-Tariah OB and Somefun OA 2007, Richard R. G and Mark R.G 2003). Our study of injury site indicated that the left ear is at a higher risk than the right ear in the ratio of 1.0:1.3 right to left which could be associated with the fact that most assailants were right handed, Thus it is likely that most of the acts of trauma such as slap occurred with the assailant and victims were facing each other making the left ear to be predominantly affected compared to the right side. Some of the causes of overpressure include slap injuries and blast injuries. Slap injuries are extremely common and can be result of either a hand or water slap and these injuries usually result in a triangular or linear tear of the TM (Mitchell K. S 2003). These slap injuries could be a product of fight or armed robbery attack. However, in our study it was found to be more common among the youth. In more than 50%of cases reviewed and those in the adult these cases were due to attack by the armed robbers or security agents. This was the highest cause of traumatic tympanic membrane perforation in our study as compared to a similar study in other regions of Nigeria where fight with spouse was the commonest aetiology recorded (da Lilly-Tariah OB and Somefun OA 2007). In contrast this type of injury made the least contribution in our study.

Slaps were the commonest type of violence seen between individuals, mostly between security agents and the offender followed by those among students. However, another study found tympanic membrane perforation resulting from slap from marital conflict between wife and husband (Mitchell K. S 2003). There is a need to educate the students and security agents on other punitive measure as there is predisposition to conductive hearing loss or an imminent chronic suppurative otitis media if not properly managed. Slap was commoner among males than in females similar to another study (Mitchell K. S 2003). Trauma to the temporal bone with fracture and leakage of cerebrospinal fluid into the middle ear causing conductive hearing losses was second common in this study and this was found to be secondary to road traffic injury. The management protocol for skull base fracture with TM perforation/CSF leakage does not require any intervention based on

Otolaryngologist perspective to avoid contamination with an ascending infection. This was also found to be higher among male subjects compared to the females, perhaps associated with the role of males in African society as the bread winners, working outside home and thus are at a higher risk of various type of traffic injuries compared to women who predominantly stay at home. Attempt at removing foreign body, ear cleaning with variety of objects including cotton bud and wax removal in an unskilled manner either by the parents or the primary care physician with TM perforation was an important cause of hearing loss found mostly among children as previously reported (Ologe FE 2002, Toner JG & Kerr AG 1997, Ladapo AA 1979, Ijaduola GTA and Okeowo PA 1986). There is a need for a primary care physician to provide patients with appropriate referral. Explosion is not a common phenomenon in our environment as the violence rate is still at a low level. Fall with perforation of tympanic membrane is an uncommon occurrence which has never been reported but was observed in a child, however the mechanism could not be explained.

Traumatic perforations often occur in healthy members of the community with generally an excellent prognosis (Toner JG & Kerr AG 1997, Ijaduola GTA 1986). Healing with formation of neomembrane was observed only in five patients (7.8%) and it is among the under five's this is not surprising as they are still growing.

5. Conclusion

Traumatic perforation of the tympanic membrane is still common in our environment. It affects all age groups, with more males affected than females. Slaps and RTI are the commonest aetiologies seen. The left ear is affected more than the right and sudden hearing loss is the most common presentation. There is a need to educate the students and security agents on alternative punitive measures and to discourage the act of unskilled removal of foreign body from the ear. Early identification, evaluation and referral of patients by primary care physician who see these patients will reduce the attendant morbidity.

6. References

[1] Bhattia, P.L. and Varughese,R. Pattern of Otolaryngological Diseases in Jos Community. Nig.Med.J. 1987; 17: 67-73.

[2] Boden LI, Galizzi M. Economic consequences of workplace injuries and illnesses: lost earnings and benefit adequacy. Am J Ind Med 1999;36:487–503.

[3] Capo JM, Lucente FE. Alkaline battery foreign bodies of the ear and nose. Arch Otolaryngol Head Neck Surg 1986;112:562–3.

[4] Challenges for the 21st century Chronic disabling conditions NATIONAL ACADEMY ON AN AGING SOCIETY 1999;2:1-6

[5] Dahiya R, Keller JD, Litofsky NS, Bankey PE, Bonassar LJ, Megerian CA. Temporal bone fractures: otic capsule sparing versus otic capsule violating clinical and radiographic considerations. . J Trauma. 1999 Dec;47(6):1079-83

[6] da Lilly-Tariah OB, Somefun AO, Traumatic perforation of the tympanic membrane in University of Port Harcourt Teaching Hospital, Port Harcourt. Nigeria., Niger Postgrad Med J. 2007; 14 (2):121-4.

[7] Ghoyareb B.Y, Yeakly J.W, Hall J.W, Jones E, Unusual complication of temporal bone fracture. Archive of otolaryngology head and Neck surgery. 1987;113: 749-53
[8] Gibson WR. Essentials of clinical electric response audiometry. Edinburgh: Churchill Livingstone, 1978: 133–56.
[9] Ijaduola, G. T.A. The Principles of Management of Deafness. Nig. Med. Pract. 1986; 12: 19-25.
[10] Ijaduola, G. T.A.; Okeowo P.A. Foreign body in the Ear and its importance: The Nigerian Experience. J. Trop. Paed. 1986; 32: 4-6
[11] Kavanagh KT, Litovitz T. Miniature battery foreign odies in auditory and nasal cavities. JAMA 1986; 255:1470–2
[12] Ladapo,A.A. Danger of foreign body in the ear Nig.Med. J. 1979; 9(1): 120-122.
[13] Lee KJ. Essential Otolaryngology- Head and neck surgery, 7th edition, Stamford. Appleton and Lange, 1995: 1- 66.
[14] Miller TR, Waehrer GM. Costs of occupational injuries to teenagers, United States. Inj Prev 1998;4:211–217.
[15] Mitchell KS 2003 Trauma to the Middle Ear, Inner Ear, and Temporal Bone in 2003: 14 ; 345-356 Ballenger's Otorhinolaryngology Head and Neck Surgery James B. Snow Jr, John Jacob Ballenger Sixteenth Edition BC Decker ISBN 1-55009-197-2 Inc Hamilton, Ontario L8N 3K7, Spain
[16] Ogren FP, Edmunds AL. Neuro-otologic findings in the lightning-injured patient. Semin Neurol 1995; 15:256–62.)
[17] Okafor, B. C. Otolaryngology in South Eastern Nigeria I: Pattern of Diseases of the Ear.Nig.Med.J. 1983; 13: 11-19.
[18] Ologe FE, Traumatic perforation of tympanic membrane in Ilorin, Nigeria Nig. J. Surg. 2002, Vol. 8 (1) :9-12
[19] Panosian MS, Dutcher PO. Transtympanic facial nerve injury in welders. Occup Med (Lond) 1994; 44:99–101).
[20] Peter JK, Paul HK, Principle of trauma in Byron J Bailey Head and Neck Surgery - Otolaryngology 3rd edition Byron J, Karen H, Gerald B, Harold C, Jonas T, M. Eugene, Robert K, Anthony Pazos, Chri Gralapp Lippincott Williams & Wilkins Publishers 2001;61 :69 of 202.
[21] Podoshin L, Fradis M, Hearing loss after head injury. Archives of Otolaryngology. 1975;101:15-8
[22] Richard R. Gacek, Mark R. Gacek, Anatomy of the Auditory and Vestibular Systems, Ballenger's Otorhinolaryngology Head and Neck Surgery Sixteenth Edition James B. Snow Jr, John Jacob Ballenger published by DC Becker Inc, Ontario, 2003; 1: 1-5.
[23] Roger FG, Maurice H. Synopsis of Otolaryngology, 5th edition, London. Butterworth-Heinemann Ltd.,1992: 3- 80.
[24] Shires GT, Thal ER, Jones RC, et al. Trauma. In: Schwartz SI, ed. Principles of surgery, 6th ed. New York: McGraw-Hill, 1994:175–224.
[25] Stanley A. Gelfand, Anatomy and Physiology of Auditory system in Essential of Audiology third edition thieme publisher, New York 2009 ;2: 77-78 google book assessed on 12/1/2012)

[26] Toner, J. G. and Kerr A. G. Ear Trauma. Scott- Brown's Otolaryngology. Otology 6th Edition Edited by J. B. Booth, General Editor Kerr, A. G. Advisory Editor Groves,J. Butterworths Meinemann, London 1997: 3/711-3/7/13.

9

Occupational Chemical-Induced Hearing Loss

Adrian Fuente[1] and Bradley McPherson[2]
[1]*The University of Queensland*
[2]*The University of Hong Kong*
[1]*Australia*
[2]*China*

1. Introduction

Exposure to chemicals in the workplace can lead to occupational chemical-induced hearing loss, as many chemicals have been internationally recognised as hazardous to hearing. A number of studies have demonstrated that, similar to noise, some chemicals not only affect the sensory organ of the auditory system (the cochlea) but also lead to adverse effects in central auditory structures. Morata and Lemasters (1995) suggested that the adverse auditory effects of chemicals such as solvents are due to a combination of oto-and neuro-toxicity. Oto-toxicity induces outer hair cell (OHC) dysfunction in the cochlea (similar to the effects of noise), whereas neuro-toxicity induces central auditory dysfunction. The main audiological sign of oto-toxicity is poorer hearing thresholds than expected relative to age. Audiological signs of neuro-toxicity may or may not include poorer hearing thresholds, in addition to difficulties discriminating sounds, such as speech, particularly in adverse listening conditions.

The aim of this review is to provide an in-depth discussion of occupational chemical-induced hearing loss, taking into consideration ototoxic agents such as solvents, pesticides and metals, and their interaction with noise. Contemporary findings from research conducted in animals and humans are included here. Also, research findings from the authors with regard to the effect of exposure to mixtures of solvents on the peripheral and central auditory system will be addressed. Finally, in the section on international legislation of occupational chemical-induced hearing loss, a review of current legislation in a number of countries is presented.

2. Solvent-induced hearing loss

2.1 Overview of solvents

A solvent is a liquid used to dissolve other substances. Most solvents are colourless liquids at room temperature that volatise easily and have strong odours. Solvents are most commonly inhaled in their volatised form and absorbed through the respiratory tract. Organic solvents are widely used around the world and many different industrial processes require their use. Table 1 summarises the main organic solvents and their common industrial uses.

Organic solvent	Industrial uses
Toluene	Electroplating, adhesive manufacture, laboratory chemicals, metal degreasing, paint manufacture, paint stripping, paper coating, pharmaceuticals manufacture, printing, rubber manufacture, wood stains and varnishes, and footwear manufacture.
Styrene	Fabrication of fibreglass boats, pulp and paper manufacture and in plastics, resins, coatings, and paint manufacture.
Xylene	Laboratory chemicals, machinery manufacture and repair, paint manufacture, paint stripping, paper coating, pesticide manufacture, pharmaceuticals manufacture, printing, rubber manufacture, and in wood stains and varnishes.
Ethyl benzene	Machinery manufacture and repair, paint manufacture, paper coating, rubber manufacture, wood stains and varnishes.
Trichloroethylene	Electroplating, integrated iron and steel manufacture, machinery manufacture and repair, metal degreasing, pulp and paper manufacture.

Table 1. Main industrial uses of some selected organic solvents.

2.2 Evidence of the adverse auditory effects of solvents from animal studies

Organic solvents such as toluene, styrene, xylene, and ethyl benzene have been identified as inducing damage to the outer hair cells (OHCs) in the cochlea of experimental animals (Campo et al., 1997; Cappaert et al., 1999; Cappaert et al., 2000; Crofton et al., 1994; Johnson & Canlon, 1994; Loquet et al., 1999; McWilliams et al., 2000; Pryor et al., 1987; Sullivan et al., 1988; Yano et al., 1992). The damage caused by these solvents in its early stages occurs in the third row of external OHCs and it then progresses toward the second and first rows. The mid-range of audible frequencies for the rat is affected first and according to some authors the damage continues toward the apical zone of the cochlea (Campo et al., 1997; Johnson & Canlon, 1994). The damage impacts mainly at the mid-frequency region of experimental animal cochleae, and this distinguishes the auditory effects induced by solvents such as toluene from those observed with ototoxic drugs such as aminoglycoside antibiotics and cisplatin (Liu et al., 1997) which mainly affect the apical region of the cochlea.

In the case of trichloroethylene, cochlear histopathology has revealed loss of spiral ganglion cells, mainly in the middle turn, and also an inconsistent loss of hair cells (Fechter et al., 1998).

Rebert et al. (1995) observed an increase in auditory brainstem response (ABR) latencies in rats after exposure by inhalation to pairs of solvents (trichloroethylene and toluene; xylene and trichloroethylene; xylene and chlorobenzene; chlorobenzene and toluene). Results of this study indicated an additive rather than a synergistic or antagonistic interaction. Other studies have also demonstrated additive ototoxic effects for styrene and trichloroethanol (Rebert et al., 1993), and styrene and ethanol (Loquet et al., 2000). This additive effect, as opposed to the synergistic effect found with combinations of solvents, implies that the mechanism of ototoxicity for these solvents may be similar.

Research has also demonstrated that rats simultaneously exposed to both toluene and noise suffer a more severe hearing loss than the summated hearing loss obtained from an equivalent exposure level to each agent alone (Brandt-Lassen et al., 2000; Lataye & Campo, 1997). The synergistic interaction between noise and toluene occurs when both agents are presented simultaneously, or when toluene is immediately followed by noise. Lataye & Campo (1997) claimed that even if the coexistence of both mechanisms (the ototoxicity induced by toluene and that induced by noise) potentiates cochlear effects, it seems nevertheless that there are no other mechanisms induced by a simultaneous exposure to noise and toluene. Combined exposure to noise and styrene in rats has also shown the existence of synergism between these two agents (Lataye et al., 2000; Makitie et al., 2003).

Evidence from Lataye et al. (2005) suggests that conditions such as level of activity of the rats may be an important factor in the mechanism of styrene-induced hearing loss. The researchers found that the same degree of styrene-induced hearing loss can be obtained by using concentrations approximately 200 ppm lower in active rats than in sedentary rats. This may explain why the studies conducted in experimental animals require higher solvent concentrations to induce hearing loss than in humans. Workers are not sedentary in the workplace. They usually are moving from one place to another, or manipulating machinery. Increased activity implies greater consumption of oxygen compared to sedentary conditions. The study of Lataye et al. (2005) has provided some explanation for the variations in concentrations that are needed to induce auditory dysfunction in experimental animals and humans. In animal models it is possible to control most of the variables; however, in humans many factors such as physical activity cannot be controlled experimentally.

Lataye et al. (2007) found a striking increase (4.2 dB) in the cochlear microphonic potential amplitude which was followed after left-carotid administration of toluene in experimental animals. An increase in the cochlear microphonic potential relates to the inhibition of the efferent control of the OHCs, and thus a lack of inhibition in the mechanical response of the OHCs to electrical signals. Lataye et al. (2007) suggested that toluene inhibits the acetylcholine (Ach) receptors located in the efferent auditory system (medial olivocochlear bundle) that mediates the contraction of the OHCs in the cochlea. Similarly, Campo et al. (2007) found that toluene may inhibit the Ach receptors of the efferent motor neurons located near the facial nerve nuclei that mediate the middle ear muscle systems. These two studies represent the first evidence from animal models that solvents may induce central auditory dysfunction at the level of the efferent auditory system.

In summary animal data demonstrates that solvents in isolation can induce OHC loss, and in the case of trichloroethylene, spiral ganglion cell loss—mainly in the middle turn of the cochlea—is observed. Also, it has been observed that solvents such as toluene adversely affect the efferent auditory system associated with the control of the contraction of the OHCs as well as with the mediation of the middle ear acoustic reflex. Synergism between solvents and noise has been observed in rats.

2.3 Evidence of the adverse effects of solvents on pure-tone thresholds: Studies on humans

Exposure to a mixture of solvents may induce hearing loss in humans (Morata, Engel et al., 1997) and, at some frequencies, solvents may damage the inner ear to a much greater extent than noise exposure (Sliwinska-Kowalska et al., 2000). Hearing loss induced by solvents has been found in workers exposed to a mixture of toluene, ethyl acetate and ethanol (Morata, Engel et al., 1997), and xylene and ethyl acetate (Sliwinska-Kowalska et al., 2000). Sliwinska-Kowalska et al. (2000) found hearing loss in 30% of workers exposed to organic solvents, in 20% of noise-exposed subjects, and in only 6% of non-exposed subjects. The relative risk value for hearing loss in workers exposed to solvents was greater (RR=9.6) in comparison to workers exposed only to noise (RR=4.2). Sulkowski et al. (2002) found high frequency sensorineural hearing loss in 42% of workers exposed to a mixture of solvents (not specified by the authors). In contrast, only 5% of the subjects in the control group (age-matched non-exposed subjects) showed hearing loss. Studies in populations of workers mainly exposed to one type of solvent have been also conducted. High frequency (8-16 kHz) hearing loss has been suggested to be associated with styrene dose exposure in humans. In the study of Muijser et al. (1988), high frequency hearing thresholds were significantly increased in those workers with the greatest exposure to styrene. Also, Morata et al. (2002) found an additive damage effect of styrene for pure-tone thresholds at 2, 3, 4 and 6 kHz. The odds ratio for hearing loss estimated by Morata et al. (2002) was 2.44 times greater for each increment of 1 mmol of mandelic acid (a biologic marker of styrene exposure) per gram of creatinine in urine. Morata et al. (2002) suggested that styrene can affect the mid-audiometric frequency of 2 kHz, which is in agreement to the findings of Sliwinska-Kowalska et al. (2001). Morata et al. (2002) also stated that styrene even below recommended values had a toxic effect on the auditory system.

Sliwinska-Kowalska et al. (2003) found a 4-fold increase in the odds of developing hearing loss in subjects exposed to styrene. In this study the mean hearing thresholds (adjusted for age, gender, and exposure to noise) were significantly higher in a solvent-exposed group than in an unexposed reference group at all frequencies tested. A positive linear relationship was observed between average working life exposure to styrene concentrations and hearing thresholds at 6 and 8 kHz. Also, the effects of carbon disulphide on hearing have been explored (Morata, 1989). Results of pure-tone audiometry indicated a 66.7% prevalence of hearing loss among exposed workers and only 6.6% of this was attributed to non-occupational causes (Morata, 1989).

The possible synergism of combined exposure to solvents and noise on hearing has not been consistently identified in human studies. Some researchers have failed to find a synergistic effect between these agents on hearing. Jacobsen et al. (1993) in a cohort study showed a dominant effect of noise and no additional hearing risk as a result of solvent exposure. However, workers exposed only to solvents had a significantly increased risk ratio for hearing loss. Sliwinska-Kowalska et al. (2001), in a study conducted involving paint and lacquer factory workers, were not able to show any additional risk of hearing loss with a combined exposure to noise and a mixture of organic solvents, when compared with isolated exposure to solvents only. However, Polizzi et al. (2003) reported a case of a painter exposed to noise and a mixture of organic solvents. The authors described an unusual pattern of hearing loss, which was characterised by a maximum loss in the low and mid-frequencies. The researchers suggested that this pattern may be induced by a possible synergistic effect of noise exposure combined with solvents. However, this finding may have limited application as the data was collected from a single subject. Other evidence supporting the claim that solvents in combination with noise may have a synergistic effect on the auditory system in humans was reported by Sliwinska-Kowalska et al. (2003). They found an increase in the odds ratio for hearing loss of 21.5 in workers exposed to styrene, toluene, and noise. These authors suggested that a synergistic action of multiple ototoxic agents with noise was evident.

A recent multicentre, cross-sectional study (Morata et al. 2011) of workers from Sweden, Finland, and Poland found an association between styrene exposure and poorer hearing thresholds than predicted by individuals' age (when compared with ANSI S3.44 annexes A and B). The effect of noise exposure, with a mean which varied across centres between 80 and 84 dBA, did not have a significant effect on hearing, except when in combination with styrene.

Hearing loss induced by simultaneous exposure to noise and mixed solvents in the aviation industry was studied by Kim et al. (2005). This study found a prevalence of hearing loss of 54.9% among workers exposed to both agents simultaneously; 17.1% among workers exposed only to noise; 27.8% among workers only exposed to a solvent mixture; and 6% among non-exposed workers. Relative risks adjusted for age were estimated to be 4.3 for the noise-only group, 8.1 for the noise and solvents group, and 2.6 for the solvents-mixture group. Also, Kaufman et al. (2005) found that subjects exposed to noise and jet fuel for three years had an increase in adjusted odds for hearing loss (RR=1.7), and in those with a history of 12 years exposed to both agents the odds for hearing loss increased to 2.41. This study found that the effects of jet fuel exposure on hearing were statistically non-significant for more than 12 years of combined noise and jet fuel exposure. The authors suggested a plateau effect for jet fuel exposure and/or that the noise-induced hearing loss may become more important for those continuing to have exposure to both agents.

All these studies provide evidence that solvents may induce peripheral hearing loss in human subjects. However, none of the previously mentioned studies provides evidence of central auditory dysfunction induced by solvent exposure or of the precise cochlear origin of such hearing losses. They only suggest poorer hearing thresholds among solvent-exposed subjects in comparison to non-exposed subjects. Next we discuss the scientific evidence for central auditory dysfunction associated with solvent exposure.

2.4 Evidence of the adverse effects of solvents on the central auditory system: Studies on humans

Many studies have found dysfunction of the central auditory nervous system (CANS) in workers exposed to a mixture of solvents (Fuente et al., 2006; Fuente & McPherson, 2007; Laukli and Hansen, 1995; Moen et al., 1999; Niklasson et al., 1998; Ödkvist et al., 1987; Ödkvist et al.,1992; Pollastrini et al., 1994; Varney et al., 1998). Fuente et al. (2006), Fuente & McPherson (2007), and Fuente (2008) have shown that workers exposed to a mixture of solvents (toluene, xylene and methyl ethyl ketone) may acquire central auditory dysfunction as evidenced by abnormal results for a set of behavioural central auditory processing tests. Varney, Kubu et al. (1998) found abnormal results for a dichotic listening test among solvent exposed subjects in comparison to previously reported norms and to a control group of subjects. The authors claimed that dichotic listening appeared to be a useful tool in the assessment of solvent-exposed workers, particularly in those who have had intermediate levels of exposure and who do not show mental status deficits of disabling severity.

Also, different studies have been conducted in workers exposed to solvents utilising electrophysiological techniques. Workers exposed to toluene obtained statistically significant higher absolute latencies and inter-peak latencies (IPL) between waves of the ABR (I-III IPL; I-V IPL; III-V IPL) than a non-exposed group of workers matched for gender and age (Abbate et al., 1993). Additional evidence of toluene-induced central auditory dysfunction in humans using ABR was shown by Vrca et al. (1996). Workers exposed to low concentrations of toluene obtained a significant decrease in all wave amplitudes of auditory evoked potentials. However, a study carried out by Schäper et al. (2003) did not find a toluene effect on ABR results in a group of workers exposed to toluene up to 50 parts per million (ppm). The authors suggested that toluene may induce central auditory dysfunction at levels above 50 ppm.

ABR abnormalities due to carbon disulphide exposure have also been studied (Hirata et al., 1992). A high percentage of workers exposed to carbon disulphide for more than 240 months obtained prolonged IPL for the ABR components III-V (Hirata et al., 1992). Other electrophysiological measures such as P300 (a long latency auditory evoked potential) have also been utilised in solvent-exposed subjects. Vrca et al. (1997) found, in a group of workers exposed to low concentrations of toluene, prolonged latencies and lower amplitudes in the P300 response in comparison to a control group. Also, Moen et al. (1999) examined the P300 component in a group of workers exposed to low levels of organic solvents in a paint factory and in a control group of non-exposed workers. The results indicated that the P300 latency was prolonged among the exposed workers compared to the control group before the summer vacation, and also, in the exposed group the P300 latency was significantly longer before the summer vacation than after. Similar results were found by Steinhauer et al. (1997).

More recently, Draper and Bamiou (2008) presented a case study of a person exposed to xylene who presented with auditory neuropathy as evidenced by abnormal ABR results and presence of otoacoustic emissions (OAEs). The patient presented with a gradual deterioration in his ability to hear in difficult acoustic environments and also to hear complex sounds such as music, over a 40-year period. His symptoms began after exposure to xylene, and in the absence of any other risk factor.

Fuente et al. (2011) conducted an investigation of central auditory functioning in normal-hearing, solvent-exposed subjects compared to normal-hearing, non-exposed subjects with a comprehensive battery of behavioural central auditory function assessment procedures. Forty-six normal-hearing, solvent-exposed subjects and 46 normal-hearing, non-exposed subjects were investigated. The test battery comprised of pure-tone audiometry (PTA), Dichotic Digits (DD), Pitch Pattern Sequence (PPS), Filtered Speech (FS), Random Gap Detection (RGD), Masking Level Difference (MLD), and Hearing-in-Noise (HINT) tests. Analyses of covariance were performed to compare the mean values of the dependent variables (results for DD, PPS, FS, RGD, MLD, and HINT) between solvent-exposed and non-exposed subjects. Age and average hearing thresholds (500-8000 Hz) were included in the analyses as covariates. Although all subjects had normal-hearing thresholds, significant differences for DD, PPS, FS, and RGD results were found between groups. Solvent-exposed participants presented with poorer results adjusted for age and hearing thresholds in comparison to non-exposed subjects.

These results are in agreement with our previous studies in which significant differences between solvent-exposed and non-exposed subjects arose for the DD, RGD, HINT, PPS, and FS tests. Fuente et al. (2008) also showed that in a group of 100 workers exposed to a mixture of solvents and 100 non-exposed workers, solvents were significantly associated with poorer pure-tone thresholds, lower amplitudes of transient evoked otoacoustic emissions (TEOAEs), and poorer results for central auditory functioning tests. Recently, in a study investigating a group of 30 medical laboratory workers exposed to xylene and a control group of non-exposed workers, Fuente (2010) found significant differences between groups for ABR results. Xylene-exposed workers presented with longer ABR latencies than non-exposed workers. Figure 1 summarises the results of our studies in different populations of workers exposed to solvents.

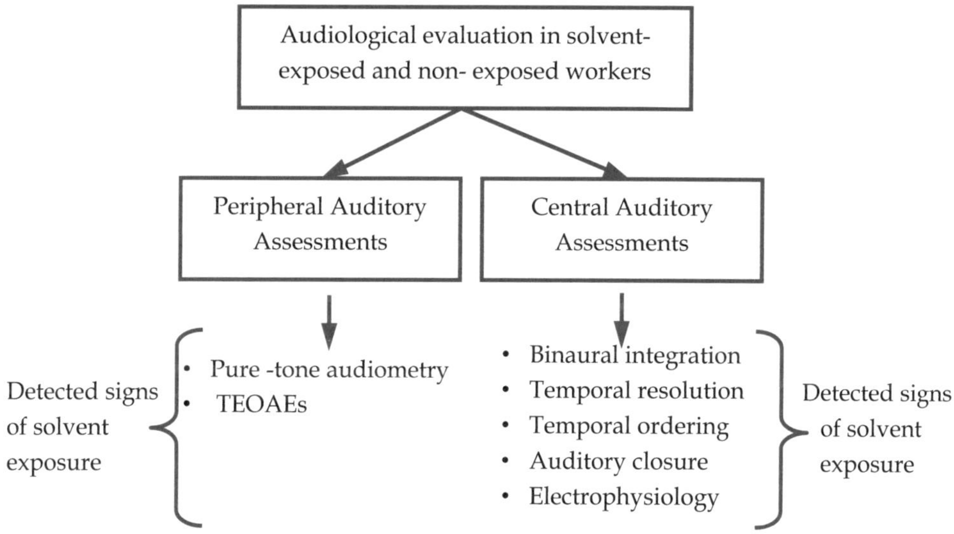

Fig. 1. Summary of audiological findings in solvent-exposed subjects from Fuente 2008, 2010) and Fuente et al. studies (2006, 2007, 2009, 2011).

From Figure 1, it is possible to observe that different procedures can be utilised to evaluate possible adverse auditory effects of solvents on the auditory system. Taking into consideration that solvents may affect a wide range of aspects of audition, an approach using a comprehensive battery of tests is required to monitor hearing in solvent-exposed individuals. Table 2 summarises the audiological procedures that can be incorporated in the test battery to evaluate solvent-induced auditory dysfunction. The tests that have been included in Table 2 are those who have been shown to be sensitive to detect differences between solvent exposed and non-exposed subjects, based on our previous studies and on the evidence provided by multiple studies, as discussed above.

Procedure	Auditory-related aspects	Procedure references
Pure-tone audiometry	Hearing thresholds from 125 Hz to 8000 Hz.	Gelfand, 2001.
OAEs	OHCs status. Differential diagnosis sensory / neural hearing loss.	Stach, 1998
ABR	Status of the brainstem auditory pathways. Differential diagnosis sensory/neural hearing loss.	Arnold, 2000
Filtered speech	Low redundancy monaural speech discrimination.	Bellis, 2003 Wilson & Mueller, 1984
Random gap detection	Temporal processes (temporal resolution).	Bellis, 2003 Keith, 2000 Keith, 2002
Pitch pattern sequence	Temporal processes.	Bellis, 2003 Musiek, 1994
Dichotic digits	Dichotic stimulation.	Bellis, 2003 Musiek, 1983 a,b
Hearing-in-noise test (HINT)	Speech discrimination in the presence of background noise. Functional assessment of hearing disability.	Nilsson et al., 1994 Laroche et al., 2003

Table 2. Recommended audiological tests for the evaluation of hearing in solvent-exposed subjects.

3. Hearing loss associated with occupational exposure to pesticides

3.1 Overview of pesticides

The Food and Agriculture Organization (FAO, 2003, Page 6) has defined pesticides as "any substance or mixture of substances intended for preventing, destroying or controlling any pest, including vectors of human or animal disease, unwanted species of plants or animals causing harm during or otherwise interfering with the production, processing, storage, transport or marketing of food, agricultural commodities, wood and wood products or animal feedstuffs, or substances which may be administered to animals for the control of insects, arachnids or other pests in or on their bodies. The term includes substances intended for use as a plant growth regulator, defoliant, desiccant or agent for thinning fruit or preventing the premature fall of fruit, and substances applied to crops either before or after harvest to protect the commodity from deterioration during storage and transport".

Most pesticides can be classified into chemical families. Table 3 summarises the four main chemical categories of pesticides according to the US Environmental Protection Agency. Pesticides are also often referred to according to the type of pest they control (e.g. fungicides, herbicides, insecticides, rodenticides).

Pesticide	Main characteristics
Organophosphates	Developed in the 19th century and extensively used in World War II as nerve agents. Most commonly used pesticides today and mainly insecticides. Affect the nervous system of the target agent.
Carbamates	First introduced in the 1950s. Affect the nervous system of the target agent.
Organochlorides	Extensively used in the past 60 years. Organochloride pesticides such as dichloro-diphenyl-trichloroethane (DDT) have been widely banned as they represent serious environmental and human health risks.
Pyrethroids	Developed for wide commercial use in the 1970s. They are used as insecticides in gardens, and with pets and livestock.

Table 3. Main chemical families of pesticides and their characteristics.

3.2 Scientific evidence of pesticide-induced auditory dysfunction

Studies on the auditory effects of exposure to pesticides are rare. Harell et al. (1978) were one of the first research groups to describe pesticide-induced hearing loss. The authors reported a case of a 27-year-old male who was referred for a re-evaluation of his bilateral hearing loss. The onset of his hearing loss was more than six years before the follow-up hearing assessment, and it developed after he sprayed several fruit trees for 15-20 minutes using a preparation containing 7.5% malathion and 15% methoxychlor. After intoxication with low levels of insecticides, the patient developed a permanent bilateral profound hearing loss with the presence of tinnitus, and also peripheral neuropathies in the extremities. Other initial signs such as renal failure and hepatic dysfunction gradually improved.

A number of cross-sectional human studies have found hearing loss associated with the use of insecticides. A study comparing two groups of individuals exposed to organophosphates with different levels of pseudocholinesterase activity reported peripheral neuropathies in the group with low values of pseudocholinesterase. Pseudocholinesterase is an enzyme involved in the breakdown of acetylcholine and it is mainly found in the plasma and liver. Reduced plasma levels of pseudocholinesterase are an indicator of excessive organophosphate absorption. Both groups of individuals with low and high levels of pseudocholinesterase had sensorineural hearing loss, ranging in severity from low to moderate (Ernest et al., 1995).

Mac Crawford et al. (2008) investigated self-reported hearing loss in licensed private pesticide applicators enrolled in the Agricultural Health Study in 1993-1997 in Iowa and North Carolina, USA. Results showed that exposure to herbicides, fungicides, or fumigants was not associated with hearing loss. However, organophosphates were associated with hearing loss, with a 17% increase in odds in the highest quartile of exposure. Carbamates, organochlorines and pyrethroids were not associated with hearing loss. The authors also found a positive association between self-reported hearing loss and several general measures of pesticide exposure such as high pesticide exposure events, pesticide poisoning and medical treatment for pesticide exposure. Additionally, the association of pesticide exposure with hearing loss was not modified or confounded by age. The authors concluded that the results of their study suggest that exposure to insecticides and, in particular, organophosphates, may contribute to hearing loss.

Guida et al. (2010) studied 40 male individuals exposed to malathion and noise and 40 individuals exposed only to noise. Individuals exposed to malathion and noise presented with significantly worse hearing thresholds for 4 kHz (both ears) and 3 kHz (left ear) than individuals exposed only to noise. Also, more than 60% of individuals exposed to malathion and noise had hearing loss in comparison to 42% of individuals exposed only to noise.

Adverse central auditory effects associated with insecticide exposure have also been found. Teixeira et al. (2002) studied a group of 98 male workers with a minimum of 3 years insecticide exposure who used organophosphate and pyrethroid compounds, and a control non-exposed group of 54 administrative workers. The insecticide-exposed workers were divided into two subgroups, insecticide-exposed only, and insecticide-and-noise-exposed (with noise levels above 90 dBA). Two procedures to evaluate central auditory function were utilised, the pitch pattern sequence (PPS) and duration pattern sequence (DPS) tests. Results showed that 56% of insecticide-exposed workers had findings for PPS and/or DPS below normal ranges, and only 7% of the control non-exposed workers had results below normal ranges, for the DPS test only. Statistically significant differences for PPS and DPS test results between insecticide only exposed workers and control non-exposed workers, and also between insecticide-and noise-exposed workers and control non-exposed workers were found. Insecticide-exposed workers performed significantly worse than non-exposed control workers in both PPS and DPS tests. Teixeira et al. (2002) concluded that chronic exposure to pyrethroid and organophosphate insecticides seems to affect central auditory function. They also suggested that central auditory functioning tests should be incorporated in the audiological evaluation of persons exposed to known neurotoxic substances.

4. Hearing loss associated with occupational exposure to metals

4.1 Overview of metals

Currently there are 86 known metals. Before the 19th century only 24 of these metals had been discovered. Metals are used in their pure forms, in the form of compounds of two or more metals (alloys), and in the form of metal salts. Table 4 summarises the industrial uses of some common selected metals.

Metal	Industrial uses
Copper	Power generation and transmission of electricity, electrical wires, roofing and plumbing, and industrial machinery.
Lead	Car batteries, ballast keel of sailboats and scuba diving weight belts, soldering and as electrodes in the process of electrolysis, polyvinyl chloride (PVC) plastic that covers electrical cords, glazing bars for stained glass or other multi-lit windows.
Mercury	Manufacture of industrial chemicals, electronic applications, cosmetics, manufacturing of thermometers and fluorescent lamps, medical applications such as dental amalgams, as part of preservatives in vaccines, and topical antiseptics.
Zinc	Galvanization, manufacturing of batteries, in copper-base alloys. Manufacture of zinc sheets to be used for sheathing or roofing.
Lithium	Manufacture of batteries, ceramics, glass and pharmaceuticals. In rubber and thermoplastics industries, air treatment and in primary aluminium production.

Table 4. Main industrial uses of some selected metals.

4.2 Scientific evidence of metal-induced auditory dysfunction

Evidence from animal studies suggests ototoxic effects may be induced by lead. Lasky et al. (1995) in a study conducted in monkeys found abnormal distortion product otoacoustic emissions and lower than normal ABR amplitudes in monkeys with the highest blood concentrations of lead.

Hirata and Kosaka (1993) studied a group of lead exposed human subjects and a control non-exposed group through ABR, among other tests. Results showed that the mean IPL between components III and V of the ABR of lead-exposed workers was significantly prolonged compared with that of the control group.

Counter and Buchanan (2002) studied ABR and pure-tone thresholds as biomarkers for neuro-ototoxicity in adult workers with chronic lead intoxication from long-term exposure in ceramic-glazing work. Blood samples collected from 30 subjects showed higher biological concentrations than the limits established by the World Health Organization (WHO). Sensorineural hearing loss for the frequencies 2, 3, 4, 6, and 8 kHz was found among lead-exposed workers. ABR results showed delayed absolute latencies consistent with sensorineural hearing loss among individuals with elevated blood lead. Counter and Buchanan (2002) concluded that noise and lead intoxication were the cause of the hearing loss observed in the sample of subjects studied.

Buchanan et al. (1999) investigated pure-tone thresholds and distortion product otoacoustic emissions (DPOAEs) in 14 children (28 ears) and 5 adults (10 ears) living in a highly lead-contaminated environment in remote villages in the Andes Mountains of Ecuador. Blood lead levels for the children were higher than the U.S. Centers for Disease Control and Prevention's toxic level. Results showed normal hearing thresholds and presence of

DPOAEs. No correlation of DPOAEs with blood lead level was found among the children. The group of adults had diminished DPOAEs which were consistent with noise-related hearing loss.

Murata et al. (1993) examined ABR and event-related potential (P300) recordings, along with non-audiological assessments in lead workers. The sample consisted of 22 gun metal foundry workers occupationally exposed to lead, zinc, and copper. Among the workers with higher blood lead concentrations, the latencies of P300 were significantly prolonged when compared with a gender- and age-matched control group. Both ABR and P300 latencies were significantly correlated with the indicators of lead absorption among these workers.

Discalzi et al. (1992) investigated the effects of industrial exposures to lead and mercury on the brainstem auditory pathway through ABR. The study included 22 workers exposed to lead, 8 workers exposed to mercury and 2 control groups of age- and gender-matched subjects never exposed to neurotoxic substances. The I-V IPL was examined. Results showed that both mercury and lead exposed workers had a significant delay for the I-V IPL. The researchers also found that those subjects with the highest level of lead in blood had a longer I-V IPL compared to workers with lower levels of lead in blood.

5. International legislation

It is well documented that workplace noise exposure is a significant health hazard that leads to permanent, occupational noise-induced hearing loss. For this reason, many countries have developed national exposure standards for occupational noise, based on levels of exposure which are considered safe for human hearing. Likewise, exposure to chemicals in the workplace can lead to occupational chemical-induced hearing loss, as many of these chemicals have been internationally recognised as being hazardous to hearing. However, unlike noise exposure, standards for permissible levels of exposure to chemicals such as solvents in the US and other countries do not consider the adverse effects of chemicals on human hearing. This is because human exposure-response relationships remain unclear and thus chemical exposure standards have not been modified to reduce the risk of hearing impairment. Currently, recommended or mandatory workplace exposure limits (OELs) have been developed in many countries for airborne exposure to gases, vapours and particulates. The most widely used limits, threshold limit values (TLVs), are those issued in the USA by the American Conference of Governmental Industrial Hygienists (ACGIH). Table 5 shows the current US permissible exposure limits for some organic solvents according to different US organisations.

Taking into consideration the ototoxicity of many chemicals, some international bodies and governments have issued guidelines or recommendations regarding the ototoxicity of chemicals alone or when combined with noise. In the WHO Special Report "Occupational exposure to noise: evaluation, prevention and control" (Goelzer, Hansen & Sehrndt, 2001), the combined exposure to noise and other factors such as solvents, vibrations and metal dust is noted and it is suggested that more stringent criteria than those specified as being standard in the document should be applied. Ototoxic properties are acknowledged on the International Chemical Safety Cards (a joint programme of the International Labour Organization, WHO, and United Nations; Obadia, 2003) only for toluene, xylene and potassium bromate.

Solvent	OSHA	NIOSH	ACGIH
Toluene	200 ppm	100 ppm	50 ppm
Styrene	100 ppm	50 ppm	20 ppm
Xylene	100 ppm	100 ppm	100 ppm
Ethyl benzene	100 ppm	100 ppm	100 ppm
Carbon disulfide	20 ppm	1 ppm	10 ppm
N-hexane	500 ppm	50 ppm	50 ppm

Table 5. Permissible exposure limits (PEL) to selected organic solvents according to different organisations in the U.S. PPM: parts per million; OSHA: Occupational Safety and Health Administration; NIOSH: National Institute for Occupational Safety and Health; ACGIH: American Conference of Industrial Hygienists.

In the United States of America, the American Conference of Industrial Governmental Hygienists (ACGIH, 2009) recommends that when exposure to noise and to carbon monoxide, lead, manganese, styrene, toluene, or xylene occurs, then periodic audiometry should be carried out and the results should be carefully reviewed. Also, the U.S. Army Fact Sheet 51-002-0903 on Occupational Ototoxins and Hearing Loss states that since the exposure threshold for ototoxic effects is not known, audiometric monitoring is necessary to determine whether the substance affects the hearing of exposed workers. It includes recommendations for annual audiometric assessment for workers whose chemical exposure (disregarding the use of respiratory protection) equals 50% of the most stringent criteria for occupational exposure limits, regardless of the noise level.

The Canadian Centre for Occupational Safety and Health (2009) has listed benzene, xylene, ethylbenze hydrogen cyanide, n-hexane, styrene, trichloroethylene, toluene, among others as chemicals associated with hearing loss.

Organic solvents such as toluene, xylenes, styrene, and trichloroethylene are considered as industrial ototoxic agents under Australian and New Zealand legislation (AS/NZS 1269.0:2005). Also, Australian government bodies such as Safe Work Australia and the Department of Commerce, have recognised solvents as ototoxic agents. Safe Work Australia (2010) indicated that some factors, such as ototoxic chemicals, may interact with noise to produce hearing loss that is greater than that associated with the effects of the individual causes. In addition, the presence of chemicals in the workplace has been suggested as being one of the possible factors leading to the maintained occurrence of noise-induced hearing loss (Safe Work Australia, 2010). In Australia (e.g., Queensland Government, 2004), it has been recommended, until revised standards are established, that the daily noise exposure of workers exposed to solvents be reduced to 80 dBA or below, and that regular audiometric testing should be carried out. Annual audiometry is highly recommended for Australian workers whose airborne exposures for some selected chemicals are at 50% or more of the exposure standards stated in the National Exposure Standards for Atmospheric

Contaminants in the Occupational Environment (NOHSC 1003, 1995), regardless of the noise level.

In Europe, the European Parliament published a noise directive (2003/10/EC), which has been adopted by all member countries since 2006. This directive calls on employers to consider the interaction of noise and work-related ototoxic substances on workers' health and safety. The European Agency for Safety and Health at Work (2009) has listed solvents such as toluene, styrene, p-xylene, among others as agents with "good evidence" about their adverse effects on hearing. In Germany, a position paper on ototoxic industrial chemicals was issued by the "Noise" and "Hazardous Substances" working groups of the Deutsche Gesetzliche Unfallversicherung (DGUV)'s committee for occupational medicine (Deutsche Gesetzliche Unfallversicherung's Occupational Medicine Committee, 2006). Among other recommendations, the position paper stated that public risk communication, including all points of contact, should be promoted, and that the ototoxicity of some chemicals should be taken into consideration when specifying occupational exposure limits.

Finally, in Brazil workers can claim compensation for hearing loss induced by occupational exposure to ototoxic chemicals, as a regulation issued in 1999 (Ministério da Previdência e Assistência Social, 1999) recognises the adverse effect of certain chemicals on hearing.

The scenario in most developing nations is very different. In many developing countries legislation is absent or under-enforced and local industrial workplace practices are performed without knowledge of the possible adverse health consequences of chemical agents. In these countries legislation requiring the safe usage of ototoxic chemicals used in industry and agriculture should be enacted, along with the establishment of adequately resourced monitoring agencies (Amedofu & Fuente, 2008).

6. Conclusion

The effects of chemical exposure on the auditory system have been studied by many authors. The findings suggest that chemicals such as solvents, pesticides and metals have both oto-and neuro-toxic properties. Studies conducted in animals have demonstrated that the outer hair cells are affected by solvents. The damage begins in the most external row of cochlear hair cells, and if the exposure continues the damage is spread to the middle and inner row of outer hair cells. A concomitant agent in many industries is noise exposure. Research conducted in animals and humans exposed to solvents and noise have found a synergism between these two agents. The ototoxicity induced by solvents appears to be different than the one induced by noise. Human studies in workers exposed to solvents have shown a higher prevalence of hearing loss among solvent-exposed workers when compared with non-exposed workers.

Additionally studies conducted in human populations exposed to pesticides have shown that these agents are associated with poorer hearing thresholds as well as with poorer performance for some central auditory functioning tests. Research conducted in human subjects exposed to metals such as lead and mercury also indicates that these agents relate to auditory dysfunction.

Current legislation in many countries establishes permissible exposure limits (PELs) for chemicals. These PELs are not based on the possible adverse auditory effects of chemicals.

Therefore, guidelines in some developed countries have emerged to reduce the risk of hearing loss/auditory dysfunction in workers exposed to chemicals alone or to chemicals in combination with noise. There is an urgent need for further studies to establish dose/response relationships. With this information legislation around the world could be modified regarding the PELs for ototoxic agents such as solvents, metals and pesticides.

Health care professionals in the field of audition must be aware of the effects of chemicals on the auditory system and understand the complexity of such effects which relate to oto- and neuro-toxic mechanisms. Chemical-exposed workers regardless of their noise exposure level should be routinely monitored with audiological procedures that investigate the peripheral and central auditory system. For these purposes, a test battery approach should be considered. There is still a lack of knowledge of the most sensitive audiological tests for the detection of chemical-induced auditory dysfunction. However, there is evidence that some tests can effectively detect some cases of central auditory dysfunction induced by solvent exposure. Such tests can be also used in populations of workers exposed to other chemicals that are known (or suspected) to have oto-and neurotoxic properties.

Current industrial processes utilise massive quantities of chemicals that may jeopardise workers' hearing health. It is the role of audiologists, other hearing health care, and occupational health and safety professionals to prevent chemical-induced hearing loss/auditory dysfunction. To assist prevention, the scientific evidence regarding chemical-induced hearing loss should be disseminated among workers, employers, health care professionals and legislators. Inside factories action to reduce exposure to these agents is essential to decrease the burden of occupational chemical-induced hearing loss. Industry-based initiatives should include the identification of populations at risk, the detection of early signs of chemical-induced hearing loss, and the delivery of hearing conservation programmes to chemical-exposed workers regardless of their noise exposure levels.

7. References

Abbate, C., Giorgianni, C., Munao, F. & Brecciaroli R. (1993). Neurotoxicity induced by exposure to toluene. An electrophysiologic study. *International Archives of Occupational and Environmental Health*, Vol.64, pp. 389-392.

ACGIH - American Conference of Governmental Industrial Hygienists. (2009). *Threshold Limit Values and Biological Exposure Indices*, ACGIH Publication, Cincinnati.

Amedofu, G. & Fuente, A. (2008). Occupational hearing loss in developing countries. In: B. McPherson & R. Brouillette (Eds.). *Audiology for Developing Countries* (pp. 189-222), Nova Scientific Publishing, New York.

Arnold, SA. (2000). The auditory brain stem response. In: R. J. Roeser, M. Valente, & H. Hosford-Dunn (Eds.). *Audiology. Diagnosis* (pp. 451-470), Thieme, New York.

Bellis, TJ. (2003). *Assessment and Management of Central Auditory Processing Disorders.* (2nd ed.), Thomson, Clifton Park, NY.

Brandt-Lassen, R., Lund, SP. & Jepsen, GB. (2000). Rats exposed to toluene and noise may develop loss of auditory sensitivity due to synergistic interaction. *Noise & Health*, Vol.3, pp. 33-44.

Ministério da Previdência e Assistência Social. (1999). *Decreto no 3048, de 12/05/1999-Aprova o regulamento da Previdência Social, e dá outras Providências*, Ministério da Previdência e Assistência Social, Brasilia.

Campo, P., Lataye, R., Cossec. B. & Placidi, V. (1997). Toluene-induced hearing loss: A mid-frequency location of the cochlear lesions. *Neurotoxicology and Teratology*, Vol.19, pp. 129-140.

Campo, P., Maguin, K. & Lataye, R. (2007). Effects of aromatic solvents on acoustic reflexes mediated by central auditory pathways. *Toxicological Sciences*, Vol.99, pp. 582-590.

Canadian Centre for Occupational Safety and Health. (2009). Chemicals and noise - a hazardous combination. *The Health and Safety Report*, Vol.7, No.10 available from http://www.ccohs.ca/newsletters/hsreport/issues/2009/10/ezine.html#inthenews

Cappaert, NL., Klis, SF., Baretta, AB., Muijser, H. & Smoorenburg, GF. (2000). Ethyl benzene-induced ototoxicity in rats: a dose-dependent mid-frequency hearing loss. *Journal of* the *Association for Research in Otolaryngology*, Vol.1, pp. 292-299.

Cappaert, NL., Klis, SF., Muijser, H., de Groot, JC., Kulig, BM. & Smoorenburg, GF. (1999). The ototoxic effects of ethyl benzene in rats. *Hearing Research*, Vol.137, pp. 91-102.

Crofton, KM., Lassiter, TL. & Rebert, CS. (1994). Solvent-induced ototoxicity in rats. An atypical selective mid-frequency hearing deficit. *Hearing Research*, Vol.80, pp. 25-30.

Deutsche Gesetzliche Unfallversicherung. (2006). *Position paper on ototoxic industrial chemicals*. Deutsche Gesetzliche Unfallversicherung's Committee for Occupational Medicine available from http://osha.europa.eu/en/publications/literature_reviews/combined-exposure-to-noise-and-ototoxic-substances

Draper, TH. & Bamiou, DE. (2009). Auditory neuropathy in a patient exposed to xylene: case report. *Journal of Laryngology and Otology*, Vol.123, pp.462-465.

European Agency for Safety and Health at Work. (2009). *Combined exposure to noise and ototoxic substances*, EU-OSHA European Agency for Safety and Health at Work, Luxembourg.

European Parliament and the Council of the European Union. (2003). Directive 2003/10/EC on the minimum health and safety requirements regarding the exposure of workers to the risks arising from physical agents (noise). *Official Journal of the European Union*, Vol.L42, 38-44.

Fechter, LD., Liu, Y., Herr, DW. & Crofton, KM. (1998). Trichloroethylene ototoxicity: evidence for a cochlear origin. *Toxicological Sciences*, Vol.42, pp. 28-31.

Food and Agriculture Organization of the United Nations. (2003). *International Code of Conduct on the Distribution and Use of Pesticides*, Food and Agriculture Organization, Rome.

Fuente, A. (2008). *Auditory damage associated with solvent exposure: evidence from a cross-sectional study*. Unpublished PhD thesis, The University of Hong Kong.

Fuente, A. (2010). Central auditory dysfunction associated with solvent exposure. *Bulletin of the American Auditory Society*, Vol.35, No.1, pp.55.

Fuente, A., Slade, MD., Taylor, T., Morata, TC., Keith, RW., Sparer, J. & Rabinowitz, PM. (2009). Peripheral and central auditory dysfunction induced by occupational exposure to organic solvents. *Journal of Occupational and Environmental Medicine*,Vol.51, pp.1202-1211.

Fuente, A. & McPherson, B. (2007). Central auditory processing effects induced by solvent exposure. *International Journal of Occupational Medicine and Environmental Health*, Vol.20, pp.271-279.

Fuente, A., McPherson, B. & Hickson, L. (2011). Central auditory dysfunction associated with exposure to a mixture of solvents. *International Journal of Audiology* (in press).

Fuente, A., McPherson, B., Muñoz, V. & Espina, JP. (2006). Assessment of central auditory processing in a group of workers exposed to solvents. *Acta Oto-Laryngologica*, Vol.126, pp.1188-1194.

Gelfand, SA. (Ed.). (2001). *Essentials of Audiology* (2nd ed), Thieme, New York.

Goelzer, B., Hansen, CH. & Sehrndt, GA. (2001). *Occupational exposure to noise: evaluation, prevention and control.* Federal Institute for Occupational Safety and Health, Dortmund, published on behalf of the World Health Organization, Geneva.

Guida, HL., Morini, RG. & Vieir-Cardoso, AC. (2010). Audiological evaluation in workers exposed to noise and pesticide. *Brazilian Journal of Otorhinolaryngology*, Vol.76, No. 4, pp. 423-427.

Harrel, M., Shea, JJ. & Emmet, JR. (1978). Bilateral sudden deafness following combined insecticide poisoning. *The Laryngoscope*, Vol. 88, pp. 1348-1351.

Hirata, M., Ogawa Y., Okayama A. & Goto S. (1992). A cross- sectional study on the brainstem auditory evoked potential among workers exposed to carbon disulfide. *International Archives of Occupational and Environmental Health*, Vol.64, pp. 321-324.

Johnson, AC. & Canlon, B. (1994). Progressive hair cell loss induced by toluene exposure. *Hearing Research*, Vol.75, pp. 1-40.

Keith, RW. (2000). *Random Gap Detection Test*, Auditec, St. Louise.

Keith, RW. (2002). Alternatives for testing the central auditory system. In: *Best practices workshop: Combined effects of chemicals and noise on hearing*, Cincinnati.

Laroche, C., Soli, S., Giguere, C., Lagace, J., Vaillancourt, V. & Fortin, M. (2003). An approach to the development of hearing standards for hearing-critical jobs. *Noise and Health*, 6, 17-37.

Lasky, RE., Maier, MM., Snodgrass, EB., Hecox, KE. & Laughlin, NK. (1995). The effects of lead on otoacoustic emissions and auditory evoked potentials in monkeys. *Neurotoxicology and Teratology*, Vol. 17, pp. 633-644.

Lataye, R. & Campo, P. (1997). Combined effects of a simultaneous exposure to noise and toluene on hearing function. *Neurotoxicology and Teratology*, Vol.19, pp. 373-382.

Liu, Y., Rao, D. & Fechter. D. (1997). Correspondence between middle frequency auditory loss in vivo and outer hair cell shortening in vitro. *Hearing Research*, Vol.112, pp. 134-140.

Lataye, R., Campo, P. & Loquet, G. (2000). Combined effects of noise and styrene exposure on hearing function in the rat. *Hearing Research*, Vol.139, pp. 86-96.

Lataye, R., Campo, P., Loquet, G. & Morel, G. (2005). Combined effects of noise and styrene on hearing: comparison between active and sedentary rats. *Noise & Health*, Vol.7, pp. 49-64.

Lataye, R., Maguin, K. & Campo, P. (2007). Increase in cochlear microphonic potential after toluene administration. *Hearing Research*, Vol.230, pp.34-42.

Laukli, E. & Hansen, PW. (1995). An audiometric test battery for the evaluation of occupational exposure to industrial solvents. *Acta Oto-laryngologica*, Vol.115, pp. 162-164.

Loquet, G., Campo, P. & Lataye, R. (1999). Comparison of toluene-induced and styrene-induced hearing losses. *Neurotoxicology and Teratology*, Vol.21, pp. 689-697.

Loquet, G., Campo, P., Lataye, R., Cossec, B. & Bonnet, P. (2000). Combined effects of exposure to styrene and ethanol on the auditory function in the rat. *Hearing Research*, Vol.148, pp. 173-180.

Mac Crawford, J., Hoppin, JA., Alavanja, MCR., Blair, A., Sandler, DP. & Kamel, F. (2008). Hearing loss among licensed pesticide applicators in the agricultural health study. *Journal of Occupational and Environmental Medicine*, Vol.50, No 7, pp. 817-826.

Makitie, AA., Pirvola U., Pyykko, I., Sakakibara, H., Riihimaki, V. & Ylikoski, J. (2003). The ototoxic interaction of styrene and noise. *Hearing Research*, Vol.179, pp. 9-20.

Moen, BE., Riise, T. & Kyvik, KR. (1999). P300 brain potential among workers exposed to organic solvents. *Norsk Epidemiologi*, Vol.9, pp. 27-31.

McWilliams, ML., Chen, GD. & Fechter, LD. (2000). Low-level toluene disrupts auditory function in guinea pigs. *Toxicology and Applied Pharmacology*, Vol.15, pp. 18-29.

Morata, TC. (1989). Study of the effects of simultaneous exposure to noise and carbon disulfide on workers hearing. *Scandinavian Audiology*, Vol.18, pp. 53-58.

Morata, TC., Engel, T., Durao, A., Costa, TRS., Krieg, EF., Dunn, DE. & Lozano, MA. (1997). Hearing loss from combined exposures among petroleum refinery workers. *Scandinavian Audiology*, Vol.26, pp. 141-149.

Morata, TC., Johnson, AC., Nylen, P., Svensson, EB., Cheng, J., Krieg, EF., Lindblad, AC., Ernstgard, L. & Franks J. (2002). Audiometric findings in workers exposed to low levels of styrene and noise. *Journal of Occupational and Environmental Medicine*, Vol.44, pp. 806-814.

Morata, TC & Lemasters, GK. (1995). Epidemiologic considerations in the evaluation of occupational hearing loss. *Occupational Medicine*, Vol.10, pp. 641-56.

Morata, TC., Sliwinska-Kowalska, M., Johnson, AC., Starck, J., Pawlas, K., Zamyslowska-Szmytke, E., Nylen, P., Toppila, E., Krieg, E., Pawlas, N. & Prasher, D. (2011). A multicenter study on the audiometric findings of styrene-exposed workers. *International Journal of Audiology* (in press).

Muijser, H., Hoogendijk, E. & Hooisma, J. (1988). The effects of occupational exposure to styrene on high-frequency hearing thresholds. *Toxicology*, Vol.49, pp. 331-340.

Murata, K., Araki, S., Yokoyama, K., Uchida, E. & Fujimura, Y. (1993). Assessment of central, peripheral, and autonomic nervous system functions in lead workers: neuroelectrophysiological studies. *Environmental Research*, Vol. 61, No. 2, pp. 323-336.

Musiek, FE. (1983a). Assessment of central auditory dysfunction: The dichotic digit test revisited. Ear and Hearing. *Ear and Hearing*,Vol. 4, pp.79-83.

Musiek, FE. (1983b). Results of three dichotic speech tests on subjects with intracranial lesions. *Ear and Hearing*, Vol.4, pp.318-323.

Musiek, FE. (1994). Frequency (pitch) and duration patterns tests. *Journal of the American Academy of Audiology*, Vol.5, pp.265-268.

National Occupational Health and Safety Commission. (1995). *Adopted National Exposure Standards for Atmospheric Contaminants in the Occupational Environment [NOHSC:1003 (1995)]*, Australian Government Publishing Service, Canberra.

Niklasson, M., Arlinger, S., Ledin, T., Müller, C., Ödkvist, L., Flodin, U. & Tham, R. (1998). Audiological disturbances caused by long-term exposure to industrial solvents.

Relation to the diagnosis of toxic encephalopathy. *Scandinavian Audiology*, Vol.27, pp. 131-136.

Nilsson, M., Soli, SD. & Sullivan, JA. (1994). Development of the Hearing In Noise Test for the measurement of speech reception thresholds in quiet and in noise. *Journal of the Acoustical Society of America*, Vol.95, pp.1085-1099.

Obadia, I. (2003). ILO activities in the area of chemical safety. *Toxicology*, Vol.190, pp. 105-115.

Ödkvist, LM., Arlinger, SD., Edling, C., Larsby, B. & Bergholtz, LM. (1987). Audiological and vestibule-oculomotor findings in workers exposed to solvents and jet fuel. *Scandinavian Audiology*, Vol.16, pp. 75-81.

Ödkvist, LM., Moller, C. & Thuomas, KA. (1992). Otoneurologic disturbances caused by solvent pollution. *Otolaryngology and Head and Neck Surgery*, Vol.106, pp. 687-692.

Pollastrini, L., Abramo, A., Cristalli, G., Baretti, F. & Greco, A. (1994). Early signs of occupational ototoxicity caused by inhalation of benzene derivative industrial solvents. *Acta Otorhinolaryngologica Italica*, Vol.14, pp. 503-512.

Pryor, GT., Rebert, CS. & Howd, RA. (1987). Hearing loss in rats caused by inhalation of mixed xylenes and styrene. *Journal of Applied Toxicology*, Vol.7, pp. 55-61.

Queensland Government. (2004). *Noise Code of Practice 2004*. Workplace Health and Safety Queensland. Queensland Government available from http://www.deir.qld.gov.au/workplace/resources/pdfs/noise_code2004.pdf

Rebert CS., Boyes, WK., Pryor, GT., Svensgaard, DJ., Kassay, KM., Gordon, GR. & Shinsky, N. (1993). Combined effects of solvents on the rat's auditory system: styrene and trichloroethylene. *International Journal of Psychophysiology*, Vol.14, pp. 49-59.

Rebert, CS., Schwartz, RW., Svendsgaard, DJ., Pryor, GT. & Boyes, WK. (1995). Combined effects of paired solvents on the rat's auditory system. *Toxicology*, Vol.105, pp. 345-354.

Safe Work Australia. (2010). Occupational noise-induced hearing loss in Australia: overcoming barriers to effective noise control and hearing loss prevention. Safe Work Australia available from http://safeworkaustralia.gov.au/AboutSafeWorkAustralia/WhatWeDo/Publications/Documents/539/Occupational_Noiseinduced_Hearing_Loss_Australia_2010.pdf

Schäper, M., Demes, P., Zupanic, M., Blaszkewicz M. & Seeber, A. (2003). Occupational toluene exposure and auditory function: results from a follow-up study. *Annals of Occupational Hygiene*, Vol.47, pp. 493-502.

Sliwinska-Kowalska, M., Zamyslowska-Szmytke, E., Szymczak, W., Kotylo, P., Fiszer, M., Dudarewicz, A., Wesolowski, W., Pawlaczyk-Luszczynska, M. & Stolarek, R. (2001). Hearing loss among workers exposed to moderate concentrations of solvents. *Scandinavian Journal of Work, Environment & Health*, Vol.27, pp. 335-342.

Sliwinska-Kowalska, M., Zamyslowska-Szmytke, E., Szymczak, W., Kotylo, P., Wesolowski, W., Dudarewicz, A., Fiszer, M., Pawlaczyk-Luszczynska, M. Politanski, P., Kucharska, M. & Bilski, B. (2000). Assessment of hearing impairment in workers exposed to mixtures of organic solvents in the paint and lacquer industry. *Medycyna pracy*, Vol.51, pp. 1-10 [in Polish].

Sliwinska-Kowalska, M., Zamyslowska-Szmytke, E., Szymczak, W., Kotylo, P., Fiszer, M., Wesolowski, W., Wesolowski, W. & Pawlaczyk-Luszczynska, M. (2003). Ototoxic effects of occupational exposure to styrene and co-exposure to styrene and noise. *Journal of Occupational and Environmental Medicine*, Vol.45, pp. 15-24.

Steinhauer, SR., Morrow, LA., Condray, R. & Dougherty, GG. (1997). Event-related potentials in workers with ongoing occupational exposure. *Biological Psychiatry*, Vol.42, pp.854-858.

Sulkowski, WJ., Kowalska, S., Matyja, W., Guzek, W., Wesolowski, W., Szymczak, W. & Kostrzewski, P. (2002). Effects of occupational exposure to a mixture of solvents on the inner ear: a field study. *International Journal of Occupational Medicine and Environmental Health*, Vol.15, pp. 247-256.

Stach, B. (1998). *Clinical Audiology: an introduction*, Singular, San Diego.

Standards Australia. (2005). *AS/NZS 1269 Occupational Noise Management*, Standards Australia, Sydney.

Sullivan, MJ., Rarey, KE. & Conolly, RB. (1988). Ototoxicity of toluene in rats. *Neurotoxicology and Teratology*, Vol.10, pp. 525-530.

Teixeira, CF., da Silva Augusto, LG. & Morata, TC. (2002). Occupational exposure to insecticides and their effects on the auditory system. *Noise & Heath*, Vol.4, No. 14 pp. 31-39.

U.S. Army Fact Sheet 51-002-0903. Occupational ototoxins and hearing loss. available from http://www.nmcphc.med.navy.mil/downloads/occmed/toolbox/occupationalototoxinfactsheet-chppm.pdf. Retrieved on 12/09/2011

Varney, NR., Morrow, LA., Pinkston, JB. & Wu, JC. (1998). PET Scan findings in a patient with a remote history of exposure to organic solvents. *Applied Neuropsychology*, Vol.5, pp.100-106.

Vrca, A., Koracic, V., Bozicevic, D. & Malinar, M. (1996). Brainstem auditory evoked potentials in individuals exposed to long-term low concentrations of toluene. *American Journal of Industrial Medicine*, Vol.30, pp. 62-66.

Vrca, A., Bozicevic, D., Bozikov, V., Fuchs, R. & Malinar, M. (1997). Brain stem evoked potentials and visual evoked potentials in relation to the length of occupational exposure to low levels of toluene. *Acta Medica Croatica*, Vol.51, pp. 215-219.

Wilson, LK. & Mueller, HG. (1984). Performance of normal hearing individuals on Auditec filtered speech tests. *ASHA*, Vol.26, pp.120.

World Health Organization. (2001). *International Classification of Functioning, Disability and Health*, World Health Organization, Geneva.

Yano, BL., Dittenber, DA., Albee, RR. & Mattsson, J. L. (1992). Abnormal auditory brainstem responses and cochlear pathology in rats induced by an exaggerated styrene exposure regimen. *Toxicologic Pathology*, Vol.20, pp. 1-6.

10

Exploration Databases on Occupational Hearing Loss

Juan Carlos Conte, Ana Isabel García,
Emilio Rubio and Ana Isabel Domínguez
Catedra de Bioestadística, Facultad de Medicina, Universidad de Zaragoza,
C/ Domingo Miral, Zaragoza
Spain

1. Introduction

Studies on occupational hearing loss have focused on noise as the primary cause. While the effect of this physical agent on hearing has been demonstrated, an analysis closer to the site of exposure confirms that the presence of other contaminants, such as chemicals, can interact with noise. This association may influence a temporal variability in the manifestation of an occupational hearing pathology.

In this respect, the term "working conditions" is too ambiguous (i.e., noise in the metal industry) as, in apparently similar conditions, several exposure environments can be identified: machining (noise+fluids, e.g. lathing), manufacture of structures (noise+fumes, e.g. welding) and surface protection (noise+solvents, e.g. painting), among others.

The European Agency for Safety and Health at Work recognises that noise-induced hearing loss is the most common occupational disorder in Europe. It advises that, in order to achieve greater efficiency in its prevention, more attention must be paid to the combined risk factors (multiple exposures) in workers exposed to high noise levels and chemical compounds associated with their work.

Similarly, recent studies conducted in the US (Agrawall et al., 2009) and New Zealand (Thorne et al., 2008) recognise noise-induced hearing loss as one of the most widespread occupational illnesses in these countries. Conclude that traditional noise monitoring and control methods have not achieved the expected results, identifying increasing prevalence in the general working population, and particularly in young people.

This study aims to test the hypothesis of interaction between various physical and chemical pollutants and their influence on hearing. It obtains a complete temporal exposure model, based on survival analysis, which covers the entire working life of an individual between t=0 (start time) and t=50 years (maximum period). The study of multiple exposures using a qualitative variable allows the prevention cost associated with hygiene risk assessment (see 2.3.1. point 1) to be sufficiently reduced. This is also the methodology used in the study of other environment related illnesses caused by prolonged exposure to different agents.

The analysis was carried out using as sample data taken from a pre-existing database on occupational health. The aim was to assess the viability of using these historical databases and the quality of the information obtained from them with regard to the interaction between noise and chemicals and the effect of this interaction on hearing.

The characteristics of the archive information determined the design of the study, the definition of the variables and the method of data analysis used. For instance, the instruments used to measure these variables in some cases may have changed over the prolonged time of this study and it is therefore difficult to maintain consistency. These instruments include: audiometers for identifying the decline in the auditory threshold; integrated sound level meters and dosimeters for the measurement of environmental noise; vacuum pumps for taking air samples, and instruments for chemical analysis used for collecting and quantifying environmental chemical contaminants. Consequently quantitative recording was avoided, defining measurements qualitatively (as binary variables) instead. This provided greater flexibility when evaluating variables, eliminating possible discrepancies associated with potential changes in technology and measurement criteria.

Using a minimum amount of information, one discrete quantitative variable (length of time exposed to noise) and the remaining qualitative variables, it was possible to estimate the influence of a particular working environment on hearing in combination with certain personal habits. The results obtained are of descriptive and explanatory interest, providing information on the interactions between the stated variables and their effects on the individual.

The analysis of the data was fast and economical, whereas obtaining pure samples of data would be less so. Furthermore, and as a corollary, average or high frequencies is required in order to give consistency to the analysis. In addition, if a classification is used to record a variable, it has to be entirely discrete. Failure to fulfil these two criteria (frequency and being discrete) can make analysis using the proposed methodology ineffective, as speculation about the data could lead to an unreliable interpretation of that data.

The results obtained show that workers exposed to noise where metalworking fluids are present show a greater delay in hearing alteration than workers exposed only to noise. By contrast, workers exposed to noise where welding fumes are present exhibited an increase in hearing alteration compared to those exposed only to noise. This thereby demonstrates the antagonistic effect of metalworking fluids with noise and the synergic effect of welding fumes.

As a preventative application, there exists a need for combined respiratory and auditory protection in processes that produce welding fumes, and the former should be effective against certain gases and metal components (use of integrated personal protection equipment). Fabric masks (a highly-used protection) do not meet this requirement, and nor do extraction systems. Environments with noise and metalworking fluids have the advantage in that the aforementioned masks can be used as respiratory protection combined with auditory protection.

Based on recognised research for the study of this problem (Gobba, 2003), the study of pathogenic mechanisms, and evaluation of new multiple-exposure thresholds. This paper focuses on the second of these aspects, the purpose being to obtain patterns that allow for the comparison of various populations of workers in multiple-exposure conditions similar to those defined by such patterns.

In view of the above, the aim of this study is to analyse the influence of the combination of different chemical agents and noise on occupational hearing loss within the metal industry, to be aware of the interrelationships between such factors for preventive purposes.

2. Material

2.1 Study design

A descriptive epidemiological study was conducted, using two types of sources: one based on the records of each individual, occupational medical examinations (OME), with a specific noise protocol (SNP), carried out on various dates during the inclusion period, providing their audiometric data, duration of exposure to noise, and personal habits.

The second type involved on-site testing of a selection of job positions, in order to ensure the type and homogeneity of the environmental exposure conditions of the individuals in the companies included in the sample during the period of study, and environmental record of exposure (ERE).

The study design presented is conceptually interpreted as longitudinal, as defined by Rothman (1986), the existence of a time interval between exposure and the onset of illness.

With two observation points, at t=0 (estimated starting point for the specified sources, after having first carried out a strict process of selection of individuals to be included in the study) and at t=n (period in which the first audiometric test was performed).

2.2 Sample collection

The Aragonese population working in the metal industry during the study period 1991-2000, was evaluated using the Industrial Companies Survey (Spanish acronym EIE) conducted by the Spanish National Statistics Institute (Spanish acronym INE), and an average population of 10,802 workers was obtained.

The data was provided by the Spanish National Institute of Safety and Hygiene at Work (Spanish acronym INSHT) and the Aragon Institute of Occupational Safety and Health (Spanish acronym ISSLA), from a list of companies in their files.

The initial sample size represented 10% of the workers, i.e. 1,080 individuals, using a systematic sampling of companies from said list.

From the initial selection, the following were eliminated: individuals not exposed to occupational noise; those who presented alterations in audiometric tests due to causes other than noise; individuals who, prior to their exposure to occupational noise (t=0), had been subjected to noise outside work over a long period of time; individuals exposed to solvents and degreasing agents and products that did not qualify for inclusion. The final study sample included 558 workers.

2.3 Description of variables

A total of six variables were used, which can be divided into two groups. The first group, characterised by not having missing values consists of three variables, which define the cause-effect relationship: time of noise exposure, the atmosphere to which individuals were exposed and the degree of hearing alteration. The second group of variables, characterised by having missing values, refers to certain personal habits (smoking, exposure to non-occupational noise and use of hearing protection). These can modify the response of the individual to the environmental factors to which they are exposed at work. These variables therefore have to be controlled to achieve the most accurate interpretation of the results.

2.3.1 Exposure or cause-effect variables (Table 1)

1. "Exposure atmosphere" (A_{EXP}). This was a nominal qualitative variable with three categories. Each category was treated as binary. The variable noise was determined using an integrated sound level meter to classify the individuals in terms of their degree of exposure and its duration. Chemicals were assessed by the presence or absence of the corresponding particles of fluids or smoke in the atmosphere at work. The classification of noise intensity, moderate or high, was adopted for this work. Each one of the three atmospheres at work considered were classified: (a) MF= mainly noise of moderate intensity [85-90) dB(A) in the presence of metalworking fluids; (b) N=only noise, of moderate or high intensity ≥ 85dB(A); (c) WF= mainly noise of high intensity ≥ 90dB(A) in the presence of welding fumes.

Variables (Cause-Effect)	n	%
EXPOSURE ATMOSPHERE (A_{EXP})	558	
Noise Only, N	177	31.7
Noise+Metalworking Fluids, MF	146	26.2
Noise+Welding Fumes, WF	235	42.1
EXPOSURE TIME (T_{EXP})	558	
0-5	57	10.2
5-10	41	7.3
10-15	36	6.5
15-20	42	7.5
20-25	85	15.2
25-30	116	20.8
30-35	106	19
35-40	50	9
40-45	22	3.9
45-50	3	0.5
DEGREE OF ALTERATION (D_{ALT})	558	
H	158	28.3
IAT	196	35.1
AAT	105	18.8
MH	70	12.5
AH	29	5.2

Table 1. Exposure variables

2. "Exposure time to noise" (T_{EXP}). This was a discrete quantitative variable expressed in years. It was an estimation of the time that the worker had been exposed to noise throughout his or her working life. It was established by consulting the individual directly. The possibility of using both the age of the workers and the length of time they were exposed to noise as the time variable was assessed. The projection of each together on a

dispersion graph illustrates the variation between them. Age was rejected as a suitable variable, since in addition to not defining the real duration of exposure effectively it had to then be transformed to achieve its lineal distribution, whereas this was not a problem when the length of time exposed to noise was used as the variable.

3. "Degree of hearing alteration" (D_{ALT}). This was an ordinal qualitative variable with five modalities. Each modality was treated as binary. The variable identified the degree of hearing alteration, defined as the decline in the auditory threshold according to acoustic frequency, measured using an audiometer. The audiometry studied at times gave rise to two types of problems in relation to the interpretation of the results. These concerned manual corrections to the audiometric profile and the impossibility of observing the audiometric profile. Therefore the degree of hearing alteration was recorded according to a diagnostic code assigned by the doctor responsible for the check-up based on the Klockhoff classification (1973): H=healthy (losses 25 dB); IAT=initial acoustic trauma (losses of between 25 and 40 dB); AAT=advanced acoustic trauma (losses of between 40 and 50 dB); MH=mild hypoacusis (losses of between 50 and 55 dB); AH=advanced hypoacusis (losses > 55 dB). The losses indicated refer to the 4000 Hz frequency. There was also a loss of adjacent frequencies as the degree of hearing alteration increases.

2.3.2 Habits or modifying variables (Table 2)

4. "Smoking habit" (SH). A nominal binary variable. Recorded whether or not the subject smoked.

5. "Noise outside work" (NOW). A nominal binary variable. Recorded whether or not noisy activities were undertaken outside of work.

6. "Hearing protection" (HP). A nominal binary variable. Recorded whether or not hearing protection was used.

Variables (Modifying)	n	%
SMOKING HABIT (SH)	558	
No	147	26.3
Yes	130	23.3
Missing values	281	50.4
NOISE OUTSIDE WORK (NOW)	558	
No	192	34.4
Yes	35	6.3
Missing values	331	59.3
HEARING PROTECTION (HP)	558	
No	103	18.5
Yes	95	17
Missing values	360	64.5

Table 2. Habit variables

The events were defined based on the "degree of hearing alteration" variable, treating this as a nominal variable of binary response. Since in reality it is an ordinal variable with five modalities, it was necessary to transform the initial variable in such a way that the code (0) represented the cases censored or in which the event did not occur, and the code (1) represented the event occurring. The system followed is represented in Table 3. This approach does not allow other reinterpretations of the type of censures to be used as they must necessarily be to the right because the exact decrease in the threshold is not available for each individual. Instead, only a diagnostic code is available, which did not allow us to define a specific decrease in dB and to relate this to the "duration of exposure" variable.

Events	Modalities	¿Event of Cox?
Event 1:		YES
Healthy (code 0)	(H)	Temporary effect (IAT)
Altered (code 1)	(IAT+AAT+MH+AH)	treated as permanent
Event 2:		YES
Recovered (code 0)	(H+IAT)	Permanent effect
Not recovered (code 1)	(AAT+MH+AH)	
Event 3:		YES
No falls in conversational freq. (code 0)	(H+IAT+AAT)	Permanent effect
With falls in conversational freq. (code 1)	(MH+AH)	

Table 3. Definition of events

3. Methods

The way of initially tackling the analysis of the data was by defining the survival functions. The main focus of this study was to identify the patterns of hearing alteration over time, related to the environmental conditions to which the individuals were exposed and their "habits". Once the survival functions were defined and examined, the data was analysed using various regression analysis techniques to identify the most suitable method.

The starting point was one quantitative variable with the remaining variables being qualitative. We are in a limiting case when applying regression theory to the data, that as indicated by Martín & Paz (2007).

Due to reason stated above the number of useful regression models was limited. Linear regression models require at least two quantitative variables. Models based on the discriminating function require the normal distribution of variables, an aspect which in this case was not satisfied as the only category contrasting with the rest (healthy) did not follow a normal distribution. The remaining categories of this variable are self-contained and as a consequence they cannot be analysed using this technique. Multivariate analysis of variance is not an alternative to discriminant analysis as it also requires at least two quantitative variables.

Specific regression techniques for the analysis of quantitative variables also present problems. Thus, logistic regression with nominal binary or polytomous response (Silva & Barroso, 2004), does not allow the quantitative variable (taken as independent) to be correlated with the others variables. Ordinal regression (Greenland, 1994) is not operational either as it is an extension of the above.

The most ideal model for the analysis of this situation is Cox's regression model, which makes it possible to work with only one quantitative variable (Cox & Snell, 1989). It also makes it possible for both the response variable and the predictor variables to establish a strong dependence relationship with the single variable, thereby obtaining suitable variants of Cox's regression model for this particular case (Cox's regression with a time dependent variable). It is true that the character of this regression applied to the data is fundamentally explanatory as the prediction must be based on the most frequently recorded samples with the objective of ensuring the accuracy of the observations.

The steps that were followed to apply Cox's model (Hosmer & Lemeshow, 1999) were: (1) Ensuring that the events defined were Cox type events: i.e. they occurred only once and after the event occurred it was set permanently; (2) Checking the proportionality and consistency of the risks. A graph was used based on the projection of the survival functions (demonstrated and not demonstrated); (3) Assessing the high multicollinearity or interdependence. Those variables defined prior to the study, with a correlation of above 0.8, were eliminated; (4) Assessing the linearity of the quantitative variable (duration of exposure). A graph was used based on the projection of the duration of exposure of each individual with respect to their partial residual plot (calculated with respect to their age); (5) Assessing the existence of influencing observations. Delta-beta values were used. (Cook's distance applied to Cox's regression). Values above 1 were rejected; (6) To identify any possible confusion and interaction between variables, the method involving changing model coefficients was used; (7) The correlation between beta coefficients was used to assess the stability of each model; (8) The fit of the models was assessed using probability reasoning; (9) The model was validated indirectly as it was not possible to obtain another, different sample with which to assess this aspect. Validation of the latent structure was used, obtained by the analysis of matches for each one of the two halves of the sample.

3.1 Nonparametric reliability models

The Kaplan-Meyer method (K-M) was used to obtain the survival function of a particular event associated with the various covariables, and for the contrast of functions and their meaning the Log-Rank test was used.

Subsequently a Cox regression model was used, with the aim of explaining the relationships between the variables.

3.2 Parametric reliability models

To obtain the reliability functions the normal distribution model was used and for their contrast a U of Mann-Whitney and t-test was used. For this each one of the binary variables was transformed into another equivalent referring to duration of exposure.

The parametric model was only used as a descriptor of the variables and for testing certain controls, hypotheses and predictions, starting with the probability distributions: (1) Tests to establish controls (regarding the population percentage, with reference to one or more alterations, which must not be exceeded). The tests concern establishing a common "cut off point" for the modalities of the variable "degree of hearing alteration"; (2) Hypothesis tests (regarding the development of hearing alteration). These involve the analysis of the differences in probabilities based on a real value and a theoretical value. An individual with a particular duration of exposure experiences a degree of hearing alteration (real value). In turn, this individual, with that duration of exposure, could experience other degrees of hearing alteration (theoretical values); (3) Tests of predictions. This involves predicting the development of certain exposed populations, based on the previous controls and hypotheses, making it possible to improve preventative management systems.

3.3 Comparison of survival models

Survival functions obtained for the data from the sample, using a parametric and non-parametric model, they were represented together in a graph to assess their equivalence. The interesting aspect of this equivalence is the complementarity of the results, allowing them to be used together i.e. where one model is not suitable, the other is. For example, for the initial data, regression is possible in a non-parametric approach but not in a parametric approach.

Factorial methods were also used with the aim of exploring the relationships between variables. The most suitable factorial method was correspondence analysis carried out using a Burt table (Benzecri, 1992). The heterogeneity of frequency distributions between the variables implies a low degree of dependency between them, above all when considering the "habits" variables with respect to the "exposure" variables. This situation makes the final solution (analogous with the regression results) more contrived than deductive, an aspect which limits the formal application of the factorial model. The problem can be solved using differential topological models (Cova, Márquez & Tovar, 2001), based on Thom's morphogenetic theory (1971), which is a future direction for this research.

4. Results

The characteristics of the sample are shown in Tables 1 and 2, which summarise its structure with respect to the various variables considered.

It is interesting to examine the categories within the "habits" variables, where the degree of personal protection, i.e. use of hearing protection, non-exposure to non-occupational noise and not smoking, is related to the atmosphere at work. It can be seen that as the noise level becomes more harmful the individuals tend to protect themselves more (Figure 1). This fact is very interesting when interpreting the effect on hearing of the noise and chemicals combination.

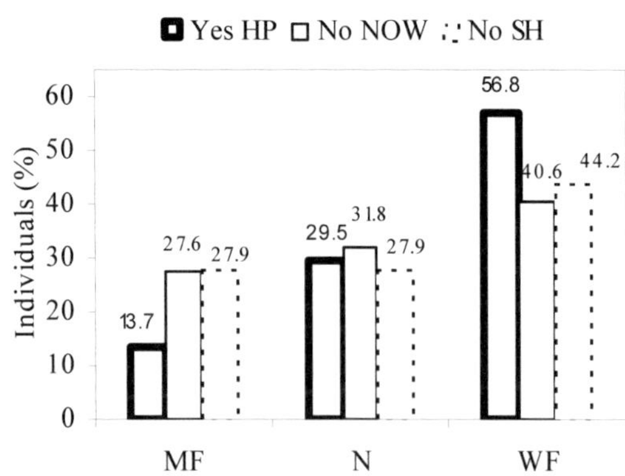

Fig. 1. Distribution of personal habits according the exposure atmosphere

As can be seen in figure 2, the survival functions obtained through the Kaplan-Meyer method define how hearing alteration appears in individuals by event and for each work atmosphere. They show clear differences between event 1 and the others.

Thus, in event 1 the "noise with metalworking fluids" atmosphere causes a delay in hearing alteration which is significant ($p<0.05$), whereas the "noise only" atmosphere and the "noise with welding fumes" atmosphere develop in unison, showing no differences between them ($p>0.05$).

For events two and three, the curves that characterise each atmosphere are separated from one another significantly ($p<0.05$), indicating the time differences that exposure to each of them represents and for the same period (see variation of the medians and contrasts, Table 4 and 5). It was demonstrated, furthermore, that the 0 to 15 years period of exposure to noise was low risk, in general presenting hearing alteration of less than 10% in the individuals exposed (Figure 2).

The percentage of individuals affected, over this period gradually decreased as the event continued. Thus, event 1 principally characterises the variations in the hearing threshold of the recoverable type (initial trauma), event 2 non-recoverable but without alteration in conversational speech (advanced trauma) and in event 3 non recoverable variations with losses in conversational speech (hypoacusis). The situation described gives a dynamic to the process of hearing alteration which is characterised by the migration of the set of survival functions to the right. This explains the existence of a lower risk in the initial periods over time, demonstrating the suitability of the model (Figure 2).

Obtaining univariate, bivariate and trivariate models (Table 6), based on the Cox regression, explains the effect of the various variables in the study, based on the hazard ratio.

In considering the "smoking habit" variable it was found that its effect was antagonistic to atmospheres with metalworking fluids, although the hazard are more or less balanced, depending on the event. This indicates uniform action over time, which is different from metalworking fluids atmosphere, which tend to intensify the effects of smoking (Figure 3.2.).

Atmosphere	Event	Sample			Percentiles						
		N	E	C	Q_{25}	SE	Q_{50}	SE	CI 95%	Q_{75}	SE
MF	1	146	91	55	38	0.94	32	1.03	(30,34)	25	1.29
N	1	177	124	53	33	0.70	28	0.75	(27,29)	21	1.65
WF	1	235	185	50	32	0.73	27	0.61	(26,28)	22	0.77
MF	2	146	35	111	44	2.43	40	1.69	(37,43)	35	1.10
N	2	177	51	126	41	2.05	34	0.88	(32,36)	29	1.37
WF	2	235	118	117	36	0.90	31	0.75	(30,32)	26	0.65
MF	3	146	12	134	45	*	44	3.60	(37,51)	40	1.15
N	3	177	25	152	45	*	41	1.72	(38,44)	32	1.62
WF	3	235	62	173	40	0.44	36	1.49	(33,39)	30	0.76

N=cases; E=events; C=censored; SE=standard error

Table 4. Characteristics of no parametric survival functions

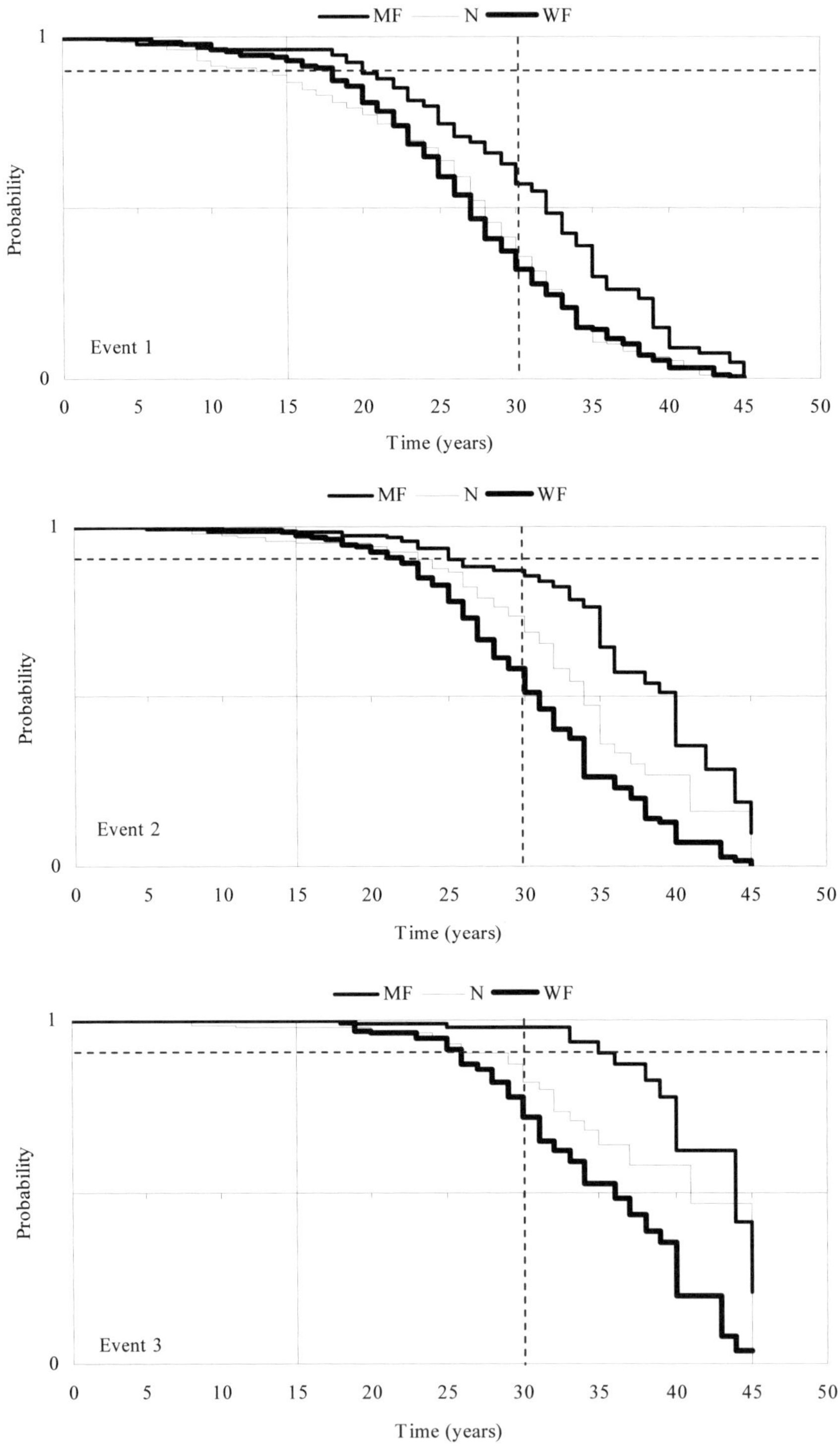

Fig. 2. No parametric survival functions, Kaplan-Meyer

Atmospheres	Event	Log Rank	df	Sig
MF / N	1	15.64	1	0.0001
WF / N	1	0.02	1	0.8904
MF / N	2	9.22	1	0.0024
WF / N	2	7.92	1	0.0049
MF / N	3	9.79	1	0.0018
WF / N	3	4.84	1	0.0279

Table 5. Contrast of no parametric survival function

Models	V_i	Event-1 Hazard	Event-1 Density CI 95%	Event-1 Wald χ^2	Event-2 Hazard	Event-2 Density CI 95%	Event-2 Wald χ^2	Event-3 Hazard	Event-3 Density CI 95%	Event-3 Wald χ^2
MF	MF	-0.524	0.467-0.748	0.000	-0.926	0.274-0.570	0.000	-1.368	0.139-0.466	0.000
WF	WF	0.389	1.208-1.801	0.001	0.816	1.686-3.034	0.000	1.159	2.031-4.998	0.000
SH	SH	0.492	1.203-2.227	0.001	0.391	0.974-2.245	0.065	-0.263	0.347-1.702	0.516
NOW	NOW	0.826	1.540-3.391	0.000	0.812	1.207-4.201	0.010	0.789	0.915-5.298	0.078
HP	HP	-0.338	0.521-0.974	0.033	-0.647	0.323-0.847	0.008	-1.058	0.172-0.701	0.003
MF / SH	MF	-0.492	0.429-0.869	0.006	-0.904	0.239-0.685	0.001	-1.582	0.072-0.584	0.003
	SH	0.473	1.179-2.185	0.002	0.347	0.930-2.151	0.105	-0.376	0.304-1.548	0.364
MF / NOW	MF	-0.269	0.542-1.075	0.123	-0.867	0.232-0.762	0.004	-1.514	0.079-0.617	0.004
	NOW	0.780	1.466-3.249	0.000	0.665	1.040-3.636	0.037	0.574	0.739-4.271	0.199
MF / HP	MF	-0.383	0.469-0.988	0.043	-0.864	0.219-0.811	0.010	-1.507	0.067-0.731	0.013
	HP	-0.271	0.554-1.048	0.095	-0.526	0.362-0.963	0.035	-0.881	0.204-0.843	0.015
WF / SH	WF	0.322	1.020-1.866	0.036	0.726	1.354-3.154	0.001	1.196	1.550-7.049	0.002
	SH	0.477	1.184-2.194	0.002	0.349	0.933-2.155	0.102	-0.371	0.308-1.548	0.369
WF / NOW	WF	0.346	1.045-1.912	0.024	1.062	1.746-4.795	0.000	1.450	1.976-9.192	0.002
	NOW	0.781	1.470-3.243	0.000	0.652	1.030-3.576	0.040	0.575	0.741-4.267	0.198
WF / HP	WF	0.411	1.076-2.117	0.017	1.134	1.735-5.571	0.000	1.432	1.686-10.39	0.002
	HP	-0.219	0.579-1.112	0.187	-0.363	0.423-1.145	0.154	-0.717	0.237-1.007	0.052
NOW / HP	NOW	0.939	1.654-3.956	0.000	0.989	1.289-5.601	0.008	1.100	1.111-8.117	0.030
	HP	-0.375	0.502-0.939	0.018	-0.692	0.308-0.813	0.005	-1.104	0.164-0.671	0.002
MF / NOW / HP	MF	-0.317	0.501-1.058	0.096	-0.805	0.232-0.863	0.016	-1.446	0.071-0.779	0.018
	NOW	0.891	1.573-3.780	0.000	0.867	1.140-4.972	0.021	0.943	0.951-6.940	0.063
	HP	-0.321	0.526-0.997	0.048	-0.583	0.341-0.913	0.020	-0.946	0.190-0.794	0.010
WF / NOW / HP	WF	0.381	1.041-2.057	0.028	1.104	1.680-5.413	0.000	1.396	1.622-10.06	0.003
	NOW	0.906	1.601-3.826	0.000	0.875	1.156-4.980	0.019	0.962	0.974-7.035	0.056
	HP	-0.259	0.555-1.071	0.121	-0.405	0.404-1.101	0.113	-0.760	0.226-0.969	0.041

Table 6. Cox regression models

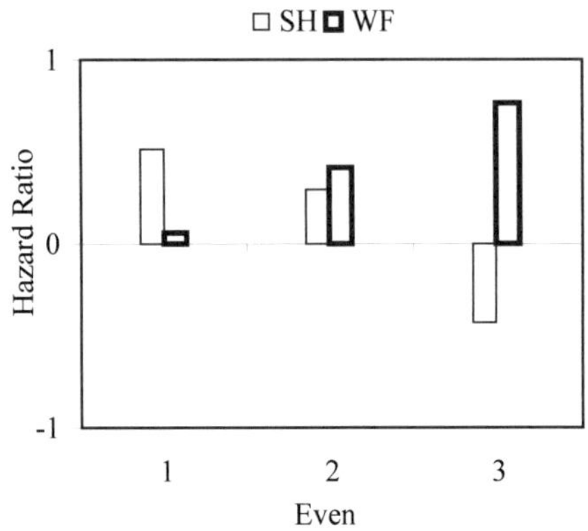

Fig. 3.1. Synergy (Competence)

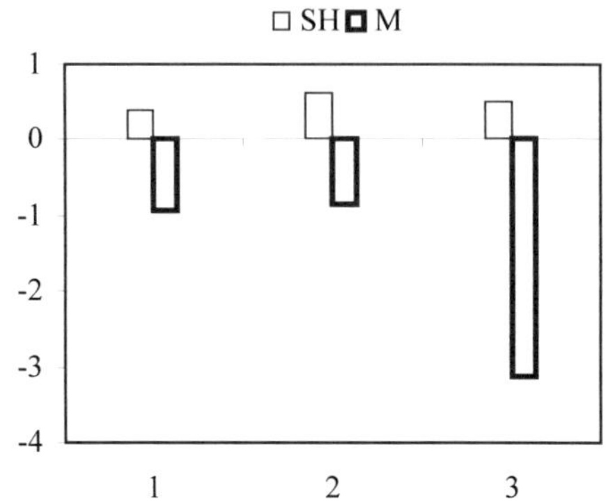

Fig. 3.2. Antagonism

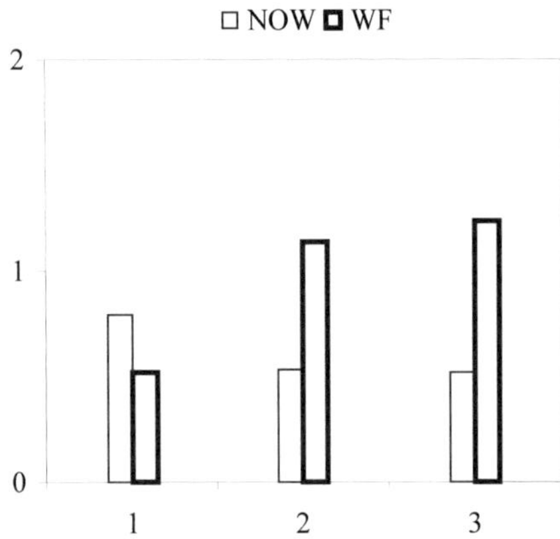

Fig. 3.3. Synergy

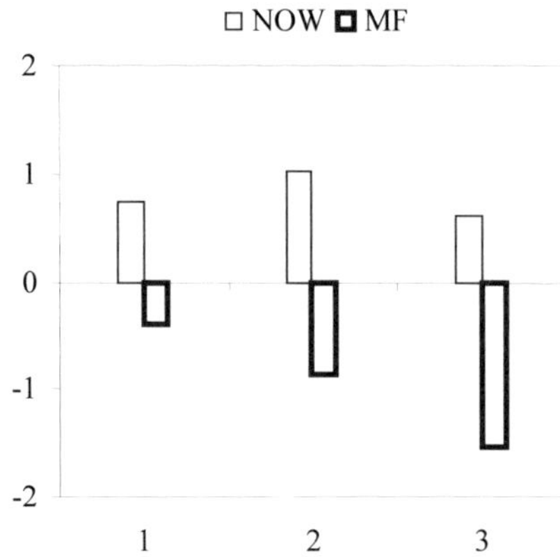

Fig. 3.4. Antagonism

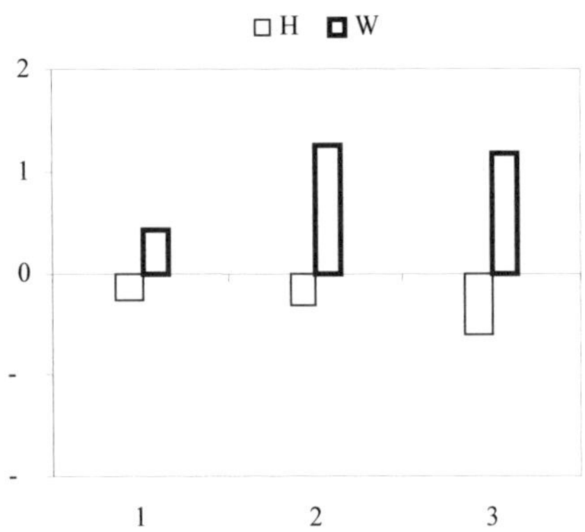

Fig. 3.5. Antagonism

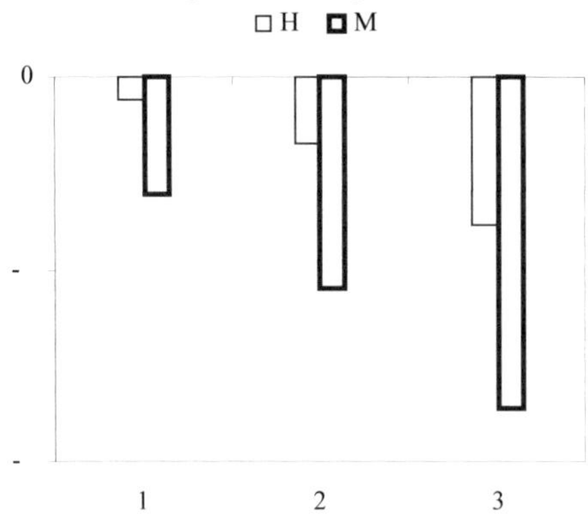

Fig. 3.6. Synergy

Fig. 3. Risk factor comparison with the personal habits through the hazard and according the event

Smoking in the WF atmosphere produces a synergistic effect, the action of which is minimised over time (Figure 3.1.). It is curious that for event 3 welding fumes and tobacco have an antagonistic effect; tobacco loses its effect in relation to welding fumes in the medium term (event 2) and long term (event 3), both with $p>0.05$.

The effect of non-occupational noise is antagonistic to that of metalworking fluids (Figure 3.4.), accelerating hearing alteration uniformly depending on the event, although it is in event 2 where it is most apparent, decreasing in the following event ($p>0.05$). By contrast, the effect of MF atmospheres strengthens over time, or to put it another way, the delay in hearing alteration increases with time $p<0.05$).

Hearing alteration	Normality					Linearity			
	μ (Xi)	σ (Xi)	VC	K-S (Z)	Sig 2 tailed	μ ln(Xi)	σ ln(Xi)	R^2 Normal	R^2 Log Normal
H	13.13	11.39	85.63%	2.076	0.0004	2.05	1.16	0.852	0.708
IAT	24.73	8.72	35.26%	1.001	0.2636	3.11	0.54	0.738	0.925
AAT	27.38	8.07	29.47%	0.959	0.3163	3.24	0.42	0.702	0.938
MH	29.31	7.92	27.02%	0.658	0.7788	3.34	0.31	0.679	0.930
AH	32.62	7.30	22.38%	0.926	0.3571	3.45	0.32	0.631	0.942

VC: Variation coefficient; K-S: Kolmogorov-Smirnov test; R^2: Determination coefficient

Table 7. Normality and linearity conditions

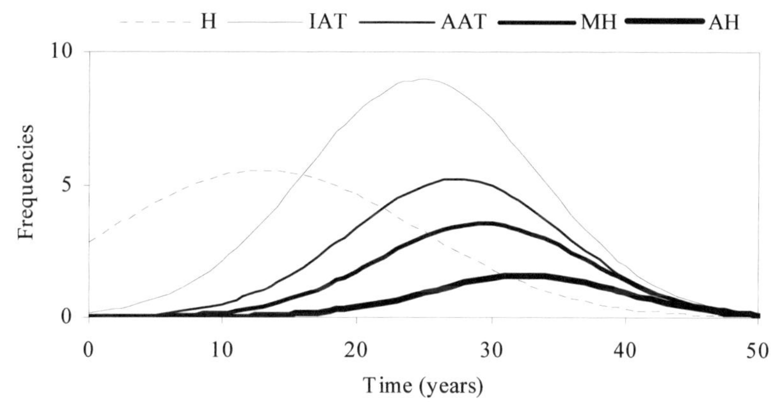

Fig. 4.1. Normal

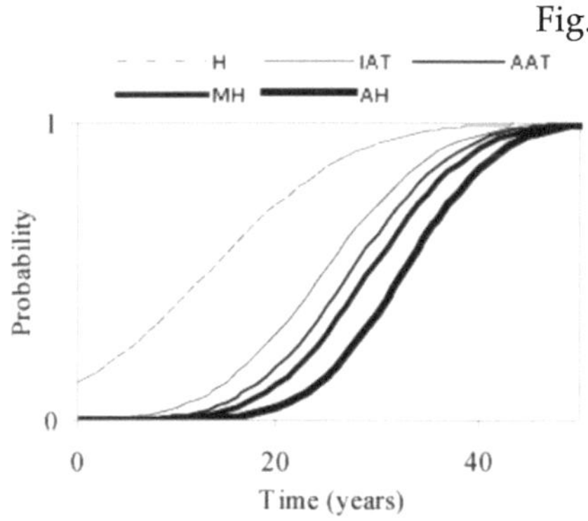

Fig. 4.2. Cumulated Normal

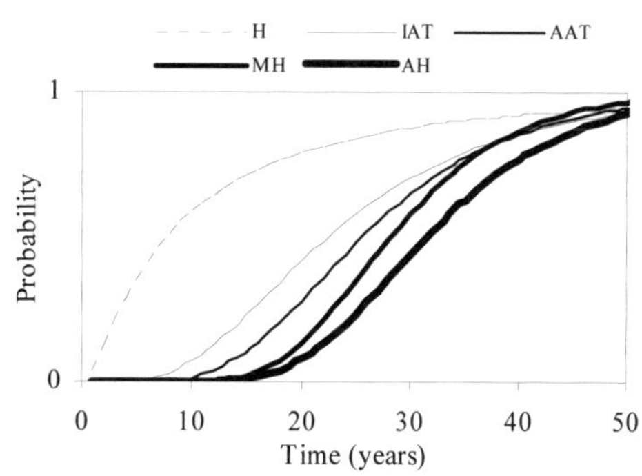

Fig. 4.3. Log Normal

Fig. 4. Parametric survival functions obtained for all atmospheres (MF+N+WF, N=558)

Categories	Normal			Log Normal		
	U	Z	Sig [1]	t	CV-t [2]	Sig
H-IAT	6811	-9.066	0.0000	3.7024	1.9839	0.0003
IAT-AAT	8349	-2.698	0.0070	0.5595	1.9804	0.5768
AAT-MH	3283	-1.193	0.2325	0.4361	1.9804	0.6635
MH-AH	715	-2.309	0.0209	0.7795	1.9802	0.4372

([1, 2]) 2 tailed; CV-t: critical value for t

Table 8. Contrast of parametric survival functions (U of Mann-Whitney and t-test)

In WF atmospheres non-occupational noise produces a uniform effect depending on the event. It plays a more active role in event 1 in hearing alteration in relation to smoke (Figure 3.3.).

The use of individual protection equipment produces an effect similar to that of metalworking fluids, although their effectiveness increases over time (Figure 3.6.). This is characteristic when the protection equipment is not used continuously. It also explains the major delay produced in MF atmospheres.

In WF atmospheres the use of individual protection equipment is clearly antagonistic (Figure 3.5.), increasing in effectiveness over time, although the action of the WF atmosphere is much more powerful than the protection equipment.

Subsequently the effect on hearing of exposure to all atmospheres in the metal industry was analysed. To do this the initial sample was subdivided into the 3 atmospheres studied and in turn each one of these was divided into the five phases of hearing alteration. In doing this the frequencies were considerably reduced and as a consequence the analysis was not very consistent. Using the combined analysis of atmospheres to study the various phases of hearing alteration was the most useful option. For this analysis a parametric model (log-normal) was used to obtain the survival functions (Figure 4.3.). This has the advantage over those non-parametric models of the probability distribution of the event using continuous functions. This gives more precision to the distribution of each degree of hearing alteration and as a consequence to the identification of the time of the event (Figure 4, Table 8).

In this case, the survival curves must be understood as the combination of individuals who present a specific hearing alteration, independently of the atmosphere to which they are exposed and their personal habits. Each function associated with a degree of hearing alteration characterises an average value i.e. a theoretical value consisting of the combination of the three atmospheres to which must be added the combination of "habits" of the individuals in the sample (Figure 4.1.).

The conditions of normality and linearity of each degree of hearing alteration, obtained according to time, were assessed (Table 7).

The similarity of the survival functions for the different degrees of hearing alteration was also assessed using parametric and non-parametric methods, with the objective of making both the results and their interpretation homogeneous (Figure 5). It should be noted that except for the group of healthy people who do not follow a normal distribution, the remaining degrees of hearing alteration do follow a normal distribution. It can also be seen that in accordance with the degree hearing alteration the mean value of the distributions are displaced to the right. This confirms the suitability of the sample, which is also corroborated by the low frequency of individuals that are affected as the degree of hearing alteration increases. The spread of hearing alteration over time can be seen. Thus, once the level of advanced acoustic trauma is reached, the individual undergoes a more rapid process of hearing alteration. This can be substantiated, because the curves tend to unite more than in the IAT / AAT transition.

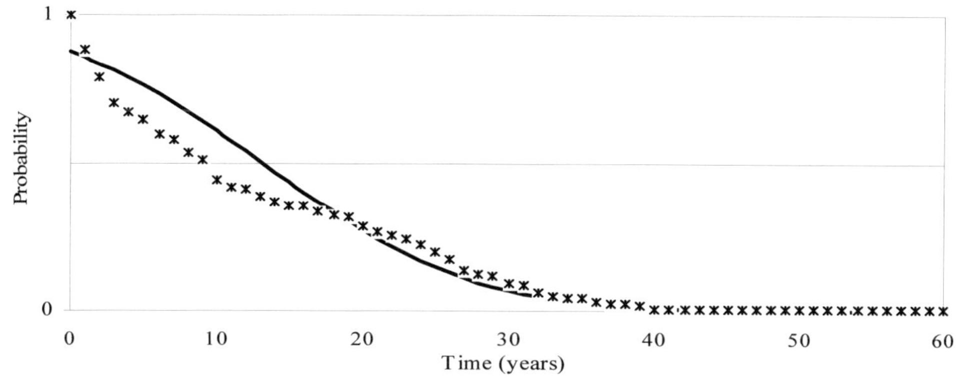

Fig. 5.1. Healthy

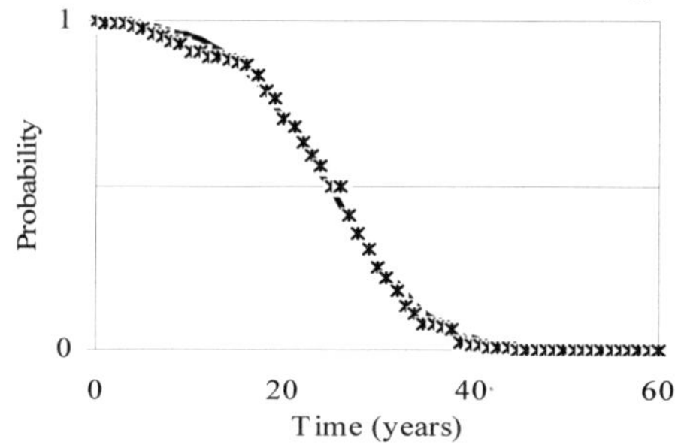

Fig. 5.2. IAT

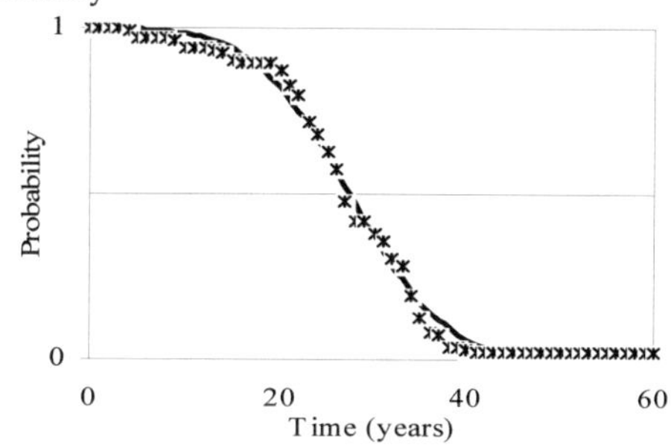

Fig. 5.3. AAT

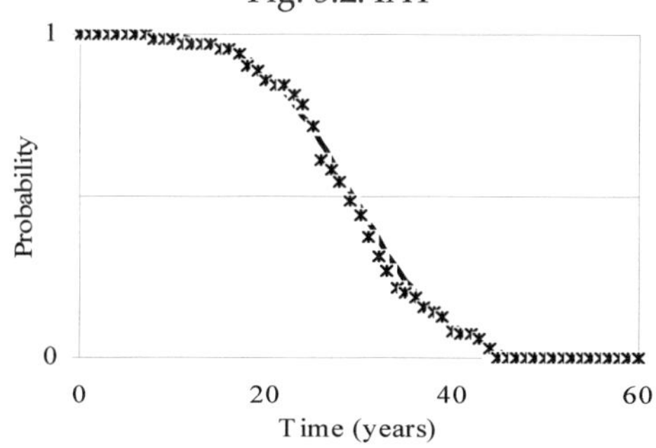

Fig. 5.4. MH

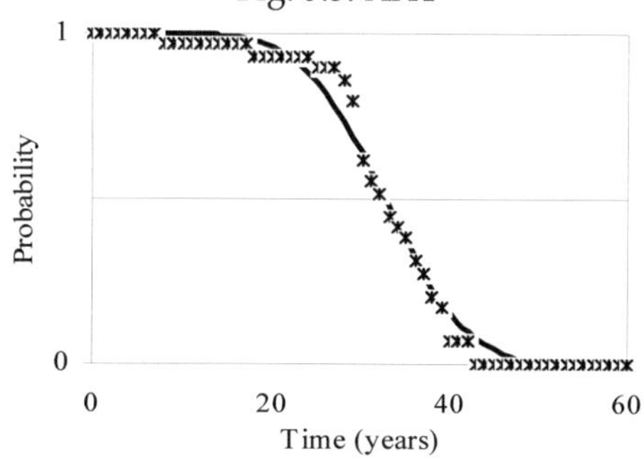

Fig. 5.5. AH

Fig. 5. Survival function equivalence obtained by parametric and no parametric models

5. Discussion

The qualitative methodology proposed for the study of the combined influence of noise and chemical pollutants on hearing loss (Conte et al., 2009) differs from that used in traditional studies on the same topic. These perform a quantitative analysis of decreases in the hearing threshold, an aspect which was replaced by an audiogram classification based on a diagnostic reference. The duration of each individual's exposure to noise was also used, instead of their age, thereby improving the linear behaviour of the temporal variable. Finally, each chemical contaminant was characterised by a binary variable, thus avoiding the use of an environmental measurement value, which provides more general and less restrictive identification than quantitative environmental measurements.

This study shows the influence of noise on hearing alteration, whether temporary (IAT) or permanent (AAT, MH, AH). This situation is consistent with studies conducted on the influence of this physical agent on hearing.

Moreover, chemical agents taken as interacting with noise (MF and WF) have been considered by various researchers as pulmonary toxins (Godderis et al., 2008; Schaller et al., 2007), due to the principal way they enter the body: by inhalation. It is nonetheless true that the influence of these agents on hearing loss, a toxic effect that can be considered indirect, has not been given due attention.

This study confirms the existence of an interaction between physical and chemical factors in the metal industry which influence the alteration of auditory function, and which can be characterised by three different exposure environments, WF with noise, MF with noise, and noise only.

The interaction of the pollutants with the individual determines whether the auditory effects caused by the main risk factor (noise) develop more quickly or slowly in the worker. Thus, it can be identified that metalworking fluids delay the development and worsening of the various stages of auditory alteration, whereas welding fumes speed up the development of same. In this respect, the behaviour of one contaminant with another is antagonistic.

The study also indicates that, in the case of welding fumes, the chemical agent is shown to be more detrimental to hearing. One of the main problems regarding welding fumes in the presence of noise is that, in general, the protection used is effective in muffling noise intensity but not in reducing the effect of the chemical agent. In this situation, cellulose masks or those of similar compounds have little effect, as their capacity to filter particles (such as charcoal) is not effective for gaseous molecules such as carbon monoxide, which is highly ototoxic (Gwin et al., 2005; Morley et al., 1999).

As regards personal habits, there is a growing tendency to use hearing protection as the harmfulness of the environment increases. The interpretation of this fact is due to an increased personal willingness to use protective equipment when the individual feels some discomfort, which may be intuitively associated with the work environment. This study verifies that the increase in using protection is not sufficiently capable of improving auditory health conditions, supporting the negative effects of welding fumes on workers.

With regard to the regression models, it has been demonstrated that the univariate models (MF and WF) are those which best, and more accurately, define each model according to the event.

Despite a loss of accuracy, the bivariate models may be more interesting as regards application. For Event1, the variable SH is shown to be the most influential and best represented of the models. For this event, NOW is also considered an acceptable model, along with WF.

For Event2 the ideal models are MF with NOW and with HP, as well as WF with NOW. There is a decline in accuracy with respect to the previous event.

For Event3 only the MF-HP model is considered suitable, with the other two habits losing significance.

This indicates the influence obtained for each habit variable: SH influences IAT; NOW influences the development of AAT; HP is influential as protection at all stages, even if it is ineffective against fumes.

The influence of smoking habits (SH) on the initial auditory alteration recognised in this study coincides with the results obtained by other authors (Pouryaghoub et al., 2007; Ferrite et al., 2005; Mizoue et al., 2003), but indicates the need for further research in order to properly assess this influence.

6. Conclusions

A methodological framework was presented which made it possible to use employment related health databases with limited information. The limitations of the data, resulting from possible changes in the way the data was obtained and recorded during the period under study, led to the use of qualitative, binary response variables and only one quantitative variable, namely the time of exposure to noise.

With this situation as the starting point, it was established that that survival analysis is one of the best ways of analysing this type of data, both in relation to defining probability-time functions and their contrasts, and for modelling using Cox regression, in relation to both the application possibilities and the results reached (descriptive-explanatory in character).

This research was aimed at the analysis of the interaction between noise and chemicals and its influence on occupational hearing loss. It was found that in the Aragonese metal sector, which was the focus of this study, there were three main atmospheres: noise with metalworking fluids, noise only and noise with welding fumes.

The analysis made it possible to establish that hearing alteration in individuals was related to the exposure atmosphere. Thus, workers exposed to noise and metalworking fluids, who protected themselves less, experienced slower hearing alteration compared to those who were exposed to only noise, and workers exposed to welding fumes, who protected themselves more, suffered hearing alterations sooner than those who were only exposed to noise.

7. References

Agrawal S, Platz EA, Niparko JK. (2009). Risk Factors for Hearing Loss in EU Adults: Data from the National Health and Nutrition Examination Survey. *Otology & Neurotology*, Vol. 30, N°2, (February 2009), pp. 139-145, ISSN 1531-7129

Benzecri J. (1992). *Correspondence Analysis Handbook*. Marcel Decker, ISBN 0824784375, New York, EEUU

Conte JC, Dominguez AI, Garcia AI, Rubio E, Perez A. (2010). Cox Regression Model of Hearing Loss in Workers Exposed to Noise and Metalworking Fluids or Welding Fumes. *Anales del Sistema Sanitario de Navarra*, Vol. 33, N° 1, (April 2010), pp. 11-21, ISSN 1137-6627

Cova LJ, Márquez JJ, Tovar R. (2001). Interpretación Catastrófica de un Análisis de Correspondencias Múltiples Aplicado a un Cultivo in vitro de Crysanthemun s.p. *Ciencia*, Vol. 9, N° 2, (April-June 2001), pp. 164-195, ISSN 1315-2076

Cox DR & Snell DJ. (1989). *Analysis of Binary Data*. Chapman & Hall, ISBN 9780412306204, London, England

Ferrite S & Santana V. (2005). Joint Effects of Smoking, Noise Exposure and Age on Hearing Loss. *Occupational Medicine*, Vol. 55, N° 1, (January 2005), pp. 48-53, ISSN 0962-7480

Gobba F. (2003). Occupational Exposure to Chemicals and Sensory Organs: a Neglected Research Field. *Neurotoxicology*, Vol. 24, N° 4-5, (August 2003), pp. 675-691, ISSN 0161-813X

Godderis L, Deschuyffeleer T, Roelandt H. (2008). Exposure to Metalworking Fluids and Respiratory and Dermatological Complains in a Secondary Aluminium Plant. *International Archives of Occupational and Environmental Health*, Vol. 81, N° 7, (July 2008), pp. 845-853, ISSN 0340-0131

Greenland S. (1994). Alternative Models for Ordinal Logistic Regression. *Statistics in Medicine*, Vol. 13, N°16, (August 1994), pp. 1665-1677, ISSN 1097-0258

Gwin KK, Wallingford KM, Morata TC, Campen LE van, Dallaire J, Alvarez FJ. (2005). Ototoxic Occupational Exposures for a Stock Car Racing Team: II. Chemical Surveys. Journal of Occupational and Environmental Hygiene, Vol. 2, N° 8, (August 2005), pp. 406-413, ISSN 1545-9264

Hosmer DW & Lemeshow S. (1999). *Applied Survival Analysis: Regression Modelling of Time to Event Data*. Wiley, ISBN 0471154105, New York, EEUU

Klockhoff I, Drettner B, Hagelin KW, Lindholm L. (1973). A Method for Computerized Classification of Pure Tone Screening Audiometry Results in Noise Exposed Groups. *Acta Oto-Laryngologica*, Vol. 75, N° 2-6, (January 1973), pp. 339-340, ISSN 0001-6489

Martín Q y de Paz YR. *Aplicación de las Redes Neuronales Artificiales a la Regresión*. (2007). La Muralla, Col. Cuadernos de Estadística, N° 35, ISBN 9788471337672, Madrid, España

Mizoue T, Miyamoto T, Shimizu T. (2003). Combined Effect of Smoking an Occupational Exposure to Noise on Hearing Loss in Steel Factory Workers. *Occupational and Environmental Medicine*, Vol. 60, N° 1, (January 2003), pp. 56-59, ISSN 1097-9212

Morley JC, Seitz T, Tubbs R. (1999). Carbon Monoxide and Noise Exposure at a Monster Truck and Motocross Show. *Applied Occupational and Environmental Hygiene*, Vol. 14, N° 10, (October 1999), pp. 645-655, ISSN 1047-322X

Pouryaghoub G, Mehrdad R, Mohammadi S. (2007). Interaction of Smoking and Occupational Noise Exposure on Hearing Loss: a Cross-Sectional Study. *BMC Public Health*, Vol. 7, N° 3, Article Number 137, (July 2007), pp. 137, ISSN 1471-2458

Rothman KJ. (1986). *Modern Epidemiology*. Little-Brown, ISBN 9780316757768, Boston, EEUU

Schaller KH, Csanady G, Filser J, Jüngert B, Drexler B. (2007). Elimination Kinetics of Metals after an Accident Exposure to Welding Fumes. *International Archives of Occupational and Environmental Health*, Vol. 80, N° 7, (July 2007), pp. 635-641, ISSN 0340-0131

Silva LC y Barroso IM. (2004). *Regresión Logística*. La Muralla / Hespérides, Col. Cuadernos de Estadística, N° 27, ISBN 847133738X, Madrid, España

Thom R. (1971). *Modéles Mathématiques de la Morphogénese*. Accademia Nazionale dei Lincei, Scuola Normale Superiore di Pisa, ISBN 9788876422928, Pisa, Italia

Thorne PR, Ameratunga SN, Stewart J, Reid N, Williams W, Purdy SC, Dodd G, Wallaart J. (2008). Epidemiology of Noise-Induced Hearing Loss in New Zealand. *New Zealand Medical Journal*, Vol. 121, N° 1280, (August 2008), pp. 33-44, ISSN 0110-7704

Part 4

Genetics

11

Genetics of Hearing Loss

Nejat Mahdieh[1,2], Bahareh Rabbani[1] and Ituro Inoue[1]
[1]*Division of Human Genetics, National Institute of Genetics, Mishima, Shizuoka,*
[2]*Medical Genetic Group, Faculty of Medicine, Ilam University of Medical Sciences, Ilam,*
[1]*Japan*
[2]*Iran*

1. Introduction

Hearing loss (HL) is the most common sensory defect in human beings, affecting 1.86 in 1000 newborns around the *world* which half of it is due to genetic causes (Morton & Nance, 2006). HL can be syndromic or nonsyndromic. Individuals affected with syndromic form have additional clinical signs whereas nonsyndromic HL is not associated with other clinical signs and symptoms. All Mendelian pattern of inheritance have been observed in nonsyndromic HL (NSHL) including autosomal dominant (AD), autosomal recessive (AR), X-linked inheritance (XL) and mitochondrial inheritance (MT); autosomal recessive is the main form of NSHL, i.e. 75-85 % of NSHL show AR pattern in affected pedigrees.

As known, ear is the organ of hearing and balance. Hearing is dependent on a series of complex events. The ear has three anatomical parts including outer, middle and inner ear. The external ear which is composed of the auricle, ear canal and eardrum membrane collects sound waves and transmits them to the eardrum. Three tiny bones of middle ear (the ossicles) act as levers and conduct the sounds to the oval window, and finally through the cochlea (a snail-shaped organ) which has the auditory receptors (the organ of Corti) in the inner ear [Raphael & Altschuler 2003]. A collagen-based extracellular matrix, called tectorial membrane on top of the hair cells is vibrated by sound waves [Richardson et al., 2008]. Within the organ of Corti, physical vibrations produce a mechanoelectrical transduction which is detected by hair cells and these cells respond by producing electrical impulses. Nerves transmit these impulses to the brain where they are interpreted. Different sound frequencies stimulate the hair cells in different parts of the organ of Corti and lead to perception of different sound frequencies. Sounds are processed in both sides of the brain but the interpretation of the sounds takes place at the left side of brain. Sounds are heard at normal hearing thresholds between 0-20 dB across the 125-8000 Hz range while loss of more than 20 dB, is said to have hearing loss which is confirmed by measuring pure tone average (PTA) (average hearing sensitivity at 500, 1000 and 2000 Hz).

Nearly one hundred and twenty million people suffer from hearing impairment around the world. History of some important events about human hereditary HL is shown in table 1 [Nance & Sweeney, 1975; Wallis et al., 1988; Kimberling et al., 1990; Leon et al., 1992;

Guilford et al., 1994; Kelsell et al., 1997; Lynch et al., 1997; Eudy et al., 1998; Gorlin, 2004; Dror & Avraham 2009].

Time	Event
Sixteenth century	Reports indicating the prevention of the deaf from marrying
Seventeenth century	The mode of recessive and dominant HL
Nineteenth century	"The most frequent causes of congenital deafness are hereditary.. ."
1968	One of the genetic forms of deafness was described
1975	The forms of HL, the need for research and genetic counseling were described
1988	An X-linked form of deafness was mapped in a large Mauritian family
1990	The first locus for syndromic HL, *USH2A*, was mapped
1992	The first locus for ADNSHL*, DFNA1, was mapped in a Costa Rican family
1994	The first and second loci for ARNSHL▪, DFNB1 and DFNB2, and DFNA2 loci were mapped
1997	*GJB2* and DIAPH1 genes were discovered for DFNB1 and DFNA1 loci, respectively

*Autosomal domiant non syndromic hearing loss, ▪Autosomal recessive nonsyndromic hearing loss

Table 1. Chronological events regarding hereditary HL.

One of the main programs of the World Health Organization (WHO) is to encourage countries for the prevention of deafness [Emery, 2003]. Understanding the molecular and genetic mechanisms of HL may lead to development of new therapy and treatment approaches. Here, we review major causes leading to either syndromic or nonsyndromic HL.

2. Classification of hearing loss

Approximately two-thirds of the HL affected children show the problem at birth and unfortunately it may not be diagnosed before the age of 3 years. HL has several classification criteria which are important for diagnosis, prognosis and treatment [Mahdieh et al., 2010a]. These criteria are summarized in table 2.

2.1 Etiology

Based on the cause of sensorineural deafness, HL is categorized into three major forms as acquired, genetic and unknown. There are many causes for hearing loss:

1. Acquired HL: infectious and pharmaceutical agents known as teratogens would affect the sense of hearing. HL could occur by physiological, biochemical or infectious factors. However, genetic background has an important effect on its occurrence. The risk factors that may affect the hearing process are as follows:

   a. factors before birth including congenital infections (e.g. toxoplasmosis, measles, syphilis, smallpox, cytomegalovirus, herpes virus), congenital deformities of aurical and ear duct [Willems, 2004; Shin et al., 2011].
   b. factors during birth including prematurity and low birth weight (less than 1500gr) and increased blood bilirubin [Willems, 2004].
   c. factors affecting after birth including infections and bacterial meningitis, mumps, otitis media, blood infection and autotxic drugs such as aminoglycosides, head injury or skull fracture which lead to anesthesia [Willems, 2004].
2. Genetic HL: the genetic basis of HL is known for more than 100 years. In the early decade of 1800s, the Irish physician William Wild explained the inheritance of HL. His theory differentiated between dominant and recessive inheritance. He also observed that men showed more X-linked transmission [Willems, 2004].

2.2 Severity

Intensity of the sound is calculated in units of decibel (dB), which is logarithm intensity of the sound wave to a reference sound intensity divided by ten [Willems, 2004]. The normal hearing threshold is 15 dB. A regular conversation occurs at level of 45 to 60 dB.

2.3 Position of damage

a. Conductive HL: Factors affecting sound transmission including aurical, ear canal, eardrum, outer and middle ear bones to the cochlea cause conductive HL. The most common causes of conductive HL are the external and middle ear congenital abnormalities such as atrophy and dysplasia, duct obstruction, impacted cerumen, otitis, middle ear and Tympanic membrane problems.
b. Sensorineural HL (SNHL): The disorder occurs in the auditory nerve or the cochlea. In other words, the abnormalities occur some place between the hair cells and auditory brain regions. The most common causes of SNHL are:
   b1. congenital causes such as rubella, syphilis, Usher syndrome, Alport Syndrome, Waardenburg syndrome and autosomal dominant and recessive sensorineural deafness [Friedman et al., 2003].
   b2. acquired factors: Infections such as measles, cytomegalovirus, bacterial meningitis, autotoxicity of drug consumption, noise pollution including long-term exposure, presbycusis and sudden idiopathic HL [Willems, 2004].
c. Mixed HL: in this type of hearing loss, conductive and sensorineural problems are observed simultaneously. Infections such as tuberculosis, some syndromes and skull fractures may also cause mixed HL.

2.4 Age of onset

On the basis of the age of onset, HL is divided into the following types:

a. Prelingual: Loss of hearing occurs before speech is acquired. If a child has a congenital hearing impairment, he would not be able to speak normally.
b. Postlingual: Loss of hearing occurs after speech is developed.
c. Presbycusis or age-related HL (ARHL): Epidemiologic studies show that nearly 25 % of 60 year olds and more than 50 % of 80 year ages undergo ARHL [Dror & Avraham, 2009; Huang & Tang, 2010].

2.5 Signs

HL may be associated with other physical problems which are called syndromic HL. Genetic HLs without any other complications is called non-syndromic genetic hearing loss [Willems, 2004]. HL loci are named with the prefix DFN, followed by the mode of inheritance which is indicated by B, A, X and Y for autosomal recessive (DFNB), autosomal dominant (DFNA), X-linked (DFNX) and Y-linked (DFNY), respectively. The order in which loci have been described is denoted by a number after these letters, e.g. DFNB1 is the first identified locus causing autosomal recessive HL [Guilford et al., 1994].

Criterion	Class	Definition and example
Age of onset	Prelingual HL	HL occurs before language acquisition
	Postlingual HL	HL occurs after language acquisition
	Presbycusis	Age-related HL
Etiology	Acquired	Caused by environmental agents such as viral and bacterial infections (prenatal, e.g., CMV, toxoplasmosis, rubella; postnatal, e.g, meningitis), hyperbilirubinemia, head trauma, anoxia, noise exposure and ototoxic drugs
	Genetic	Caused by gene mutation
	Idiopathic	Unexplained cause
Clinical phenotypes	Syndromic	associated with other symptoms
	Nonsyndromic	Deafness is the only defect
Position of damage	Conductive HL	Caused by a problem transferring sound waves through the external ear, tympanic membrane or middle ear
	Sensorineural HL	Caused by damage to the inner ear (vestibulocochlear nerve)
	Mixed HL	Caused by a combination of sensorineural and conductive HL
Severity	Mild	Difficulty in hearing of 26–40 dB sounds
	Moderate	41–55 dB
	Moderately severe	56–70 dB
	Severe	71–90 dB
	Profound	>90 dB
Mode of inheritance	Autosomal dominant	DFNA loci (DFNA1-64)
	Autosomal recessive	DFNB loci (DFNB1-96)
	Sex-linked	DFNX loci (DFN1-8)
	Y-linked	DFNY loci (DFNY1)
	Mitochondrial	12SrRNA (MT-RNR1), $tRNA^{Ser(UCN)}$ (MT-TS1)

Table 2. Various criteria for the classification of hearing loss.

3. The frequency of genetic HL

Genetic HL occurs 1 in 2000 to 1 in 650 live births [Morton & Nance, 2006]. About 70% of the cases are nonsyndromic [Tekin et al., 2001]. Studies show that 75% of nonsyndromic HL are inherited as autosomal recessive [Tekin et al., 2001]. 10-20% of cases are inherited as autosomal dominant and 1-5% are X-linked recessive. Approximately, 1% of human genes, i.e 200 to 250 genes are responsible for hereditary HL [Finsterer & Fellinger, 2005]. So far, more than one hundred loci and 55 genes have identified which are involved in nonsyndromic HL (http://hereditaryhearingloss.org).

4. Non-syndromic HL

A high frequency of genetic HL occurs without any abnormality in other organs classified as non-syndromic HL. Different patterns of inheritance have been observed in NSHL.

4.1 Different types of NSHL

Variety of protein coding genes such as gap junctions (connexin encoding genes), motor proteins (myosins) cytoskeletal (e.g. actin), ion channels, structural proteins (Tectorin alpha, Otoancorin, Stereocilin, etc), transcription factors (POU3F4, POU4F3 and Eyes absent 4 or EYA4), and additionally microRNA genes are involved in HL [Willems, 2004; Mencia et al., 2009; Mahdieh et al., 2010a]. *GJB2* mutations are seen in 50% of autosomal recessive HL in the Caucasians [Kelsell et al., 1997; Tekin et al., 2001]. Some genes e.g. *GJB2* gene is expressed in a variety of organs of the body while others such as *OTOA*ncorin is only expressed in the inner ear.

4.1.1 Autosomal recessive non-syndromic HL

Autosomal recessive non-syndromic HL (ARNSHL) was first described in 1846. It is the severest form of congenital HL in which there is a defect in cochlea in nearly all cases. Loci of ARNSHL are designated as the DFNB; DF stands for Deafness and B indicates the autosomal recessive pattern of inheritance. Up to date, 46 genes and nearly 100 loci have been identified for HL (Table 3). Regarding different studies, connexin 26 gene mutations differ depending on geographical place and ethnicity [Zelante et al., 1997; Morell et al., 1998; Mahdieh & Rabbani, 2009]. Here, we discuss the most common genes causing ARNSHL.

4.1.1.1 *GJB2* and *GJB6* genes and connexins

The first locus of ARNSHL designated as DFNB1 was identified by Guilford and colleagues in 1994. These researches confirmed linkage to chromosome 13q12-q13 in two consanguineous families [Guilford et al., 1994]. More consanguineous families of different ethnic groups were linked to the DFNB1 locus [Morle et al., 2000]. Phenotypic differences were observed within different families which indicated that allelic heterogeneity may be present in the locus DFNB1.

GJB2 is a small gene encompassing 5.5 Kb. It has two exons encoding a 4.2Kb mRNA and a protein of 226 amino acids. A six repeat of G is located at position 30 to 35 of coding region of *GJB2* gene from which deletion of one G is known as 35delG or 30delG (Figure 1) [Kelley et al., 1998]. 35delG is the most common mutation in the Caucasians and may cause up to 70% of all *GJB2* gene mutations. Profound HL caused by *GJB2* gene mutations is found in 50% of the cases; 30% are severe, 20% moderate and 1-2% are mild cases [Smith & Hone, 2003]. Other *GJB2* mutations have been reported with higher frequencies in some ethnic groups [Morell et al., 1998; Mahdieh & Rabbani, 2009]. A large number of studies have been reported about *GJB2* mutations including genotype-phenotype correlations, phenotypic variability, de novo mutations, dominant mutations, ethnic-specific distribution of mutations, digenic inheritance and allelic heterogeneity [del Castillo et al., 2002; Smith & Hone, 2003; Mahdieh et al., 2009; 2010b, 2010c]. Also, a modifier gene has been suggested because of intrafamilial phenotypic variability of the cases [Higert et al., 2009a; Mahdieh et al., 2010b].

GJB2 and *GJB6* genes are about 35 kb apart from each other. *GJB6* gene encodes a protein called Connexin 30 (MIM 604418) which has 261 amino acids. Connexin 30 is produced in different tissues of the body such as the cochlea, brain and thyroid [Grifa et al., 1999]. The importance of this gene was evident when some families had a mutated allele of *GJB2* and the second mutant allele was in the *GJB6* (digenic inheritance) [del Castillo et al., 2002].

Locus	Location	Gene	references
		X-Linked	
DFNX1	Xq22	*PRPS1*	Liu et al., 2010
DFNX2	Xq21.1	*POU3F4*	De Kok et al., 1995
DFNX4	Xp22	*SMPX*	del Castillo et al., 1996
		Autosomal Dominant	
DFNA1	5q31	DIAPH1	Lynch et al., 1997
DFNA2A	1p34	*KCNQ4*	Kubisch et al., 1999
DFNA2B	1p35.1	GJB3	Xia et al., 1998
DFNA3A	13q11-q12	*GJB2*	Kelsell et al., 1997
DFNA3B	13q12	*GJB6*	Grifa et al., 1999
DFNA4	19q13	*MYH14*	Donaudy et al, 2004
DFNA5	7p15	*DFNA5*	Van Laer et al., 1998
DFNA6	4p16.3	*WFS1*	Bespalova et al., 2001
DFNA9	14q12-q13	*COCH*	Robertson et al., 1998
DFNA10	6q22-q23	*EYA4*	Wayne et al., 2001
DFNA11	11q12.3-q21	*MYO7A*	Liu et al., 1997
DFNA12	11q22-24	*TECTA*	Verhoeven et al., 1998
DFNA13	6p21	*COL11A2*	McGuirt et al., 1999
DFNA15	5q31	*POU4F3*	Vahava et al., 1998
DFNA17	22q	*MYH9*	Lalwani et al., 2000
DFNA20	17q25	*ACTG1*	Zhu et al., 2003,
DFNA22	6q13	*MYO6*	Melchionda et al.,
DFNA28	8q22	*GRHL2*	Peters et al., 2002
DFNA36	9q13-q21	*TMC1*	Kurima et al., 2002
DFNA39	4q21.3	*DSPP*	Xiao et al., 2001
DFNA44	3q28-29	*CCDC50*	Modamio-Hoybjor et al., 2007
DFNA48	12q13-q14	*MYO1A*	Donaudy et al., 2003
DFNA50	7q32.2	*MIR96*	Mencia et al., 2009
DFNA51	9q21	*TJP2*	Walsh et al., 2010
DFNA64	12q24.31-12q24.32	*SMAC/DIABLO*	Cheng et al., 2011

Locus	Location	Gene	references
		Autosomal Recessive	
DFNB1	13q12	*GJB2*	Kelsell et al., 1997
DFNB2	11q13.5	*MYO7A*	Liu et al., 1997
DFNB3	17p11.2	*MYO15A*	Wang et al., 1998
DFNB4	7q31	*SLC26A4*	Li et al., 1998
DFNB6	3p14-p21	*TMIE*	Naz et al, 2002
DFNB7/11	9q13-q21	*TMC1*	Kurima et al., 2002
DFNB8/10	21q22	*TMPRSS3*	Scott et al., 2001
DFNB9	2p22-p23	*OTOF*	Yasunaga et al., 1999
DFNB12	10q21-q22	*CDH23*	Bork et al., 2001
DFNB15	19p13	*GIPC3*	Charizopoulou et al., 2011
DFNB16	15q21-q22	*STRC*	Verpy et al., 2001
DFNB18	11p14-15.1	*USH1C*	Ouyang et al., 2002
DFNB21	11q	*TECTA*	Mustapha et al., 1999
DFNB22	16p12.2	*OTOA*	Zwaenepoel et al ., 2002
DFNB23	10p11.2-q21	*PCDH15*	Ahmed et al, 2003
DFNB24	11q23	*RDX*	Khan et al., 2007
DFNB25	4p13	*GRXCR1*	Schraders et al., 2010
DFNB28	22q13	*TRIOBP*	Riazuddin et al, 2006
DFNB29	21q22	*CLDN14*	Wilcox et al., 2001
DFNB30	10p11.1	*MYO3A*	Walsh et al., 2002
DFNB31	9q32-q34	*WHRN*	Mburu et al., 2003
DFNB32	1p13.3-22.1	*GPSM2*	Walsh et al., 2010
DFNB35	14q24.1-24.3	*ESRRB*	Collin et al., 2008
DFNB36	1p36.3	*ESPN*	Naz et al., 2004
DFNB37	6q13	*MYO6*	Ahmed et al., 2003
DFNB39	7q21.1	*HGF*	Schultz et al., 2009
DFNB42	3q13.31-q22.3	*ILDR1*	Borck et al., 2011
DFNB49	5q12.3-q14.1.	*MARVELD2*	Riazuddin et al., 2006
DFNB53	6p21.3	*COL11A2*	Chen et al., 2005
DFNB59	2q31.1-q31.3	*PJVK*	Delmaghani et al., 2006
DFNB61	7q22.1	*SLC26A5*	Liu et al., 2003
DFNB63	11q13.2-q13.4	*LRTOMT/ COMT2*	Ahmed et al., 2008
DFNB66	6p21.2-22.3	*LHFPL5*	Shabbir et al., 2006
DFNB72	19p13.3	*GIPC3*	Rehman et al., 2011
DFNB73	1p32.3	*BSND*	Riazuddin et al., 2009
DFNB74	12q14.2-q15	*MSRB3*	Ahmed et al., 2011
DFNB77	18q12-q21	*LOXHD1*	Grillet et al., 2009
DFNB79	9q34.3	*TPRN*	Rehman et al., 2010
DFNB84	12q21.2	*PTPRQ*	Schraders er al., 2010
DFNB91	6p25	*SERPINB6*	Sirmaci et al., 2010
DFNB95	19p13	*GIPC3*	Charizopoulou et al., 2011

Table 3. Non-syndromic genes responsible for HL up to 2011.

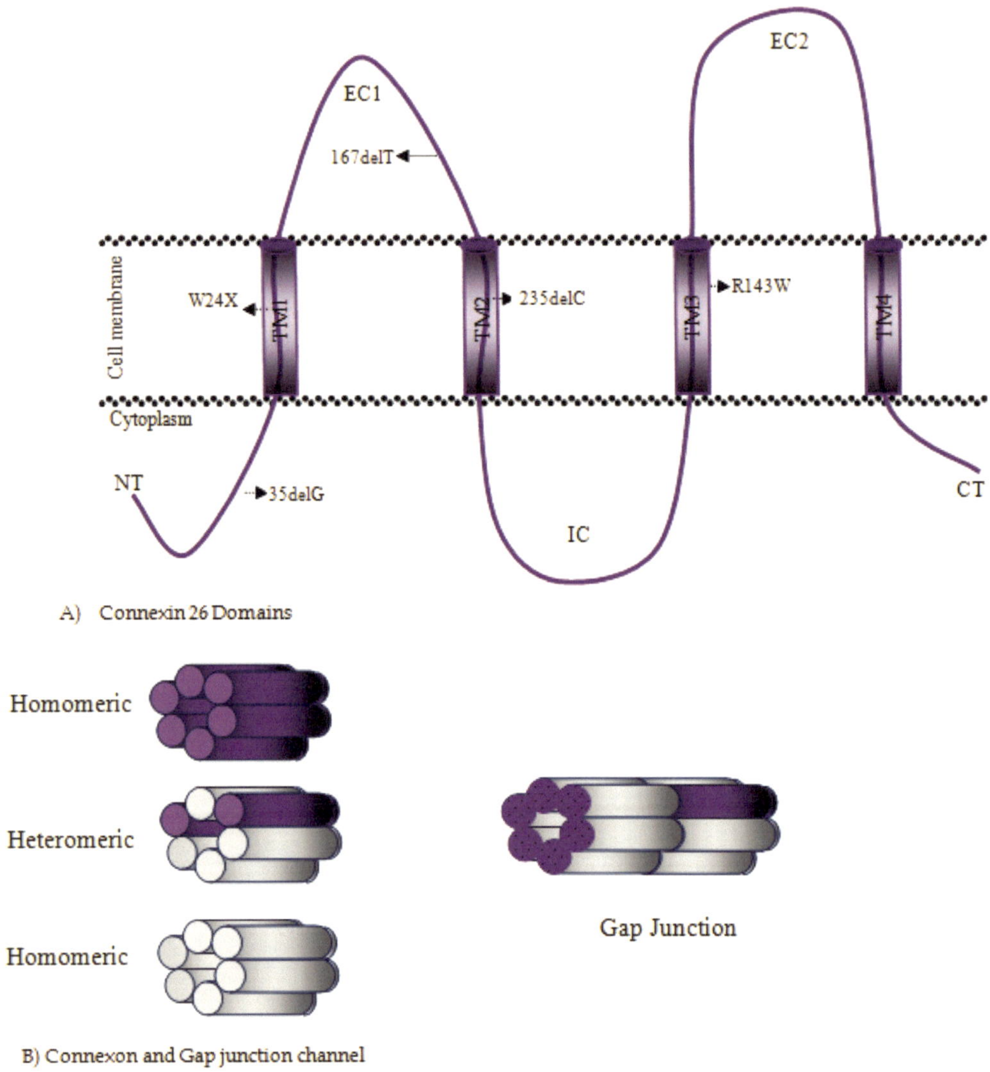

Fig. 1. Schematic structure and domains of Connexin 26 protein, Connexon and Gap Junction channel. A) The most common mutations in specific populations (35delG, 167delT, 235delC, R143W and W24X mutations in the Caucasian, Ashkenazi Jewish, Japanese, Ghanian and Indian populations, respectively) are shown. 35delG, W24X, 167delT, 235delC and R143W located on NT, TM1, EC1, TM2 and TM3 domains, respectively. TM1-TM4 denotes transmembrane domains, EC1-2 denotes extracellular domains, IC denotes cytoplasmic domain, NT denotes amino (NH2) terminus and CT denotes carboxyl (COOH) terminus. B) Six connexins can oligomerize to form hemichannels named connexons. Connexons then pass throughout the membrane to make the gap junction channels. Homomeric and heteromeric channels can be formed as connexins selectively interact with each other.

A few point mutations have also been reported in *GJB6* as the cause of ARNSHL *GJB6* [del Castillo et al., 2005; Pallares-Ruiz et al., 2002]. Later studies determined that *GJB6* mutations in cis state, not in trans, would destroy the *GJB2* expression. Therefore, the digenic hypothesis may not be correct. Four large deletions have been recognized in *GJB6* gene including del(*GJB6*-D13S1830), del(*GJB6*-D13S1854), del(chr13:19,837,344-19, 968,698) and 920 Kb deletion [del Castillo et al., 2002, 2005; Wilch et al., 2010]. The deletions may include more than 10% of DFNB1alleles [Stevenson et al., 2003]. So far, del (*GJB6*-D13S1830) has not been seen in many populations [Mahdieh et al., 2004, 2011]. The del (*GJB6*-D13S1830) and del (*GJB6*-D13S1854) mutations not only truncate the synthesis of *GJB6* gene but also destroy *GJB2* gene expression.

Connexins encoded by GJ genes are members of transmembrane family proteins that have 20 members in humans [Holms & Steel, 1999]. These proteins were classified in three groups of alpha, beta and gamma proteins. Common nomenclature system is based on molecular weight of proteins e.g. Cx26 and Cx32. Despite the differences in the size and primary amino acid composition, connexins have similar topology. These proteins have four transmembrane domains which are connected by two extracellular and one intracellular loop. The carboxyl and amino terminals are located at the cytoplasmic side. Most cells express more than one type of connexin. Gap junctions show different permeability and conductance which may create channels with specific characteristics. Also, in order to compensate for the decrease in the expression of some of the connexins, other connexins may be produced at an enhanced rate [Kumar & Kilula, 1996]. Hemi-channels (connexons) are composed of six connexin subunits and two hemi-channels make the channel forming the gap junctions [Kelley et al., 1998]. The important role of these channels is transportation of potassium ions [Kelley et al., 1998] and glutamate released from hair cells to initiate action potential. Different connexins may be made up of hemi channels with homomer or heteromer subunits.

4.1.1.2 *MYO15A* gene in DFNB3 locus

In 1995, a report showed that 2% of rural individuals in the north coast of Bali, Indonesia were affected with a profound sensorineural non-syndromic HL. Due to high percentage of deaf people in this village a local sign language had been created for communication [Wang et al., 1998].

The locus was mapped on chromosome 17p11.2 by whole genome study. *MYO15A* gene has 66 exons and 71097 bp, encoding a 11863 bp transcript [Liang et al., 1999]. Myosin gene was identified by positional and functional cloning approaches [Wang et al., 1998]. Mutations in the gene are responsible for 5% of severe to profound deafness cases in Pakistan [Friedman et al., 2003]. *MYO15A* gene mutations were reported in families from Turkey, Brazil and India [Kalay et al., 2007; Nal et al., 2007; Lezirovitz et al., 2008]. The role of myosin filaments can be traced in a variety of cellular functions including cell motility, muscle contraction, synaptic transmission, cytokenesis, endocytosis, exocytosis and probably in gene expression as a modulator [Craig & Woodhead, 2006; Loikkanen et al., 2009]. As the organism gets more complex, there may be more myosin isoforms found in the organism [Oliver et al., 1999; Friedman et al., 1999]. The heavy chain of XV myosin has 3531 amino acids. There is a unique proline-rich region at the amino terminal of myosin which weighs 140KDa and has no similarity to any of the known proteins. Next to this domain exists a motor domain and a tail domain [Belyantseva et al., 2003]. In addition to the sensory cells of cochlear, myosin is expressed in the pituitary gland, neuroendocrine cells, parathyroid and pancreas [Llyod et al., 2001]. It is also found in stereocilia of hair cells [Belyantseva et al., 2003].

4.1.1.3 *SLC26A4* gene in DFNB4 locus

DFNB4 locus, located at chromosome 7q31, was first reported to be linked to recessive non-syndromic deafness in a large Middle-Eastern Druze family. In 1997, the *SLC26A4* (Penderin coding protein) was identified by positional cloning at the pendred syndrome locus (Everett et al. 1997) and was later also shown to be the gene mutated in DFNB4 [Li et al., 1998]. Pendred syndrome was identified in 1896 as neurosensory HL and goiter. HL in Pendred syndrome is the most common cause of deafness due to defect of cochlea such as dilation sac and duct of endolyph and enlarged vestibular duct [Everett et al., 1997].

Mutations of *SLC26A4* gene are the second leading cause of ARNSHL. So far, more than 140 mutations have been reported for Pendred syndrome. Phenotypic spectrum of *SLC26A4* gene mutations varies from Pendred syndrome to nonsyndromic HL. Four mutations are common in northern Europeans i.e L236P, T416P, E384G, IVS8 +1 G> A) [Hilgert et al., 2008]. In a study conducted in Spanish population 27% had homozygous *SLC26A4* mutations [Pera et al., 2008]. Mutations of *SLC26A4* gene have been observed in several ethnic populations [Albert et al., 2006; Hu et al., 2007; Yoon et al., 2008]. The prevalence of *SLC26A4* gene mutation is about 40% in Caucasians of which 24% are bi-allelic [Albert et al., 2006].

SLC26A4 gene has 21 exons within 57175 bp of DNA sequence. Its transcript is about 5 Kb encoding into a 87KDa protein having 780 amino acids. The gene is expressed in lining cells of endolymph duct as well as non-sensory cells of utricle, saccule, kidney and thyroid. Various models have been reported for the structure of Pendrin protein. New model suggests that pendrin protein is a transmembrane protein traversing fifteen times throughout the membrane [Dossena et al., 2009]. The protein in involved in anion exchange of HCO-, Cl-, I-and OH- ions [Mount & Romero, 2004].

4.1.1.4 *TMC1* gene in DFNB7/11 locus

DFNB7 and DFNB11 were determined as the cause of HL on chromosome 9q13-q21 in two Indian and two inbred Israeli families, respectively [Jian et al., 1995]. In 2002, eight different mutations in *TMC1* gene were linked to one DFNA36 family and eleven DFNB7/11 families [Kurima et al., 2002]. More than twenty different point mutations and two deletions have been identified in different families. It seems that c.100C>T mutation includes appromximately 40% of all *TMC1* mutations in Turkey [Hilgert et al., 2008, 2009b]. In a survey of 51 Turkish families, 5 patients had mutations of *TMC1* gene [Hilgert et al., 2008]. Mutations of *TMC1* are responsible for at least 6% of all cases of ARNSHL in northeast and eastern part of Turkey [Kalay et al., 2005]. Three mutations c.100C> T (R34X), c.77611G> A and g.94615A> C have been reported in Iranian families [Hilgert et al., 2009b].

Based on sequence homology studies, eight TMC genes exist in vertebrates. *TMC1* gene has 24 exons and encodes a 3201 nucleotide RNA. It expresses a complete transmembrane protein with six membrane passing domain which has no similarity to proteins of known function. Mouse ortholog transcript (*TMC1*) is expressed in cochlea and vestibular hair cells [Kurima et al., 2002].

4.1.1.5 *TMPRSS3* gene in DFNB8/10 locus

DFNB8/10 locus was separately mapped on chromosome 21q22.3 in two consanguineous Pakistani (DFNB8) and Palestinian families (DFNB10) [Bonné-Tamir et al., 1996; Veske et al., 1996]. Haplotype analysis and sequencing analysis of the families resulted in detection of mutations in *TMPRSS3* [Scott et al., 2001]. The gene belongs to a subfamily of trans-membrane serine proteases type III protein [Szabo et al., 2003] expressed in supporting cells of the organ of Corti [Guipponi et al., 2002]. Although, the specific role of *TMPRSS3* protein in growth, development and survival of auditory apparatus has not been found but it activates the epithelial sodium channel (ENaC) in vitro [Guipponi et al., 2002]. The mutated alleles of the gene may inactivate the serine protease catalytic activitiy. Therefore, *TMPRSS3* proteolytic function may be important during the development of inner ear [Guipponi et al., 2002, 2008].

TMPRSS3 gene has 13 exons within 24 Kb, encoding a 2468 bp mRNA which encodes a protein with 454 amino acids [Guipponi et al., 2008]. In 2009, 16 mutations in *TMPRSS3* have been reviwed and reported by a study [Hilgert et al., 2009b]. From 25 studied Turkish families, three had mutations of *TMPRSS3* gene [Wattenhofer et al., 2005; Sahin-Calapoglu et al., 2005]. Mutations of *TMPRSS3* gene account for 1% of hearing loss in Caucasian children with non-syndromic HL [Wattenhofer et al., 2005]. Mutations of *TMPRSS3* gene have been reported in 4 of 290 Pakistani families [Ahmed et al., 2004].

4.1.1.6 *OTOF* gene in DFNB9 locus

OTOF gene contains 48 exons encoding a 1997 amino acid polypeptide called otoferlin which is member of Ferlin family of proteins [Mirghomizadeh et al., 2002]. Ferlin family of proteins have a domain called C2. These proteins contain a transmembrane C-terminal domain [Yasunaga et al., 1999]. C2 domain is a structural domain in some proteins that are involved in directing proteins to the cell membrane [Davletov & Südhof, 1993].

Otoferlin is expressed in the brain and cochlea. This protein plays an important role in releasing neurotransmitters in the auditory nerve cells [Yasunaga et al., 1999]. Mutations of the gene can lead to auditory neuropathy in which the sound from inner ear is not transferred to the brain. Q829X mutation is very common in the Hispanic which is the third cause of ARNSHL [Migliosi et al., 2002]. Mutations of the gene have been found in families of Lebanese origin [Yasunaga et al., 1999]. Varga *et al.* reported 8 mutations in 65 studied families with ARNSHL [Varga et al., 2006]. OTOF mutations have been found in Pakistani families; gene mutations may account for deafness in 2.3% of this population [Choi et al., 2009].

4.1.1.7 *CDH23* gene in DFNB12 locus

The superfamily of cadherin has about 100 members with a variety of roles in cell adhesion, growth and developmental signaling, maintenance and function of the tissues [Jamora & Fuchs, 2002; Nelson & Nusse, 2004; Gumbiner, 2005; Halbleib & Nelson, 2006]. Cadherin 23 protein has a role in connection of developing stereocilia [Siemens et al., 2004]. In 1996, DFNB12 was mapped to chromosome 10q21-q22 in a consanguineous Syrian family [Chaib et al., 1996]. Usher syndrome type 1 D (USH1D) was also mapped to the same position. Allelic mutations of the *CDH23* gene encoding cadherin 23 cause DFNB12 HL and USH1D [Bolz et al., 2001; Bork et al., 2001]. Missense mutations usually cause DFNB12 HL but nonsense and premature stop codon mutations cause Usher syndrome type 1D although this relationship is not definite. No single gene mutation is common in this gene [Hilgert 2009b]. In 64 Japanese families, five mutations were found in *CDH23* [Wagatsuma et al., 2007].

4.1.1.8 *TMHS* or LHFPL5 genes in DFNB67 locus

Non syndromic HL in a Pakistani family linked to a new region on chromosome 6p21.1-p22.3 defining a new locus, DFNB67 in 2006; *TMHS* or *LHFPL5* gene was mapped in this region [Shabbir et al., 2006]. *LHFPL5* has 4 exons and encodes a 2162 nucleotide mRNA and translates into a protein of 219 amino acids. The proposed structure of the protein is a four pass transmembrane domain. Mutations of this gene have been reported in patients from Pakistan and Turkey (C161F, Y127C, P83fsX84). *TMHS* is important for the transmission of sound.

4.1.2 Autosomal dominant non- syndromic hearing loss

Late onset, mild and progressive forms of HL are the usual phenotypes associated with autosomal dominant form of deafness. About 25 genes and more than 60 loci have been reported for autosomal dominant non- syndromic hearing loss (ADNSHL). There is no frequent gene mutated in ADNSHL but mutations in some genes including *WFS1*, *KCNQ4*, *COCH* and *GJB2* have been suggested to be common (Kelsell et al., 1997; Nie 2008; Higert et al., 2009).

4.1.2.1 *WFS1* gene and its protein

The *WFS1* (Wolfram) gene at DFNA6 locus, located on 4p16, consists of 8 exons and has a length of about 33.4 kb and a 3.6 kb transcript. It codes for a polypeptide of 890 amino acids [Hofmann et al., 2003]. The Wolframin protein is a resident component of the endoplasmic reticulum (ER) and may be involved in membrane trafficking, processing and/or regulation of ER calcium homeostasis [Fonseca et al., 2010]. In the inner ear, however, this protein may be helpful to maintain the appropriate levels of calcium ions and/or other charged particles required for hearing process [Cryns et al., 2003].

Dominant mutations in *WFS1* can cause a characteristic type of HL which affects the low frequencies and less loss in hearing in the high frequencies [Bespalova et al., 2001; Fukuoka et al., 2007]. It has been shown that dominant mutations are usually located in the C-terminal domain. The recessive Wolfram syndrome is caused by numerous mutations distributed along the entire gene. Two mutations c.424_425ins16 and c.1362_1377del16 have a high frequency in some specific populations including Spanish patients and Italians, respectively [Gómez-Zaera et al., 2001; Colosimo et al., 2003]. It is hypothesized that, inactivating mutations may lead to Wolfram syndrome and missense mutations occurring in the C-terminal domain can cause the characteristic low-frequency ADNSHL [Cryns et al., 2003].

4.1.2.2 *KCNQ4* gene and its protein

The *KCNQ4* gene at DFNA2 locus, located on 1p34, consists of 14 exons and codes for a polypeptide of 695 amino acids, a voltage-gated potassium channel. It is a member of the KCNQ voltage-gated K+ channel family [Coucke et al., 1999]. It has an important role in K^+

secretion into the endolymph by strial marginal cells. Ten missense mutations, two small deletions and one splice mutation in *KCNQ4* have been reported so far. It is believed that a dominant-negative effect of the missense mutations in this gene lead to interference of the mutant protein with the normal channel subunit, affecting the pore structure of the channels. Therefore, hearing loss with a lower age of onset is observed at all frequencies [Coucke et al., 1999; Akita et al., 2001]. Deletion mutations which have a haploinsufficiency effect lead to a milder HL with an older age of onset at high frequencies [Coucke et al., 1999; Akita et al., 2001].

4.1.2.3 *COCH* gene and its protein

The DFNA9 causative gene, *COCH* located on 14q12-q13, consists of 11exons and encodes a 550 amino acid extracellular matrix protein named cochlin. This protein has several domains including two von Willebrand factor A-like domains (vWFA1 and 2) and a LCCL domain (a region homologous to a domain in factor C of Limulus). To date, eleven missense mutations and one small deletion in *COCH* gene have been reported. Most of the missense mutations are located within exon 4 and 5 which encode the LCCL domain (Figure 2) [Robertson et al., 1998; Collin et al., 2006].

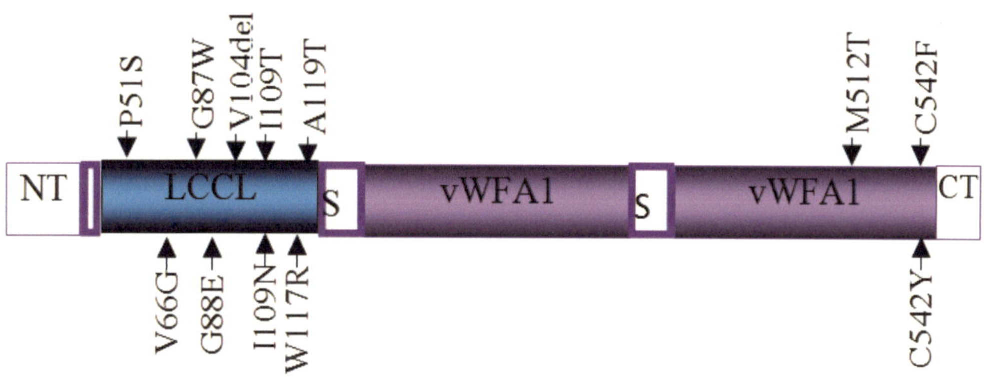

Fig. 2. Schematic structure of cochlin and distribution of the mutations along its domains. The NT signal peptide is followed by a LCCL domain and two vWF domains. S indicates several cysteine residues, NT denotes amino (NH2) terminus and CT denotes carboxyl (COOH) terminus.

4.1.3 X and Y linked HL

There are fewer X-linked forms of HL (DFNX) than ARNSHL and ADNSHL. X-linked form of deafness has been reported as prelingual or progressive in different families. Five loci and three genes (POU3F4, *SMPX* and *PRPS1*) have been reported for X-linked HL (http://hereditaryhearingloss.org/).

To date, only one locus has been linked to chromosome Y (DFNY1) that was found in a very large Chinese family (seven generations) [Wang et al., 2004]. They reported that the ages of onset for the patrilineal relatives were from 7 to 27 years. *PCDH11Y*, encoding a protocadherin, was suggested to be the causality [Wang et al., 2004].

4.1.4 Mitochondrial HL

In healthy individuals, only one type of mitochondrial DNA genotype (homoplasmy) exists, but in many mitochondrial diseases, mitochondrial genome has mixed genotype (heteroplasmy). Heteroplasmy differs from one tissue to another and can even differ within the cells of a tissue. A few genes contribute to mitochondrial HL [Fischel-Ghodsian, 2003]. Due to the important function of mitochondria in producing chemical energy through oxidative phosphorylation, mitochondrial DNA mutations can cause systemic neuromascular disorders such as HL. mtDNA mutations may be inherited or acquired (Table 4); the inherited mitochondrial mutations can cause many clinical features including myopathy, neuropathy, diabetes mellitus and sensorineural HL [Finsterer & Fellinger, 2005; Guan 2011]. Acquired mitochondrial mutations may be associated with aging and age-related HL or presbycusis [Fischel-Ghodsian, 1999, 2003]. Multiorganic mitochondrial syndromes are often lethal in homoplasmic state. Mitochondrial homoplasmy exists in LHON (Leber Hereditary Optic Neuropathy) and maternal inherited HL [Fischel-Ghodsian, 2003]. Myoclonic epilepsy and ragged red fibers (MERRF), Kearns-Sayre syndrome (KSS) and mitochondrial encephalomyopathy with lactic acidosis and stroke-like episodes are associated with progressive HL [Zeviani et al., 1998; Goto et al., 1990].

Gene	Mutation	Phenotype	Reference
MTRNR1 (12S rRNA)	1555A->G	NSHL/Aminoglycoside induced/worsened	Estivill et al., 1998
	1494C->T	NSHL/Aminoglycoside induced/worsened	Zhao et al., 2004
	961 (mutations)	NSHL/Aminoglycoside induced/worsened	Bacino et al., 1995
	1095T>C	NSHL/Aminoglycoside induced/ parkinsonism, and neuropathy	Zhao et al., 2004
	827A>G	NSHL/Aminoglycoside induced	Li et al., 2005
MTTS1 (tRNA$^{Ser(UCN)}$)	7444G>A	NSHL/Aminoglycoside induced	Pandya et al., 1999;
	7445A->G	NSHL/Palmoplantar keratoderma	Fischel-Ghodsian, 2003
	7472insC	NSHL/Neurological dysfunction, including ataxia, dysarthria and myoclonus	Jaksch et al., 1998
	7510T->C	NSHL/no additional symptoms	Hutchin et al.2000
	7511T->C	NSHL/no additional symptoms	Friedman et al., 1999
	7512T>C	HL/Progressive myoclonic epilepsy and ataxia	Jaksch et al., 1998
MTTL1 (tRNA$^{Leu(UUR)}$)	3243A>G	maternally inherited diabetes and deafness/MELAS	Goto et al., 1990
tRNA^{Lys}	8296A>G	maternally inherited diabetes and deafness	Kameoka et al., 1998
	8332A>G	dystonia, stroke-like episodes and HL	Gal et al., 2010
tRNA^{Glu}	14709T>C	maternally inherited diabetes and deafness	Rigoli et al., 2001

Table 4. Identified mitochondrial DNA mutations in HL.

5. Age-related HL

Biological changes accumulate in people during life as individuals age. About one hundred thousand individuals die each day of age-related causes around the world [de Grey, 2007]. Age-related HL (ARHL) or presbycusis is the most frequent sensory defect in the elderly people. It occurs due to accumulation of environmental and genetic changes i.e. gradual deleterious changes in the ear gives rise hearing impairment in older people. Approximately 25 % of 60 year olds and more than 50 % of 80 year ages suffer from ARHL [Dror & Avraham, 2009; Huang & Tang, 2010]. Many heterogeneous factors including family history, exposure to loud noises, ototoxic medication, exposure to chemicals, free radical (reactive oxygen species) chronic medical conditions, malnutrition, mtDNA mutations, alcohol abuse and smoking etc. may cause this type of HL [Van Eyken et al., 2007b; Huang & Tang, 2010].

Some common deletions and acquired mtDNA point mutations due to reactive oxygen spicies (ROS) have also been suggested to cause prebyscusis. Although genetic studies on ARHL are increasing in the recent years, there is a little information about the role of genes to its etiology. Two basic approaches have been used to identify susceptibility genes for ARHL: the linkage study and the association study [Van Eyken et al., 2007b]. Several single nucleotide polymorphisms (SNPs) have been reported to correlate with presbycusis; variants in *GRHL2*, *GRM7*, *KCNQ4* and N-acetyltransferase 2 are involved (Table 5) [Van Eyken et al., 2006, 2007a; Van Laer et al., 2008; Friedman et al., 2009]. Mutations in cadherin 23 coded by *CDH23* gene may also cause ARHL [Johnson et al., 2010]. More recently, a genome-wide association scan was conducted on ARHL in the genetically isolated Finnish Saami population. This study confirmed, and also provided further evidence for the role of the previous reported gene, *GRM7* in ARHL. *IQGAP2* gene was also proposed to be involved in presbycusis [van Laer et al., 2010]. Mechanism of ARHL is not well understood. However, new promising technology and strategies may help to discover the exact role of genetic mutations in presbycusis. Finding of the genetic variants causing ARHL will ultimately lead to discovery of new pharmaceutical interventions and the development of new approaches to identify at risk individuals.

SNP (RS number)	Gene	Protein or Function	
SNP9 (rs727146) SNP12 (rs2149034) SNP18 (rs12143503)	*KCNQ4*	Potassium channel (voltage-gated)	Van Eyken et al., 2006
NAT2*6A (rs1799930)	N-acetyltransferase 2	metabolism of cytotoxic, carcinogenic compounds and ROS	Unal et al., 2005
36738A>G (rs10955255) 42731C>T (rs2127034) 53110C>T (rs1981361)	*GRHL2*	transcription factor cellular promoter 2-like 3	Van Laer et al., 2008
7155702T>A (rs11928865)	*GRM7*	glutamate receptor, metabotropic,7	Friedman et al., 2009
75920972A>G (rs457717) 75922504C>T (rs1697845)	*IQGAP2*	IQ motif-containing GTPase-activating-like protein	Van Laer et al., 2010

Table 5. SNPs associated with ARHL.

6. Syndromic genetic deafness

More than 400 syndromes have been described in OMIM. Here, genetic aspects of common syndromes which are associted with HL are briefly explained.

Usher Syndrome: Usher syndrome, named after Charles Usher (1914) a British ophthalmologist, is the most prevalent cause of autosomal recessive HL, accounting for nearly 3-5 per 100,000 in the general population and 1-10% among profoundly deaf children [Boughman et al., 1983]. Several clinical subtypes have been distinguished based on its characterized features i. e. severity of the HL and the onset of retinitis pigmentosa [Yan & Liu, 2010]. Type 1 patients have profound HL, vestibular dysfunction and the onset of retinitis pigmentosa in childhood [Hope et al., 1997]. The type 2 patients have normal vestibular response, mild to moderate HL and RP begins in the second decade of life [Hope et al., 1997]. Progressive HL and variable vestibular response characterize type 3 patients and the onset of retinitis pigmentosa is variable as well [Smith et al., 1995]. Usher syndrome has a heterogeneous causality (Table 6); to date, 12 different loci and 10 genes have been reported (http://hereditaryhearingloss.org/). One of these identified genes, *MYO7A*, encoding myosin 7A, is a unique molecular motor for hair cells [Weil et al., 1995]. Cadherin 23, an adhesion molecule, coded by *CDH23* gene may have an important role in crosslinking of stereocilia [Bolz et al., 2001; Bork et al., 2001].

Locus	Gene	Ref.
USH1B (11q13.5)	*MYO7A*	Weil et al.,1995
USH1C (11p15.1)	*USH1C*	Smith et al., 1992
USH1D (10q22.1)	*CDH23*	Bork et al., 2001
USH1F (10q21-22)	*PCDH15*	Ahmed et al., 2001
USH1G (17q24-25)	*SANS*	Mustapha et al., 2002
USH2A (1q41)	*USH2A*	Kimberling et al., 1990
USH2C (5q14.3-q21.3)	*VLGR1*	Weston et al., 2004
USH2D (9q32)	*WHRN*	Ebermann et al., 2007
USH3 (3q21-q25)	*USH3A*	Joensuu et al., 2001
10q24.31	*PDZD7*	Ebermann et al., 2010

Table 6. Reported genes for Usher syndrome.

Pendred syndrome: Pendred syndrome, named after Vaughan Pendred (1896) a British physician, is the most common syndromic form of HL and associated with abnormal iodine metabolism (goiter). It is an autosomal recessive disorder which accounts for 4-10% of deaf cases [Fraser 1965]. The defective organic binding of iodine in the thyroid gland may distinguished by a positive potassium perchlorate discharge test; however the test is not specific and its sensitivity is unclear. HL is usually bilateral, severe to profound and may be present at birth, and sloping in the higher frequencies [Kopp et al., 2008]. The casual gene is *SLC26A4* (PDS) on chromosome 7q31 encoding a protein named pendrin (Figure 3). It regulates transportation of iodine and chloride/ bicarbonate ions in the inner ear, thyroid, and kidney. Mutations of this gene can cause NSHL DFNB4 and enlarged vestibular aqueduct syndrome as well [Everett et al., 1997].

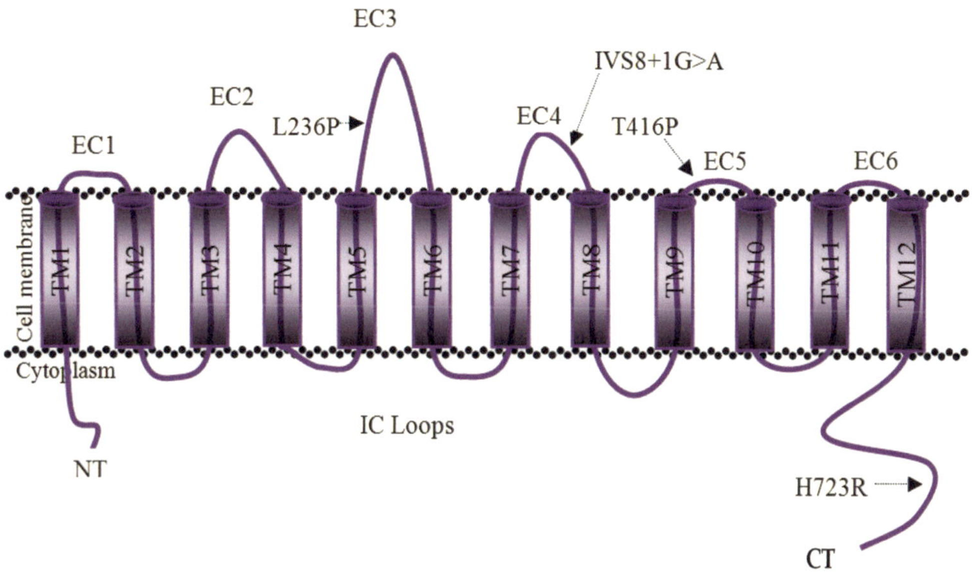

Fig. 3. Hypothetic structure and domains of Pendrin protein. The most common mutations (L236P, IVS8+1G>A, T416P, and H723R) accounting for approximately 60% of the total PS genetic load are shown. TM1-TM12 denotes transmembrane domains, EC1-6 denotes extracellular domains, IC denotes cytoplasmic domain, NT denotes amino (NH2) terminus and CT denotes carboxyl (COOH) terminus.

Alport syndrome: Alport syndrome, a hereditary disorder of basement membranes, is characterized by renal abnormalities including glomerulonephritis, hematuria ("red diaper") and renal failure, and ocular problems as well as progressive sensorineural HL [Wester et al., 1995]. Mutations in various genes encoding type 4 collagen (COL4A3, COL4A4 and COL4A5) have been reported to cause Alport syndrome [Lemmink et al., 1994; Hudson et al., 2003]; nearly 85% of the cases are due to COL4A5 mutations [Hudson et al., 2003]. These collagens are components of the basilar membranes, the spiral ligament and stria vascularis. X-linked pattern of inheritance is observed in the majority (80 %); the remaining shows autosomal recessive [Lemmink et al., 1994] and autosomal dominant [van der Loop et al., 2000], inheritance patterns. It is estimated that 10% to 15% of X-linked patients represent de novo mutations in *COL4A5* [Gubler et al., 2007]. Since uremia leads to death in males prior to 30 years of age, it is essential to diagnose it early in men. Symptoms are usually more severe than women. The progressive sensorineural HL usually begins in the adolescent years [Wester et al., 1995]. The mechanism of HL has not been explained exactly yet, although the basement membrane damages are suggested to affect adhesion of the cells of the organ of Corti and basilar membrane leading to HL [Merchant et al., 2004].

Waardenburg syndrome: Waardenburg disease, named after Petrus Johannes Waardenburg (1886-1979), accounts for 1-3% of congenital HL [Read & Newton, 1997]. In addition, the disease shows other clinical features. Four types of syndrome can be distinguished on the basis of accompanying abnormalities [Read & Newton, 1997]: In type 1, patients show dystopia canthorum, iris heterochromy, brilliant blue eyes, broad nasal root, premature graying of hair, white forelock, and vestibular dysfunction. Type 2 patients have similar phenotype but not dystopia canthorum. In type 3 (so called Klein-Waardenburg syndrome) [Klein, 1983], upper extremity abnormalities other Type 1 clinical features and dystopia canthorum and are observed. In type 4 (so called Shah-Waardenburg syndrome) [Shah et al., 1981] patients demonstrate all findings shown in Type 2 with the addition of pigmentation abnormalities and Hirschsprung's disease. Sensorineural hearing loss is observed in 60 % and 90 % of type 1 and type 2 patients, respectively [Newton, 1990].

Types 1 and 3 of Waardenburg syndrome occur due to mutations in the *PAX3* gene encoding a DNA-binding protein essential for determining the fate of neural crest cells [Baldwin et al., 1994]. Type 2 is due to mutations in MITF gene [Tassabehji et al., 1994]. Mutations in three genes, *EDN3*, *SOX10* and *EDNRB* genes, can lead to Type 4 [Edery et al., 1996; Hofstra et al., 1996; Pingault et al., 1998]. *SOX10* mutations, account for approximately half of type 4 patients and are likely responsible for about 15% of Type 2 as well [Bondurand et al., 2007]. *In vitro* studies have shown that *EDN3* plays as a stimulation factor of proliferation and melanogenesis of neural crest cells. *EDNRB* is suggested to have an important role in the development of epidermal melanocytes and enteric neurons. *SOX10* is a DNA-binding transcription factor and involved in promoting cell survival prior to lineage commitment [Kapur, 1999]. There is a wide range of variation in HL phenotype so that some patients may not exhibit HL.

Branchio-oto-renal syndrome: Branchio-oto-renal syndrome (BOR) is an autosomal dominant disorder, accounting for 2% of profoundly deaf children and is characterized by branchial derived anomalies, otologic anomalies (Mondini's dysplasia and stapes fixation) and renal malformation. HL may affect 70-93% of the BOR patients but there is a high variability in age of onset and severity [Chen et al., 1995]. HL can be sensorineural, conductive or mixed, stable or progressive and mild or profound. Mutations in *EYA1* gene have been identified to cause BOR syndrome (BOR1) [Abdelhak et al., 1997]. It has been shown that this gene has a role in development of the inner ear and kidney [Abdelhak et al., 1997]. Studies of transgenic mice have indicated that EYA1 homozygous knockouts have not developed ears and kidneys. In addition to *EYA1*, mutations in two genes named SIX1 and SIX5 have been reported to cause BOR3 and BOR2, respectively [Ruf et al., 2004; Hoskins et al., 2007].

Stickler Syndrome: Stickler Syndrome (STL), named after Stickler (1965), follows an autosomal dominant pattern of inheritance and is characterized by progressive sensorineural HL, cleft palate, abnormal development of the epiphysis, vertebral abnormalities and osteoarthritis. On the basis of clinical features, four types of STL exist. Type 1 patients have typical features of the disease including progressive myopia leading to retinal detachment, midface hypoplasia, cleft palate, variable sensorineural HL and vitreoretinal degeneration. Mutations in *COL2A1* gene encoding a fibrillar collage type 2 subunitA1 can cause the classic phenotype [Ahmad et al., 1991]. There is no retinal detachment in Type 2 andthe phenotype is caused by *COL11A1* gene mutations [Richards et al., 1996]. Facial abnormalities seen in Type 1 are not observed in Type 3. Mutations of *COL11A2* lead to STL Type 3 [Vikkula et al., 1995]. Recently, mutations in *COL9A1* have been identified to cause an autosomal recessive form of STL, Type 4 [Van Camp et al., 2006].

7. Genetic evaluation

The main problem in the diagnosis of disorders such as deafness is its heterogenicity. Genetic study of HL has considerable benefits for patients which are as follows:

a. Identifying the medical and non medical decisions e.g cochlear implant
b. Carrier testing and prenatal diagnosis
c. Prediction for the progressive state of the disease
d. Eliminating unnecessary tests and investigations
e. Providing appropriate genetic counseling before marriage, especially when they have heterogeneous conditions that carry different mutated genes.

Genetic evaluation should be considered for children with newly diagnosed loss of hearing especially if no specific cause is determined. For example, there is no need for genetic evaluation of the family of a child with HL due to meningitis; although, they may need assurance of not transmitting the disease to the next generation. Genetic evaluation includes several steps:

1. Reviewing the complete history of prenatal, neonatal and medical history of growth and development
2. Complete physical examination of patients and other family members
3. Evaluating the genetics, molecular and cellular diagnosis

Based on previous studies, deaf people have positive assortive marriage; it is estimated that 90% of deaf individuals marry deaf. Depending on the pattern of inheritance they might have a deaf child. For example if both parental recessive alleles are similar, there is 100% chance of having a deaf child; and if one of the parents carry a dominant form of HL and the other carry the recessive form of HL the chance would be 50% for the dominant gene.

Early diagnosis of HL is important in gaining speech progression and social skills of the children which would lead to better life of these individuals and would later help them in cochlea implant. Hereditary or genetic understanding of the causes of HL is important. The benefits of this understanding and knowledge, not only allows physicians to help the families of at risk but also may help in treatment and control of HL. Sometimes it is possible to prevent hearing loss from worsening. HL may be one of the clinical signs of a syndrome and if the genetic cause of HL is determined it may help to predict and treat other clinical complications [Extivill et al., 1998].

8. Conclusion

HL is the most common sensory defect affecting human beings. It is categorized on the basis of several criteria. Genetic factors can be traced in half of the cases. Nonsyndromic HL can follow any of the Mendelian inheritance patterns, but the majority are ARNSHL. Approximately fifty genes have been reported to be involved in HL, and based on an estimation nearly 200 to 250 genes may cause HL. Genetic understanding of the causes of HL and finding the molecular mechanism of hearing process are valuable for genetic counseling, prevention and development of new therapeutic approaches. Many studies have been published about finding new genes causing prelingual nonsyndromic HL. Presbycusis is very common among eldely people and research on this phenotype needs more attention.

New technology and strategies such as next generation sequencing can help to discover new genes for deafness in future.

9. References

Abdelhak S, Kalatzis V, Heilig R, Compain S, Samson D, Vincent C, Levi-Acobas F, Cruaud C, Le Merrer M, Mathieu M, König R, Vigneron J, Weissenbach J, Petit C & Weil D. Clustering of mutations responsible for branchio-oto-renal (BOR) syndrome in the eyes absent homologous region (eyaHR) of *EYA1*. Hum Mol Genet. 1997;6(13):2247-55.

Ahmad NN, Ala-Kokko L, Knowlton RG, Jimenez SA, Weaver EJ, Maguire JI, Tasman W & Prockop DJ. Stop codon in the procollagen II gene (*COL2A1*) in a family with the Stickler syndrome (arthro-ophthalmopathy). Proc Natl Acad Sci U S A. 1991;88(15):6624-7.

Ahmed ZM, Li XC, Powell SD, Riazuddin S, Young TL, Ramzan K, Ahmad Z, Luscombe S, Dhillon K, MacLaren L, Ploplis B, Shotland LI, Ives E, Riazuddin S, Friedman TB, Morell RJ & Wilcox ER. Characterization of a new full length *TMPRSS3* isoform and identification of mutant alleles responsible for nonsyndromic recessive deafness in Newfoundland and Pakistan. BMC Med Genet. 2004;5:24.

Ahmed ZM, Masmoudi S, Kalay E, Belyantseva IA, Mosrati MA, Collin RW, Riazuddin S, Hmani-Aifa M, Venselaar H, Kawar MN, Tlili A, van der Zwaag B, Khan SY, Ayadi L, Riazuddin SA, Morell RJ, Griffith AJ, Charfedine I, Caylan R, Oostrik J, Karaguzel A, Ghorbel A, Riazuddin S, Friedman TB, Ayadi H & Kremer H. Mutations of *LRTOMT*, a fusion gene with alternative reading frames, cause nonsyndromic deafness in humans. Nat Genet. 2008;40(11):1335-40.

Ahmed ZM, Riazuddin S, Ahmad J, Bernstein SL, Guo Y, Sabar MF, Sieving P, Riazuddin S, Griffith AJ, Friedman TB, Belyantseva IA & Wilcox ER. *PCDH15* is expressed in the neurosensory epithelium of the eye and ear and mutant alleles are responsible for both USH1F and DFNB23. Hum Mol Genet. 2003;12(24):3215-23.

Ahmed ZM, Riazuddin S, Bernstein SL, Ahmed Z, Khan S, Griffith AJ, Morell RJ, Friedman TB, Riazuddin S & Wilcox ER. Mutations of the protocadherin gene *PCDH15* cause Usher syndrome type 1F. Am J Hum Genet. 2001;69(1):25-34.

Ahmed ZM, Yousaf R, Lee BC, Khan SN, Lee S, Lee K, Husnain T, Rehman AU, Bonneux S, Ansar M, Ahmad W, Leal SM, Gladyshev VN, Belyantseva IA, Van Camp G, Riazuddin S, Friedman TB & Riazuddin S. Functional null mutations of *MSRB3* encoding methionine sulfoxide reductase are associated with human deafness DFNB74. Am J Hum Genet. 2011;88(1):19-29.

Akita J, Abe S, Shinkawa H, Kimberling WJ & Usami S. Clinical and genetic features of nonsyndromic autosomal dominant sensorineural hearing loss: *KCNQ4* is a gene responsible in Japanese. J Hum Genet. 2001;46(7):355-61.

Albert S, Blons H, Jonard L, Feldmann D, Chauvin P, Loundon N, Sergent-Allaoui A, Houang M, Joannard A, Schmerber S, Delobel B, Leman J, Journel H, Catros H, Dollfus H, Eliot MM, David A, Calais C, Drouin-Garraud V, Obstoy MF, Tran Ba Huy P, Lacombe D, Duriez F, Francannet C, Bitoun P, Petit C, Garabédian EN, Couderc R, Marlin S & Denoyelle F. *SLC26A4* gene is frequently involved in nonsyndromic hearing impairment with enlarged vestibular aqueduct in Caucasian populations. Eur J Hum Genet. 2006;14(6):773-9.

Bacino C, Prezant TR, Bu X, Fournier P & Fischel-Ghodsian N. Susceptibility mutations in the mitochondrial small ribosomal RNA gene in aminoglycoside induced deafness. Pharmacogenetics. 1995 Jun;5(3):165-72.

Baldwin CT, Lipsky NR, Hoth CF, Cohen T, Mamuya W & Milunsky A. Mutations in *PAX3* associated with Waardenburg syndrome type I. Hum Mutat. 1994;3(3):205-11.

Baldwin CT, Weiss S, Farrer LA, De Stefano AL, Adair R, Franklyn B, Kidd KK, Korostishevsky M & Bonné-Tamir B. Linkage of congenital, recessive deafness (DFNB4) to chromosome 7q31 and evidence for genetic heterogeneity in the Middle Eastern Druze population. Hum Mol Genet. 1995;4(9):1637-42.

Belyantseva IA, Boger ET & Friedman TB. Myosin XVa localizes to the tips of inner ear sensory cell stereocilia and is essential for staircase formation of the hair bundle. Proc Natl Acad Sci U S A. 2003;100(24):13958-63.

Bespalova IN, Van Camp G, Bom SJ, Brown DJ, Cryns K, DeWan AT, Erson AE, Flothmann K, Kunst HP, Kurnool P, Sivakumaran TA, Cremers CW, Leal SM, Burmeister M & Lesperance MM. Mutations in the Wolfram syndrome 1 gene (*WFS1*) are a common cause of low frequency sensorineural hearing loss. Hum Mol Genet. 2001;10(22):2501-8.

Bolz H, von Brederlow B, Ramírez A, Bryda EC, Kutsche K, Nothwang HG, Seeliger M, del C-Salcedó Cabrera M, Vila MC, Molina OP, Gal A & Kubisch C. Mutation of *CDH23*, encoding a new member of the cadherin gene family, causes Usher syndrome type 1D. Nat Genet. 2001;27(1):108-12.

Bondurand N, Dastot-Le Moal F, Stanchina L, Collot N, Baral V, Marlin S, Attie-Bitach T, Giurgea I, Skopinski L, Reardon W, Toutain A, Sarda P, Echaieb A, Lackmy-Port-Lis M, Touraine R, Amiel J, Goossens M & Pingault V. Deletions at the *SOX10* gene locus cause Waardenburg syndrome types 2 and 4. Am J Hum Genet. 2007;81(6):1169-85.

Bonné-Tamir B, DeStefano AL, Briggs CE, Adair R, Franklyn B, Weiss S, Korostishevsky M, Frydman M, Baldwin CT & Farrer LA. Linkage of congenital recessive deafness (gene DFNB10) to chromosome 21q22.3. Am J Hum Genet. 1996;58(6):1254-9.

Borck G, Ur Rehman A, Lee K, Pogoda HM, Kakar N, von Ameln S, Grillet N, Hildebrand MS, Ahmed ZM, Nürnberg G, Ansar M, Basit S, Javed Q, Morell RJ, Nasreen N, Shearer AE, Ahmad A, Kahrizi K, Shaikh RS, Ali RA, Khan SN, Goebel I, Meyer NC, Kimberling WJ, Webster JA, Stephan DA, Schiller MR, Bahlo M, Najmabadi H, Gillespie PG, Nürnberg P, Wollnik B, Riazuddin S, Smith RJ, Ahmad W, Müller U, Hammerschmidt M, Friedman TB, Riazuddin S, Leal SM, Ahmad J & Kubisch C. Loss-of-function mutations of *ILDR1* cause autosomal-recessive hearing impairment DFNB42. Am J Hum Genet. 2011;88(2):127-37.

Bork JM, Peters LM, Riazuddin S, Bernstein SL, Ahmed ZM, Ness SL, Polomeno R, Ramesh A, Schloss M, Srisailpathy CR, Wayne S, Bellman S, Desmukh D, Ahmed Z, Khan SN, Kaloustian VM, Li XC, Lalwani A, Riazuddin S, Bitner-Glindzicz M, Nance WE, Liu XZ, Wistow G, Smith RJ, Griffith AJ, Wilcox ER, Friedman TB & Morell RJ. Usher syndrome 1D and nonsyndromic autosomal recessive deafness DFNB12 are caused by allelic mutations of the novel cadherin-like gene *CDH23*. Am J Hum Genet. 2001;68(1):26-37.

Boughman JA, Vernon M & Shaver KA. Usher syndrome: definition and estimate of prevalence from two high-risk populations. J Chronic Dis. 1983;36(8):595-603.

Chaib H, Place C, Salem N, Dodé C, Chardenoux S, Weissenbach J, el Zir E, Loiselet J & Petit C. Mapping of DFNB12, a gene for a non-syndromal autosomal recessive deafness, to chromosome 10q21-22. Hum Mol Genet. 1996;5(7):1061-4.

Charizopoulou N, Lelli A, Schraders M, Ray K, Hildebrand MS, Ramesh A, Srisailapathy CR, Oostrik J, Admiraal RJ, Neely HR, Latoche JR, Smith RJ, Northup JK, Kremer H, Holt JR & Noben-Trauth K. *GIPC3* mutations associated with audiogenic seizures and sensorineural hearing loss in mouse and human. Nat Commun. 2011;2:201.

Chen A, Francis M, Ni L, Cremers CW, Kimberling WJ, Sato Y, Phelps PD, Bellman SC, Wagner MJ & Pembrey M. Phenotypic manifestations of branchio-oto-renal syndrome. Am J Med Genet. 1995;58(4):365-70.

Chen W, Kahrizi K, Meyer NC, Riazalhosseini Y, Van Camp G, Najmabadi H & Smith RJ. Mutation of *COL11A2* causes autosomal recessive non-syndromic hearing loss at the DFNB53 locus. J Med Genet. 2005 Oct;42(10):e61.

Cheng J, Zhu Y, He S, Lu Y, Chen J, Han B, Petrillo M, Wrzeszczynski KO, Yang S, Dai P, Zhai S, Han D, Zhang MQ, Li W, Liu X, Li H, Chen ZY & Yuan H. Functional mutation of *SMAC/DIABLO*, encoding a mitochondrial proapoptotic protein, causes human progressive hearing loss DFNA64. Am J Hum Genet. 2011;89(1):56-66.

Choi BY, Ahmed ZM, Riazuddin S, Bhinder MA, Shahzad M, Husnain T, Riazuddin S, Griffith AJ & Friedman TB. Identities and frequencies of mutations of the otoferlin gene (OTOF) causing DFNB9 deafness in Pakistan. Clin Genet. 2009;75(3):237-43.

Collin RW, Kalay E, Tariq M, Peters T, van der Zwaag B, Venselaar H, Oostrik J, Lee K, Ahmed ZM, Caylan R, Li Y, Spierenburg HA, Eyupoglu E, Heister A, Riazuddin S, Bahat E, Ansar M, Arslan S, Wollnik B, Brunner HG, Cremers CW, Karaguzel A, Ahmad W, Cremers FP, Vriend G, Friedman TB, Riazuddin S, Leal SM & Kremer H. Mutations of *ESRRB* encoding estrogen-related receptor beta cause autosomal-recessive nonsyndromic hearing impairment DFNB35. Am J Hum Genet. 2008;82(1):125-38.

Collin RW, Pauw RJ, Schoots J, Huygen PL, Hoefsloot LH, Cremers CW & Kremer H. Identification of a novel *COCH* mutation, G87W, causing autosomal dominant hearing impairment (DFNA9). Am J Med Genet A. 2006;140(16):1791-4.

Colosimo A, Guida V, Rigoli L, Di Bella C, De Luca A, Briuglia S, Stuppia L, Salpietro DC & Dallapiccola B. Molecular detection of novel *WFS1* mutations in patients with Wolfram syndrome by a DHPLC-based assay. Hum Mutat. 2003;21(6):622-9.

Coucke PJ, Van Hauwe P, Kelley PM, Kunst H, Schatteman I, Van Velzen D, Meyers J, Ensink RJ, Verstreken M, Declau F, Marres H, Kastury K, Bhasin S, McGuirt WT, Smith RJ, Cremers CW, Van de Heyning P, Willems PJ, Smith SD & Van Camp G. Mutations in the *KCNQ4* gene are responsible for autosomal dominant deafness in four DFNA2 families. Hum Mol Genet. 1999;8(7):1321-8.

Craig R & Woodhead JL. Structure and function of myosin filaments. Curr Opin Struct Biol. 2006;16(2):204-12.

Cryns K, Sivakumaran TA, Van den Ouweland JM, Pennings RJ, Cremers CW, Flothmann K, Young TL, Smith RJ, Lesperance MM & Van Camp G. Mutational spectrum of the *WFS1* gene in Wolfram syndrome, nonsyndromic hearing impairment, diabetes mellitus, and psychiatric disease. Hum Mutat. 2003;22(4):275-87.

Davletov BA & Südhof TC. A single C2 domain from synaptotagmin I is sufficient for high affinity Ca2+/phospholipid binding. J Biol Chem 1993;268(35):26386-90.

de Grey ADNJ. Life Span Extension Research and Public Debate: Societal Considerations. Studies in Ethics, Law, and Technology 1 2007.doi:10.2202/1941-6008.1011.

de Kok YJ, van der Maarel SM, Bitner-Glindzicz M, Huber I, Monaco AP, Malcolm S, Pembrey ME, Ropers HH & Cremers FP. Association between X-linked mixed deafness and mutations in the POU domain gene *POU3F4*. Science 1995;267(5198):685-8.

del Castillo FJ, Rodríguez-Ballesteros M, Alvarez A, Hutchin T, Leonardi E, de Oliveira CA, Azaiez H, Brownstein Z, Avenarius MR, Marlin S, Pandya A, Shahin H, Siemering KR, Weil D, Wuyts W, Aguirre LA, Martín Y, Moreno-Pelayo MA, Villamar M, Avraham KB, Dahl HH, Kanaan M, Nance WE, Petit C, Smith RJ, Van Camp G, Sartorato EL, Murgia A, Moreno F & del Castillo I. A novel deletion involving the connexin-30 gene, del(*GJB6*-d13s1854), found in trans with mutations in the *GJB2* gene (connexin-26) in subjects with DFNB1 non-syndromic hearing impairment. J Med Genet. 2005;42(7):588-94.

del Castillo I, Villamar M, Moreno-Pelayo MA, del Castillo FJ, Alvarez A, Tellería D, Menéndez I & Moreno F. A deletion involving the connexin 30 gene in nonsyndromic hearing impairment. N Engl J Med. 2002;346(4):243-9.

del Castillo I, Villamar M, Sarduy M, Romero L, Herraiz C, Hernández FJ, Rodríguez M, Borrás I, Montero A, Bellón J, Tapia MC & Moreno F. A novel locus for non-syndromic sensorineural deafness (DFN6) maps to chromosome Xp22. Hum Mol Genet. 1996;5(9):1383-7.

Delmaghani S, del Castillo FJ, Michel V, Leibovici M, Aghaie A, Ron U, Van Laer L, Ben-Tal N, Van Camp G, Weil D, Langa F, Lathrop M, Avan P & Petit C. Mutations in the gene encoding pejvakin, a newly identified protein of the afferent auditory pathway, cause DFNB59 auditory neuropathy. Nat Genet. 2006;38(7):770-8.

Di Palma F, Pellegrino R & Noben-Trauth K. Genomic structure, alternative splice forms and normal and mutant alleles of cadherin 23 (*CDH23*). Gene. 2001;281(1-2):31-41.

Donaudy F, Ferrara A, Esposito L, Hertzano R, Ben-David O, Bell RE, Melchionda S, Zelante L, Avraham KB & Gasparini P. Multiple mutations of *MYO1A*, a cochlear-expressed gene, in sensorineural hearing loss. Am J Hum Genet. 2003;72(6):1571-7.

Donaudy F, Snoeckx R, Pfister M, Zenner HP, Blin N, Di Stazio M, Ferrara A, Lanzara C, Ficarella R, Declau F, Pusch CM, Nürnberg P, Melchionda S, Zelante L, Ballana E, Estivill X, Van Camp G, Gasparini P & Savoia A. Nonmuscle myosin heavy-chain gene *MYH14* is expressed in cochlea and mutated in patients affected by autosomal dominant hearing impairment (DFNA4). Am J Hum Genet. 2004;74(4):770-6.

Dossena S, Rodighiero S, Vezzoli V, Nofziger C, Salvioni E, Boccazzi M, Grabmayer E, Bottà G, Meyer G, Fugazzola L, Beck-Peccoz P & Paulmichl M. Functional characterization of wild-type and mutated pendrin (*SLC26A4*), the anion transporter involved in Pendred syndrome. J Mol Endocrinol. 2009;43(3):93-103.

Dror AA & Avraham KB. Hearing loss: mechanisms revealed by genetics and cell biology. Annu Rev Genet. 2009;43:411-37.

Ebermann I, Phillips JB, Liebau MC, Koenekoop RK, Schermer B, Lopez I, Schäfer E, Roux AF, Dafinger C, Bernd A, Zrenner E, Claustres M, Blanco B, Nürnberg G, Nürnberg P, Ruland R, Westerfield M, Benzing T & Bolz HJ. *PDZD7* is a modifier of retinal disease and a contributor to digenic Usher syndrome. J Clin Invest. 2010;120(6):1812-23.

Ebermann I, Scholl HP, Charbel Issa P, Becirovic E, Lamprecht J, Jurklies B, Millán JM, Aller E, Mitter D & Bolz H. A novel gene for Usher syndrome type 2: mutations in the long isoform of whirlin are associated with retinitis pigmentosa and sensorineural hearing loss. Hum Genet. 2007;121(2):203-11.

Edery P, Attié T, Amiel J, Pelet A, Eng C, Hofstra RM, Martelli H, Bidaud C, Munnich A & Lyonnet S. Mutation of the endothelin-3 gene in the Waardenburg-Hirschsprung disease (Shah-Waardenburg syndrome). Nat Genet. 1996;12(4):442-4.

Emery A. Hereditary. Rimoin DL, Connor JM, Pyeritz RE, Korf BR. In: Emery and Rimom's principles and practice of Medical Genetics. Churchill Livingstone, 5th edition. 2003; 1:243-244.

Estivill X, Fortina P, Surrey S, Rabionet R, Melchionda S, D'Agruma L, Mansfield E, Rappaport E, Govea N, Milà M, Zelante L & Gasparini P. Connexin-26 mutations in sporadic and inherited sensorineural deafness. Lancet. 1998;351: 394-398.

Eudy JD, Weston MD, Yao S, Hoover DM, Rehm HL, Ma-Edmonds M, Yan D, Ahmad I, Cheng JJ, Ayuso C, Cremers C, Davenport S, Moller C, Talmadge CB, Beisel KW, Tamayo M, Morton CC, Swaroop A, Kimberling WJ & Sumegi J. Mutation of a gene encoding a protein with extracellular matrix motifs in Usher syndrome type IIa. Science. 1998;280(5370):1753-7.

Everett LA, Glaser B, Beck JC, Idol JR, Buchs A, Heyman M, Adawi F, Hazani E, Nassir E, Baxevanis AD, Sheffield VC & Green ED. Pendred syndrome is caused by mutations in a putative sulphate transporter gene (PDS). Nat Genet. 1997;17(4):411-22.

Finsterer J & Fellinger J. Nuclear and mitochondrial genes mutated in nonsyndromic impaired hearing. Int J Pediatr Otorhinolaryngol. 2005;69(5):621-47.

Fischel-Ghodsian N. Mitochondrial deafness mutations reviewed. Hum Mutat. 1999;13:261-270.

Fonseca SG, Ishigaki S, Oslowski CM, Lu S, Lipson KL, Ghosh R, Hayashi E, Ishihara H, Oka Y, Permutt MA, Urano F. Wolfram syndrome 1 gene negatively regulates ER stress signaling in rodent and human cells. J Clin Invest. 2010;120(3):744-55.

Fraser Gr. Association of congenital deafness with gitre (Pendred's syndrome) a study of 207 families. Ann Hum Genet. 1965;28:201-49.

Friedman RA, Van Laer L, Huentelman MJ, Sheth SS, Van Eyken E, Corneveaux JJ, Tembe WD, Halperin RF, Thorburn AQ, Thys S, Bonneux S, Fransen E, Huyghe J, Pyykkö I, Cremers CW, Kremer H, Dhooge I, Stephens D, Orzan E, Pfister M, Bille M, Parving A, Sorri M, Van de Heyning PH, Makmura L, Ohmen JD, Linthicum FH Jr, Fayad JN, Pearson JV, Craig DW, Stephan DA & Van Camp G. *GRM7* variants confer susceptibility to age-related hearing impairment. Hum Mol Genet. 2009;18(4):785-96

Friedman TB, Schultz JM, Ben-Yosef T, Pryor SP, Lagziel A, Fisher RA, Wilcox ER, Riazuddin S, Ahmed ZM, Belyantseva IA & Griffith AJ. Recent advances in the understanding of syndromic forms of hearing loss. Ear Hear 2003;24(4):289-302.

Friedman TB, Sellers JR & Avraham KB. Unconventional myosins and the genetics of hearing loss. Med Genet. 1999;89:147-157.

Fukuoka H, Kanda Y, Ohta S & Usami S. Mutations in the *WFS1* gene are a frequent cause of autosomal dominant nonsyndromic low-frequency hearing loss in Japanese. J Hum Genet. 2007;52(6):510-5.

Gal A, Pentelenyi K, Remenyi V, Pal Z, Csanyi B, Tomory G, Rasko I & Molnar MJ. Novel heteroplasmic mutation in the anticodon stem of mitochondrial tRNA(Lys) associated with dystonia and stroke-like episodes. Acta Neurol Scand. 2010;122(4):252-6.

Gómez-Zaera M, Strom TM, Rodríguez B, Estivill X, Meitinger T & Nunes V. Presence of a major *WFS1* mutation in Spanish Wolfram syndrome pedigrees. Mol Genet Metab. 2001;72(1):72-81.

Gorlin RJ. Genetic hearing loss—a brief history. Toriello HV, Reardon W, Gorlin RJ. In: Hereditary Hearing Loss and Its Syndromes. Second Edition, Oxf University Press, Baltimore 2004.

Goto Y, Nonaka I & Horai S. A mutation in the tRNALeu(UUR) gene associated with the MELAS subgroup of mitochondrial encephalomyopathies. Nature. 1990; 348:651-653.

Greinwald JH Jr, Scott DA, Marietta JR, Carmi R, Manaligod J, Ramesh A, Zbar RI, Kraft ML, Elbedour K, Yairi Y, Musy M, Skvorak AB, Van Camp G, Srisailapathy CR, Lovett M, Morton CC, Sheffield VC & Smith RJ. Construction of P1-derived artificial chromosome and yeast artificial chromosome contigs encompassing the DFNB7 and DFNB11 region of chromosome 9q13-21. Genome Res. 1997;7(9):879-86.

Grifa A, Wagner CA, D'Ambrosio L, Melchionda S, Bernardi F, Lopez-Bigas N, Rabionet R, Arbones M, Monica MD, Estivill X, Zelante L, Lang F & Gasparini P. Mutations in *GJB6* cause nonsyndromic autosomal dominant deafness at DFNA3 locus. Nat Genet. 1999;23(1):16-8.

Grillet N, Schwander M, Hildebrand MS, Sczaniecka A, Kolatkar A, Velasco J, Webster JA, Kahrizi K, Najmabadi H, Kimberling WJ, Stephan D, Bahlo M, Wiltshire T, Tarantino LM, Kuhn P, Smith RJ & Müller U. Mutations in *LOXHD1*, an evolutionarily conserved stereociliary protein, disrupt hair cell function in mice and cause progressive hearing loss in humans. Am J Hum Genet. 2009;85(3):328-37.

Guan MX. Mitochondrial 12S rRNA mutations associated with aminoglycoside ototoxicity. Mitochondrion. 2011;11(2):237-45.

Gubler MC, Heidet L & Antignac C. Alport's syndrome, thin basement membrane nephropathy, nail-patella syndrome, and type III collagen glomerulopathy. In: Jennette JC, Olson JL, Schwartz MM, Silva FG, eds. Heptinstall's Pathology of the Kidney. 6th ed. Philadelphia, Pa: LippincottWilliams & Wilkins; 2007:487–515.

Guilford P, Ben Arab S, Blanchard S, Levilliers J, Weissenbach J, Belkahia A & Petit C. A non-syndrome form of neurosensory, recessive deafness maps to the pericentromeric region of chromosome 13q. Nat Genet. 1994;6(1):24-8.

Guipponi M, Antonarakis SE & Scott HS. *TMPRSS3*, a type II transmembrane serine protease mutated in non-syndromic autosomal recessive deafness. Front Biosci. 2008;13:1557-67.

Guipponi M, Vuagniaux G, Wattenhofer M, Shibuya K, Vazquez M, Dougherty L, Scamuffa N, Guida E, Okui M, Rossier C, Hancock M, Buchet K, Reymond A, Hummler E, Marzella PL, Kudoh J, Shimizu N, Scott HS, Antonarakis SE & Rossier BC. The transmembrane serine protease (*TMPRSS3*) mutated in deafness DFNB8/10 activates the epithelial sodium channel (ENaC) in vitro. Hum Mol Genet. 2002;11(23):2829-36.

Gumbiner BM. Regulation of cadherin-mediated adhesion in morphogenesis. Nat Rev Mol Cell Biol 2005;6:622-634.

Hilgert N, Alasti F, Dieltjens N, Pawlik B, Wollnik B, Uyguner O, Delmaghani S, Weil D, Petit C, Danis E, Yang T, Pandelia E, Petersen MB, Goossens D, Favero JD, Sanati MH, Smith RJ & Van Camp G. Mutation analysis of *TMC1* identifies four new mutations and suggests an additional deafness gene at loci DFNA36 and DFNB7/11. Clin Genet. 2008;74(3):223-32.

Hilgert N, Huentelman MJ, Thorburn AQ, Fransen E, Dieltjens N, Mueller-Malesinska M, Pollak A, et al. Phenotypic variability of patients homozygous for the GJB2 mutation 35delG cannot be explained by the influence of one major modifier gene. Eur J Hum Genet. 2009a Apr;17(4):517-24.

Hilgert N, Smith RJ & Van Camp G. Forty-six genes causing nonsyndromic hearing impairment: which ones should be analyzed in DNA diagnostics? Mutat Res 2009b;681(2-3):189-96.

Hofmann S, Philbrook C, Gerbitz KD & Bauer MF. Wolfram syndrome: structural and functional analyses of mutant and wild-type wolframin, the *WFS1* gene product. Hum Mol Genet. 2003;12(16):2003-12.

Hofstra RM, Osinga J, Tan-Sindhunata G, Wu Y, Kamsteeg EJ, Stulp RP, van Ravenswaaij-Arts C, Majoor-Krakauer D, Angrist M, Chakravarti A, Meijers C, Buys CH. A homozygous mutation in the endothelin-3 gene associated with a combined Waardenburg type 2 and Hirschsprung phenotype (Shah-Waardenburg syndrome). Nat Genet. 1996;12(4):445-7.

Holms RH & Steel KP. Genes involved in deafness. Curr opin Gene Dev. 1999; 9:309-314.

Hope CI, Bundey S, Proops D & Fielder AR. Usher syndrome in the city of Birmingham--prevalence and clinical classification. Br J Ophthalmol. 1997;81(1):46-53.

Hoskins BE, Cramer CH, Silvius D, Zou D, Raymond RM, Orten DJ, Kimberling WJ, Smith RJ, Weil D, Petit C, Otto EA, Xu PX & Hildebrandt F. Transcription factor SIX5 is mutated in patients with branchio-oto-renal syndrome. Am J Hum Genet. 2007;80(4):800-4.

Hu H, Wu L, Feng Y, Pan Q, Long Z, Li J, Dai H, Xia K, Liang D, Niikawa N & Xia J. Molecular analysis of hearing loss associated with enlarged vestibular aqueduct in the mainland Chinese: a unique *SLC26A4* mutation spectrum. J Hum Genet. 2007;52(6):492-7.

Huang Q & Tang J. Age-related hearing loss or presbycusis. Eur Arch Otorhinolaryngol. 2010;267(8):1179-91.

Hudson BG, Tryggvason K, Sundaramoorthy M & Neilson EG. Alport's syndrome, Goodpasture's syndrome, and type IV collagen. N Engl J Med. 2003;348(25):2543-56.

Jaksch M, Klopstock T, Kurlemann G, et al. Progressive myoclonus epilepsy and mitochondrial myopathy associated with mutations in the tRNASer(UCN)) gene. Ann Neurol. 1998; 44:635- 640.

Jamora C & Fuchs E. Intercellular adhesion, signalling and the cytoskeleton. Nat Cell Biol. 2002;4(4):E101-8.

Joensuu T, Hämäläinen R, Yuan B, Johnson C, Tegelberg S, Gasparini P, Zelante L, Pirvola U, Pakarinen L, Lehesjoki AE, de la Chapelle A & Sankila EM. Mutations in a novel gene with transmembrane domains underlie Usher syndrome type 3. Am J Hum Genet. 2001;69(4):673-84.

Johnson KR, Yu H, Ding D, Jiang H, Gagnon LH & Salvi RJ. Separate and combined effects of Sod1 and *CDH23* mutations on age-related hearing loss and cochlear pathology in C57BL/6J mice. Hear Res. 2010;268(1-2):85-92.

Kalay E, Uzumcu A, Krieger E, Caylan R, Uyguner O, Ulubil-Emiroglu M, Erdol H, Kayserili H, Hafiz G, Başerer N, Heister AJ, Hennies HC, Nürnberg P, Başaran S, Brunner HG, Cremers CW, Karaguzel A, Wollnik B & Kremer H. *MYO15A* (DFNB3) mutations in Turkish hearing loss families and functional modeling of a novel motor domain mutation. Am J Med Genet A. 2007;143A(20):2382-9.

Kameoka K, Isotani H, Tanaka K, et al. Novel mitochondrial DNA mutation in tRNA(Lys) (8296A→G) associated with diabetes. Biochem Biophys Res Commun. 1998;245:523-527.

Kapur RP. Early death of neural crest cells is responsible for total enteric aganglionosis in *SOX10*(Dom)/*SOX10*(Dom) mouse embryos. Pediatr Dev Pathol. 1999;2(6):559-69.

Kelley PM, Harris DJ, Comer BC, Askew JW, Fowler T, Smith SD & Kimberling WJ. Novel mutations in the connexin 26 gene (*GJB2*) that cause autosomal recessive (DFNB1) hearing loss. Am J Hum Genet. 1998; 62: 792-799.

Kelsell DP, Dunlop J, Stevens HP, Lench NJ, Liang JN, Parry G, Mueller RF & Leigh IM. Connexin 26 mutations in hereditary non-syndromic sensorineural deafness. Nature. 1997;387(6628):80-3.

Khan SY, Ahmed ZM, Shabbir MI, Kitajiri S, Kalsoom S, Tasneem S, Shayiq S, Ramesh A, Srisailpathy S, Khan SN, Smith RJ, Riazuddin S, Friedman TB & Riazuddin S. Mutations of the *RDX* gene cause nonsyndromic hearing loss at the DFNB24 locus. Hum Mutat. 2007;28(5):417-23.

Kimberling WJ, Weston MD, Möller C, Davenport SL, Shugart YY, Priluck IA, Martini A, Milani M & Smith RJ. Localization of Usher syndrome type II to chromosome 1q. Genomics. 1990;7(2):245-9.

Klein D. Historical background and evidence for dominant inheritance of the Klein-Waardenburg syndrome (type III). Am J Med Genet. 1983;14(2):231-9.

Kopp P, Pesce L & Solis-S JC. Pendred syndrome and iodide transport in the thyroid. Trends Endocrinol Metab. 2008;19(7):260-8.

Kubisch C, Schroeder BC, Friedrich T, Lütjohann B, El-Amraoui A, Marlin S, Petit C & Jentsch TJ. *KCNQ4*, a novel potassium channel expressed in sensory outer hair cells, is mutated in dominant deafness. Cell 1999;96(3):437-46.

Kumar NM & Gilula NB. The gap Junction communication channel. Cell. 1996; 84:381-388.

Kurima K, Peters LM, Yang Y, Riazuddin S, Ahmed ZM, Naz S, Arnaud D, Drury S, Mo J, Makishima T, Ghosh M, Menon PS, Deshmukh D, Oddoux C, Ostrer H, Khan S, Riazuddin S, Deininger PL, Hampton LL, Sullivan SL, Battey JF Jr, Keats BJ, Wilcox ER, Friedman TB & Griffith AJ. Dominant and recessive deafness caused by mutations of a novel gene, *TMC1*, required for cochlear hair-cell function. Nat Genet. 2002;30(3):277-84.

Lalwani AK, Goldstein JA, Kelley MJ, Luxford W, Castelein CM & Mhatre AN. Human nonsyndromic hereditary deafness DFNA17 is due to a mutation in nonmuscle myosin *MYH9*. Am J Hum Genet. 2000;67(5):1121-8.

Lemmink HH, Mochizuki T, van den Heuvel LP, Schröder CH, Barrientos A, Monnens LA, van Oost BA, Brunner HG, Reeders ST & Smeets HJ. Mutations in the type IV collagen alpha 3 (*COL4A3*) gene in autosomal recessive Alport syndrome. Hum Mol Genet. 1994;3(8):1269-73.

Leon PE, Raventos H, Lynch E, Morrow J & King MC. The gene for an inherited form of deafness maps to chromosome 5q31. Proc Natl Acad Sci U S A. 1992;89(11):5181-4.

Lezirovitz K, PardonoE, de Mello Auricchio MTB, de Carvalho e Silva FL, Lopes JJ, Abreu-Silva RS, Romanos J, Batissoco AC & Mingroni-Netto RC. Unexpected genetic heterogeneity in a large consanguineous Brazilian pedigree presenting deafness. Eur J Hum Genet. 2008;16:89–96.

Li XC, Everett LA, Lalwani AK, Desmukh D, Friedman TB, Green ED & Wilcox ER. A mutation in PDS causes non-syndromic recessive deafness. Nat Genet. 1998;18(3):215-7.

Li Z, Li R, Chen J, et al. Mutational analysis of the mitochondrial 12S rRNA gene in Chinese pediatric subjects with aminoglycoside- induced and nonsyndromic hearing loss. Hum Genet. 2005; 117:9-15.

Liang Y, Wang A, Belyantseva IA, Anderson DW, Probst FJ, Barber TD, Miller W, Touchman JW, Jin L, Sullivan SL, Sellers JR, Camper SA, Lloyd RV, Kachar B, Friedman TB & Fridell RA. Characterization of the human and mouse unconventional myosin XV genes responsible for hereditary deafness DFNB3 and shaker 2. Genomics. 1999;61:243-258.

Liu X, Han D, Li J, Han B, Ouyang X, Cheng J, Li X, Jin Z, Wang Y, Bitner-Glindzicz M, Kong X, Xu H, Kantardzhieva A, Eavey RD, Seidman CE, Seidman JG, Du LL, Chen ZY, Dai P, Teng M, Yan D & Yuan H. Loss-of-function mutations in the *PRPS1* gene cause a type of nonsyndromic X-linked sensorineural deafness, DFN2. Am J Hum Genet. 2010;86(1):65-71.

Liu XZ, Ouyang XM, Xia XJ, Zheng J, Pandya A, Li F, Du LL, Welch KO, Petit C, Smith RJ, Webb BT, Yan D, Arnos KS, Corey D, Dallos P, Nance WE & Chen ZY. Prestin, a cochlear motor protein, is defective in non-syndromic hearing loss. Hum Mol Genet. 2003;12(10):1155-62.

Liu XZ, Walsh J, Tamagawa Y, Kitamura K, Nishizawa M, Steel KP & Brown SD. Autosomal dominant non-syndromic deafness caused by a mutation in the myosin VIIA gene. Nat Genet. 1997;17(3):268-9.

Loikkanen I, Toljamo K, Hirvikoski P, Väisänen T, Paavonen TK & Vaarala MH. Myosin VI is a modulator of androgen-dependent gene expression. Oncol Rep. 2009;22(5):991-5.

Lynch ED, Lee MK, Morrow JE, Welcsh PL, León PE & King MC. Nonsyndromic deafness DFNA1 associated with mutation of a human homolog of the Drosophila gene diaphanous. Science. 1997;278(5341):1315-8.

Mahdieh N & Rabbani B. Statistical study of 35delG mutation of *GJB2* gene: a meta-analysis of carrier frequency. Int J Audiol. 2009;48(6):363-70.

Mahdieh N, Bagherian H, Shirkavand A, Sharafi M & Zeinali S. High level of intrafamilial phenotypic variability of non-syndromic hearing loss in a Lur family due to delE120 mutation in *GJB2* gene. Int J Pediatr Otorhinolaryngol. 2010b;74:1089-1091.

Mahdieh N, Nishimura C, Ali-Madadi K, Riazalhosseini Y, Yazdan H, Arzhangi S, Jalalvand K, Ebrahimi A, Kazemi S, Smith RJ & Najmabadi H. The frequency of *GJB2* mutations and the Delta (*GJB6*-D13S1830) deletion as a cause of autosomal recessive non-syndromic deafness in the Kurdish population. Clin Genet. 2004;65(6):506-8.

Mahdieh N, Rabbani B, Shirkavand A, Bagherian H, Movahed ZS, Fouladi P, Rahiminejad F, Masoudifard M, Akbari MT & Zeinali S. Impact of consanguineous marriages in *GJB2*-related hearing loss in the Iranian population: a report of a novel variant. Genet Test Mol Biomarkers. 2011;15(7-8):489-93.

Mahdieh N, Rabbani B, Wiley S, Akabari MT & Zeinali S. Genetic causes of nonsyndromic hearing loss in Iran in comparison with other populations. J Hum Genet. 2010a;55(10):639-48.

Mahdieh N, Shirkavand A, Raeisi M, Akbari MT & Zeinali S. Unexpected heterogeneity due to recessive and de novo dominant mutations of *GJB2* in an Iranian family with nonsyndromic hearing loss: implication for genetic counseling. Biochem Biophys Res Commun 2010c;402(2):305-7.

Mburu P, Mustapha M, Varela A, Weil D, El-Amraoui A, Holme RH, Rump A, Hardisty RE, Blanchard S, Coimbra RS, Perfettini I, Parkinson N, Mallon AM, Glenister P, Rogers MJ, Paige AJ, Moir L, Clay J, Rosenthal A, Liu XZ, Blanco G, Steel KP, Petit C & Brown SD. Defects in whirlin, a PDZ domain molecule involved in stereocilia elongation, cause deafness in the whirler mouse and families with DFNB31. Nat Genet. 2003;34(4):421-8.

McGuirt WT, Prasad SD, Griffith AJ, Kunst HP, Green GE, Shpargel KB, Runge C, Huybrechts C, Mueller RF, Lynch E, King MC, Brunner HG, Cremers CW, Takanosu M, Li SW, Arita M, Mayne R, Prockop DJ, Van Camp G & Smith RJ. Mutations in *COL11A2* cause non-syndromic hearing loss (DFNA13). Nat Genet. 1999 Dec;23(4):413-9.

Melchionda S, Ahituv N, Bisceglia L, Sobe T, Glaser F, Rabionet R, Arbones ML, Notarangelo A, Di Iorio E, Carella M, Zelante L, Estivill X, Avraham KB & Gasparini P. *MYO6*, the human homologue of the gene responsible for deafness in Snell's waltzer mice, is mutated in autosomal dominant nonsyndromic hearing loss. Am J Hum Genet. 2001;69(3):635-40.

Mencia A, Modamio-Høybjør S, Redshaw N, Morín M, Mayo-Merino F, Olavarrieta L, Aguirre LA, del Castillo I, Steel KP, Dalmay T, Moreno F & Moreno-Pelayo MA. Mutations in the seed region of human miR-96 are responsible for nonsyndromic progressive hearing loss. Nat Genet. 2009;41(5):609-13.

Merchant SN, Burgess BJ, Adams JC, Kashtan CE, Gregory MC, Santi PA, Colvin R, Collins B & Nadol JB Jr.Temporal bone histopathology in alport syndrome. Laryngoscope. 2004;114(9):1609-18.

Migliosi V, Modamio-Høybjør S, Moreno-Pelayo MA, Rodríguez-Ballesteros M, Villamar M, Tellería D, Menéndez I, Moreno F & Del Castillo I. Q829X, a novel mutation in the gene encoding *OTOF*erlin (*OTOF*), is frequently found in Spanish patients with prelingual non-syndromic hearing loss. J Med Genet. 2002;39(7):502-6.

Mirghomizadeh F, Pfister M, Apaydin F, Petit C, Kupka S, Pusch CM, Zenner HP & Blin N. Substitutions in the conserved C2C domain of *OTOF*erlin cause DFNB9, a form of nonsyndromic autosomal recessive deafness. Neurobiol Dis. 2002;10(2):157-64.

Modamio-Hoybjor S, Mencia A, Goodyear R, del Castillo I, Richardson G, Moreno F & Moreno-Pelayo MA. A mutation in *CCDC50*, a gene encoding an effector of epidermal growth factor-mediated cell signaling, causes progressive hearing loss. Am J Hum Genet. 2007;80(6):1076-89.

Morell RJ, Kim HJ, Hood LJ, Goforth L, Friderici K, Fisher R, Van Camp G, Berlin CI, Oddoux C, Ostrer H, Keats B & Friedman TB. Mutations in the connexin 26 gene (GJB2) among Ashkenazi Jews with nonsyndromic recessive deafness. N Engl J Med. 1998 Nov 19;339(21):1500-5.

Morle L, Bozon M, Alloisio N, Latour P, Vandenberghe A, Plauchu H, Collet L, Edery P, Godet J & Lina-Granade G. A novel C202F mutation in the connexin26 gene (*GJB2*) associated with autosomal dominant isolated hearing loss. J Med Genet. 2000; 37: 368-370.

Morton CC & Nance WE. Newborn hearing screening--a silent revolution. N Engl J Med. 2006;354(20):2151-64.

Mount DB & Romero MF. The SLC26 gene family of multifunctional anion exchangers. Pflugers Archiv 2004;447:710-721.

Mustapha M, Chouery E, Torchard-Pagnez D, Nouaille S, Khrais A, Sayegh FN, Mégarbané A, Loiselet J, Lathrop M, Petit C & Weil D. A novel locus for Usher syndrome type I, USH1G, maps to chromosome 17q24-25. Hum Genet. 2002;110(4):348-50.

Mustapha M, Weil D, Chardenoux S, Elias S, El-Zir E, Beckmann JS, Loiselet J & Petit C. An alpha-tectorin gene defect causes a newly identified autosomal recessive form of sensorineural pre-lingual non-syndromic deafness, DFNB21. Hum Mol Genet. 1999;8(3):409-12.

Nal N, Ahmed ZM, Erkal E, Alper OM, Lüleci G, Dinç O, Waryah AM, Ain Q, Tasneem S, Husnain T, Chattaraj P, Riazuddin S, Boger E, Ghosh M, Kabra M, Riazuddin S, Morell RJ & Friedman TB. Mutational spectrum of *MYO15A*: the large N-terminal extension of myosin XVA is required for hearing. Hum Mutat. 2007;28(10):1014-9.

Nance WE & Sweeney A. Symposium on sensorineural hearing loss in children: early detection and intervention. Genetic factors in deafness of early life. Otolaryngol Clin North Am. 1975;8(1):19-48.

Naz S, Giguere CM, Kohrman DC, Mitchem KL, Riazuddin S, Morell RJ, Ramesh A, Srisailpathy S, Deshmukh D, Riazuddin S, Griffith AJ, Friedman TB, Smith RJ & Wilcox ER. Mutations in a novel gene, *TMIE*, are associated with hearing loss linked to the DFNB6 locus. Am J Hum Genet. 2002;71(3):632-6.

Naz S, Griffith AJ, Riazuddin S, Hampton LL, Battey JF Jr, Khan SN, Riazuddin S, Wilcox ER & Friedman TB. Mutations of *ESPN* cause autosomal recessive deafness and vestibular dysfunction. J Med Genet. 2004;41(8):591-5.

Nelson WJ & Nusse R. Convergence of Wnt, beta-catenin, and cadherin pathways. Science. 2004;303(5663):1483-7.

Newton V. Hearing loss and Waardenburg's syndrome: implications for genetic counselling. J Laryngol Otol. 1990;104(2):97-103.

Nie L. *KCNQ4* mutations associated with nonsyndromic progressive sensorineural hearing loss. Curr Opin Otolaryngol Head Neck Surg. 2008;16(5):441-4.

Oliver TN, Berg JS & Cheney RE. Tails of unconventional myosins. Cell Mol Life Sci. 1999;56:243-257.

Ouyang XM, Xia XJ, Verpy E, Du LL, Pandya A, Petit C, Balkany T, Nance WE & Liu XZ. Mutations in the alternatively spliced exons of *USH1C* cause non-syndromic recessive deafness. Hum Genet. 2002 Jul;111(1):26-30.

Pallares-Ruiz N, Blanchet P, Mondain M, Claustres M & Roux AF. A large deletion including most of *GJB6* in recessive non syndromic deafness: a digenic effect? Eur J Hum Genet. 2002;10(1):72-6.

Pandya A, Xia XJ, Erdenetungalag R, et al. Heterogenous point mutations in the mitochondrial tRNASer(UCN) precursor coexisting with the A1555G mutation in deafness students from Mongolia. Am J Hum Genet. 1999;65:1803-1806.

Peters LM, Anderson DW, Griffith AJ, Grundfast KM, San Agustin TB, Madeo AC, Friedman TB & Morell RJ. Mutation of a transcription factor, TFCP2L3, causes progressive autosomal dominant hearing loss, DFNA28. Hum Mol Genet. 2002;11(23):2877-85.

Pingault V, Bondurand N, Kuhlbrodt K, Goerich DE, Préhu MO, Puliti A, Herbarth B, Hermans-Borgmeyer I, Legius E, Matthijs G, Amiel J, Lyonnet S, Ceccherini I, Romeo G, Smith JC, Read AP, Wegner M & Goossens M. *SOX10* mutations in patients with Waardenburg-Hirschsprung disease. Nat Genet. 1998;18(2):171-3.

Raphael Y & Altschuler RA. Structure and innervation of the cochlea. Brain Res Bull. 2003;60(5-6):397-422.

Read AP & Newton VE. Waardenburg syndrome. J Med Genet 1997;34:656–665.

Rehman AU, Gul K, Morell RJ, Lee K, Ahmed ZM, Riazuddin S, Ali RA, Shahzad M, Jaleel AU, Andrade PB, Khan SN, Khan S, Brewer CC, Ahmad W, Leal SM, Riazuddin S & Friedman TB. Mutations of *GIPC3* cause nonsyndromic hearing loss DFNB72 but not DFNB81 that also maps to chromosome 19p. Hum Genet. 2011 Jun 10. [Epub ahead of print]

Rehman AU, Morell RJ, Belyantseva IA, Khan SY, Boger ET, Shahzad M, Ahmed ZM, Riazuddin S, Khan SN, Riazuddin S & Friedman TB. Targeted capture and next-generation sequencing identifies C9orf75, encoding taperin, as the mutated gene in nonsyndromic deafness DFNB79. Am J Hum Genet. 2010;86(3):378-88.

Riazuddin S, Ahmed ZM, Fanning AS, Lagziel A, Kitajiri S, Ramzan K, Khan SN, Chattaraj P, Friedman PL, Anderson JM, Belyantseva IA, Forge A, Riazuddin S & Friedman TB. Tricellulin is a tight-junction protein necessary for hearing. Am J Hum Genet. 2006;79(6):1040-51.

Riazuddin S, Anwar S, Fischer M, Ahmed ZM, Khan SY, Janssen AG, Zafar AU, Scholl U, Husnain T, Belyantseva IA, Friedman PL, Riazuddin S, Friedman TB & Fahlke C. Molecular basis of DFNB73: mutations of *BSND* can cause nonsyndromic deafness or Bartter syndrome. Am J Hum Genet. 2009;85(2):273-80.

Riazuddin S, Khan SN, Ahmed ZM, Ghosh M, Caution K, Nazli S, Kabra M, Zafar AU, Chen K, Naz S, Antonellis A, Pavan WJ, Green ED, Wilcox ER, Friedman PL, Morell RJ, Riazuddin S& Friedman TB. Mutations in *TRIOBP*, which encodes a putative cytoskeletal-organizing protein, are associated with nonsyndromic recessive deafness. Am J Hum Genet. 2006;78(1):137-43.

Richards AJ, Yates JR, Williams R, Payne SJ, Pope FM, Scott JD & Snead MP.A family with Stickler syndrome type 2 has a mutation in the *COL11A1* gene resulting in the substitution of glycine 97 by valine in alpha 1 (XI) collagen.Hum Mol Genet. 1996;5(9):1339-43.

Richardson GP, Lukashkin AN & Russell IJ. The tectorial membrane: one slice of a complex cochlear sandwich. Curr Opin Otolaryngol Head Neck Surg. 2008;16(5):458-64.

Rigoli L, Prisco F, Caruso RA, Iafusco D, Ursomanno G, Zuccarello D, Ingenito N, Rigoli M & Barberi I. Association of the T14709C mutation of mitochondrial DNA with maternally inherited diabetes mellitus and/or deafness in an Italian family. Diabet Med. 2001;18(4):334-6.

Robertson NG, Lu L, Heller S, Merchant SN, Eavey RD, McKenna M, Nadol JB Jr, Miyamoto RT, Linthicum FH Jr, Lubianca Neto JF, Hudspeth AJ, Seidman CE, Morton CC & Seidman JG. Mutations in a novel cochlear gene cause DFNA9, a human nonsyndromic deafness with vestibular dysfunction. Nat Genet. 1998;20(3):299-303.

Ruf RG, Xu PX, Silvius D, Otto EA, Beekmann F, Muerb UT, Kumar S, Neuhaus TJ, Kemper MJ, Raymond RM Jr, Brophy PD, Berkman J, Gattas M, Hyland V, Ruf EM, Schwartz C, Chang EH, Smith RJ, Stratakis CA, Weil D, Petit C & Hildebrandt F. SIX1 mutations cause branchio-oto-renal syndrome by disruption of *EYA1*-SIX1-DNA complexes. Proc Natl Acad Sci U S A. 2004;101(21):8090-5.

Sahin-Calapoglu N, Calapoglu M & Karaguzel A. Non-syndromic recessive hearing loss linkaged *TMPRSS3* gene in the Turkish population. SDÜ Týp Fak Derg. 2005;12(3):31-35.

Schraders M, Lee K, Oostrik J, Huygen PL, Ali G, Hoefsloot LH, Veltman JA, Cremers FP, Basit S, Ansar M, Cremers CW, Kunst HP, Ahmad W, Admiraal RJ, Leal SM & Kremer H. Homozygosity mapping reveals mutations of *GRXCR1* as a cause of autosomal-recessive nonsyndromic hearing impairment. Am J Hum Genet. 2010;86(2):138-47.

Schraders M, Oostrik J, Huygen PL, Strom TM, van Wijk E, Kunst HP, Hoefsloot LH, Cremers CW, Admiraal RJ & Kremer H. Mutations in *PTPRQ* are a cause of autosomal-recessive nonsyndromic hearing impairment DFNB84 and associated with vestibular dysfunction. Am J Hum Genet. 2010;86(4):604-10.

Schultz JM, Khan SN, Ahmed ZM, Riazuddin S, Waryah AM, Chhatre D, Starost MF, Ploplis B, Buckley S, Velásquez D, Kabra M, Lee K, Hassan MJ, Ali G, Ansar M, Ghosh M, Wilcox ER, Ahmad W, Merlino G, Leal SM, Riazuddin S, Friedman TB & Morell RJ. Noncoding mutations of *HGF* are associated with nonsyndromic hearing loss, DFNB39. Am J Hum Genet. 2009;85(1):25-39.

Scott HS, Kudoh J, Wattenhofer M, Shibuya K, Berry A, Chrast R, Guipponi M, Wang J, Kawasaki K, Asakawa S, Minoshima S, Younus F, Mehdi SQ, Radhakrishna U, Papasavvas MP, Gehrig C, Rossier C, Korostishevsky M, Gal A, Shimizu N, Bonne-Tamir B & Antonarakis SE. Insertion of beta-satellite repeats identifies a transmembrane protease causing both congenital and childhood onset autosomal recessive deafness. Nat Genet. 2001;27(1):59-63.

Shabbir MI, Ahmed ZM, Khan SY, Riazuddin S, Waryah AM, Khan SN, Camps RD, Ghosh M, Kabra M, Belyantseva IA, Friedman TB & Riazuddin S. Mutations of human *TMHS* cause recessively inherited non-syndromic hearing loss. J Med Genet. 2006;43(8):634-40.

Shah KN, Dalal SJ, Desai MP, Sheth PN, Joshi NC & Ambani LM. White forelock, pigmentary disorder of irides, and long segment Hirschsprung disease: possible variant of Waardenburg syndrome. J Pediatr. 1981;99(3):432-5.

Sheffield VC, Kraiem Z, Beck JC, Nishimura D, Stone EM, Salameh M, Sadeh O & Glaser B. Pendred syndrome maps to chromosome 7q21-34 and is caused by an intrinsic defect in thyroid iodine organification. Nat Genet. 1996;12:424-426.

Shin JJ, Keamy DG Jr & Steinberg EA. Medical and surgical interventions for hearing loss associated with congenital cytomegalovirus: a systematic review. Otolaryngol Head Neck Surg. 2011;144(5):662-75.

Siemens J, Lillo C, Dumont RA, Reynolds A, Williams DS, Gillespie PG & Müller U. Cadherin 23 is a component of the tip link in hair-cell stereocilia. Nature. 2004;428(6986):950-5.

Sirmaci A, Erbek S, Price J, Huang M, Duman D, Cengiz FB, Bademci G, Tokgöz-Yilmaz S, Hişmi B, Ozdağ H, Oztürk B, Kulaksizoğlu S, Yildirim E, Kokotas H, Grigoriadou M, Petersen MB, Shahin H, Kanaan M, King MC, Chen ZY, Blanton SH, Liu XZ, Zuchner S, Akar N & Tekin M. A truncating mutation in *SERPINB6* is associated with autosomal-recessive nonsyndromic sensorineural hearing loss. Am J Hum Genet. 2010;86(5):797-804.

Smith RJ & Hone S. Genetic screening for deafness. Pediatr Clin North Am. 2003;50(2):315-29.

Smith RJ, Berlin CI, Hejtmancik JF, Keats BJ, Kimberling WJ, Lewis RA, Möller CG, Pelias MZ & Tranebjaerg L. Clinical diagnosis of the Usher syndromes. Usher Syndrome Consortium. Am J Med Genet. 1994;50(1):32-8.

Smith RJ, Lee EC, Kimberling WJ, Daiger SP, Pelias MZ, Keats BJ, Jay M, Bird A, Reardon W, Guest M, et al. Localization of two genes for Usher syndrome type I to chromosome 11. Genomics. 1992;14(4):995-1002.

Stevenson VA, Ito M & Milunsky JM. Connexin-30 deletion analysis in connexin-26 heterozygotes. Genet Test. 2003;7:151-4.

Szabo R, Wu Q, Dickson RB, Netzel-Arnett S, Antalis TM & Bugge TH. Type II transmembrane serine proteases. Thromb Haemost. 2003; 90(2):185-93.

Tassabehji M, Newton VE & Read AP. Waardenburg syndrome type 2 caused by mutations in the human microphthalmia (MITF) gene. Nat Genet. 1994;8(3):251-5.

Tekin M, Arnos KS & Pandya A. Advances in hereditary deafness. Lancet 2001;358(9287):1082-90.

Unal M, Tamer L, Doğruer ZN, Yildirim H, Vayisoğlu Y & Camdeviren H. N-acetyltransferase 2 gene polymorphism and presbycusis. Laryngoscope. 2005;115(12):2238-41.

Vahava O, Morell R, Lynch ED, Weiss S, Kagan ME, Ahituv N, Morrow JE, Lee MK, Skvorak AB, Morton CC, Blumenfeld A, Frydman M, Friedman TB, King MC & Avraham KB. Mutation in transcription factor *POU4F3* associated with inherited progressive hearing loss in humans. Science. 1998;279(5358):1950-4.

Van Camp G, Snoeckx RL, Hilgert N, van den Ende J, Fukuoka H, Wagatsuma M, Suzuki H, Smets RM, Vanhoenacker F, Declau F, Van de Heyning P & Usami S. A new autosomal recessive form of Stickler syndrome is caused by a mutation in the *COL9A1* gene. Am J Hum Genet. 2006;79(3):449-57.

van der Loop FT, Heidet L, Timmer ED, van den Bosch BJ, Leinonen A, Antignac C, Jefferson JA, Maxwell AP, Monnens LA, Schröder CH & Smeets HJ. Autosomal dominant Alport syndrome caused by a *COL4A3* splice site mutation. Kidney Int. 2000;58(5):1870-5.

Van Eyken E, Van Camp G & Van Laer L. The complexity of age-related hearing impairment: contributing environmental and genetic factors. Audiol Neurootol. 2007b;12(6):345-58.

Van Eyken E, Van Camp G, Fransen E, Topsakal V, Hendrickx JJ, Demeester K, Van de Heyning P, Mäki-Torkko E, Hannula S, Sorri M, Jensen M, Parving A, Bille M, Baur M, Pfister M, Bonaconsa A, Mazzoli M, Orzan E, Espeso A, Stephens D, Verbruggen K, Huyghe J, Dhooge I, Huygen P, Kremer H, Cremers CW, Kunst S, Manninen M, Pyykkö I, Lacava A, Steffens M, Wienker TF & Van Laer L. Contribution of the N-acetyltransferase 2 polymorphism NAT2*6A to age-related hearing impairment. J Med Genet. 2007a;44(9):570-8.

Van Eyken E, Van Laer L, Fransen E, Topsakal V, Lemkens N, Laureys W, Nelissen N, Vandevelde A, Wienker T, Van De Heyning P & Van Camp G. *KCNQ4*: a gene for age-related hearing impairment? Hum Mutat. 2006;27(10):1007-16

Van Laer L, Huizing EH, Verstreken M, van Zuijlen D, Wauters JG, Bossuyt PJ, Van de Heyning P, McGuirt WT, Smith RJ, Willems PJ, Legan PK, Richardson GP & Van Camp G. Nonsyndromic hearing impairment is associated with a mutation in DFNA5. Nat Genet. 1998;20(2):194-7.

Van Laer L, Huyghe JR, Hannula S, Van Eyken E, Stephan DA, Mäki-Torkko E, Aikio P, Fransen E, Lysholm-Bernacchi A, Sorri M, Huentelman MJ & Van Camp G. A genome-wide association study for age-related hearing impairment in the Saami. Eur J Hum Genet. 2010;18(6):685-93.

Van Laer L, Van Eyken E, Fransen E, Huyghe JR, Topsakal V, Hendrickx JJ, Hannula S, Mäki-Torkko E, Jensen M, Demeester K, Baur M, Bonaconsa A, Mazzoli M, Espeso A, Verbruggen K, Huyghe J, Huygen P, Kunst S, Manninen M, Konings A, Diaz-Lacava AN, Steffens M, Wienker TF, Pyykkö I, Cremers CW, Kremer H, Dhooge I, Stephens D, Orzan E, Pfister M, Bille M, Parving A, Sorri M, Van de Heyning PH & Van Camp G. The grainyhead like 2 gene (*GRHL2*), alias TFCP2L3, is associated with age-related hearing impairment. Hum Mol Genet. 2008;17(2):159-69.

Varga R, Avenarius MR, Kelley PM, Keats BJ, Berlin CI, Hood LJ, Morlet TG, et al. *OTOF* mutations revealed by genetic analysis of hearing loss families including a potential temperature sensitive auditory neuropathy allele. J Med Genet. 2006; 43(7):576-81.

Verhoeven K, Van Laer L, Kirschhofer K, Legan PK, Hughes DC, Schatteman I, Verstreken M, Van Hauwe P, Coucke P, Chen A, Smith RJ, Somers T, Offeciers FE, Van de Heyning P, Richardson GP, Wachtler F, Kimberling WJ, Willems PJ, Govaerts PJ & Van Camp G. Mutations in the human alpha-tectorin gene cause autosomal dominant non-syndromic hearing impairment. Nat Genet. 1998;19(1):60-2.

Verpy E, Masmoudi S, Zwaenepoel I, Leibovici M, Hutchin TP, Del Castillo I, Nouaille S, Blanchard S, Lainé S, Popot JL, Moreno F, Mueller RF & Petit C. Mutations in a new gene encoding a protein of the hair bundle cause non-syndromic deafness at the DFNB16 locus. Nat Genet. 2001;29(3):345-9.

Veske A, Oehlmann R, Younus F, Mohyuddin A, Müller-Myhsok B, Mehdi SQ & Gal A. Autosomal recessive non-syndromic deafness locus (DFNB8) maps on chromosome 21q22 in a large consanguineous kindred from Pakistan. Hum Mol Genet. 1996;5(1):165-8.

Vikkula M, Mariman EC, Lui VC, Zhidkova NI, Tiller GE, Goldring MB, van Beersum SE, de Waal Malefijt MC, van den Hoogen FH, Ropers HH, Mayne R, Cheah KE, Olsen BR, Warman ML & Brunner HG. Autosomal dominant and recessive osteochondrodysplasias associated with the *COL11A2* locus. Cell 1995;80(3):431-7.

Wagatsuma M, Kitoh R, Suzuki H, Fukuoka H, Takumi Y, Usami S. Distribution and frequencies of *CDH23* mutations in Japanese patients with non-syndromic hearing loss. Clin Genet. 2007;72(4):339-44.

Wallis C, Ballo R, Wallis G, Beighton P & Goldblatt J. X-linked mixed deafness with stapes fixation in a Mauritian kindred: linkage to Xq probe pDP34. Genomics. 1988;3(4):299-301.

Walsh T, Pierce SB, Lenz DR, Brownstein Z, Dagan-Rosenfeld O, Shahin H, Roeb W, McCarthy S, Nord AS, Gordon CR, Ben-Neriah Z, Sebat J, Kanaan M, Lee MK, Frydman M, King MC & Avraham KB. Genomic duplication and overexpression of *TJP2/ZO-2* leads to altered expression of apoptosis genes in progressive nonsyndromic hearing loss DFNA51. Am J Hum Genet. 2010;87(1):101-9.

Walsh T, Walsh V, Vreugde S, Hertzano R, Shahin H, Haika S, Lee MK, Kanaan M, King MC & Avraham KB. From flies' eyes to our ears: mutations in a human class III myosin cause progressive nonsyndromic hearing loss DFNB30. Proc Natl Acad Sci U S A. 2002;99(11):7518-23.

Wang A, Liang Y, Fridell RA, Probst FJ, Wilcox ER, Touchman JW, Morton CC, Morell RJ, Noben-Trauth K, Camper SA & Friedman TB. Association of unconventional myosin MYO15 mutations with human nonsyndromic deafness DFNB3. Science. 1998; 280 (5368):1447-51.

Wang QJ, Lu CY, Li N, Rao SQ, Shi YB, Han DY, Li X, Cao JY, Yu LM, Li QZ, Guan MX, Yang WY & Shen Y. Y-linked inheritance of non-syndromic hearing impairment in a large Chinese family. J Med Genet. 2004;41(6):e80.

Wattenhofer M, Sahin-Calapoglu N, Andreasen D, Kalay E, Caylan R, Braillard B, Fowler-Jaeger N, Reymond A, Rossier BC, Karaguzel A & Antonarakis SE. A novel *TMPRSS3* missense mutation in a DFNB8/10 family prevents proteolytic activation of the protein. Hum Genet. 2005;117(6):528-35.

Wayne S, Robertson NG, DeClau F, Chen N, Verhoeven K, Prasad S, Tranebjärg L, Morton CC, Ryan AF, Van Camp G & Smith RJ. Mutations in the transcriptional activator EYA4 cause late-onset deafness at the DFNA10 locus. Hum Mol Genet. 2001;10(3):195-200.

Weil D, Blanchard S, Kaplan J, Guilford P, Gibson F, Walsh J, Mburu P, Varela A, Levilliers J, Weston MD, Kelley PM, Kimberling WJ, Wagenaar M, Levi-Acobas F, Larget-Piet D, Munnich A, Steel KP, Brown SM & Petit C. Defective myosin VIIA gene responsible for Usher syndrome type 1B. Nature. 1995;374(6517):60-1.

Wester DC, Atkin CL, Gregory MC. Alport syndrome: clinical update. J Am Acad Audiol. 1995;6(1):73-9.

Weston MD, Luijendijk MW, Humphrey KD, Möller C, Kimberling WJ. Mutations in the *VLGR1* gene implicate G-protein signaling in the pathogenesis of Usher syndrome type II. Am J Hum Genet. 2004;74(2):357-66.

Wilch E, Azaiez H, Fisher RA, Elfenbein J, Murgia A, Birkenhäger R, Bolz H, Da Silva-Costa SM, Del Castillo I, Haaf T, Hoefsloot L, Kremer H, Kubisch C, Le Marechal C, Pandya A, Sartorato EL, Schneider E, Van Camp G, Wuyts W, Smith RJ, Friderici KH. A novel DFNB1 deletion allele supports the existence of a distant cis-regulatory region that controls *GJB2* and *GJB6* expression. Clin Genet. 2010;78(3):267-74.

Wilcox ER, Burton QL, Naz S, Riazuddin S, Smith TN, Ploplis B, Belyantseva I, Ben-Yosef T, Liburd NA, Morell RJ, Kachar B, Wu DK, Griffith AJ, Riazuddin S & Friedman TB. Mutations in the gene encoding tight junction claudin-14 cause autosomal recessive deafness DFNB29. Cell. 2001;104(1):165-72.

Willems PJ. Gene localization and isolation in nonsyndromic hearing loss. Willems PJ. In: Genetic Hearing Loss. Marcel Dekker Inc. New York, 2004;203.

Xia JH, Liu CY, Tang BS, Pan Q, Huang L, Dai HP, Zhang BR, Xie W, Hu DX, Zheng D, Shi XL, Wang DA, Xia K, Yu KP, Liao XD, Feng Y, Yang YF, Xiao JY, Xie DH & Huang JZ. Mutations in the gene encoding gap junction protein beta-3 associated with autosomal dominant hearing impairment. Nat Genet. 1998;20(4):370-3.

Xiao S, Yu C, Chou X, Yuan W, Wang Y, Bu L, Fu G, Qian M, Yang J, Shi Y, Hu L, Han B, Wang Z, Huang W, Liu J, Chen Z, Zhao G & Kong X. Dentinogenesis imperfecta 1 with or without progressive hearing loss is associated with distinct mutations in *DSPP*. Nat Genet. 2001;27(2):201-4.

Yan D & Liu XZ. Genetics and pathological mechanisms of Usher syndrome. J Hum Genet. 2010;55(6):327-35.

Yasunaga S, Grati M, Cohen-Salmon M, El-Amraoui A, Mustapha M, Salem N, El-Zir E, Loiselet J & Petit C. A mutation in *OTOF*, encoding *OTOF*erlin, a FER-1-like protein, causes DFNB9, a nonsyndromic form of deafness. Nat Genet. 1999;21(4):363-9.

Yoon JS, Park HJ, Yoo SY, Namkung W, Jo MJ, Koo SK, Park HY, Lee WS, Kim KH & Lee MG. Heterogeneity in the processing defect of *SLC26A4* mutants. J Med Genet. 2008;45(7):411-9.

Zelante L, Gasparini P, Estivill X, Melchionda S, D'Agruma L, Govea N, Milá M, Monica MD, Lutfi J, Shohat M, Mansfield E, Delgrosso K, Rappaport E, Surrey S & Fortina P. Connexin 26 mutations associated with the most common form of nonsyndromic neurosensory autosomal recessive deafness (DFNB1) in Mediterraneans. Hum Mol Genet 1997;6:1605–1609.

Zeviani M, Moraes CT, DiMauro S, Nakase H, Bonilla E, Schon EA, Rowland LP. Deletions of mitochondrial DNA in Kearns-Sayre syndrome. Neurology. 1998;51(6):1525-33.

Zhao L, Young WY, Li R, Wang Q, Qian Y, Guan MX. Clinical evaluation and sequence analysis of the complete mitochondrial genome of three Chinese patients with hearing impairment associated with the 12S rRNA T1095C mutation. Biochem Biophys Res Commun. 2004;325(4):1503-8.

Zhu M, Yang T, Wei S, DeWan AT, Morell RJ, Elfenbein JL, Fisher RA, Leal SM, Smith RJ & Friderici KH. Mutations in the gamma-actin gene (*ACTG1*) are associated with dominant progressive deafness (DFNA20/26). Am J Hum Genet. 2003;73(5):1082-91.

Zwaenepoel I, Mustapha M, Leibovici M, Verpy E, Goodyear R, Liu XZ, Nouaille S, Nance WE, Kanaan M, Avraham KB, Tekaia F, Loiselet J, Lathrop M, Richardson G & Petit C. *OTOA*ncorin, an inner ear protein restricted to the interface between the apical surface of sensory epithelia and their overlying acellular gels, is defective in autosomal recessive deafness DFNB22. Proc Natl Acad Sci U S A. 2002;99(9):6240-5.

12

Genetics of Nonsyndromic Recessively Inherited Moderate to Severe and Progressive Deafness in Humans

Sadaf Naz
*School of Biological Sciences,
University of the Punjab, Lahore
Pakistan*

1. Introduction

Nonsyndromic deafness in humans involves hearing loss as the only presenting feature in contrast to syndromes in which hearing loss is accompanied by other abnormalities. The majority of nonsyndromic deafness is recessively inherited which involves mutations of both alleles of a gene.

Deafness is a sensory impairment which results in a partial or total loss in reception of sound. The intensity of sound can be measured in decibels (dB). It is usual to assess hearing thresholds at frequencies of 0.25, 0.5, 1, 2, 4 and 8 KHz. Sounds of each frequency are presented at different intensities to a subject and the response is recorded graphically as an audiogram. A loss in hearing is indicated if the threshold for perception of sound for any frequency is elevated by 10 dB or greater as compared to the defined standard value for each frequency. Like visual foveae, organisms also have acoustic foveae, in which a certain frequency occupies greater space and is resolved more than other frequencies. In humans, the frequencies of 2 to 4 KHz are finely resolved. The frequencies of 0.5-2 KHz are the most important for hearing conversations. Therefore, individuals can have usable hearing if deafness does not impair these frequencies to a profound degree. A hearing loss of >91 dB constitutes profound deafness while those between 41 to 90 dB are defined as moderate (41-55 dB), moderate to severe (56-70 dB) or severe hearing loss (71-90 dB), respectively. Progressive deafness involves a gradual loss in the ability to hear over time.

The genetics and biology of moderate to severe and progressive hearing loss in humans has been understudied. More than 65 loci have been mapped for nonsyndromic recessively inherited deafness. Notably, mutations of only some of these genes are associated with stable moderate to severe hearing loss (Chishti et al., 2009; Naz et al., 2003; Villamar et al., 1999; Zwaenepoel et al., 2002). The past few years have revealed mutations in more than 10 genes and loci which can cause variable degrees of hearing loss or progressive deafness in humans. Additionally, the observation of intra- and inter- familial variability in the degree of deafness associated with identical mutations in a few genes has also implicated a role for specific additional epistatic interactions which can modify the hearing loss in some instances.

2. Molecular genetics

Most individuals with inherited hearing loss suffer from profound deafness. It is hypothesized that the degree of hearing loss is profound when mutations affect genes which cause hair cell loss while it may be less severe or progressive in nature when mutations disrupt genes which affect hair cell function or that of the tectorial membrane (Grillet et al., 2009). In other instances, presence of missense or nonsense mutations in the same gene have been associated with variability in degree of hearing loss (Pennings et al., 2004). Additionally, some mutations creating new cryptic splice sites within genes have also been associated with intra-familial variability of hearing loss (Lopez-Bigas et al., 1999). However, in some instances there are no genotype-phenotype correlations. For example individuals who are homozygous for the c.35delG mutation in *GJB2* have phenotypes ranging from congenital and profound to early onset and mild hearing loss (Denoyelle et al., 1997; Snoeckx et al., 2005). There are a few other reports of identical mutations in the same gene in different subjects causing a significantly dissimilar hearing loss. This is illustrated by individuals with mutations in *CDH23*, *CLDN14* or *TRIC*. Individuals who are homozygous for identical mutations in *CDH23*, *CLDN14* or *TRIC* exhibit different degrees of hearing loss (Bashir, Fatima & Naz, 2010b; Riazuddin et al., 2006; Schultz et al., 2005).

Less severe degree of hearing loss may also result when mutations create hypomorphic alleles or affect particular domains of proteins. For example, a hypomorphic allele is hypothesized to be responsible for the moderate to profound hearing loss in affected individuals at the *DFNB73* locus (Riazuddin et al., 2009). It has also been shown that mutations that specifically disrupt the long isofrom of MYO15A cause less severe hearing loss in contrast to mutations which disrupt function of both isoforms (Bashir et al., in press, Cengiz et al., 2010; Nal et al., 2010).

Intra- or inter- familal phenotypic variability is also observed due to progression of hearing loss (*DFNB7, DFNB8, DFNB25, DFNB30, DFNB59, DFNB72/95, DFNB77, DFNB79, DFNB84* and *DFNB91*) (Charizopoulou et al., 2011; de Heer et al., 2011; Ebermann et al., 2007b; Grillet et al., 2009; Li et al., 2010; Rehman et al., 2011; Schraders et al., 2010a; Schraders et al., 2010b; Sirmaci et al., 2010; Walsh et al., 2002; Weegerink et al., 2011). Younger individuals with mutations in *BSND* (*DFNB73*) also have a less severe degree of hearing loss which suggests a progressive nature of their hearing loss (Riazuddin et al., 2009). Other loci for which hearing loss is reported as less than profound are based on data from single families and the causative genes are unknown (*DFNB32, DFNB33, DFNB71, DFNB89, DFNB93*) (Basit et al., 2011; Belguith et al., 2009; Chishti et al., 2009; Masmoudi et al., 2003; Medlej-Hashim et al., 2002; Mustapha et al., 1998; Tabatabaiefar et al., 2011). For some deafness loci the degree of hearing loss was reported to be moderate to severe or severe in degree, but audiograms were not provided (*DFNB13, DFNB22, DFNB32, DFNB33* and *DFNB89*) (Basit et al., 2011; Belguith et al., 2009; Masmoudi et al., 2004; Masmoudi et al., 2003; Zwaenepoel et al., 2002). The known instances in which the degree of hearing loss is less than profound or can progress to different degrees are summarized in Table 1.

LOCUS	GENE	PHENOTYPE	REFERENCE
DFNB1	*GJB2*	Mild to profound HL, No genotype-phenotype correlation	(Snoeckx et al., 2005)
*DFNB2**	*MYO7A*	A missense mutations may cause a less severe degree of HL	(Hildebrand et al., 2010)
DFNB3	*MYO15A*	Mutations affecting N-terminal extension domain cause less severe degree of HL	(Cengiz et al., 2010; Nal et al., 2007)
DFNB4	*SLC26A4*	Splice site and some missesnse mutations cause less severe degree of HL which may be progressive	(Kitamura et al., 2000; Lopez-Bigas et al., 1999; Luxon et al., 2003)
DFNB7	*TMC1*	Progressive HL in one family	(de Heer et al., 2011)
DFNB8	*TMPRSS3*	Hypomorphic alleles cause progressive HL	(Hutchin et al., 2005; Scott et al., 2001; Veske et al., 1996; Weegerink et al., 2011)
DFNB12	*CDH23*	Compound heterozygous mutations may cause progressive HL	(Astuto et al., 2002)
DFNB13	Unknown	Progressive or Severe HL (No audiograms provided)	(Masmoudi et al., 2004; Mustapha et al., 1998)
DFNB16	*STRC*	Moderate to severe HL (One audiogram provided)	(Villamar et al., 1999)
DFNB20	Unknown	Moderate to profound HL, progressive inferred	(Moynihan et al., 1999)
DFNB21	*TECTA*	Moderate to severe HL (Flat or U-shaped audiograms)	(Meyer et al., 2007; Naz et al., 2003)
DFNB22	*OTOA*	Moderate to severe HL (No audiogram provided)	(Zwaenepoel et al., 2002)
DFNB25	*GRXCR1*	Progressive HL	(Schraders et al., 2010a)
DFNB29	*CLDN14*	Moderate to profound HL, No genotype-phenotype correlation	(Bashir et al., 2010b)
DFNB30	*MYO3A*	Progressive HL	(Walsh et al., 2002)
DFNB32	Unknown	Severe HL (No audiograms provided)	(Masmoudi et al., 2003)
DFNB33	Unknown	Severe HL (No audiograms provided)	(Belguith et al., 2009; Medlej-Hashim et al., 2002)
DFNB42	*ILDR1*	Moderate to profound HL	(Aslam et al., 2005; Borck et al., 2011b)
DFNB49	*TRIC*	Moderately severe to profound HL, No genotype-phenotype correlation	(Riazuddin et al., 2006)
DFNB59	*PJVK*	Progressive HL in two families	(Ebermann et al., 2007b)

LOCUS	GENE	PHENOTYPE	REFERENCE
DFNB71	Unknown	Severe HL (One audiogram provided)	(Chishti et al., 2009)
DFNB72/95	*GIPC3*	2 families with mild to severe HL, Individuals with a C terminal mutation have progressive HL	(Charizopoulou et al., 2011; Rehman et al., 2011)
DFNB73	*BSND*	Younger individuals have less severe degree of HL	(Riazuddin et al., 2009)
DFNB77	*LOXHD1*	Progressive HL in one family	(Grillet et al., 2009)
DFNB79	*TPRN*	Progressive HL in one family, Moderate to severe HL in another	(Li et al., 2010)
DFNB84	*PTPRQ*	Progressive HL or Moderate to severe HL	(Schraders et al., 2010a; Shahin et al., 2010a)
DFNB89	Unknown	Moderate to severe HL, no audiograms provided	(Basit et al., 2011)
DFNB91	*SERPINB6*	Progressive HL	(Sirmaci et al., 2010)
DFNB93	Unknown	Moderate to Severe HL	(Tabatabaiefar et al., 2011)

Table 1. List of nonsyndromic recessive deafness loci associated with less than profound deafness

The table lists autosomal nonsyndromic recessive deafness loci for which at least two individuals are reported to have a less severe hearing loss (<80 dB). HL, Hearing loss. * Only one patient has a dramatically less severe degree of hearing loss.

2.1a Genes involved in moderate to severe hearing loss

Three genes have been identified in which mutations exclusively cause recessively inherited moderate to severe hearing loss in humans. Interestingly, they are either part of the tectorial membrane, or are in direct contact with it. The tectorial membrane acts as the cochlear amplifier and results in gain in sound intensity by 30 dB. No progression has been documented for hearing loss due to mutations in the three genes, *STRC, TECTA* and *OTOA*, although some variability in degree of auditory thresholds is observed in affected individuals with identical mutations in these genes.

STRC (DFNB16)

Mutations in *STRC* encoding stereocilin are reported to cause mild to severe deafness in humans with an onset in childhood at 3-5years with increased involvement of high frequencies (Verpy et al., 2001; Villamar et al., 1999). Additionally, mice with a targeted deletion of *Strc* become progressively deaf by P60 (Verpy et al., 2008). The DPOAE cannot be recorded at P14 in *Strc*$^{-/-}$ mice though hearing thresholds are almost normal at that age. *Strc*$^{-/-}$ mice lack horizontal top connectors of outer hair cells' stereocilia. It is interesting to note that stereocilin may establish contact with tectorial membrane as inferred by lack of characteristic ring like staining of STRC from tallest row of outer hair cell stereocilia in *Tecta*$^{\Delta ENT/\Delta ENT}$ mice which have disrupted tectorial membranes due to loss of TECTA (Verpy et al., 2008).

TECTA (DFNB21)

Inactivating mutations of *TECTA* lead to moderate to severe recessively inherited hearing loss in humans which can be more severe in the mid frequencies leading to a flat or U shaped audiogram (Meyer et al., 2007; Naz et al., 2003). *TECTA* is the major protein of the tectorial membrane which lies over the organ of Corti within the cochlea. The tectorial membrane is in contact with the tallest stereocilia of the outer hair cells and acts as a cochlear amplifier which was elegantly shown in mice with a targeted mutation in *Tecta* (Legan et al., 2000). $Tecta^{\Delta ENT/\Delta ENT}$ mice have detached tectorial membranes and the noncollagenous matrix is missing. $Tecta^{\Delta ENT/\Delta ENT}$ mutants are 35 dB less sensitive to sound. However DPOAE can be elicited at high threshold sounds of 65 dB SPL in $Tecta^{\Delta ENT/\Delta ENT}$ mice (Lukashkin et al., 2004) though these are absent in humans with homozygous inactivating *TECTA* mutations (Naz et al. 2003, unpublished data).

OTOA (DFNB22)

Two Palestinian families have been reported in which the affected individuals had hearing loss due to deleterious mutations in the gene encoding otoancorin, *OTOA* (Shahin et al., 2010b; Zwaenepoel et al., 2002). The hearing loss was reported to be moderate to severe in one family while it was profound in the other. One of the families had a splice site mutation in *OTOA* (Zwaenepoel et al., 2002) while the second family with members affected with profound deafness had a complete deletion of the gene (Shahin et al., 2010b; Zwaenepoel et al., 2002). *OTOA* has sequence similarity to *STRC* (Jovine, Park & Wassarman, 2002) although its expression pattern is different. Both OTOA and STRC are predicted to be superhelical lectins which can bind the carbohydrate moieties of extracellular glycoproteins (Sathyanarayana et al., 2009). In mice, *Otoa* expression is restricted to specific regions between sites of attachment of tectorial membrane and underlying sensory epithelia.

2.1b Loci involved in moderate to severe or severe hearing loss

There are five chromosomal regions which have been implicated in genetics of moderate to severe hearing loss and the genes are currently unknown. Although *DFNB32* and *DFNB82* were mapped to overlapping regions on chromosome 1, the identification of *GPSM2* mutations for the latter (Walsh et al., 2010) excluded this as the causative gene for the former since it lies outside the linkage interval of *DFNB32* (Masmoudi et al., 2003).

DFNB32, DFNB33, DFNB71, DFNB89, DFNB93

Five loci for less severe hearing loss have been mapped to chromosomes 1p13.3-22.1, 10p11.23-q21.1, 8p22-21.3, 16q21-q23.2 and 11q12.3-13.3 respectively (Belguith et al., 2009; Chishti et al., 2009; Masmoudi et al., 2003; Tabatabaiefar et al., 2011). All loci have been described in single families except for *DFNB89* for which two families were reported. Deafness was described to be moderate to severe in degree in all affected individuals in these two families but no audiometric data was provided. Similarly, hearing loss is described as being severe in degree for families linked to both *DFNB32* and *DFNB33* without provision of audiometric data. Patients in families described for *DFNB71* and *DFNB93* have severe and moderate to severe hearing loss respectively as documented by 1 and 4 audiograms respectively. The identification of genes involved in pathogenesis due to mutations at these loci will shed light on their essential functions in the auditory pathways.

2.2 Genes involved in Intra- or inter- familial variability of hearing loss

GJB2 (DFNB1)

In the cochlea, gap junctions are proposed to maintain K^+ homeostasis by transporting K^+ away from the hair cells during auditory transduction (Kikuchi et al., 1995). *GJB2* encodes connexin 26 which oligomerizes to form a connexon (a hemichannel) which binds to a connexon from adjacent cell to form a functional gap junction in many tissues including the inner ear. *GJB2* is expressed in the supporting cells and the stria vascularis in the cochlea. The important function of *GJB2* in normal hearing is shown by the large number of mutations which have been reported in this gene from most diverse human populations which cause deafness. Although most individuals who are homozygous for c.35delG mutation in *GJB2* have severe to profound deafness, many individuals with the identical mutation have a mild or a less severe hearing loss (Murgia et al., 1999). Additionally, patients who are compound heterozygous for one truncating mutation together with a missense mutation in *GJB2* usually have a less severe hearing impairment (Liu et al., 2005; Snoeckx et al., 2005).

MYO7A (DFNB2)

MYO7A encodes a protein classified as an unconventional myosin which plays a role in intracellular trafficking. Unconventional myosins are actin-activated motor proteins with structurally conserved heads important for movement along actin filaments. The tails are highly divergent and are presumed to interact with different macromolecular components in the cell. All mutations in *MYO7A* except one cause severe to profound deafness. However, an individual with a missense mutation affecting the motor domain of MYO7A had a dramatically reduced hearing loss as compared to all other cases with *MYO7A* mutations, including those in his own family (Hildebrand et al., 2010). The onset of deafness was delayed to seven years of age and the degree of hearing loss was moderate to severe at the age of 31.

MYO7A is present in cytoplasm of hair cells and in the stereocilia including the upper tip-link density (Grati & Kachar, 2011). Different mutations of *Myo7a* result in profound deafness in mice (Gibson et al., 1995). However, one missense mutation affecting the kinesin and MyTH4 domains of myosin 7a leads to a severe deafness phenotype in contrast to other mice with mutations in *Myo7a* (Mburu et al., 1997).

MYO15A (DFNB3)

Mutations in *MYO15A* are a significant cause of deafness in many world populations. All pathogenic mutations in *MYO15A* except three which are located in exon 2 cause profound deafness. The four mutations were identified in three Pakistani and one Turkish families and are associated with hearing loss which can range from moderate to severe or moderate to profound in degree (Bashir et al., in press, Cengiz et al., 2010; Nal et al., 2010). The mutations in alternatively spliced exon 2 affect the class 1 isoform of MYO15A which has a long N-terminal extension. The presence of residual hearing in affected individuals who have mutations in exon 2 of *MYO15A* is probably due to the availability of normally functioning short isoform of MYO15A which remains unaffected by the mutations in exon 2 (Nal et al., 2007).

MYO15A is a motor protein present in hair cells in a cap like structure at top of the stereocilia where it is known to interact with WHRN (Belyantseva et al., 2005). It is interesting to note that mutations affecting the long isoform of WHRN (Ebermann et al., 2007a) also cause a less severe hearing loss in contrast to mutations which disrupt the short isoform (Mburu et al., 2003).

Currently, no corresponding mouse carrying a mutation affecting the long N terminal extension domain has been reported. However, in *shaker 2* mice, a missense mutation affects the motor domain of MYO15A and the mice are profoundly deaf (Probst et al., 1998) . The stereocilia are extremely short and this defect can be fully rescued by transfecting *shaker 2* hair cells with MYO15A isoform 2 (Belyantseva et al., 2005). No specific role is known for MYO15A isoform 1 and its function remains to be elucidated.

SLC26A4 (DFNB4/PDS)

SLC26A4 mutations may cause Pendred syndrome or non-syndromic deafness with enlarged vestibular aqueducts. Considerable residual hearing is present in some affected individuals who are homozygous for mutations creating new splice sites in *SLC26A4* (Lopez-Bigas et al., 1999; Naz, 2001). These two described mutations create splice sites a few nucleotides away from the canonical donor sites, and support the hypothesis that variable degree of hearing loss in *SLC26A4* linked families may indicate splice site mutations. Additionally, a few missense mutations of *SLC26A4* also cause a significantly less severe hearing loss (Kitamura et al., 2000). Some mutations of *SLC26A4* result in development of a progressive hearing loss (Luxon et al., 2003).

SlC26A4 or pendrin is expressed in endolymphatic duct and sac as well as in the external sulcus in the cochlea (Everett et al., 1999). SLC26A4 plays a significant role in the maintenance of the ionic balance within the inner ear and is involved in bicarbonate secretion (Wangemann et al., 2007). There are three different mouse mutants of *Slc26a4* which lack pendrin but none of them model the less severe hearing loss observed in humans (Dror et al., 2010; Everett et al., 2001; Lu et al., 2011). However, recently, transgenic mice with *Slc26a4* expression inducible by doxycycline on a background of mice lacking endogenous pendrin expression were generated. It was demonstrated that expression of pendrin at early embryonic stages of E0-E17.5 was necessary and sufficient to restore normal hearing in Tg[E];Tg[R];$Slc26a4^{\Delta/\Delta}$ mice (Choi et al., 2011). Ablating expression of *Slc26A4* at this critical time results in complete or partial hearing loss in these mice, recapitulating the phenotypes documented for many patients with mutations in *SLC26A4* (Choi et al., 2011).

CLDN14 (DFNB29)

CLDN14 is an integral part of the tight junctions in the sensory epithelium within the inner ear. Only two mutations have been reported in this gene in four Pakistani families which cause hearing loss. The usual phenotype associated with the two mutations is severe to profound deafness (Wilcox et al., 2001). However members of one family with p.V85D mutation in *CLDN14* have hearing loss which varies from moderately severe to severe in degree (Bashir et al., 2010b). It is interesting to note that mice with a targeted deletion of *Cldn14* are profoundly deaf and no variability of hearing loss was observed in these mice (Ben-Yosef et al., 2003).

ILDR1 (DFNB42)

ILDR1 is a membrane protein with an Immunoglobulin-like extracellular domain, and has different motifs for interaction with other proteins. Additionally, soluble isoforms of ILDR1 also exist which may be involved in lipoprotein transport (Borck et al., 2011b). Hearing loss due to mutations of this gene varies from moderate to profound in different individuals while it is severe in degree for one family with a mutation affecting the start codon of *ILDR1* (Borck et al., 2011b). *Ildr1* is expressed in the developing mouse cochlea but the expression is low at birth. It increases gradually by P4 and P10. The pillar and Hensen cells have the highest expression of *Ildr1* while it can also be detected in other cells in organ of Corti including the hair cells (Borck et al., 2011b).

TRIC (DFNB49)

TRIC or *MARVELD2* encodes a tight junction protein with a ubiquitous expression in the epithelial junctions throughout the body tissues. In the inner ear, TRIC is specifically expressed in the tricellular junctions of sensory epithelia as well as those between supporting cells and the hair cells (Riazuddin et al., 2006). Affected individuals with identical mutations in *TRIC* show a wide range of variability in severity of deafness ranging from moderate to severe hearing loss to profound deafness (Chishti et al., 2008; Riazuddin et al., 2006). All mutations described in *TRIC* are predicted to produce truncated proteins and consequent inability to bind several scaffolding proteins.

2.3 Genes involved in Progressive Hearing Loss

There are a few genes mutations in which have been described to cause progressive loss in hearing (*MYO3A, LOXHD1, PTPRQ* and *SERPINB6*). Additionally, some mutations in genes which cause stable and profound deafness, for example *TMC1* and *TMPRSS3* also cause progressive hearing loss. Many different mutations have been described in *TMC1, TMPRSS3, GRXRC1, PJVK, GIPC3, TPRN* and *PTPRQ* in affected individuals from different countries. However, it is noteworthy that apart from *DFNB8* (*TMPRSS3*), *DFNB59* (*PJVK*)) and *DFNB84* (*PTPRQ*) only one family is reported to have progression of deafness for each locus. All other mutations in these genes have been described to cause stable, moderate to profound deafness. This could be due to either of two reasons; the hearing loss associated with other mutations in these genes may also be progressive (slow or rapid progression) and has not been documented since many patients undergo audiometry at the time of enrollment in a genetic study. Alternatively, some mutations affecting a gene may cause a progressive hearing loss due to the type of mutation as for example those in *TMPRSS3*. Identical mutations may also cause stable or progressive hearing loss depending on the genetic background of the individuals.

TMC1 (DFNB7)

Homozygous inactivating mutations in *TMC1* cause severe to profound prelingual hearing impairment at the *DFNB7* locus. However, a Dutch family with autosomal recessive hearing loss was reported in which affected individuals had a postlingual onset, progressive hearing loss due to a mutation near the donor splice site of intron 19 (c.1763+3A→G) in *TMC1* (de Heer et al., 2011). The hearing loss initially affected the high frequencies and by second decade of life the hearing loss progressed to profound degree. This was documented as a "corner audiogram". Both normally spliced and aberrantly spliced *TMC1* transcripts were detected in blood of the patients. The presence of some wild type protein may account for the late onset of deafness and residual hearing in the patients, or alternately, the truncated mutant protein may have residual function (de Heer et al., 2011).

TMC1 is a transmembrane protein present in hair cells and may be involved in intracellular protein trafficking. Additionally it is also proposed to play a role in differentiation of hair cells into functional auditory receptors. The *deafness* mice mutants carry a homozygous genomic deletion in *Tmc1* and are profoundly deaf (Kurima et al., 2002). Currently there is no mouse model which mimics the recessively inherited progressive hearing loss due to mutations in *Tmc1* though a model, *Beethoven* exists for dominant deafness *DFNA36* and the mice have a missense mutation in *Tmc1* (Vreugde et al., 2002).

TMPRSS3 (DFNB8)

The gene encoding serine protease, TMRSS3 is expressed in supporting cells, stria vasularis as well as in the spiral ganglion in the inner ear. Mutations in *TMPRSS3* are responsible for deafness at the *DFNB8* locus. Most mutations in *TMPRSS3* result in severe to profound deafness in many world populations. However there are many mutations in *TMPRSS3* causing less severe hearing loss which is progressive in nature. The first family with progression in hearing loss due to a *TMPRSS3* mutation was reported from Pakistan. Affected members in this family suffered from progressive deafness with onset of hearing loss in childhood and had a mutation at a splice acceptor site in intron 4 (Scott et al., 2001; Veske et al., 1996). This is predicted to create an alternative splice acceptor site which on use introduces a frameshift in the open reading frame of *TMPRSS3*. It is hypothesized that this mutation may allow limited normal splicing since the actual splice site remains unchanged. Thus some normal TMPRSS3 could be produced accounting for progressive hearing loss observed in the affected individuals.

There are other reports of mutations in *TMPRSS3* causing post-lingual progressive deafness in British, Turkish, German and Dutch families (Elbracht et al., 2007; Hutchin et al., 2005; Wattenhofer et al., 2005; Weegerink et al., 2011). One of the first studies reported a British family with two affected individuals who were homozygous for a missense mutation in *TMPRSS3* and suffered from moderate to severe hearing loss (Hutchin et al., 2005). A recent study involved 8 small nuclear families from Holland and affected individuals were compound heterozygous for different mutations of *TMPRSS3* including missense and frameshift mutations (Weegerink et al., 2011). The higher frequencies were affected first resulting in a distinctive "ski-slope" audiometric configuration followed by low frequency hearing loss resulting in a flat audiogram (Weegerink et al., 2011). It was hypothesized that some mutations in *TMPRSS3* result in creation of hypomorphic alleles accounting for the less severe loss in hearing and progression of deafness observed in affected individuals (Weegerink et al., 2011).

Tmprss3 was shown to be important for hearing in mice as well since mutants homozygous for a nonsense mutation in the gene suffer from deafness. The hair cells start to degenerate at P12 from basal to apical turn of the cochlea and the degeneration is complete by P14 (Fasquelle et al., 2011). However, no mouse model has been reported which mimics the progressive hearing loss as observed in humans.

CDH23 (DFNB12)

Most mutations of *CDH23* cause severe phenotypes of deafness or *USH1D*. However, a few missense mutations in *CDH23* when present together in compound heterozygosity are reported to cause moderate to severe hearing loss or severe to profound deafness which is progressive in nature (Astuto et al., 2002). In two German siblings with deafness, the age of onset was also different, with onset of hearing loss at 4 and 6 years respectively. The degree of hearing loss was variable and there was asymmetric hearing loss in the older sibling.

In the inner ear, *CDH23* is expressed in the hair cells and Reissner's membrane. Mice lacking CDH23 are profoundly deaf and suffer from developmental defects of the stereocilia (Di Palma et al., 2001). In contrast, ENU induced *salsa* mutants have a recessively inherited missense mutation in *Cdh23* which affects the tip links of the stereocilia (Schwander et al., 2009). These mice have a progressive hearing loss which increases from severe in degree to profound deafness by three months of age as a consequence of gradual loss of tip links and eventual hair cell death (Schwander et al., 2009).

GRXCR1 (DFNB25)

Splice site mutations were identified in *GRXCR1* in two Dutch families while three missense and a nonsense mutation were identified in *GRXRC1* in families from Pakistan and Iran which segregated with hearing loss (Odeh et al., 2010; Schraders et al., 2010a). Two mutations create alternative splice sites within *GRXCR1* which on usage are predicted to create frameshifts in the open reading frame of the gene. The presence of alternatively spliced transcripts was demonstrated for one of the splice site mutations by an *in vivo* assay on lymphoblastoid cell lines derived from patients' blood.

The single affected individual in one of the Dutch families with a splice site mutation had a significantly milder phenotype of moderate to severe hearing loss which was not progressive in nature. Additionally, the hearing loss in affected members of another Dutch family and Pakistani families varied from moderate to profound in degree. The loss in hearing was progressive from moderate to profound in the Dutch family, while it was severe in the two families from Pakistan (Schraders et al., 2010a). The audiometric profile varied from flat to a slight U-shape and was down-sloping (Schraders et al., 2010a). Data was not provided about the audiometric profile of affected individuals in families from Iran, although hearing loss was reported to be severe to profound in degree (Odeh et al., 2010).

GRXCR1 is predicted to contain a GRX-like domain. These domains take part in reversible S-glutathionylation of proteins by which they are predicted to control activity or localization of the proteins. In the inner ear, *Grxcr1* is expressed in the hair cells and is localized along the lengths of stereocilia exhibiting a differential pattern in levels of expression in young and adult mice (Odeh et al., 2010). There are five mutant alleles of *Grxcr1* which cause profound deafness in the *pirouette* mice (Odeh et al., 2010). The absence of GRXCR1 results in formation of relatively short and thin stereocilia and cytocauds indicating actin abnormalities. This suggests that GRXCR1 plays an active role in development of actin architecture in the stereocilia (Beyer et al., 2000; Odeh et al., 2010).

MYO3A (DFNB30)

A class III myosin, *MYO3A* is required for normal hearing as shown by a single family originating from Iraq in which affected individuals had a progressive hearing loss with onset in second decade of life (Walsh et al., 2002). Interestingly, three different mutations were identified in this family which were either present in homozygosity or individuals were compound heterozygous for any of the mutations. The hearing loss first affected high frequencies. By the age of 50 there was moderate hearing loss at low frequencies while the high and middle frequencies were severely affected. All individuals were equally affected by the sixth decade of life. The three mutations identified in *MYO3A* included a nonsense and two splice site mutations. Hearing loss was significantly worse in affected individuals homozygous for the nonsense mutation than those who were compound heterozygous for a nonsense and a splice site mutation.

MYO3A is present in the hair cells stereocilia at the tips in a characteristic pattern described as "thimble-like" (Schneider et al., 2006) with presence at the stereocilia tip and also extending further down into the shaft of the stereocilia. Mice created as models for *DFNB30* mimic the hearing loss phenotype observed in humans. *Myo3a*$^{KI/KI}$ mice have an engineered nonsense mutation in the gene and they exhibit a hearing loss which progresses from mild to moderate, and to moderate to severe between ages of 2.5 months to 13 months. More severe loss in hearing is observed for sounds of high frequencies. In *Myo3a*$^{KI/KI}$ mice, development of hair cells stereocilia is normal which is followed by a gradual loss of hair cells from basal to apical turn of the cochlea (Walsh et al., 2011). It is hypothesized that loss of MYO3A may result in failure of transport of essential components within stereocilia (Walsh et al., 2011). This affects signal transduction in the inner ear, leading to loss of function and ultimate degeneration of hair cells.

PJVK (DFNB59)

Mutations in *PJVK* cause hearing loss with or without auditory neuropathy. The hearing loss is severe to profound and stable in all individuals reported so far except in members of one Moroccan, one Iranian and three Arab families (Borck et al., 2011a; Ebermann et al., 2007b; Schwander et al., 2007). Three affected individuals in the Moroccan family had deafness with onset by age of 4 in one individual and congenital hearing loss was observed in the other two individuals. The loss in hearing is severe in degree in the former and profound in the latter two individuals. Audiometry performed over a period of three years revealed a progressive nature of hearing loss for all three affected individuals. Unlike other families with *PJVK* mutations which have missense mutations in the gene, this family had a frameshift mutation in exon 2 of the 7 exon gene and the mutation is predicted to severely truncate the protein. Hearing loss is also reported to be progressive in nature and moderate to profound in degree in a family from Iran with a frameshift mutation of *PJVK* but audiometric profiles were not provided (Schwander et al., 2007). Additionally, deafness due to a nonsense mutation in three Arab families is reported to cause stable moderate to severe hearing loss but no audiograms were provided (Borck et al., 2011a).

PJVK exhibits 32% identity and 54% similarity over a stretch of 250 amino acids to DFNA5 protein. It is expressed in the hair cells and spiral ganglion. Mice with a targeted knock-in missense mutation in *Pjvk*, *Dfnb59*$^{tm1Ugds/tm1Ugd}$ have a moderate to severe non-progressive hearing loss which is elevated at high frequencies (Delmaghani et al., 2006) unlike *sirtaki* mice which have a nonsense mutation in *Pjvk* (Schwander et al., 2007). The *sirtaki* mice have outer hair cell functional defects as apparent by absent DPOAE and also suffer from progressive deafness. No morphological defects are apparent in the ears of the *sirtaki* or knock-in mutant mice. It is hypothesized that that functional null allele of *Pjvk* inactivates protein function in both hair cells and neurons, while the missense mutation affect its function only in the neurons.

GIPC3 (DFNB72/15/95)

GIPC3 encodes a PDZ domain containing protein which is important in peripheral auditory signal transmission. Mutations in this gene cause both profound deafness and progressive hearing loss. In a small Dutch hearing loss followed a different course in the two affected siblings. In the oldest affected individual, the loss in hearing was 70 dB HL at 11 months which progressed to 110 dB HL by 12 years of age. The hearing loss in second individual was 80 dB HL at 3 months which seemed to be stable as it only progressed to 90 dB HL by age of 14 years. (Charizopoulou et al., 2011). The mutation in *GIPC3* identified in the Dutch family introduces a stop codon in exon 6 (p.W301X) truncating the C-terminal. It is hypothesized that since this mutation is in the last exon it will not cause nonsense mediated decay and will allow production of a mutant protein retaining some function.

GIPC3 mutations have also been reported in seven other large families from Pakistan which include one framsehift and and six missense mutations (Rehman et al., 2011). The younger affected individuals in these families (7 and 9 years old) had better hearing as compared to the older affected individuals (20 and 25 years old). However, information is not available as yet whether hearing loss in any of the affected individuals is stable or progressive.

A mutation affecting PDZ domain of GIPC3 has also been reported in mice which causes progressive hearing loss, *ahl5* (Charizopoulou et al., 2011). The mice have a moderate hearing loss at one month of age which progresses to profound in degree by 1 year of age. The higher frequencies are affected first with eventual involvement of all frequencies. DPOAE and the endocochlear potential are gradually affected as well. The stereocilia are defective and degenerate together with the spiral ganglion cells.

BSND (DFNB73)

BSND encodes barttin which is an essential subunit for two chloride channels. Heteromeric channels formed by barttin and the chloride channels play an important role in potassium recycling in the inner ear (Estevez et al., 2001). A missense mutation, p.I12Tof BSND segregates with hearing loss in three families from Pakistan while in a fourth family it is present with a nonsense mutation in compound heterozygosity (Riazuddin et al., 2009). The younger individuals have a less severe hearing loss as compared to the older affected individuals suggesting that *BSND* may be involved in aetiology of progressive deafness. Functional analysis of the p.I12T mutation of *BSND* in HEK293T cells have demonstrated that function of the channels is unaffected. However, the number of channels on the surface membrane is reduced which results in a decreased current amplitude (Riazuddin et al., 2009).

LOXHD1 (DFNB77)

The 15 PLAT (polycystin/lipoxygenase/a-toxin) domains encoding gene *LOXHD1* was found to be mutated in an Iranian family with postlingual onset of hearing loss at ages ranging from 7 to 8 years. Affected individuals in the family had preserved hearing at low frequencies in the beginning. The loss was mild to moderate at frequencies of 0.5 to 2 KHz. Hearing loss worsened during childhood and adolescence to moderate to severe at mid and high frequencies. All frequencies were affected eventually (Grillet et al., 2009). A nonsense mutation, p.R670X was identified which introduces a premature stop codon at the C-terminal end of f the fifth PLAT domain. This could either lead to a protein lacking 10 PLAT domains or nonsense mediated decay of the transcript could lead to absence of LOXHD1. In contrast, the only other mutation reported in *LOXHD1* is a founder mutation, p.R1572X, in the Ashkenazi Jews and causes prelingual profound degree of deafness (Edvardson et al., 2011).

Normally LOXHD1 is present along the lengths of hair cell stereocilia plasma membrane while it cannot be detected at the tips of the stereocilia (Grillet et al., 2009). Interestingly, the hair cells bodies have no expression of *LOXHD1*. ENU induced *samba* mutants homozygous for a missense mutation in *Loxhd1* acquire hearing loss by 3 weeks of age and are completely deaf by eight weeks. The stereocilia develop normally. However, the hair cells have functional defects and DPOAE cannot be elicited from ears of *samba* mutants. Morphological defects are also observed in the inner ears of *samba* mutants with fused stereocilia and ruffled membranes at the apical cell surfaces. Additional degenerative changes are visible by post natal day 90 which include hair cell loss (Grillet et al., 2009).

TPRN (DFNB79)

Mutations of *TPRN* cause different degrees of hearing loss in humans. In a Dutch family, hearing loss is documented as moderate to severe in degree till 11 years of age and by 15 years it progresses to profound deafness (Li et al., 2010). In contrast, hearing loss in a Moroccan family is severe in degree even in the third decade of life (Li et al., 2010). Affected members of the Dutch family had a nonsense mutation in exon 1 of *TPRN* while the affected individuals in the Moroccan family were homozygous for a frameshift mutation in exon 1. It is interesting to note that the same frameshift mutation as observed in the Moroccan family was also identified in a Pakistani family. However, individuals in this family had profound degree of deafness (Khan et al., 2009; Rehman et al., 2010).

TPRN is present in the supporting cells as well as at the base of hair cells' stereocilia in the organ of Corti at the taper region of each stereocilium just above the cuticular plate (Rehman et al., 2010).

PTPRQ (DFNB84)

Congenital hearing loss which has been shown to be progressive in nature is associated with mutations in *PTPRQ*, a gene which encodes a phosphatase specific for phoshatidyl inositol, $PI(4,5)_{P2}$ (Schraders et al., 2010b; Seifert et al., 2003). $PI(4,5)_{P2}$ plays an important part in actin remodeling. Hearing loss due to mutations *PTPRQ* is severest in a Dutch family with a p.Y497X mutation and hearing loss was self reported to have progressed to profound by the third to fourth decade of life. However in affected individuals of a Moroccan family, a p.R457G mutation in PTPRQ caused a less severe loss in hearing. The loss in hearing was moderate which had deteriorated with age (Schraders et al., 2010b). Otoacoustic emissions were normal at the age of 13 months. The 1 to 2 KHz frequencies seemed to be more affected comparable to that observed in members of a Palestinian family with moderate to severe hearing loss also with a mutation of *PTPRQ* (Shahin et al., 2010a). In the Palestinian family, there were four affected individuals with considerable variation of hearing loss. A nonsense mutation, p.Q429X, was observed in *PTPRQ* for this family (Shahin et al., 2010a). Data is not available about progression of deafness in the Palestinian family.

Ptprq is transiently expressed over a period of first three weeks in mouse hair cells at the basal turn of the cochlea (Goodyear et al., 2003). MYO6 plays a role in localization of PTPRQ in plasma membranes (Sakaguchi et al., 2008). PTPRQ has been shown to be required for formation of shaft connectors and the taper of the stereocilia (Goodyear et al., 2003; Sakaguchi et al., 2008). Two transgenic mouse mutants, *Ptprq-TM-KO* and *Ptprq-CAT-KO* were generated in which the alleles encode proteins lacking transmembrane and catalytic domains of PTPRQ respectively (Goodyear et al., 2003). Cochlear development was normal in both mice and there was progressive deterioration of the sensory epithelium. Inner hair cells abnormalities were apparent by P1. Some stereocilia were misaligned or missing in the basal turn of cochlea. Stereocilia eventually fused and ultimately the organ of Corti disappeared in some mice by the age of three months (Goodyear et al., 2003).

SERPINB6 (DFNB91)

A single Turkish family has been described in which affected individuals have a mutation in *SERPINB6* segregating with hearing loss. The nonsense mutation, p.E245X was shown to substantially decrease the amount of the mutant transcript in blood of affected individuals (Sirmaci et al., 2010). The degree of hearing loss is moderate to severe with some residual hearing in all affected individuals. The 54 year old individual was the oldest and had the severest degree of hearing loss with greater degree of loss at high frequencies. The two younger individuals 24 and 23 years respectively, presented with moderate to severe hearing loss which was more severe in the 23 year old patient. Progressive nature of hearing loss was self reported by affected individuals but had not been documented by audiometry.

SERPINB6 is present in the hair cells in the organ of Corti as well as the greater epithelial ridge and may function as an inhibitor of proteases. It is hypothesized that SERPINB6 prevents non-specific tissue damage to inner ear tissue by inhibiting proteases. A transgenic mouse line lacking *Serpinb6* was created (Scarff et al., 2004) but the hearing status of the mice and inner ear structure was not evaluated. It will be interesting to identify if *Serpinb6*$^{-/-}$ mice have deafness at onset of hearing or whether they exhibit progressive deafness.

So far the results of genetic studies have revealed that although moderate to severe hearing loss is the usual finding for individuals with mutations in *STRC, TECTA* and *OTO* and in some individuals with mutations which cause progressive deafness, some individuals with mutations in other genes, for example *GJB2, CLDN14* or *TRIC* also have similarly milder phenotypes. Additionally, identical mutations in a gene may cause either progressive or stable hearing loss (Bashir et al. manuscript in preparation). Research has also shown that genes involved in progressive hearing loss may also have implications for age related hearing loss. For example, a polymorphism in *Cdh23* has been associated with age related hearing loss in different mice strains (Noben-Trauth, Zheng & Johnson, 2003).

2.4a Moderate to severe or progressive deafness in Usher Syndrome

Usher syndrome (USH) is a common syndrome of deafness-blindness and can be easily misdiagnosed as nonsyndromic hearing loss since onset of retinitis pigmentosa is gradual and the early manifestation can be very mild in some cases. So far mutations in 4 genes have been identified which cause the less severe phenotypes of hearing loss in Usher syndrome (*USH2A, GPR98, WHRN* and *CLRN1*). Additionally, some mutations of genes which cause Usher type 1 can also cause phenotypes termed as atypical usher syndromes.

Hearing loss for USH2 can vary from mild to severe in degree and may also show interfamilial variation (Abadie et al., 2011). The four Usher genes are expressed in hair cells where except for CLRN1, all proteins interact at the ankle link in the stereocilia and form a complex.

USH2A (USH2A)

Usher type 2A is the most frequent cause of Usher syndrome. A large number of missense, nonsense, insertion and deletion mutations have been identified in *USH2A*. The mutations were first described in North European, Spanish and African American patients (Eudy et al., 1998). *USH2A* encodes a large transmembrane protein, usherin, with an intracellular PDZ binding domain. Usherin is present in both outer and inner hair cells stereocilia and cannot be detected by 2 months of age in mice (Liu et al., 2007). *Ush2a*$^{-/-}$ transgenic mice have a moderate, non-progressive hearing loss which is more noticeable at high frequencies, mimicking the phenotype observed in humans (Liu et al., 2007). In the ears of the *Ush2a*$^{-/-}$ mice the inner hair cells and stereocilia are intact in all but at the basal turn of the cochlea where widespread loss of outer hair cells is observed.

GPR98 (USH2C)

Mutations of *GPR98* or *VLGR1* were first described in USH2 patients from United States and Sweden (Weston et al., 2004). *Gpr98* is expressed transiently during the first week in mice and is no longer detectable by P11. GPR98 forms the ankle links that connect the stereocilia of hair cells at their base in the developing hair cell bundles. Transgenic *Vlgr1/del7TM* mice which lack transmembrane and cytoplasmic domains of the protein are severely deaf by third week of life and lack ankle links (McGee et al., 2006). The stereocilia are arranged in a more rounded shape as compared to the "V" like pattern present in the wild type mice. A gradual loss of both type of hair cells and pillar cells is observed at the base of the cochlea (McGee et al., 2006).

WHRN (USH2D)

The description of *USH2D (WHRN)* is based on only two families from Germany and Portugal. The patients in the German family had mild to moderate hearing loss (Ebermann et al., 2007a) while the Portuguese family had variable degree of hearing loss with post lingual onset which was progressive in nature (Audo et al., 2011). In the German family two mutations in *WHRN* were detected in compound heterozygosity, involving a nonsense mutation in exon 1 and a splice site mutation in intron 2. The splice site mutation causes an in-frame skipping of the second exon and is predicted to result in production of an aberrant protein (Ebermann et al., 2007a). In the Portuguese family a deletion mutation was detected in exon 2 which is predicted to truncate the protein or mark the message for nonsense mediated decay (Audo et al., 2011). These mutations disrupt only the long isoform of WHRN.

Mice with a targeted deletion of the long isoform of whirlin have some partial hearing (75 dB SPL) which is non-progressive in nature (Yang et al., 2010) . The inner hair cells stereocilia are unaffected while the outer hair cells stereocilia loose their characteristic "V" shaped formation and assume a "U" shape. Some of the stereocilia are missing from the innermost row in outer hair cells. However, unlike *whirler* mutant mice who are deaf due to a deletion in *Whrn* disrupting both isoforms of the protein, mice with targeted ablation of the long isoform of whirlin do not have abnormally short stereocilia.

CLRN1 (USH3A)

The deafness phenotype associated with USH3 involves postlingual, progressive hearing loss. The time of onset and severity of hearing loss can be highly variable (Ness et al., 2003). So far only one gene, *CLRN1* has been identified which causes an USH3 phenotype (Joensuu et al., 2001). In contrast to other world populations, mutations in *CLRN1* are a frequent cause of Usher syndrome in the Finnish population. *Clrn1*$^{-/-}$ mice have early onset hearing loss and are profoundly deaf by P30 (Geng et al., 2009). *Clrn1*$^{-/-}$ mice have demonstrated that CLRN1 is important for normal maturation of hair cells as well as the afferent nerve synapses. Absence of CLRN1 in mice leads to gradual loss of outer hair cells and supporting cells which is most severe at the basal turn of the cochlea (Geng et al., 2009).

CLRN1 is a small 232 amino acid transmembrane protein which is present at both the basal and apical poles of the hair cells with expression being higher in outer hair cells as compared to the inner hair cells (Geng et al., 2009; Zallocchi et al., 2009). *Clrn1* is also expressed in the spiral ganglion (Geng et al., 2009; Zallocchi et al., 2009). In mice, CLRN1 cannot be detected at the apex of hair cells at P1 and continues to be expressed in both the pre- and post-synaptic regions of outer hair cell type I afferent ribbon synapses (Zallocchi et al., 2009). Additionally, CLRN1 may also have a role in actin assembly (Tian et al., 2009) and intracellular vesicle transport (Zallocchi et al., 2009).

2.4b Atypical manifestations of hearing loss in Usher syndrome

Atypical USH is genetically heterogeneous. Two different mutations of *SANS* (*USH1G*) have been reported to cause a USH2 like phenotype in two consanguineous families from Turkey and Pakistan (Bashir, Fatima & Naz, 2010a; Kalay et al., 2005). Similarly, some mutations in *MYO7A* (*USH1B*) cause an USH3 phenotype (Liu et al., 1998). Additionally, two mutations in *CDH23* (*USH1D*), result in an atypical phenotype of milder USH3. These involve a missense and an intronic mutation which are compound heterozygous in a German family with two affected siblings (Astuto et al., 2002). Some USH2A mutations also cause atypical manifestations and the phenotype resembles that of USH3 (Liu et al., 1999). On the converse, it is interesting to note that though majority of the mutations in CLRN1 cause a USH3 phenotype, some mutations in the same gene cause a more severe USH1 phenotype (Aller et al., 2004; Pennings et al., 2003) or in some cases an USH2 phenotype (Sadeghi et al., 2005). The finding of identical mutations in some cases which cause both the less severe or the more profound USH phenotype suggest the importance of genetic background in manifestation of the disorder and a role of modifiers in its aetiology.

2.5 Modifiers in less severe hearing loss

To date a single modifier, *DFNM1*, has been mapped to chromosome 1 which completely ameliorates hearing loss (Riazuddin et al., 2000) but the gene is currently unknown. Targeted sequencing of the linked region from DNA of both affected and unaffected individuals using massively parallel sequencing technology may identify the causative change in future.

A role of modifier genes in reducing severity of hearing loss is suspected for many other deafness loci as well, especially those showing a wide phenotypic variation in presence of identical genetic mutations. However, currently no locus has been mapped or any gene identified as a potential modifier. Usually each family has few individuals with sufficiently different phenotypes to make gene mapping studies feasible. Using whole genome sequencing approaches in either a small subset of such individuals or in larger families may identify genetic modifiers in future.

GJB2 is the most widely sequenced deafness genes and mutations in this gene are associated with deafness which is mild in degree to more profound losses. However, it has not been possible to map a genetic modifier which reduces severity of hearing loss using either traditional linkage analysis or association studies. A whole genome association study on DNA of more than a thousand *GJB2* c.35delG homozygous individuals living across Europe and North America regions failed to identify a single locus as a modifier in individuals with mild phenotypes of hearing loss. However, some SNPs with smaller modifying effects on the phenotype were identified (Hilgert et al., 2009). It is possible that a more stringent ethnic definition and data re-analysis in a smaller group may succeed in mapping a single locus for at least a subset of the participants.

The unavailability of different cell types derived from inner ear tissues in humans have inhibited direct evaluation of modifier genes in hearing loss by transcriptional analysis as for other disorders such as spinal muscular atrophy (Oprea et al., 2008). However, induced pluripotent stem cell lines can be derived from more and less severely affected deaf individuals respectively. These could be then differentiated *in vitro* into the relevant cochlear cell types followed by comparison of their mRNA expression profiles. This may help in identification of genetic modifiers in future.

Modifiers of hearing loss identified in mice may also be eventually found to be implicated in humans. Currently, only two genes have been identified which result in complete rescue of hearing defects in mice. For example alleles of *Cdh23* and *Mtap1a* can rescue hearing loss in mice with mutations in *Atp2b2* and *Tub* respectively (reviewed by Yan & Liu, 2010). Targeted sequencing of these genes in humans may also identify comparable variants important for modification of hearing loss.

3. Conclusions

Genes and loci continue to be identified in aetiology of moderate to severe and progressive deafness. Current research has revealed that different alleles of a deafness gene can cause less severe hearing loss or more profound deafness. Further work needs to be carried out to identify additional loci and genes for progressive deafness and those for less severe hearing loss phenotypes as well as modifiers in the genetic background that suppress or enhance hearing loss. The contribution of different genes to moderate to severe and progressive hearing loss also needs to be studied in different world populations. Additionally, it remains important to document hearing loss in families which have already been described to suffer from moderate to severe hearing loss in order to check for progression of hearing loss in future. Strategies need to be evolved for identification of modifiers which will elucidate molecular pathways involved in normal hearing. This may be of help in designing strategies to treat and cure deafness in future.

4. Acknowledgements

I thank Dr. Thomas B Friedman for helpful comments and critical overview of the manuscript. Supported by Fogarty International Center and National Institute on Deafness and other Communication Disorders, National Institutes of Health, USA, (R01TW007608).

5. References

Abadie, C., Blanchet, C., Baux, D., Larrieu, L., Besnard, T., Ravel, P., Biboulet, R., Hamel, C., Malcolm, S., Mondain, M., Claustres, M. & Roux, A. F. (2011). Audiological findings in 100 USH2 patients. *Clin Genet.*

Aller, E., Jaijo, T., Oltra, S., Alio, J., Galan, F., Najera, C., Beneyto, M. & Millan, J. M. (2004). Mutation screening of USH3 gene (clarin-1) in Spanish patients with Usher syndrome: low prevalence and phenotypic variability. *Clin Genet* 66, 525-9.

Aslam, M., Wajid, M., Chahrour, M. H., Ansar, M., Haque, S., Pham, T. L., Santos, R. P., Yan, K., Ahmad, W. & Leal, S. M. (2005). A novel autosomal recessive nonsyndromic hearing impairment locus (DFNB42) maps to chromosome 3q13.31-q22.3. *Am J Med Genet A* 133A, 18-22.

Astuto, L. M., Bork, J. M., Weston, M. D., Askew, J. W., Fields, R. R., Orten, D. J., Ohliger, S. J., Riazuddin, S., Morell, R. J., Khan, S., Riazuddin, S., Kremer, H., van Hauwe, P., Moller, C. G., Cremers, C. W., Ayuso, C., Heckenlively, J. R., Rohrschneider, K., Spandau, U., Greenberg, J., Ramesar, R., Reardon, W., Bitoun, P., Millan, J., Legge, R., Friedman, T. B. & Kimberling, W. J. (2002). CDH23 mutation and phenotype heterogeneity: a profile of 107 diverse families with Usher syndrome and nonsyndromic deafness. *Am J Hum Genet* 71, 262-75.

Audo, I., Bujakowska, K., Mohand-Said, S., Tronche, S., Lancelot, M. E., Antonio, A., Germain, A., Lonjou, C., Carpentier, W., Sahel, J. A., Bhattacharya, S. & Zeitz, C. (2011). A novel DFNB31 mutation associated with Usher type 2 syndrome showing variable degrees of auditory loss in a consanguineous Portuguese family. *Mol Vis* 17, 1598-606.

Bashir, R., Fatima, A. & Naz, S. (2010a). A frameshift mutation in SANS results in atypical Usher syndrome. *Clin Genet* 78, 601-3.

Bashir, R., Fatima, A. & Naz, S. (2010b). Mutations in CLDN14 are associated with different hearing thresholds. *J Hum Genet* 55, 767-70.

Bashir R., Fatima, A. & Naz, S. Prioritized sequencing of the second exon of MYO15A reveals a new mutation segregating in a Pakistani family with moderate to severe hearing loss. *Eur J Med Genet* (in press DOI: 10.1016/j.ejmg.2011.12.003)

Basit, S., Lee, K., Habib, R., Chen, L., Umm e, K., Santos-Cortez, R. L., Azeem, Z., Andrade, P., Ansar, M., Ahmad, W. & Leal, S. M. (2011). DFNB89, a novel autosomal recessive nonsyndromic hearing impairment locus on chromosome 16q21-q23.2. *Hum Genet* 129, 379-85.

Belguith, H., Masmoudi, S., Medlej-Hashim, M., Chouery, E., Weil, D., Ayadi, H., Petit, C. & Megarbane, A. (2009). Re-assigning the DFNB33 locus to chromosome 10p11.23-q21.1. *Eur J Hum Genet* 17, 122-4.

Belyantseva, I. A., Boger, E. T., Naz, S., Frolenkov, G. I., Sellers, J. R., Ahmed, Z. M., Griffith, A. J. & Friedman, T. B. (2005). Myosin-XVa is required for tip localization of whirlin and differential elongation of hair-cell stereocilia. *Nat Cell Biol* 7, 148-56.

Ben-Yosef, T., Belyantseva, I. A., Saunders, T. L., Hughes, E. D., Kawamoto, K., Van Itallie, C. M., Beyer, L. A., Halsey, K., Gardner, D. J., Wilcox, E. R., Rasmussen, J., Anderson, J. M., Dolan, D. F., Forge, A., Raphael, Y., Camper, S. A. & Friedman, T. B. (2003). Claudin 14 knockout mice, a model for autosomal recessive deafness DFNB29, are deaf due to cochlear hair cell degeneration. *Hum Mol Genet* 12, 2049-61.

Beyer, L. A., Odeh, H., Probst, F. J., Lambert, E. H., Dolan, D. F., Camper, S. A., Kohrman, D. C. & Raphael, Y. (2000). Hair cells in the inner ear of the pirouette and shaker 2 mutant mice. *J Neurocytol* 29, 227-40.

Borck, G., Rainshtein, L., Hellman-Aharony, S., Volk, A., Friedrich, K., Taub, E., Magal, N., Kanaan, M., Kubisch, C., Shohat, M. & Basel-Vanagaite, L. (2011a). High frequency of autosomal-recessive DFNB59 hearing loss in an isolated Arab population in Israel. *Clin Genet*.

Borck, G., Ur Rehman, A., Lee, K., Pogoda, H. M., Kakar, N., von Ameln, S., Grillet, N., Hildebrand, M. S., Ahmed, Z. M., Nurnberg, G., Ansar, M., Basit, S., Javed, Q., Morell, R. J., Nasreen, N., Shearer, A. E., Ahmad, A., Kahrizi, K., Shaikh, R. S., Ali, R. A., Khan, S. N., Goebel, I., Meyer, N. C., Kimberling, W. J., Webster, J. A., Stephan, D. A., Schiller, M. R., Bahlo, M., Najmabadi, H., Gillespie, P. G., Nurnberg, P., Wollnik, B., Riazuddin, S., Smith, R. J., Ahmad, W., Muller, U., Hammerschmidt, M., Friedman, T. B., Riazuddin, S., Leal, S. M., Ahmad, J. & Kubisch, C. (2011b). Loss-of-function mutations of ILDR1 cause autosomal-recessive hearing impairment DFNB42. *Am J Hum Genet* 88, 127-37.

Cengiz, F. B., Duman, D., Sirmaci, A., Tokgoz-Yilmaz, S., Erbek, S., Ozturkmen-Akay, H., Incesulu, A., Edwards, Y. J., Ozdag, H., Liu, X. Z. & Tekin, M. (2010). Recurrent and private MYO15A mutations are associated with deafness in the Turkish population. *Genet Test Mol Biomarkers* 14, 543-50.

Charizopoulou, N., Lelli, A., Schraders, M., Ray, K., Hildebrand, M. S., Ramesh, A., Srisailapathy, C. R., Oostrik, J., Admiraal, R. J., Neely, H. R., Latoche, J. R., Smith, R. J., Northup, J. K., Kremer, H., Holt, J. R. & Noben-Trauth, K. (2011). Gipc3 mutations associated with audiogenic seizures and sensorineural hearing loss in mouse and human. *Nat Commun* 2, 201.

Chishti, M. S., Bhatti, A., Tamim, S., Lee, K., McDonald, M. L., Leal, S. M. & Ahmad, W. (2008). Splice-site mutations in the TRIC gene underlie autosomal recessive nonsyndromic hearing impairment in Pakistani families. *J Hum Genet* 53, 101-5.

Chishti, M. S., Lee, K., McDonald, M. L., Hassan, M. J., Ansar, M., Ahmad, W. & Leal, S. M. (2009). Novel autosomal recessive non-syndromic hearing impairment locus (DFNB71) maps to chromosome 8p22-21.3. *J Hum Genet* 54, 141-4.

Choi, B. Y., Kim, H. M., Ito, T., Lee, K. Y., Li, X., Monahan, K., Wen, Y., Wilson, E., Kurima, K., Saunders, T. L., Petralia, R. S., Wangemann, P., Friedman, T. B. & Griffith, A. J. (2011). Mouse model of enlarged vestibular aqueducts defines temporal requirement of Slc26a4 expression for hearing acquisition. *J Clin Invest* 121, 4516-25.

de Heer, A. M., Collin, R. W., Huygen, P. L., Schraders, M., Oostrik, J., Rouwette, M., Kunst, H. P., Kremer, H. & Cremers, C. W. (2011). Progressive sensorineural hearing loss and normal vestibular function in a Dutch DFNB7/11 family with a novel mutation in TMC1. *Audiol Neurootol* 16, 93-105.

Delmaghani, S., del Castillo, F. J., Michel, V., Leibovici, M., Aghaie, A., Ron, U., Van Laer, L., Ben-Tal, N., Van Camp, G., Weil, D., Langa, F., Lathrop, M., Avan, P. & Petit, C. (2006). Mutations in the gene encoding pejvakin, a newly identified protein of the afferent auditory pathway, cause DFNB59 auditory neuropathy. *Nat Genet* 38, 770-8.

Denoyelle, F., Weil, D., Maw, M. A., Wilcox, S. A., Lench, N. J., Allen-Powell, D. R., Osborn, A. H., Dahl, H. H., Middleton, A., Houseman, M. J., Dode, C., Marlin, S., Boulila-ElGaied, A., Grati, M., Ayadi, H., BenArab, S., Bitoun, P., Lina-Granade, G., Godet, J., Mustapha, M., Loiselet, J., El-Zir, E., Aubois, A., Joannard, A., Petit, C. & et al. (1997). Prelingual deafness: high prevalence of a 30delG mutation in the connexin 26 gene. *Hum Mol Genet* 6, 2173-7.

Di Palma, F., Holme, R. H., Bryda, E. C., Belyantseva, I. A., Pellegrino, R., Kachar, B., Steel, K. P. & Noben-Trauth, K. (2001). Mutations in Cdh23, encoding a new type of cadherin, cause stereocilia disorganization in waltzer, the mouse model for Usher syndrome type 1D. *Nat Genet* 27, 103-7.

Dror, A. A., Politi, Y., Shahin, H., Lenz, D. R., Dossena, S., Nofziger, C., Fuchs, H., Hrabe de Angelis, M., Paulmichl, M., Weiner, S. & Avraham, K. B. (2010). Calcium oxalate stone formation in the inner ear as a result of an Slc26a4 mutation. *J Biol Chem* 285, 21724-35.

Ebermann, I., Scholl, H. P., Charbel Issa, P., Becirovic, E., Lamprecht, J., Jurklies, B., Millan, J. M., Aller, E., Mitter, D. & Bolz, H. (2007a). A novel gene for Usher syndrome type 2: mutations in the long isoform of whirlin are associated with retinitis pigmentosa and sensorineural hearing loss. *Hum Genet* 121, 203-11.

Ebermann, I., Walger, M., Scholl, H. P., Charbel Issa, P., Luke, C., Nurnberg, G., Lang-Roth, R., Becker, C., Nurnberg, P. & Bolz, H. J. (2007b). Truncating mutation of the DFNB59 gene causes cochlear hearing impairment and central vestibular dysfunction. *Hum Mutat* 28, 571-7.

Edvardson, S., Jalas, C., Shaag, A., Zenvirt, S., Landau, C., Lerer, I. & Elpeleg, O. (2011). A deleterious mutation in the LOXHD1 gene causes autosomal recessive hearing loss in Ashkenazi Jews. *Am J Med Genet A* 155A, 1170-2.

Elbracht, M., Senderek, J., Eggermann, T., Thurmer, C., Park, J., Westhofen, M. & Zerres, K. (2007). Autosomal recessive postlingual hearing loss (DFNB8): compound heterozygosity for two novel TMPRSS3 mutations in German siblings. *J Med Genet* 44, e81.

Estevez, R., Boettger, T., Stein, V., Birkenhager, R., Otto, E., Hildebrandt, F. & Jentsch, T. J. (2001). Barttin is a Cl- channel beta-subunit crucial for renal Cl- reabsorption and inner ear K+ secretion. *Nature* 414, 558-61.

Eudy, J. D., Weston, M. D., Yao, S., Hoover, D. M., Rehm, H. L., Ma-Edmonds, M., Yan, D., Ahmad, I., Cheng, J. J., Ayuso, C., Cremers, C., Davenport, S., Moller, C., Talmadge, C. B., Beisel, K. W., Tamayo, M., Morton, C. C., Swaroop, A., Kimberling, W. J. & Sumegi, J. (1998). Mutation of a gene encoding a protein with extracellular matrix motifs in Usher syndrome type IIa. *Science* 280, 1753-7.

Everett, L. A., Belyantseva, I. A., Noben-Trauth, K., Cantos, R., Chen, A., Thakkar, S. I., Hoogstraten-Miller, S. L., Kachar, B., Wu, D. K. & Green, E. D. (2001). Targeted disruption of mouse Pds provides insight about the inner-ear defects encountered in Pendred syndrome. *Hum Mol Genet* 10, 153-61.

Everett, L. A., Morsli, H., Wu, D. K. & Green, E. D. (1999). Expression pattern of the mouse ortholog of the Pendred's syndrome gene (Pds) suggests a key role for pendrin in the inner ear. *Proc Natl Acad Sci U S A* 96, 9727-32.

Fasquelle, L., Scott, H. S., Lenoir, M., Wang, J., Rebillard, G., Gaboyard, S., Venteo, S., Francois, F., Mausset-Bonnefont, A. L., Antonarakis, S. E., Neidhart, E., Chabbert, C., Puel, J. L., Guipponi, M. & Delprat, B. (2011). Tmprss3, a transmembrane serine protease deficient in human DFNB8/10 deafness, is critical for cochlear hair cell survival at the onset of hearing. *J Biol Chem* 286, 17383-97.

Geng, R., Geller, S. F., Hayashi, T., Ray, C. A., Reh, T. A., Bermingham-McDonogh, O., Jones, S. M., Wright, C. G., Melki, S., Imanishi, Y., Palczewski, K., Alagramam, K. N. & Flannery, J. G. (2009). Usher syndrome IIIA gene clarin-1 is essential for hair cell function and associated neural activation. *Hum Mol Genet* 18, 2748-60.

Gibson, F., Walsh, J., Mburu, P., Varela, A., Brown, K. A., Antonio, M., Beisel, K. W., Steel, K. P. & Brown, S. D. (1995). A type VII myosin encoded by the mouse deafness gene shaker-1. *Nature* 374, 62-4.

Goodyear, R. J., Legan, P. K., Wright, M. B., Marcotti, W., Oganesian, A., Coats, S. A., Booth, C. J., Kros, C. J., Seifert, R. A., Bowen-Pope, D. F. & Richardson, G. P. (2003). A receptor-like inositol lipid phosphatase is required for the maturation of developing cochlear hair bundles. *J Neurosci* 23, 9208-19.

Grati, M. & Kachar, B. (2011). Myosin VIIa and sans localization at stereocilia upper tip-link density implicates these Usher syndrome proteins in mechanotransduction. *Proc Natl Acad Sci U S A* 108, 11476-81.

Grillet, N., Schwander, M., Hildebrand, M. S., Sczaniecka, A., Kolatkar, A., Velasco, J., Webster, J. A., Kahrizi, K., Najmabadi, H., Kimberling, W. J., Stephan, D., Bahlo, M., Wiltshire, T., Tarantino, L. M., Kuhn, P., Smith, R. J. & Muller, U. (2009). Mutations in LOXHD1, an evolutionarily conserved stereociliary protein, disrupt hair cell function in mice and cause progressive hearing loss in humans. *Am J Hum Genet* 85, 328-37.

Hildebrand, M. S., Thorne, N. P., Bromhead, C. J., Kahrizi, K., Webster, J. A., Fattahi, Z., Bataejad, M., Kimberling, W. J., Stephan, D., Najmabadi, H., Bahlo, M. & Smith, R. J. (2010). Variable hearing impairment in a DFNB2 family with a novel MYO7A missense mutation. *Clin Genet.*

Hilgert, N., Huentelman, M. J., Thorburn, A. Q., Fransen, E., Dieltjens, N., Mueller-Malesinska, M., Pollak, A., Skorka, A., Waligora, J., Ploski, R., Castorina, P., Primignani, P., Ambrosetti, U., Murgia, A., Orzan, E., Pandya, A., Arnos, K., Norris, V., Seeman, P., Janousek, P., Feldmann, D., Marlin, S., Denoyelle, F., Nishimura, C. J., Janecke, A., Nekahm-Heis, D., Martini, A., Mennucci, E., Toth, T., Sziklai, I., Del Castillo, I., Moreno, F., Petersen, M. B., Iliadou, V., Tekin, M., Incesulu, A., Nowakowska, E., Bal, J., Van de Heyning, P., Roux, A. F., Blanchet, C., Goizet, C., Lancelot, G., Fialho, G., Caria, H., Liu, X. Z., Xiaomei, O., Govaerts, P., Gronskov, K., Hostmark, K., Frei, K., Dhooge, I., Vlaeminck, S., Kunstmann, E., Van Laer, L., Smith, R. J. & Van Camp, G. (2009). Phenotypic variability of patients homozygous for the GJB2 mutation 35delG cannot be explained by the influence of one major modifier gene. *Eur J Hum Genet* 17, 517-24.

Hutchin, T., Coy, N. N., Conlon, H., Telford, E., Bromelow, K., Blaydon, D., Taylor, G., Coghill, E., Brown, S., Trembath, R., Liu, X. Z., Bitner-Glindzicz, M. & Mueller, R.

(2005). Assessment of the genetic causes of recessive childhood non-syndromic deafness in the UK - implications for genetic testing. *Clin Genet* 68, 506-12.

Joensuu, T., Hamalainen, R., Yuan, B., Johnson, C., Tegelberg, S., Gasparini, P., Zelante, L., Pirvola, U., Pakarinen, L., Lehesjoki, A. E., de la Chapelle, A. & Sankila, E. M. (2001). Mutations in a novel gene with transmembrane domains underlie Usher syndrome type 3. *Am J Hum Genet* 69, 673-84.

Jovine, L., Park, J. & Wassarman, P. M. (2002). Sequence similarity between stereocilin and otoancorin points to a unified mechanism for mechanotransduction in the mammalian inner ear. *BMC Cell Biol* 3, 28.

Kalay, E., de Brouwer, A. P., Caylan, R., Nabuurs, S. B., Wollnik, B., Karaguzel, A., Heister, J. G., Erdol, H., Cremers, F. P., Cremers, C. W., Brunner, H. G. & Kremer, H. (2005). A novel D458V mutation in the SANS PDZ binding motif causes atypical Usher syndrome. *J Mol Med (Berl)* 83, 1025-32.

Khan, S. Y., Riazuddin, S., Shahzad, M., Ahmed, N., Zafar, A. U., Rehman, A. U., Morell, R. J., Griffith, A. J., Ahmed, Z. M., Riazuddin, S. & Friedman, T. B. (2009). DFNB79: reincarnation of a nonsyndromic deafness locus on chromosome 9q34.3. *Eur J Hum Genet* 18, 125-9.

Kikuchi, T., Kimura, R. S., Paul, D. L. & Adams, J. C. (1995). Gap junctions in the rat cochlea: immunohistochemical and ultrastructural analysis. *Anat Embryol (Berl)* 191, 101-18.

Kitamura, K., Takahashi, K., Noguchi, Y., Kuroishikawa, Y., Tamagawa, Y., Ishikawa, K., Ichimura, K. & Hagiwara, H. (2000). Mutations of the Pendred syndrome gene (PDS) in patients with large vestibular aqueduct. *Acta Otolaryngol* 120, 137-41.

Kurima, K., Peters, L. M., Yang, Y., Riazuddin, S., Ahmed, Z. M., Naz, S., Arnaud, D., Drury, S., Mo, J., Makishima, T., Ghosh, M., Menon, P. S., Deshmukh, D., Oddoux, C., Ostrer, H., Khan, S., Riazuddin, S., Deininger, P. L., Hampton, L. L., Sullivan, S. L., Battey, J. F., Jr., Keats, B. J., Wilcox, E. R., Friedman, T. B. & Griffith, A. J. (2002). Dominant and recessive deafness caused by mutations of a novel gene, TMC1, required for cochlear hair-cell function. *Nat Genet* 30, 277-84.

Legan, P. K., Lukashkina, V. A., Goodyear, R. J., Kossi, M., Russell, I. J. & Richardson, G. P. (2000). A targeted deletion in alpha-tectorin reveals that the tectorial membrane is required for the gain and timing of cochlear feedback. *Neuron* 28, 273-85.

Li, Y., Pohl, E., Boulouiz, R., Schraders, M., Nurnberg, G., Charif, M., Admiraal, R. J., von Ameln, S., Baessmann, I., Kandil, M., Veltman, J. A., Nurnberg, P., Kubisch, C., Barakat, A., Kremer, H. & Wollnik, B. (2010). Mutations in TPRN Cause a Progressive Form of Autosomal-Recessive Nonsyndromic Hearing Loss. *Am J Hum Genet* 86, 479-484.

Liu, X., Bulgakov, O. V., Darrow, K. N., Pawlyk, B., Adamian, M., Liberman, M. C. & Li, T. (2007). Usherin is required for maintenance of retinal photoreceptors and normal development of cochlear hair cells. *Proc Natl Acad Sci U S A* 104, 4413-8.

Liu, X. Z., Hope, C., Liang, C. Y., Zou, J. M., Xu, L. R., Cole, T., Mueller, R. F., Bundey, S., Nance, W., Steel, K. P. & Brown, S. D. (1999). A mutation (2314delG) in the Usher syndrome type IIA gene: high prevalence and phenotypic variation. *Am J Hum Genet* 64, 1221-5.

Liu, X. Z., Hope, C., Walsh, J., Newton, V., Ke, X. M., Liang, C. Y., Xu, L. R., Zhou, J. M., Trump, D., Steel, K. P., Bundey, S. & Brown, S. D. (1998). Mutations in the myosin

VIIA gene cause a wide phenotypic spectrum, including atypical Usher syndrome. *Am J Hum Genet* 63, 909-12.

Liu, X. Z., Pandya, A., Angeli, S., Telischi, F. F., Arnos, K. S., Nance, W. E. & Balkany, T. (2005). Audiological features of GJB2 (connexin 26) deafness. *Ear Hear* 26, 361-9.

Lopez-Bigas, N., Rabionet, R., de Cid, R., Govea, N., Gasparini, P., Zelante, L., Arbones, M. L. & Estivill, X. (1999). Splice-site mutation in the PDS gene may result in intrafamilial variability for deafness in Pendred syndrome. *Hum Mutat* 14, 520-6.

Lu, Y. C., Wu, C. C., Shen, W. S., Yang, T. H., Yeh, T. H., Chen, P. J., Yu, I. S., Lin, S. W., Wong, J. M., Chang, Q., Lin, X. & Hsu, C. J. (2011). Establishment of a knock-in mouse model with the SLC26A4 c.919-2A>G mutation and characterization of its pathology. *PLoS One* 6, e22150.

Lukashkin, A. N., Lukashkina, V. A., Legan, P. K., Richardson, G. P. & Russell, I. J. (2004). Role of the tectorial membrane revealed by otoacoustic emissions recorded from wild-type and transgenic Tecta(deltaENT/deltaENT) mice. *J Neurophysiol* 91, 163-71.

Luxon, L. M., Cohen, M., Coffey, R. A., Phelps, P. D., Britton, K. E., Jan, H., Trembath, R. C. & Reardon, W. (2003). Neuro-otological findings in Pendred syndrome. *Int J Audiol* 42, 82-8.

Masmoudi, S., Charfedine, I., Rebeh, I. B., Rebai, A., Tlili, A., Ghorbel, A. M., Belguith, H., Petit, C., Drira, M. & Ayadi, H. (2004). Refined mapping of the autosomal recessive non-syndromic deafness locus DFNB13 using eight novel microsatellite markers. *Clin Genet* 66, 358-64.

Masmoudi, S., Tlili, A., Majava, M., Ghorbel, A. M., Chardenoux, S., Lemainque, A., Zina, Z. B., Moala, J., Mannikko, M., Weil, D., Lathrop, M., Ala-Kokko, L., Drira, M., Petit, C. & Ayadi, H. (2003). Mapping of a new autosomal recessive nonsyndromic hearing loss locus (DFNB32) to chromosome 1p13.3-22.1. *Eur J Hum Genet* 11, 185-8.

Mburu, P., Liu, X. Z., Walsh, J., Saw, D., Jr., Cope, M. J., Gibson, F., Kendrick-Jones, J., Steel, K. P. & Brown, S. D. (1997). Mutation analysis of the mouse myosin VIIA deafness gene. *Genes Funct* 1, 191-203.

Mburu, P., Mustapha, M., Varela, A., Weil, D., El-Amraoui, A., Holme, R. H., Rump, A., Hardisty, R. E., Blanchard, S., Coimbra, R. S., Perfettini, I., Parkinson, N., Mallon, A. M., Glenister, P., Rogers, M. J., Paige, A. J., Moir, L., Clay, J., Rosenthal, A., Liu, X. Z., Blanco, G., Steel, K. P., Petit, C. & Brown, S. D. (2003). Defects in whirlin, a PDZ domain molecule involved in stereocilia elongation, cause deafness in the whirler mouse and families with DFNB31. *Nat Genet* 34, 421-8.

McGee, J., Goodyear, R. J., McMillan, D. R., Stauffer, E. A., Holt, J. R., Locke, K. G., Birch, D. G., Legan, P. K., White, P. C., Walsh, E. J. & Richardson, G. P. (2006). The very large G-protein-coupled receptor VLGR1: a component of the ankle link complex required for the normal development of auditory hair bundles. *J Neurosci* 26, 6543-53.

Medlej-Hashim, M., Mustapha, M., Chouery, E., Weil, D., Parronaud, J., Salem, N., Delague, V., Loiselet, J., Lathrop, M., Petit, C. & Megarbane, A. (2002). Non-syndromic recessive deafness in Jordan: mapping of a new locus to chromosome 9q34.3 and prevalence of DFNB1 mutations. *Eur J Hum Genet* 10, 391-4.

Meyer, N. C., Alasti, F., Nishimura, C. J., Imanirad, P., Kahrizi, K., Riazalhosseini, Y., Malekpour, M., Kochakian, N., Jamali, P., Van Camp, G., Smith, R. J. & Najmabadi,

H. (2007). Identification of three novel TECTA mutations in Iranian families with autosomal recessive nonsyndromic hearing impairment at the DFNB21 locus. *Am J Med Genet A* 143A, 1623-9.

Moynihan, L., Houseman, M., Newton, V., Mueller, R. & Lench, N. (1999). DFNB20: a novel locus for autosomal recessive, non-syndromal sensorineural hearing loss maps to chromosome 11q25-qter. *Eur J Hum Genet* 7, 243-6.

Murgia, A., Orzan, E., Polli, R., Martella, M., Vinanzi, C., Leonardi, E., Arslan, E. & Zacchello, F. (1999). Cx26 deafness: mutation analysis and clinical variability. *J Med Genet* 36, 829-32.

Mustapha, M., Chardenoux, S., Nieder, A., Salem, N., Weissenbach, J., el-Zir, E., Loiselet, J. & Petit, C. (1998). A sensorineural progressive autosomal recessive form of isolated deafness, DFNB13, maps to chromosome 7q34-q36. *Eur J Hum Genet* 6, 245-50.

Nal, N., Ahmed, Z. M., Erkal, E., Alper, O. M., Luleci, G., Dinc, O., Waryah, A. M., Ain, Q., Tasneem, S., Husnain, T., Chattaraj, P., Riazuddin, S., Boger, E., Ghosh, M., Kabra, M., Riazuddin, S., Morell, R. J. & Friedman, T. B. (2007). Mutational spectrum of MYO15A: the large N-terminal extension of myosin XVA is required for hearing. *Hum Mutat* 28, 1014-9.

Naz, S. (2001). Study of non-syndromic recessive deafness by linkage analysis. *PhD thesis*.University of the Punjab, Lahore, Pakistan.

Naz, S., Alasti, F., Mowjoodi, A., Riazuddin, S., Sanati, M. H., Friedman, T. B., Griffith, A. J., Wilcox, E. R. & Riazuddin, S. (2003). Distinctive audiometric profile associated with DFNB21 alleles of TECTA. *J Med Genet* 40, 360-3.

Ness, S. L., Ben-Yosef, T., Bar-Lev, A., Madeo, A. C., Brewer, C. C., Avraham, K. B., Kornreich, R., Desnick, R. J., Willner, J. P., Friedman, T. B. & Griffith, A. J. (2003). Genetic homogeneity and phenotypic variability among Ashkenazi Jews with Usher syndrome type III. *J Med Genet* 40, 767-72.

Noben-Trauth, K., Zheng, Q. Y. & Johnson, K. R. (2003). Association of cadherin 23 with polygenic inheritance and genetic modification of sensorineural hearing loss. *Nat Genet* 35, 21-3.

Odeh, H., Hunker, K. L., Belyantseva, I. A., Azaiez, H., Avenarius, M. R., Zheng, L., Peters, L. M., Gagnon, L. H., Hagiwara, N., Skynner, M. J., Brilliant, M. H., Allen, N. D., Riazuddin, S., Johnson, K. R., Raphael, Y., Najmabadi, H., Friedman, T. B., Bartles, J. R., Smith, R. J. & Kohrman, D. C. (2010). Mutations in Grxcr1 are the basis for inner ear dysfunction in the pirouette mouse. *Am J Hum Genet* 86, 148-60.

Oprea, G. E., Krober, S., McWhorter, M. L., Rossoll, W., Muller, S., Krawczak, M., Bassell, G. J., Beattie, C. E. & Wirth, B. (2008). Plastin 3 is a protective modifier of autosomal recessive spinal muscular atrophy. *Science* 320, 524-7.

Pennings, R. J., Fields, R. R., Huygen, P. L., Deutman, A. F., Kimberling, W. J. & Cremers, C. W. (2003). Usher syndrome type III can mimic other types of Usher syndrome. *Ann Otol Rhinol Laryngol* 112, 525-30.

Pennings, R. J., Topsakal, V., Astuto, L., de Brouwer, A. P., Wagenaar, M., Huygen, P. L., Kimberling, W. J., Deutman, A. F., Kremer, H. & Cremers, C. W. (2004). Variable clinical features in patients with CDH23 mutations (USH1D-DFNB12). *Otol Neurotol* 25, 699-706.

Probst, F. J., Fridell, R. A., Raphael, Y., Saunders, T. L., Wang, A., Liang, Y., Morell, R. J., Touchman, J. W., Lyons, R. H., Noben-Trauth, K., Friedman, T. B. & Camper, S. A.

(1998). Correction of deafness in shaker-2 mice by an unconventional myosin in a BAC transgene. *Science* 280, 1444-7.

Rehman, A. U., Gul, K., Morell, R. J., Lee, K., Ahmed, Z. M., Riazuddin, S., Ali, R. A., Shahzad, M., Jaleel, A. U., Andrade, P. B., Khan, S. N., Khan, S., Brewer, C. C., Ahmad, W., Leal, S. M., Riazuddin, S. & Friedman, T. B. (2011). Mutations of GIPC3 cause nonsyndromic hearing loss DFNB72 but not DFNB81 that also maps to chromosome 19p. *Hum Genet*.

Rehman, A. U., Morell, R. J., Belyantseva, I. A., Khan, S. Y., Boger, E. T., Shahzad, M., Ahmed, Z. M., Riazuddin, S., Khan, S. N., Riazuddin, S. & Friedman, T. B. (2010). Targeted Capture and Next-Generation Sequencing Identifies C9orf75, Encoding Taperin, as the Mutated Gene in Nonsyndromic Deafness DFNB79. *Am J Hum Genet* 86, 378-388.

Riazuddin, S., Ahmed, Z. M., Fanning, A. S., Lagziel, A., Kitajiri, S., Ramzan, K., Khan, S. N., Chattaraj, P., Friedman, P. L., Anderson, J. M., Belyantseva, I. A., Forge, A., Riazuddin, S. & Friedman, T. B. (2006). Tricellulin is a tight-junction protein necessary for hearing. *Am J Hum Genet* 79, 1040-51.

Riazuddin, S., Anwar, S., Fischer, M., Ahmed, Z. M., Khan, S. Y., Janssen, A. G., Zafar, A. U., Scholl, U., Husnain, T., Belyantseva, I. A., Friedman, P. L., Riazuddin, S., Friedman, T. B. & Fahlke, C. (2009). Molecular basis of DFNB73: mutations of BSND can cause nonsyndromic deafness or Bartter syndrome. *Am J Hum Genet* 85, 273-80.

Riazuddin, S., Castelein, C. M., Ahmed, Z. M., Lalwani, A. K., Mastroianni, M. A., Naz, S., Smith, T. N., Liburd, N. A., Friedman, T. B., Griffith, A. J., Riazuddin, S. & Wilcox, E. R. (2000). Dominant modifier DFNM1 suppresses recessive deafness DFNB26. *Nat Genet* 26, 431-4.

Sadeghi, M., Cohn, E. S., Kimberling, W. J., Tranebjaerg, L. & Moller, C. (2005). Audiological and vestibular features in affected subjects with USH3: a genotype/phenotype correlation. *Int J Audiol* 44, 307-16.

Sakaguchi, H., Tokita, J., Naoz, M., Bowen-Pope, D., Gov, N. S. & Kachar, B. (2008). Dynamic compartmentalization of protein tyrosine phosphatase receptor Q at the proximal end of stereocilia: implication of myosin VI-based transport. *Cell Motil Cytoskeleton* 65, 528-38.

Sathyanarayana, B. K., Hahn, Y., Patankar, M. S., Pastan, I. & Lee, B. (2009). Mesothelin, Stereocilin, and Otoancorin are predicted to have superhelical structures with ARM-type repeats. *BMC Struct Biol* 9, 1.

Scarff, K. L., Ung, K. S., Nandurkar, H., Crack, P. J., Bird, C. H. & Bird, P. I. (2004). Targeted disruption of SPI3/Serpinb6 does not result in developmental or growth defects, leukocyte dysfunction, or susceptibility to stroke. *Mol Cell Biol* 24, 4075-82.

Schneider, M. E., Dose, A. C., Salles, F. T., Chang, W., Erickson, F. L., Burnside, B. & Kachar, B. (2006). A new compartment at stereocilia tips defined by spatial and temporal patterns of myosin IIIa expression. *J Neurosci* 26, 10243-52.

Schraders, M., Lee, K., Oostrik, J., Huygen, P. L., Ali, G., Hoefsloot, L. H., Veltman, J. A., Cremers, F. P., Basit, S., Ansar, M., Cremers, C. W., Kunst, H. P., Ahmad, W., Admiraal, R. J., Leal, S. M. & Kremer, H. (2010a). Homozygosity mapping reveals mutations of GRXCR1 as a cause of autosomal-recessive nonsyndromic hearing impairment. *Am J Hum Genet* 86, 138-47.

Schraders, M., Oostrik, J., Huygen, P. L., Strom, T. M., van Wijk, E., Kunst, H. P., Hoefsloot, L. H., Cremers, C. W., Admiraal, R. J. & Kremer, H. (2010b). Mutations in PTPRQ are a cause of autosomal-recessive nonsyndromic hearing impairment DFNB84 and associated with vestibular dysfunction. *Am J Hum Genet* 86, 604-10.

Schultz, J. M., Yang, Y., Caride, A. J., Filoteo, A. G., Penheiter, A. R., Lagziel, A., Morell, R. J., Mohiddin, S. A., Fananapazir, L., Madeo, A. C., Penniston, J. T. & Griffith, A. J. (2005). Modification of human hearing loss by plasma-membrane calcium pump PMCA2. *N Engl J Med* 352, 1557-64.

Schwander, M., Sczaniecka, A., Grillet, N., Bailey, J. S., Avenarius, M., Najmabadi, H., Steffy, B. M., Federe, G. C., Lagler, E. A., Banan, R., Hice, R., Grabowski-Boase, L., Keithley, E. M., Ryan, A. F., Housley, G. D., Wiltshire, T., Smith, R. J., Tarantino, L. M. & Muller, U. (2007). A forward genetics screen in mice identifies recessive deafness traits and reveals that pejvakin is essential for outer hair cell function. *J Neurosci* 27, 2163-75.

Schwander, M., Xiong, W., Tokita, J., Lelli, A., Elledge, H. M., Kazmierczak, P., Sczaniecka, A., Kolatkar, A., Wiltshire, T., Kuhn, P., Holt, J. R., Kachar, B., Tarantino, L. & Muller, U. (2009). A mouse model for nonsyndromic deafness (DFNB12) links hearing loss to defects in tip links of mechanosensory hair cells. *Proc Natl Acad Sci U S A* 106, 5252-7.

Scott, H. S., Kudoh, J., Wattenhofer, M., Shibuya, K., Berry, A., Chrast, R., Guipponi, M., Wang, J., Kawasaki, K., Asakawa, S., Minoshima, S., Younus, F., Mehdi, S. Q., Radhakrishna, U., Papasavvas, M. P., Gehrig, C., Rossier, C., Korostishevsky, M., Gal, A., Shimizu, N., Bonne-Tamir, B. & Antonarakis, S. E. (2001). Insertion of beta-satellite repeats identifies a transmembrane protease causing both congenital and childhood onset autosomal recessive deafness. *Nat Genet* 27, 59-63.

Seifert, R. A., Coats, S. A., Oganesian, A., Wright, M. B., Dishmon, M., Booth, C. J., Johnson, R. J., Alpers, C. E. & Bowen-Pope, D. F. (2003). PTPRQ is a novel phosphatidylinositol phosphatase that can be expressed as a cytoplasmic protein or as a subcellularly localized receptor-like protein. *Exp Cell Res* 287, 374-86.

Shahin, H., Rahil, M., Abu Rayan, A., Avraham, K. B., King, M. C., Kanaan, M. & Walsh, T. (2010a). Nonsense mutation of the stereociliar membrane protein gene PTPRQ in human hearing loss DFNB84. *J Med Genet* 47, 643-5.

Shahin, H., Walsh, T., Rayyan, A. A., Lee, M. K., Higgins, J., Dickel, D., Lewis, K., Thompson, J., Baker, C., Nord, A. S., Stray, S., Gurwitz, D., Avraham, K. B., King, M. C. & Kanaan, M. (2010b). Five novel loci for inherited hearing loss mapped by SNP-based homozygosity profiles in Palestinian families. *Eur J Hum Genet* 18, 407-13.

Sirmaci, A., Erbek, S., Price, J., Huang, M., Duman, D., Cengiz, F. B., Bademci, G., Tokgoz-Yilmaz, S., Hismi, B., Ozdag, H., Ozturk, B., Kulaksizoglu, S., Yildirim, E., Kokotas, H., Grigoriadou, M., Petersen, M. B., Shahin, H., Kanaan, M., King, M. C., Chen, Z. Y., Blanton, S. H., Liu, X. Z., Zuchner, S., Akar, N. & Tekin, M. (2010). A truncating mutation in SERPINB6 is associated with autosomal-recessive nonsyndromic sensorineural hearing loss. *Am J Hum Genet* 86, 797-804.

Snoeckx, R. L., Huygen, P. L., Feldmann, D., Marlin, S., Denoyelle, F., Waligora, J., Mueller-Malesinska, M., Pollak, A., Ploski, R., Murgia, A., Orzan, E., Castorina, P., Ambrosetti, U., Nowakowska-Szyrwinska, E., Bal, J., Wiszniewski, W., Janecke, A.

R., Nekahm-Heis, D., Seeman, P., Bendova, O., Kenna, M. A., Frangulov, A., Rehm, H. L., Tekin, M., Incesulu, A., Dahl, H. H., du Sart, D., Jenkins, L., Lucas, D., Bitner-Glindzicz, M., Avraham, K. B., Brownstein, Z., del Castillo, I., Moreno, F., Blin, N., Pfister, M., Sziklai, I., Toth, T., Kelley, P. M., Cohn, E. S., Van Maldergem, L., Hilbert, P., Roux, A. F., Mondain, M., Hoefsloot, L. H., Cremers, C. W., Lopponen, T., Lopponen, H., Parving, A., Gronskov, K., Schrijver, I., Roberson, J., Gualandi, F., Martini, A., Lina-Granade, G., Pallares-Ruiz, N., Correia, C., Fialho, G., Cryns, K., Hilgert, N., Van de Heyning, P., Nishimura, C. J., Smith, R. J. & Van Camp, G. (2005). GJB2 mutations and degree of hearing loss: a multicenter study. *Am J Hum Genet* 77, 945-57.

Tabatabaiefar, M. A., Alasti, F., Shariati, L., Farrokhi, E., Fransen, E., Nooridaloii, M. R., Chaleshtori, M. H. & Van Camp, G. (2011). DFNB93, a novel locus for autosomal recessive moderate-to-severe hearing impairment. *Clin Genet* 79, 594-8.

Tian, G., Zhou, Y., Hajkova, D., Miyagi, M., Dinculescu, A., Hauswirth, W. W., Palczewski, K., Geng, R., Alagramam, K. N., Isosomppi, J., Sankila, E. M., Flannery, J. G. & Imanishi, Y. (2009). Clarin-1, encoded by the Usher Syndrome III causative gene, forms a membranous microdomain: possible role of clarin-1 in organizing the actin cytoskeleton. *J Biol Chem* 284, 18980-93.

Verpy, E., Masmoudi, S., Zwaenepoel, I., Leibovici, M., Hutchin, T. P., Del Castillo, I., Nouaille, S., Blanchard, S., Laine, S., Popot, J. L., Moreno, F., Mueller, R. F. & Petit, C. (2001). Mutations in a new gene encoding a protein of the hair bundle cause non-syndromic deafness at the DFNB16 locus. *Nat Genet* 29, 345-9.

Verpy, E., Weil, D., Leibovici, M., Goodyear, R. J., Hamard, G., Houdon, C., Lefevre, G. M., Hardelin, J. P., Richardson, G. P., Avan, P. & Petit, C. (2008). Stereocilin-deficient mice reveal the origin of cochlear waveform distortions. *Nature* 456, 255-8.

Veske, A., Oehlmann, R., Younus, F., Mohyuddin, A., Muller-Myhsok, B., Mehdi, S. Q. & Gal, A. (1996). Autosomal recessive non-syndromic deafness locus (DFNB8) maps on chromosome 21q22 in a large consanguineous kindred from Pakistan. *Hum Mol Genet* 5, 165-8.

Villamar, M., del Castillo, I., Valle, N., Romero, L. & Moreno, F. (1999). Deafness locus DFNB16 is located on chromosome 15q13-q21 within a 5-cM interval flanked by markers D15S994 and D15S132. *Am J Hum Genet* 64, 1238-41.

Vreugde, S., Erven, A., Kros, C. J., Marcotti, W., Fuchs, H., Kurima, K., Wilcox, E. R., Friedman, T. B., Griffith, A. J., Balling, R., Hrabe De Angelis, M., Avraham, K. B. & Steel, K. P. (2002). Beethoven, a mouse model for dominant, progressive hearing loss DFNA36. *Nat Genet* 30, 257-8.

Walsh, T., Shahin, H., Elkan-Miller, T., Lee, M. K., Thornton, A. M., Roeb, W., Abu Rayyan, A., Loulus, S., Avraham, K. B., King, M. C. & Kanaan, M. (2010). Whole exome sequencing and homozygosity mapping identify mutation in the cell polarity protein GPSM2 as the cause of nonsyndromic hearing loss DFNB82. *Am J Hum Genet* 87, 90-4.

Walsh, T., Walsh, V., Vreugde, S., Hertzano, R., Shahin, H., Haika, S., Lee, M. K., Kanaan, M., King, M. C. & Avraham, K. B. (2002). From flies' eyes to our ears: mutations in a human class III myosin cause progressive nonsyndromic hearing loss DFNB30. *Proc Natl Acad Sci U S A* 99, 7518-23.

Walsh, V. L., Raviv, D., Dror, A. A., Shahin, H., Walsh, T., Kanaan, M. N., Avraham, K. B. & King, M. C. (2011). A mouse model for human hearing loss DFNB30 due to loss of function of myosin IIIA. *Mamm Genome* 22, 170-7.

Wangemann, P., Nakaya, K., Wu, T., Maganti, R. J., Itza, E. M., Sanneman, J. D., Harbidge, D. G., Billings, S. & Marcus, D. C. (2007). Loss of cochlear HCO3- secretion causes deafness via endolymphatic acidification and inhibition of Ca2+ reabsorption in a Pendred syndrome mouse model. *Am J Physiol Renal Physiol* 292, F1345-53.

Wattenhofer, M., Sahin-Calapoglu, N., Andreasen, D., Kalay, E., Caylan, R., Braillard, B., Fowler-Jaeger, N., Reymond, A., Rossier, B. C., Karaguzel, A. & Antonarakis, S. E. (2005). A novel TMPRSS3 missense mutation in a DFNB8/10 family prevents proteolytic activation of the protein. *Hum Genet* 117, 528-35.

Weegerink, N. J., Schraders, M., Oostrik, J., Huygen, P. L., Strom, T. M., Granneman, S., Pennings, R. J., Venselaar, H., Hoefsloot, L. H., Elting, M., Cremers, C. W., Admiraal, R. J., Kremer, H. & Kunst, H. P. (2011). Genotype-Phenotype Correlation in DFNB8/10 Families with TMPRSS3 Mutations. *J Assoc Res Otolaryngol* 12, 753-66.

Weston, M. D., Luijendijk, M. W., Humphrey, K. D., Moller, C. & Kimberling, W. J. (2004). Mutations in the VLGR1 gene implicate G-protein signaling in the pathogenesis of Usher syndrome type II. *Am J Hum Genet* 74, 357-66.

Wilcox, E. R., Burton, Q. L., Naz, S., Riazuddin, S., Smith, T. N., Ploplis, B., Belyantseva, I., Ben-Yosef, T., Liburd, N. A., Morell, R. J., Kachar, B., Wu, D. K., Griffith, A. J., Riazuddin, S. & Friedman, T. B. (2001). Mutations in the gene encoding tight junction claudin-14 cause autosomal recessive deafness DFNB29. *Cell* 104, 165-72.

Yan, D. & Liu, X. Z. (2010). Modifiers of hearing impairment in humans and mice. *Curr Genomics* 11, 269-78.

Yang, J., Liu, X., Zhao, Y., Adamian, M., Pawlyk, B., Sun, X., McMillan, D. R., Liberman, M. C. & Li, T. (2010). Ablation of whirlin long isoform disrupts the USH2 protein complex and causes vision and hearing loss. *PLoS Genet* 6, e1000955.

Zallocchi, M., Meehan, D. T., Delimont, D., Askew, C., Garige, S., Gratton, M. A., Rothermund-Franklin, C. A. & Cosgrove, D. (2009). Localization and expression of clarin-1, the Clrn1 gene product, in auditory hair cells and photoreceptors. *Hear Res* 255, 109-20.

Zwaenepoel, I., Mustapha, M., Leibovici, M., Verpy, E., Goodyear, R., Liu, X. Z., Nouaille, S., Nance, W. E., Kanaan, M., Avraham, K. B., Tekaia, F., Loiselet, J., Lathrop, M., Richardson, G. & Petit, C. (2002). Otoancorin, an inner ear protein restricted to the interface between the apical surface of sensory epithelia and their overlying acellular gels, is defective in autosomal recessive deafness DFNB22. *Proc Natl Acad Sci U S A* 99, 6240-5.

13

Genetic Hearing Loss Associated with Craniofacial Abnormalities

S. Lunardi[1,2], F. Forli[3], A. Michelucci[4], A. Liumbruno[3], F. Baldinotti[4], A. Fogli[4], V. Bertini[4], A. Valetto[4], B. Toschi[4], P. Simi[4], A. Boldrini[1], S. Berrettini[3] and P. Ghirri[1,2]

University Hospital of Pisa, Pisa

Italy

1. Introduction

It is estimated that hereditary hearing loss accounts for 60% of deafness in the developed countries. About 30% of hereditary hearing impairment is syndromic which involves other presenting abnormalities along with deafness. There are more than 400 syndromes which include various degrees of hearing impairment with different phenotypes. (Barlow Stewart et al., 2007; Berrettini et al., 2008). Abnormalities of different systems or suggestive clinical findings have been associated with syndromic hearing loss. These include craniofacial malformations, dental abnormalities, ocular abnormalities, renal defects, cardiac abnormalities, endocrine dysfunction, neurologic dysfunction, skeletal abnormalities, integumentary abnormalities, metabolic disease, chromosomal abnormalities.

Treacher Collins, Goldenhar and Charge syndrome, Pierre Robin sequence, Stickler, Apert, Crouzon, Pfeiffer and velocardiofacial syndrome are just few conditions in which hearing loss is associated with craniofacial abnormalities. Most of these conditions are related to first and second branchial arches development abnormalities. The first and second branchial arches contribute to the development of skeletal (e.g. mandibula, maxilla, middle ear ossicules), muscular (facial muscles) and nervous (e.g. facial nerve) structures of the face. That explains why, due to the abnormal development of first and second branchial arches, midface malformations are usually the typical findings in these patients. (Gorlin et al., 1995; Johnson et al., 2011)

We describe some of these disorders underlining the main characteristic impairments and the observed hearing loss. We also report our observations on some clinical cases seen at Neonatology Unity of Santa Chiara University Hospital of Pisa (Table 2).

---

[1]*Neonatology Unit and NICU, Italy*

[2]*Section of Neonatal Endocrinology and Dysmorphology, Mother and Child Department, Italy*

[3]*Division of ENT, Department of Neuroscience, Italy*

[4]*Cytogenetics and Molecular Genetics Unit, Mother and Child Department, Italy*

2. Clinical syndromes

2.1 Goldenhar syndrome

Hemifacial microsomia (or Goldenahr syndrome or oculo-auricolar-vertebral syndrome) is usually a sporadic disorder even if there is evidence of familial transmission. In some cases autosomal recessive and autosomal dominant inheritance have also been described. The incidence of Goldenhar syndrome is reported to be approximately 1 in 5,000-25,000 live births (Editorial Team Orphanet, 2005). Genetic heterogenity is frequently observed . Kelberman et al performed a genome search for linkage in two families with features of hemifacial microsomia and identified data highly suggestive of linkage to a region of approximately 10.7 cM on chromosome 14q32 for one family (Kelberman et al., 2001).

During embryogenesis the correct development of the 1st or the 2nd branchial arches are hypothesized to be interrupted resulting in Goldenhar Syndrome. Clinical features mainly consist of a hemifacial microsomia. Maxillary, temporal, malar and skull bones can also be involved. Auricular malformations range from mild abnormalities in the external ears (such as preauricular tags or pinnae hypoplasia of various degrees) to anotia. Vertebrae abnormalities (e.g. hemivertebrae and fused vertebrae) as well as facial cleft or ocular abnormalities (epibulbar dermoid, eyelid coloboma, microphtalmia, retinal anomalies) are described. Mouth opening can be modified by mandibular hypoplasia. Congenital heart diseases of various degrees (e.g. ventricular septal defect of Tetralogy of Fallot) or a wide range of CNS malformations can be associated too. Bony involvement can cause weakness of cranial nerves. Mental retardation is described in 5-15% patients. Kidney, pulmonary or gastrointestinal abnormalities can also be associated less frequently. (OMIM 164210; Toriello et al., 2004)

Hearing loss in Goldenhar syndrome usually ranges from mild to moderate conductive impairment and severe to profound sensorineural hearing loss (Skarzynski et al., 2009). Deformity of the auricle, external auditory canal atresia and malformation of the tympanic cavity or ossicles may be the main cause of conductive hearing impairment. Abnormalities of the stria vascularis and the semicircular canals have also been reported (Scholtz et al., 2001). Sensorineural hearing loss and facial nerve disfunction is often underestimated. In the study by Carvalho et al (Carvalho et a.l, 1999) 11% of the patients with Hemifacial microsomia had sensorineural hearing loss.

2.2 Charge syndrome

In 1981 Pagon et al. first introduced the acronym "CHARGE" to define a nonrandom association of the following features: **C**oloboma, **H**eart defect, **A**tresia choanae, **R**etarded growth and development, **G**enital hypoplasia and **E**ar anomalies/deafness.

Charge syndrome (OMIM 214800) is a rare disorder with an incidence of about 1 in every 8500–10000 births (Issekutz et al., 2005). CHARGE syndrome is an autosomal dominant disorder. Mutations in *CHD7* have been detected in more than 75% of CHARGE patients. *CHD7* belongs to the gene family coding for ChromodomainHelicase DNA binding proteins. During early human development, *CHD7* is expressed in the undifferentiated neuroepithelium and in mesenchyme of neural crest origin. It is thought to play a role in regulating the expression of important developmental genes in mesenchymal cells derived from the cephalic neural crest, by chromatin remodeling. The phenotype of CHARGE syndrome can also be caused by mutation in the semaphorin-3E gene. (Michelucci et al., 2010).Patients with Charge syndrome have a typical square-flattened face, usually asymmetric, with a bulbous nasal tip, long philtrum, low-set and dysplastic ears, antimongoloid slant of palpebral fissures, anteverted nares and malar hypoplasia. Ptosis and cleft lip or palate can also be associated findings. (OMIM 214800). Based on Blake et al definition, individuals with all four major characteristics (the classical 4C's: Choanal atresia, Coloboma, Characteristic ears and Cranial nerve anomalies) or three major and three minor characteristics (Cardiovascular malformations, Genital hypoplasia, Cleft lip/palate, Tracheoesophageal fistula, Distinctive CHARGE facies, Growth deficiency, Developmental delay) are highly likely to have CHARGE syndrome. Nevertheless any infant with one or two major criteria and several minor characteristics is highly suspected to have CHARGE. (Blake et al). Based on Verloes criteria the presence of three major findings (Coloboma of the iris or choroid, with or without microphthalmia, Atresia of Choanae, Hypoplastic semi-circular Canals) are necessary and sufficient to make a diagnosis of CHARGE, even if no other features are present. Patients with "borderline phenotypes" are classified in two groups: partial (or incomplete) CHARGE and atypical CHARGE. Partial CHARGE are those individuals who have two major signs but only one minor sign (minor signs for Verloes are Rhombencephalic dysfunction, Hypothalamo-hypophyseal dysfunction, Abnormal middle or external ear, Malformation of mediastinal organs, Mental retardation), whereas individuals with atypical CHARGE are those who have two major signs and no minor sign, or one major sign and at least three minor signs of CHARGE. (Verloes et al., 2005) Coloboma is uni-lateral or bilateral, involving iris, retina and/or disc.

Heart defects in CHARGE syndrome are mainly conotruncal defects or aortic arch anomalies. Urinary defects range from abnormalities of kidney (or genitourinary tract) size or position to renal agenesis, genital hypoplasia, which is typically recognized only in males (micropenis/cryptorchidism). Almost every part of the audiologic system can be involved in Charge association. External ears are typically low-set and malformed. Unusually shaped and floppy external Pinnae can cause difficulties in placing behind-ear- hearing aids. Ear canals may be stenotic. The most common audiological features are severe-to-profound asymmetric mixed losses. (Edwards et al., 2002). Ossicular anomalies (eg stapes or incus abnormalities), absence of oval window or absence of the stapedium muscle and middle ear effusion (eustachian tube dysfunction from craniofacial malformation is a common finding) cause conductive hearing loss which is often asymmetrical and fluctuating in nature, usually greater on low frequencies. (Dhooge et al., 1998) . Cochlear malformations such as Mondini's Displasia can contribute to hearing loss. Cochlear involvement is greatest for high frequencies (Thelin et al., 1986). Abnormalities of the semicircular canals can be found in most patients (Morimoto et al., 2006). Auditory neural pathway abnormalities (such as hypoplasia or absence of the auditory nerve) may be involved as well.

2.3 Pierre Robin sequence

This condition is commonly defined Pierre Robin "sequence" instead of "syndrome" because the major clinical features have a common origin. The mandibular hypoplasia starts being evident in the first period of gestation and causes an anomalous position of the tongue. This prevents the correct development of the palate. At birth micrognathia, glossoptosis and cleft palate are the main signs. Consequently, respiratory, feeding and swallowing problems are the major problems in these patients. (Evans et al., 2011)

Pierre Robin sequence is usually a sporadic event with an estimated prevalence of about 1/10.000. In about 10% of patients a familial transmission has been described although the involved genes have not been identified.

Hearing loss is typically conductive and bilateral patients with Pierre Robin sequence. In Middle ear effusion is a finding in most patients. Therefore the use of tympanostomy (ventilation) tubes is the therapy of choice in patients with Pierre Robin Sequence. In a study by Handzic et al the mean hearing loss at speech frequencies was 24.5 dB (Handzić J et al., 1995, 1996). Pierre Robin Sequence is also a risk factor for sensorineural Hearing Loss: the 30% of the Pierre Robin patients in a study (Medard et al., 1999) had congenital permanent sensorineural evolutive hearing loss.

Another study revealed multiple architectural anomalies involving the entire ear such as abnormal auricles or ossicles, aplasia of the lateral semicircular canals or a large vestibual aqueduct (Gruen et al., 2005).

2.4 Stickler syndrome

Stickler syndrome affects about 1 in every 7.500/9.000 newborns. Mutations in the *COL2A1, COL9A1, COL11A1*, and *COL11A2* genes impairing collagen production have been identified as the cause of this disorder. Except for *COL9A1* mutations which are transmitted in an autosomal recessive fashion, the syndrome is autosomal dominantly inherited. The affected patients show a typical long and flat face with malar and mandibular hypoplasia (midface hypoplasia). The nose is small with a depressed nasal bridge and anteverted nares. The flatness of the face gives the appearance of large eyes. Vision is altered: myopia, cataracts, glaucoma and retinal detachment can be some of the associated findings. Cleft palate, bifid uvula and macroglossia may also occur.

Joint problems are presented by the patients from an early age. This involves arthritis which causes joint pain and stiffness. Flattened vertebrae and spine deformity such as scoliosis or kyphosis vertebral may also be present. Additionally, the prevalence of mitral valve prolapse in this syndrome has been reported to be higher than that in the general population.

Hearing loss can be both sensorineural and conductive. The conductive hearing loss in Stickler syndrome type I (*COL2A1*) can be due to the stapedial fixation. It can therefore be improved by stapes surgery. (Baijens et al., 2004)

Mutations in the fibrillar collagen genes *COL11A1* and *COL11A2* can cause sensorineural hearing loss probably due to the essential role these two genes have in the function of the basilar or tectorial membranes. There seems to be a correlation of hearing loss severity, onset, progression and affected frequencies with the underlying mutated collagen gene (Shpargel et al, 2004). In the study by Admiraal et al the mean sensorineural hearing threshold in Stickler patients with *COL11A2* mutation was about 40 dB HL and was liable to increase at the highest frequencies. (Admiraal et al., 2000)

In the study conducted by Szymko-Bennett (Szymko-Bennett et al., 2001) most of the 46 adults with Stickler syndrome had a sensorineural hearing loss, affecting high frequencies. Additionally, hearing loss was not more progressive as compared to age-related hearing loss.

2.5 Brachio-Oto-renal (BOR) syndrome

Branchio-oto-renal syndrome (OMIM 113650) is a genetic condition with a prevalence of 1/40.000 births and has an autosomal dominant mode of inheritance. *EYA1, SIX1,* and *SIX5* are three genes which are known to be mutated in this syndrome. The syndrome is called "Branchio-oto-renal" because malformations of the second branchial arch are associated with ears and renal abnormalities. The face is typically long and narrow with a constricted palate. (Alkis et al., 2002)Kidney and urinary tract show various degree of involvement. Shape or position abnormalities can be isolated or associated with an impaired renal function. Abnormalities in the development of the second branchial arch lead to neck malformations such as branchial cleft, cysts or fistulae.

Auditory system involvement ranges from pinnae abnormalities such as microtia, abnormally shaped ears, pre-auricular tags or pits to inner ear or middle ear malformations leading to sensorineural, conductive or mixed hearing loss. Hearing impairment occurs in 75%-93% of patients with BOR syndrome and ranges from mild to profound. Age of onset varies from early childhood to adult age. Younger patients manifest greater threshold fluctuation. Inner and middle ear anomalies ranges from cochlear hypoplasia, semicircular canals hypoplasia, ossicular anomalies, external auditory canal stenosis or atresia, vestibular displasia, enlarged aqueductus or endolymphatic sac (the last seems to predispose to more severe hearing impairment), absence of stapedium muscle or Eustachian tube dilation and cochlear nerve deficiency. (Huang et al., 2011; Kemperman et al., 2004)

2.6 Treacher-Collins syndrome

Treacher Collins syndrome (TCS) is an autosomal dominant disorder of craniofacial development with an incidence of 1 in 50.000 live births. It shows genetic heterogeneity: Treacher Collins syndrome-1 (TCS-1) (OMIM 154500) is caused by a heterozygous mutation in *TCOF-1* located on chromosome 5q32 (Wise et al., 1997). Treacher Collins syndrome-2 (OMIM 613717) is caused by an heterozygous mutation in *POLR1D* on chromosome 5q3213q12.2, while TCS-3 (OMIM 248390) is caused by an heterozygous mutation in the *POLR1C* gene on chromosome 6. However, about 60% of TCS patients have *de novo* gene mutations. Some authors hypothesize that these genetic mutations lead to an aberrant expression of a nuclear protein critically required during human craniofacial development.

Facial abnormalities are usually bilateral in TCS. They involve facial bones showing zygomatic arches hypoplasia, hypoplasia of supraorbital rims and micrognathia. The face is narrow with an antimongoloid slant of the eyes and hypertelorism. Coloboma of the lower lid can be present with deficiency of cilia medial to the coloboma. Ophthalmologic defects such as vision loss or refractive errors require specialistic evaluation: Preauricular hair displacement is a typical finding.

External ear show abnormalities ranging from various degree of pinnae malformations to microtia. About 40-50% of the patients with Treacher Collins have conductive **hearing loss** (often compounded by a high-frequency sensory component) mainly caused by hypoplasia of the middle ear or malformations of the ossicles. Inner ear is usually normal. Pron et al. reported on the hearing loss and computerized tomography (CT) assessments of ear malformations in a large pediatric series of patients with Treacher Collins. Of the 23 subjects assessed the external ear abnormalities were largely symmetric, with a stenotic atresic canal. In most cases, the middle ear cavity was hypoplastic and dysmorphic with aberrants ossicles while inner ear structures were normal. The majority of patients had asymmetric conductive hearing loss of various degrees. Hearing loss was bilateral and mixed in three patients. (Pron et al., 1993; Jahrsdoerfer et al., 1995).

2.7 Apert syndrome

Apert syndrome (or Acrocephalosyndactyly) (OMIM 101200) occurs in about 1 every 65.000-88.000 newborns. It is usually sporadic but some familial cases with an autosomal dominant way of inheritance have been observed. Mutations in *FGFR2* (fibroblast growth factor receptor-2) increase the number of precursor cells involved in the osteogenic process leading to increased subperiosteal bone matrix and premature ossification. Consequent premature skull bone ossification leads to craniosynostosis (especially affecting the coronal sutures) which is the main clinical pattern in Apert syndrome (Rice et al., 2008). Patients with this condition have a typical back to front flat skull with frontal bossing which is longer than usual. Eyes are wide set and the midface is typically hypoplastic with a retrusion of supraorbital wings which make proptosis evident, eyebrows interruption, a beaked nose and a small upper jaw causing crowded upper teeth projecting back to the lower teeth.

Cranial abnormalities are quite directly related to brain development: mental status ranges from normal intelligence to various degree of mental retardation. Hydrocephalus and malformations of corpum callosum or septum pellucidum are common findings. Craniofacial abnormalities are associated to finger or toes webbing: syndactyly of at least three finger or three toes typically involves bones structure. When vertebral abnormalities occur, C5-C6 fusion is typically observed. Hyperhidrosis is frequently reported as is also skin with acne.

Vision and auditory problems are usual findings in Apert syndrome.

Hearing loss is a common diagnosis in these patients. The conductive hearing loss, usually bilateral, may be due to ossicular chain fixation or otitis media with effusion. Hearing loss is rarely present at birth. In about 50% of the cases hearing loss is acquired by the age of 20. It ranges from mild to moderate, predominantly affecting the lower frequencies. The incidence of congenital hearing loss is low (3–6%) (Rajenderkumar et al., 2005).

In a study by Zhou et al. hearing loss was found in 90% of the 20 pediatric patients with Apert syndrome and 80% of them had conductive hearing loss. Air-bone gaps were found at all frequencies, maximum at the low ones. Inner ear anomalies were found in all patients at CT scans of the temporal bones. The most frequent anomalies were dilated vestibule, malformed lateral semicircular canal and cochlear dysplasia (Zhou et al., 2009)

2.8 Crouzon syndrome

Crouzon syndrome (OMIM 123500) was first described in 1912 by Crouzon. It is a condition which is inherited in an autosomal dominant way. In Europe it occurs in 1 child every 50.000 live births. The syndrome is caused by mutation in the fibroblast growth factor receptor 2. Mutations in this gene lead to the production of an abnormal protein which overstimulates immature cells to form mature bone cells. The premature fusion of skull sutures causes the typical synostosis which begins in the first year of life and is completed by 2-3 years from birth. Different patterns of skull growth depend on which suture is mainly involved (Harroop et al., 2006; Kirman et al., 2005).Increased intracranial pressure can occur, mainly when treatment is delayed.

The face is typically huge with a high forehead, proptosis which causes external strabismus, hypertelorism, prognathism and hypoplastic upper jaw which leads to dental problems. The nose is usually beak shaped. Cleft lips or palate have sometimes been observed.

Hearing loss is mainly conductive and is due to auditory canal abnormalities such as middle ear effusions, intratympanic bony masses, ossicular or oval window malformations. Sensorineural hearing loss may rarely occur.

In the study by De Jong et al. mild or moderate hearing loss (mostly conductive) was found in 28.5% of patients with Crouzon syndrome (De Jong et al., 2011).

In the study by Orvidas et al 8 of the 19 patients with Crouzon syndrome had ear anomalies ranging from pinna malformations to auditory canal atresia while 10 had proper hearing impairment: in 4 of them conductive hearing loss was found (mainly due to ossicular fixation and otitis media) in 4 of them hearing loss was sensorineural while in 2 was mixed (Orvidas et al., 1999)

A particular variant of Crouzon syndrome caused by a mutation in *FGFR3* has been described in association to Acanthosis Nigrigans. In these patients hydrocephalus, coanal stenosis or atresia and Chiari malformation have been described. (Arnaud-López et al., 2007)

2.9 Pfeiffer syndrome

Crouzon syndrome and Pfeiffer syndrome (OMIM 101600) are allelic disorders with overlapping features. Pfeiffer syndrome is an autosomal dominant condition which occurs in 1 every 100.000 live births. It is caused by mutations in *FGFR1* or *FGFR2* which cause prolonged signaling which over stimulates premature cells in the developing embryo. This causes the premature fusion of skull bones. Early fusion of the coronal and lambdoid sutures and occasionally of the sagittal sutures leads to an abnormal skull shape.

The face is usually broad with midface hypoplasia, prognatism, high forehead, flat occiput, hypertelorism and swallowing orbits which cause proptosis. Upperways obstruction can follow midface hypoplasia and nasal obstruction (Vogels et al., 2006).

Skull malformation is associated to limb abnormalities such as short and broad deviating thumbs, big toes and syndactyly of the second and third fingers.

Three different subtypes of this condition have been described. In type 1 patients, mild skull and facial abnormalities such as brachycephaly and midface hypoplasia are associated with fingers and toes malformations while neurological development is usually normal. In type 2 patients trilobated skull deformity is associated with neurological problems such as underdeveloped brain or increased intracranial pressure. Proptosis is evident and causes visual problems. Other limb defects such as elbow ankylosis are associated to fingers and toes abnormalities. Kidney malformations can also occur. Type 3 patients are similar to type 2 patients without cloverleaf skull.

Otologic malformations and **hearing loss** are common features in Pfeiffer syndrome. They are mainly due to external auditory canal or middle ear malformation. For example atresic or stenotic auditory canal, hypoplasic ossicules or fixed ossicular chain, hypoplasic or enlarged middle ear cavity can be common findings. The inner ear is usually normal though an enlarged internal acoustic meatus may be present. (Cremers et al., 1981)

In a study by Vallino et al. hearing loss, mostly moderate to severe, was present in eight of the nine patients with Pfeiffer syndrome. Seven patients had conductive hearing loss and one had mixed loss (Vallino-Napoli et al., 1996).

Sensorineural hearing loss is less common and may be related to the effect of *FGFR* mutations on cranial nerve or inner-ear development. (Desai et al., 2010)

2.10 Saethre-Chotzen syndrome

This is a genetic condition with an incidence which ranges from 1:25.000 to 1:50.000 births (OMIM 101400). It is inherited in an autosomal dominant way and it is caused by mutation of *TWIST1*. Patients with Saethre-Chotzen syndrome typically show an abnormal fusion in the skull's bones causing the typical appearance: brachycephaly, low frontal hair line, flattened nasofrontal angle with a beaked nose, widely spaced eyes, ptosis, facial asymmetry. Fingers and Toes defects such as mild syndactyly and a broad or duplicated thumb or hallux are typical; vertebral anomalies and short stature can also be associated.

Mild external ear anomalies can be additional findings. The hearing defect is usually conductive (Clauser et al., 2004) and can be due to stapes ankylosis, fixed ossicular chain, microtia or enlarged vestibules (sometimes associated to a small epitympanum and small or even absent mastoids) (Ensink et al., 1996). Mixed hearing loss due to brain stem anomalies has also been described (Lamonica et al., 2010).

2.11 Townes-Brocks syndrome

Townes-Brocks syndrome (OMIM 107480) is a genetic condition showing an incidence of about 1 in 250.000 live births. It is caused by mutations in *SALL1* causing abnormal production of transcription factors. It is inherited in an autosomal dominant pattern. Patients with this syndrome typically show the triad: anus imperforatus (in about the 82% of the patients) with rectovaginal or rectoperineal fistula, external ear anomalies (85%) usually associated with thumbs malformation (89%) such as thumb duplication or hypoplasia.

In 65%of cases sensorineural or conductive hearing loss are part of the clinical presentation. External ear anomalies range from overfolded superior helices which cause the typical satyr form, to microtia, preauricolar tags or pits and can be associated to middle ear anomalies (e.g. ossicular abnormalities, hypoplastic malleus head and abnormally shaped oval window andincus. (Toriello et al., 2004; Powell et al., 1999). The hearing loss is predominantly sensorineural and slowly progressive (from mild during early childhood to moderate in early adulthood), it affects high-frequency thresholds more than the low-frequency ones and has a variable, but usually small, conductive component. (Rossmiller et al., 1994)

Renal and genitourinary abnormalities, congenital heart disease, foot malformation and mental retardation have also been described in Townes-Brocks syndrome.

2.12 Miller syndrome

Miller syndrome or postaxial acrofacial dysostosis (OMIM 263750) is a rare condition which affects fewer than 1 in 1 million of newborns. It has an autosomal recessive mode of inheritance. Mutations in *DHODH* cause this syndrome disrupting the development of the first and second pharyngeal arch. Patients with this syndrome typically show craniofacial abnormalities such as malar hypoplasia, micrognathia, down-slanting eyes with drooping of the lower eyelids (which becomes more evident with age) and coloboma, cleft palate, long philtrum and small, protruding "cup-shaped" ears.

Craniofacial abnormalities are associated with limb defects such as syndactyly, hypoplasia or absence of fingers or toes (eg the fifth digits), hypoplasia of forearms or lower legs.

Extra nipples, vertebrae or ribs deformities have been described while abnormalities of the heart, kidneys, genitalia, or gastrointestinal tract are less common.

Hearing loss is usually caused by defects in the middle ear (various degree conductive hearing loss). (Toriello et al., 2004)

2.13 Nager acrofacial dysostosis

Nager syndrome (OMIM 154400) is a rare condition (about 70 cases have been described) and the involved genes are unknown. Both autosomal and recessive cases have been described. Facial malformation is associated with limbs abnormalities. The face shows maxillar hypoplasia and micrognatia. The eyes have typical downslanting fissures with ptosis of the upper lids, lack or absence of the lower eyelashes and occasionally coloboma of the lower lids.

Ears can show various degree of malformations which range from abnormal positioning to microtia. Auditory canal or middle ear can be involved leading to conductive **hearing loss**. Otitis media is a common problem. In a study by Herrmann et al. 8 over 10 patients with Nager syndrome had pure conductive hearing loss (> 30 db HL in 90% of cases, between 55 and 70 dB HL in 40% of patients) while in 2 cases hearing impairment was mixed. In the last two cases the sensorineural deficit was progressive and developed later in childhood. A Choleasteatoma has been described in some cases.

Limb malformations consist of hypoplasia or absence of radius, radioulnar synostosis, and hypoplasia or absence of the thumbs. Phocomelia is rare. Renal and genital abnormalities occasionally occur. (Opitz et al., 2003)

Syndrome	Main Clinical Features	Genetics	Hearing loss
Goldenhar syndrome	• Hemifacial microsomia • Auricular malformations • Vertebrae abnormalities • Facial cleft • Ocular abnormalities • Congenital heart diseases	Genetic heterogeneity	Ranges from mild to moderate conductive impairment and severe to profound sensorineural hearing loss

Syndrome	Main Clinical Features	Genetics	Hearing loss
Charge syndrome	• Choanal atresia • Coloboma • Characteristic ears • Cranial nerve anomalie • Cardiovascular malformations • Genital hypoplasia • Cleft lip/palate • Tracheoesophageal fistula • Growth deficiency • Developmental delay	Mutations in *CHD7* are detected in more than 75% of CHARGE patients	Severe-to-profound asymmetrical mixed losses.
Pierre Robin Sequence	• Micrognathia • Glossoptosis • Cleft palate	Genetic heterogeneity	Typically conductive and bilateral
Stickler syndrome	• Long and flat face • Malar and mandibular hypoplasia • Small nose with a depressed nasal bridge and anteverted nares • Altered vision • Joint problems	Mutations in *COL2A1*, *COL9A1*, *COL11A1*, and *COL11A2* genes	Both sensorineural and conductive
BOR syndrome	• Branchial cleft, cysts or fistulae • Ear abnormalities • Kidney abnormalities	*EYA1*, *SIX1*, and *SIX5* mutations	Sensorineural, conductive or mixed hearing loss
Treacher-Collins syndrome	• Zygomatic arches hypoplasia • Hypoplasia of supraorbital rims • Micrognathia • Narrow face • Antimongoloid slant of the eyes and hypertelorism • Coloboma of the lower lid with deficiency of cilia medial to the coloboma • Large nose is with hypoplastic alae • Down-turning mouth • Cleft palate • External ear abnormalities	Genetic heterogeneity: TCS-1, TCS-2 and TCS- 3 have been related to mutations in *TCOF-1*, *POLR1D* and *POLR1C* respectively	About 40-50% of patients with Treacher Collins have conductive hearing loss. Few cases of mixed hearing loss have been described.
Apert syndrome	• Craniosynostosis • Frontal bossing • Wide set eyes • Hypoplastic midface	*FGFR2* mutations	Mild to moderate conductive hearing loss

Syndrome	Main Clinical Features	Genetics	Hearing loss
Crouzon syndrome	• Proptosis • Small upper jaw • Syndactyly • Synostosis • High forehead • Proptosis • External strabismus • Hypertelorism • Prognathism • Hypoplastic upper jaw	*FGFR2*	Conductive hearing loss
Saethre-Chotzen syndrome	• Brachycephaly • Low frontal hair line • Flattened nasofrontal angle • Widely spaced eyes • Ptosis • Facial asymmetry • Syndactyly • Broad or duplicated thumb or hallux	*TWIST1*	Conductive or mixed
Pfeiffer syndrome	• Broad face is midface hypoplasia • Prognatism • High forehead, flat occiput, hypertelorism • Swallowing orbits which cause proptosis • Skull malformation • Limb abnormalities	*FGFR1* & *FGFR2*	Conductive
Townes-Brock syndrome	• Anus imperforatus • Rectovaginal • Rectoperineal fistula • External ear anomalies • Thumbs malformation	It is caused by mutations in *SALL1*	Sensorineural or conductive hearing loss
Miller syndrome	• Malar hypoplasia • Micrognathia • Down-slanting eyes • Coloboma • Cleft palate • Limb defects	*DHODH*	Conductive hearing loss- mainly due to anomalies of middle ear
Nager syndrome	• Limbs abnormalities • Maxillar hypoplasia • Micrognatia	Not known	Conductive or mixed hearing loss

Table 1. Main craniofacial syndromes associated with hearing loss

3. Imaging

Imaging studies of middle and inner ear are required for better management of the craniofacial syndromes. They are necessary for a correct diagnosis of anatomical aberrations and for the planning of the surgical intervention.

MRI is the first-choice of imaging technique for craniofacial syndromes, midface masses and brain abnormalities; it is important in showing the anatomy of the brain and the soft tissue structures and in detecting any associated cerebral malformations.

	Case 1	Case 2	Case 3	Case 4
Gender	M	M	F	F
Family History	First son of a non-consaguineous gypsy couple. The mother was 17-yrs old and father was 18. Un-remarkable family history.	Unremarkable family history. Non-consaguineous parents.	Unremarkable family history. Non-consaguineous parents.	High percentage of in-utero deaths in mother's family history.
Gravidic History	No exposure to known teratogens during pregnancy. Gravidic history was unremarkable until 34 weeks of GA when a spontaneous vaginal delivery occurred	Pregnancy was complicated by polhydramnios	Unremarkable gravidic history	Unremarkable gravidic history
Neonatal Outcome	Soon after the delivery, the newborn required ventilation support because of bradycardia, irregular breathing, hypotonia, and hyporeactivity	Term delivery at 42 weeks of gestational age (GA)	Spontaneous vaginal delivery at 41 weeks of GA. At birth ventilation support was required because of bradycardia and irregular breathing.	Spontaneous vaginal delivery at 41 weeks of GA
Physical Examination	The weight at birth was 2035 g (10th-25th percentile), length was 46,5 cm (50th -75th),	Birth Weight 3400 g (10th-50th percentile); Birth length 50 cm (10th-50th). He had bilateral	At birth she weighed 2680 g (3th-10th centile), length was 47 cm (3th-10th), and her head circumference was 33.5 cm (10th-50th). She was pale and had petecchiae at	At birth she weighed 2670 g (3th-10th percentile). She showed hyperemic and

	Case 1	Case 2	Case 3	Case 4
Gender	M	M	F	F
	and head circumference was 29.5 cm (3 th percentile). He had microcephaly and trigonocephaly, prominent forehead, flat occiput, narrow palpebral fissures, big and rounded nose with hypoplasic alae, small mouth, with the inferior dental arch lying behind the superior one, low-set ears, micropenis, talipes and metatarsus varus. A single umbical artery was found.	coloboma, atresia of the right choana, characteristic external ears and hypoplasia of the cochlea. Characteristic facial features with square-shaped facies, narrow bifrontal diameter, broad nasal bridge, small mouth and inverted V-shaped upper lip. He had bilateral cryptorchidism, hypoplastic genitalia and orofacial cleft	upper limbs, neck, head, axillae and inguinal region. She showed mild hypotonia and characteristic facial features: plagiocephaly, with flat occiput, frontal bossing, head bent to the left, left eyelid ptosis; thin upper lip with long filtrum and short tongue frenulum. Clinodactily of the fifth fingers. Bilteral shortness of ulna and radius with carpal bones relatively longer than fore-arm. Mild enlargement of cardiac profile.	edematous eyelids and atresia of the left choana, Characteristic facial features: hypertelorism, bilateral frontal bossing, large anterior fontanel, bilateral hypoplasic elix and low-set ears, right eye ptosis, rounded nose with flat origin, hypoplasic alae and micrognatia. The fifth finger was bilateral curved with nails abnormalities.
Main problems	Breathing problems and chronic tirage due to laryngomalacia was found. Feeding difficulties (poor sucking, gastric stagnation, regurgitation, vomiting) with subsequent failure to thrive due to gastro-oesophageal reflux and hypertrophic pyloric stenosis surgically	Transposition of the great arteries surgically corrected during the first week of life. At 21 months growth deficiency was apparent. He showed delayed motor milestones, hypotonia, and delayed development of social and emotional skills. He was fed via percutaneous endoscopic	Low platelets count (16.000/mmc). Cranial USS showed mild dilation of lateral ventricles, hyperechogenic areas in the basal ganglia and candelabrum-like appearance of the thalamus. Echocardiography showed mild increasing pulmonary transvalvular gradient and atrial septum defect (ostium secundum). Growth deficiency with delayed motor milestones and delayed development of social and emotional skills	Growth deficiency with delayed motor milestones and delayed development of social and emotional skills were apparent

	Case 1	Case 2	Case 3	Case 4
Gender	M	M	F	F
	treated at 7 months of age. Echocardiogram showed pulmonary valve stenosis. Brain magnetic resonance imaging (BMRI) revealed dysmature brain in a trigonocephalic skull.	gastrostomy (PEG) from the age of 4 months and required surgery for gastroesophageal reflux. He also required a tracheostomy between ages of 2 and 5 months.		
Hearing Loss	Bilateral sensorineural hypoacusia: average threshold of 50 dB HL on the right side and 70 dB HL on the left side (2000-4000 Hz)	Moderate bilateral sensorineural hypoacusia (bilateral average threshold of 55 dB on the left and 45 dB HL on the right at 2000-4000 Hz).	Profound bilateral sensorineural hypoacusia (bilateral average threshold above 80 dB at 2000-4000 Hz)	Sensorineural bilateral hypoacusia (bilateral average threshold above 90 dB on the left and 75 dB HL on the right at 2000-4000 Hz). Partially corrected by a Cochlear implant.
Genetic Findings	High resolution chromosome analysis on PHA-cultured lymphocyte pointed out a male karyotype with a partial 5q duplication and pericentric inversion of chromosome 9 (46,XY, inv9qh, dup(5)(q11.2-q13). Parents did not authorize any cytogenetic studies on themselves	The patient met all the four major and six minor Blake criteria for CHARGE syndrome. Direct sequencing of exon 2 of CHD7 gene revealed the presence of a nonsense mutation: a C→T transition at the nucleotide 925 (c.925C>T) causing a premature stop codon (p.Q309X).	Chromosome analysis revealed a female karyotype with a chromosome deriving from a paternal traslocation: 46XX-11,+der11t(6;11) (11pter→11q24.2::6p22.3→6pter). CGH array revealed a microduplication at region 6pter → 6p22.3 in the short arm of chromosome 6 and a microdeletion at the region 11q24.2 →11qter in the long arm of chromosome 11.	Genetic studies showed a female Karyotype with an interstitial deletion at the long arm of chromosome 9. CGH-Array and FISH pointed out a 10 Mb de novo interstitial deletion in the regionq31.1-9q31.3.

Table 2. Some clinical cases observed at Neonatology Unity of Santa Chiara University Hospital of Pisa

CT (best of all three dimensional CT) is the referral technique for studying syndromes of the first and second branchial arch: the resolution provided by this technique for the fine bony craniofacial structures is unmatched by other modalities. It is useful for example in diagnosing early suture fusion and in detecting any underlying abnormality of the brain. It is also useful when choanal stenosis or pyriform cavity or nasolacrimal ductus abnormalities are present as well as when anomalies of the temporal bone, osseous labyrinth, or internal and external acoustic canal are involved. The choice between techniques depends on the anatomical or functional damage which causes the hearing loss but often only the combined use of MRI and CT is able to give a complete imaging of craniofacial malformations. (Lowe et al., 2000; Johnson et al., 2001; Tokumaru et al., 2006)

4. Conclusion

The knowledge of clinical characteristics of syndromes is still the first and most important step for reaching a correct diagnosis. The clinical appearance leads the clinician to suggest various genetic tests to make a definitive diagnosis. Although many syndromes with craniofacial malformations and hearing loss are known, there are many patients with craniofacial abnormalities and deafness whose disorder cannot be currently classified into any syndrome (Table 2). These patients may have detectable genetic aberrations (e.g. chromosomal abnormalities such as deletions or duplications). The imaging aid to the diagnosis and for intervention in hearing loss associated with these syndromes is certain. The choice between CT o MRI depends on the anatomical/functional damage which causes the hearing.

5. References

Admiraal RJ, Brunner HG, Dijkstra TL, Huygen PL, Cremers CW.Hearing loss in the nonocular Stickler syndrome caused by a COL11A2 mutation. Laryngoscope. 2000 Mar;110(3 Pt 1):457-61

Ahmad N, Richards AJ, Murfett HC, Shapiro L, Scott JD, Yates JR, Norton J, Snead MP. Prevalence of mitral valve prolapse in Stickler syndrome. Am J Med Genet A. 2003 Jan 30;116A(3):234-7

Alkis M. Pierides, Yiannis Athanasiou, Kyproula Demetriou et al. A family with the branchio-oto-renal syndrome: clinical and genetic correlations. Nephrol Dial Transplant 2002; 17 (6): 1014-1018

Arnaud-López L, Fragoso R, Mantilla-Capacho J, Barros-Núñez P. Crouzon with acanthosis nigricans. Further delineation of the syndrome.Clin Genet. 2007 Nov;72(5):405-10.

Baijens LW, De Leenheer EM, Weekamp HH, Cruysberg JR, Mortier GR, Cremers CW. Stickler syndrome type I and Stapes ankylosis. Int J Pediatr Otorhinolaryngol. 2004 Dec;68(12):1573-80

Barlow-Stewart K and Mona Sale. Centre for Genetics Education . Deafness and Hearing Loss - Genetic Aspects. The Australasian Genetics Resource Book, 2007

Berrettini S. Linee guida per la conduzione dello screening audiologico neonatale nella Regione Toscana,.2008 http://www.fimp.org

Blake K D, Prasad Chitra. CHARGE syndrome. Orphanet Journal of Rare Diseases 2006, 1:34

Blake K.D., Davenport S.L., Hall B.D., Hefner M.A., Pagon R.A., Williams M.S., et al.,CHARGE association: an update and review for the primary paediatrician, Clin. Pediatr. (Phila.) 37 (1998) 159–173
Carvalho GJ, Song CS, Vargervik K, Lalwani AK.Auditory and facial nerve dysfunction in patients with hemifacial microsomia. Arch Otolaryngol Head Neck Surg. 1999 Feb;125(2):209-12
Clauser L et al. Saethre-Chotzen syndrome. Orphanet encyclopedia. July 2004
Cremers C W. Hearing loss in Pfeiffer's syndrome. Int J Pediatr Otorhinolaryngol 3(4):343-53 (1981)
De Jong T, Toll MS, de Gier HH, Mathijssen IM. Audiological profile of children and young adults with syndromic and complex craniosynostosis. Arch Otolaryngol Head Neck Surg. 2011 Aug;137(8):775-8.
Desai U, Rosen H, Mulliken JB, Gopen Q, Meara JG, Rogers GF. Audiologic findings in Pfeiffer syndrome. J Craniofac Surg. 2010 Sep;21(5):1411-8
Dhooge I, Lemmerling M, Lagache M, Standaert L, Govaert P, Mortier G. Otological manifestations of CHARGE association. Ann Otol Rhinol Laryngol. 1998;107:935–41
Editorial Team Orphanet, 2005. http://www.orpha.net
Edwards BM, Kileny PR, Van Riper LA. CHARGE syndrome: a window of opportunity for audiologic intervention. Pediatrics. 2002;110:119–26.
Ensink RJ, Marres HA, Brunner HG, Cremers CW. Hearing loss in the Saethre-Chotzen syndrome. J Laryngol Otol. 1996 Oct;110(10):952-7
Evans KN, Sie KC, Hopper RA, Glass RP, Hing AV, Cunningham ML. Robin sequence: from diagnosis to development of an effective management plan. Pediatrics. 2011 May;127(5):936-48. Epub 2011 Apr 4
Evidence of progression and fluctuation of hearing impairment in branchio-oto-renal syndrome. Int J Audiol. 2004 Oct;43(9):523-32
Gorlin RJ., Helga V. Toriello, Meyer Michael Cohen. Hereditary hearing loss and its syndromes. Oxford University Press,1995.
Gruen PM, Carranza A, Karmody CS, Bachor E. Anomalies of the ear in the Pierre Robin triad. Ann Otol Rhinol Laryngol. 2005 Aug;114(8):605-13
Handzić J, Bagatin M, Subotić R, Cuk V.Hearing levels in Pierre Robin syndrome. Cleft Palate Craniofac J. 1995 Jan;32(1):30-6
Handzić-Cuk J, Cuk V, Risavi R, Katić V, Katusić D, Bagatin M, Stajner-Katusić S, Gortan D.Pierre Robin syndrome: characteristics of hearing loss, effect of age on hearing level and possibilities in therapy planning. J Laryngol Otol. 1996 Sep;110(9):830-5
Harroop Kaur, Harmeet Singh Waraich and Chander Mohan Sharma.CLINICAL REPORT Crouzon syndrome: A case report and review of literature. INDIAN JOURNAL OF OTOLARYNGOLOGY AND HEAD & NECK SURGERY; 2006; Volume 58, Number 4, 381-382
Herrmann B W., Karzon R, Molter D W.. Otologic and audiologic features of Nager acrofacial dysostosis. International Journal of Pediatric Otorhinolaryngology, 2005; 69(vol 8): 1053-1059
Huang BY, Zdanski C, Castillo M. Pediatric Sensorineural Hearing Loss, Part 2: Syndromic and Acquired Causes. AJNR Am J Neuroradiol. 2011 May 19. [Epub ahead of print]
Issekutz K.A., Graham Jr J.M.., Prasad C., Smith I.M., Blake KD, An epidemiological analysis of CHARGE syndrome: preliminary results from a Canadian study, Am. J.Med. Genet. A 133 (2005) 309–317

Jahrsdoerfer RA, Jacobson JT.Treacher Collins syndrome: otologic and auditory management. J Am Acad Audiol. 1995 Jan;6(1):93-102
Johnson JM et al. Syndromes of the first and second branchial arches, part 1: embryology and characteristics defects- Am J Neuroradiol 32: 14-19; 2011
Johnson JM, G. Moonis, G.E. Green, R. Carmody, H.N. Burbank. Syndromes of the First and Second Branchial Arches, Part 1: Embryology and Characteristic Defects.Am J Neuroradiol 2011; 32:14 –19
Kelberman, D., Tyson, J., Chandler, D. C., McInerney, A. M., Slee, J., Albert, D., Aymat, A., Botma, M., Calvert, M., Goldblatt, J., Haan, E. A., Laing, N. G., Lim, J., Malcolm, S., Singer, S. L., Winter, R. M., Bitner-Glindzicz, M. Hemifacial microsomia: progress in understanding the genetic basis of a complex malformation syndrome. Hum. Genet. 109: 638-645, 2001
Kemperman MH, Koch SM, Kumar S, Huygen PL, Joosten FB, Cremers CW.
Kirman CN, Tran B, Sanger C, Railean S, Glazier SS, David LR.Difficulties of delayed treatment of craniosynostosis in a patient with Crouzon, increased intracranial pressure, and papilledema. J Craniofac Surg. 2011 Jul;22(4):1409-12.
Lamônica DA, Maximino LP, Feniman MR, Silva GK, Zanchetta S, Abramides DV, Passos-Bueno MR, Rocha K, Richieri-Costa A. Saethre-Chotzen Syndrome, Pro136His TWIST Mutation, Hearing Loss, and External and Middle Ear Structural Anomalies: Report on a Brazilian Family. Cleft Palate Craniofac J. 2010 Sep;47(5):548-52
Lowe Lisa H., Timothy N. Booth, Jeanne M. Joglar, Nancy K. Rollins. Midface Anomalies in Children. RadioGraphics 2000; 20:907–922
Medard C, François M, Narcy P. Hearing status of Robin sequence patients. Ann Otolaryngol Chir Cervicofac. 1999 Dec;116(6):317-21
Michelucci A, Ghirri P, Iacopetti P, Conidi M E, Fogli A, Baldinotti F, Lunardi S et al. Identification of three novel mutations in the CHD7 gene in patients with clinical signs of typical or atypical CHARGE syndrome International Journal of Pediatric Otorhinolaryngology 74 (2010) 1441–1444
Morimoto AK, Wiggins RH, Hudgins PA, Hedlund GL, Hamilton B, Mukherji SK, Telian SA, Harnsberger HR. Absent semicircular canals in CHARGE
OMIM 113650
Online Mendelian Inheritance in Man: 164210
Online Mendelian Inheritance in Man: 214800
Opitz JM. Acrofacial Dysostosis 1, Nager type. Orphanet Encyclopedia, May 2003
Orvidas LJ, Fabry LB, Diacova S, McDonald TJ. Hearing and otopathology in Crouzon syndrome. Laryngoscope. 1999 Sep;109(9):1372-5.
Powell CM, Michaelis RC.Townes-Brocks syndrome. J Med Genet 1999;36:89–9
Pron G, Galloway C, Armstrong D Posnick J. Ear Malformation and Hearing Loss in Patients with Treacher Collins Syndrome. The Cleft Palate-Craniofacial Journal: January 1993, Vol. 30, No. 1, pp. 97-103
Rajenderkumar D Bamiou, D-E, Sirimanna T. Audiological profile in Apert syndrome. Arch Dis Child 2005;90:592–593. doi: 10.1136/adc.2004.06729
Rice D P.. Craniofacial sutures: development, disease and treatment. Karger Publishers, 2008
Rossmiller DR, Pasic TR.Hearing loss in Townes-Brocks syndrome. Otolaryngol Head Neck Surg. 1994 Sep;111(3 Pt 1):175-80

Scholtz AW, Fish JH 3rd, Kammen-Jolly K, Ichiki H, Hussl B, Kreczy A, Schrott-Fischer A. Goldenhar's syndrome: congenital hearing deficit of conductive or sensorineural origin? Temporal bone histopathologic study. Otol Neurotol. 2001 Jul;22(4):501-5

Shpargel KB, Makishima T, Griffith AJ.Col11a1 and Col11a2 mRNA expression in the developing mouse cochlea: implications for the correlation of hearing loss phenotype with mutant type XI collagen genotype. Acta Otolaryngol. 2004 Apr;124(3):242-8

Skarzyński H, Porowski M, Podskarbi-Fayette R. Treatment of otological features of the oculoauriculovertebral dysplasia (Goldenhar syndrome). Int J Pediatr Otorhinolaryngol. 2009 Jul;73(7):915-21

Szymko-Bennett YM, Mastroianni MA, Shotland LI, Davis J, Ondrey FG, Balog JZ, Rudy SF, McCullagh L, Levy HP, Liberfarb RM, Francomano CA, Griffith AJ. Auditory dysfunction in Stickler syndrome. Arch Otolaryngol Head Neck Surg. 2001 Sep;127(9):1061-8

Thelin JW, Mitchell JA, Hefner MA, Davenport SL. CHARGE syndrome. Part II. Hearing loss. Int J Pediatr Otorhinolaryngol. 1986 Dec;12(2):145-63

Tokumaru Aya M., Barkovich A. James, Ciricillo Samuel F., and Edwards Michael S. B.. Skull Base and Calvarial Deformities: Association with Intracranial Changes in Craniofacial Syndromes. Am J Neuroradiol 1996; 17:619–630

Toriello HV, Reardon W, Gorlin R J. Hereditary Hearing Loss and Its Syndromes. Oxford University Press,2004

Vallino-Napoli LD. Audiologic and otologic characteristics of Pfeiffer syndrome.Cleft Palate Craniofac J. 1996 Nov;33(6):524-9

Verloes A. Updated Diagnostic Criteria for CHARGE Syndrome:A Proposal. American Journal of Medical Genetics 133A:306–308 (2005)

Vogels Annick and Fryns Jean-Pierre.Pfeiffer syndrome. Orphanet Journal of Rare Diseases 2006, 1:19

Wise CA, Chiang LC, Paznekas WA et al.TCOF1 gene encodes a putative nuclear phosphoprotein that exhibits mutations in Treacher Collins syndrome throughout its coding region. Proc Nat Acad Sci 94:3110-3115,1997

Zhou G, Schwartz LT, Gopen Q. Inner ear anomalies and conductive hearing loss in children with Apert syndrome: an overlooked otologic aspect. Otol Neurotol. 2009 Feb;30(2):184-9.

14

Usher Syndrome: Genes, Proteins, Models, Molecular Mechanisms, and Therapies

Jun Yang
Department of Ophthalmology and Visual Sciences, Moran Eye Center, University of Utah
USA

1. Introduction

Usher syndrome (USH) is an autosomal recessive genetic disease, characterized by both deafness and blindness. It was first described by Albrecht von Grafe, a German ophthalmologist, in 1858 (von Graefe, 1858) and then named after Charles Usher, a British ophthalmologist, who reported the inheritance of this disease on the basis of 69 cases in 1914 (Usher, 1914). USH is clinically heterogeneous and is categorized into three types, according to the severity of its hearing and vestibular symptoms (Smith et al., 1994; Petit, 2001). Type I (USH1) patients have congenital severe to profound deafness as well as vestibular dysfunction; Patients with USH2 exhibit congenital moderate degree of hearing loss and normal vestibular function; and those with USH3 display progressive hearing impairment and occasional vestibular dysfunction. The vision problem of all three types is manifested as retinitis pigmentosa (Hartong et al., 2006; Sadeghi et al., 2006; Fishman et al., 2007; Sandberg et al., 2008; Malm et al., 2011), showing early night and peripheral vision loss and eventual central vision loss.

USH is the most common genetic cause of combined blindness and deafness, occurring in about 1 in 23,000 people worldwide (Boughman et al., 1983; Keats and Corey, 1999; Hartong et al., 2006). It represents 50% of the blindness-deafness cases, 5% of all congenital deafness and 18% of retinitis pigmentosa (Millan et al., 2011). In Europe, USH1, USH2 and USH3 generally account for 25-44%, 56-75%, and 2% of all USH cases, respectively (Grondahl, 1987; Hope et al., 1997; Rosenberg et al., 1997; Spandau and Rohrschneider, 2002). Due to the regional founder effect, USH3 is much more common in Birmingham and Finland (Pakarinen et al., 1995; Hope et al., 1997). To date, there is no cure for this disease. USH patients mainly rely on early diagnosis and early education to adapt themselves to their dual sensory loss.

2. USH genes

USH is genetically diverse besides its clinical heterogeneity. Currently, eleven loci have been identified (Hereditary hearing loss homepage and Hmani-Aifa et al., 2009), and nine genes on these loci are known. Among these genes, five are involved in USH1, three in USH2 and one in USH3 (Reiners et al., 2006; Williams, 2008; Millan et al., 2011). Although the functions of some USH genes are relatively clear now in the inner ear (see section 6), extensive work is still necessary to elucidate the functions of USH genes in both the inner ear and the retina.

2.1 USH1 genes

In the past 20 years, seven loci have been assigned to USH1. They are *USH1B-H*. *USH1A* was first localized on 14a32.1 from a study in nine USH1 families in the Poitou-Charentes region of France, and was recently withdrawn due to the discovery that most of these families in fact carry mutations on the *USH1B* locus (Gerber et al., 2006). The genes underlying *USH1B*, *USH1C*, *USH1D*, *USH1F*, and *USH1G* have been identified as *MYO7A* (myosin VIIa) (Weil et al., 1995), *USH1C* (harmonin) (Bitner-Glindzicz et al., 2000; Verpy et al., 2000), *CDH23* (cadherin 23) (Bolz et al., 2001; Bork et al., 2001), *PCDH15* (protocadherin 15) (Ahmed et al., 2001; Alagramam et al., 2001b), and *USH1G* (SANS) (Weil et al., 2003), respectively. Among them, *MYO7A*, *USH1C*, *CDH23* and *PCDH15* are also the causative genes for nonsyndromic deafness, *DFNB2/DFNA11* (Liu et al., 1997; Weil et al., 1997), *DFNB18* (Ahmed et al., 2002), *DFNB12* (Bork et al., 2001), and *DFNB23* (Ahmed et al., 2003), respectively. The *USH1E* and *USH1H* loci were mapped to chromosome 21q21 and 15q22-23 (Chaib et al., 1997; Ahmed et al., 2009). However, the genes at these loci have not yet been pinpointed.

MYO7A is the most prevalent gene causing USH1 (Astuto et al., 2000). It encodes an unconventional actin-based motor protein with the conserved motor domain and five IQ motifs (Figure 1A). These domains are responsible for binding to actin, ATP, and myosin light chain. Therefore, MYO7A may move its cargos along the actin filaments using the energy generated from the hydrolysis of ATP. However, the motor domain of MYO7A shows a strong affinity to ADP and, thus, stays bound to actin filament for a long time (Heissler and Manstein, 2011). In this case, MYO7A may be involved in generating tensions between two proteins or cellular structures. The tail of MYO7A has a series of protein-protein interaction domains, including a single α-helix (SAH), a coiled-coil domain (CC), two myosin tail homology 4 domains (MyTH4), two band 4.1, ezrin, radixin, moesin domains (FERM), and a src homology 3 domain (SH3) (Figure 1A). These domains are thought to be engaged in binding to cargos and/or anchoring to proteins.

Harmonin (also known as AIE-75 or PDZ-73) is expressed in many different tissues (Kobayashi et al., 1999; Scanlan et al., 1999). Nine transcripts have so far been discovered (Verpy et al., 2000; Reiners et al., 2003). They are categorized into three groups, isoforms a, b and c (Figure 1B). All these isoforms have multiple PDZ (postsynaptic density 95; discs large; zonula occludens-1) domains and at least one CC domain. The CC domain is reported to participate in harmonin dimerization (Adato et al., 2005b), and the PDZ domain is well known to interact with PDZ-binding motifs (PBMs) in other proteins (Sheng and Sala, 2001). Isoform b specifically has a proline, serine and threonine-rich (PST) domain. This domain has been demonstrated to bind and bundle actin filaments (Boeda et al., 2002). In summary, harmonin may organize a multi-protein complex and attach this complex to actin filaments.

CDH23 and PCDH15 both have multiple transcripts and are grouped into isoforms a, b and c for CDH23 (Lagziel et al., 2005; Lagziel et al., 2009) and isoforms CD1, CD2, CD3 and SI for PCDH 15 (Ahmed et al., 2006) (Figures 1C and 1D). As the distant members of the classical cadherin superfamily, the proteins of these two genes have various repeats of extracellular cadherin (EC) domains in their extracellular regions. Accordingly, it has been proposed and supported by many studies in hair cells (see below) that the two proteins function in cell adhesion through their homophilic and heterophilic interactions. The two proteins probably anchor to the intracellular structures through the PBMs in their cytoplasmic regions (Figures 1C and 1D).

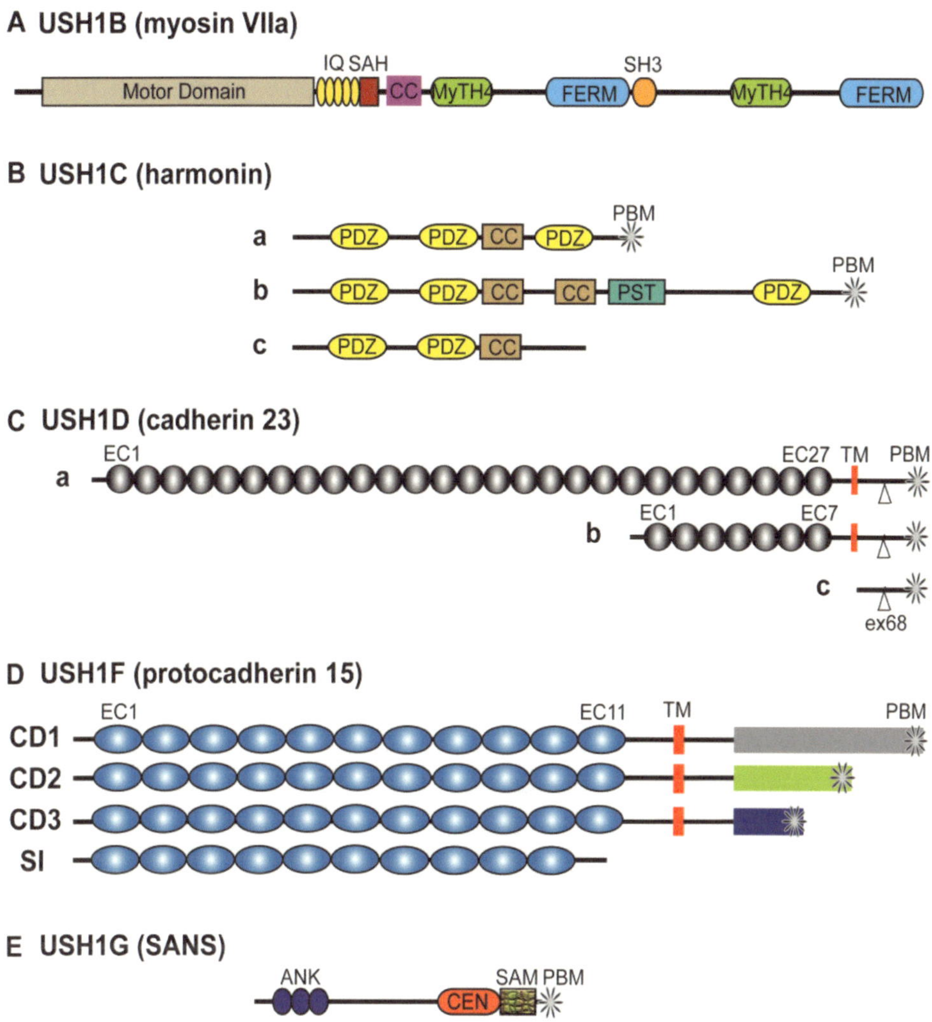

Fig. 1. Domain structures of USH1 proteins

Mutations in SANS are rare in USH1 patients. Some mutations, such as c.1373 A>T and c.163_164 + 13del15, cause the clinical symptoms close to USH2 (Kalay et al., 2005; Bashir et al., 2011). The protein of this gene consists of several putative protein-protein interaction domains, including three ankyrin -like (ANK) repeats, a central (CEN) domain, a sterile alpha motif (SAM) and a PBM (Figure 1E). Therefore, like harmonin, SANS is believed to be a putative scaffold protein.

2.2 USH2 genes

Four USH2 loci were originally defined, *USH2A-D*. The genes responsible for *USH2A*, *USH2C*, and *USH2D* are *USH2A* (usherin) (Eudy et al., 1998), *GPR98* (G Protein-coupled Receptor 98) (Weston et al., 2004), and *WHRN* (whirlin) (Ebermann et al., 2006), respectively. The gene for *USH2B* was once considered to be *NBC3* (sodium bicarbonate cotransporter)

(Bok et al., 2003). However, further study of the consanguineous Tunisian family carrying the *USH2B* locus demonstrates that mixed mutations in the *GPR98* and *PDE6B* genes are responsible for the disease manifestation in the family and, thus, the *USH2B* locus was withdrawn (Hmani-Aifa et al., 2009). Moreover, a novel USH2 locus has recently been localized on the chromosome 15q, though the underlying gene has not been identified so far (Ben Rebeh et al., 2008). '

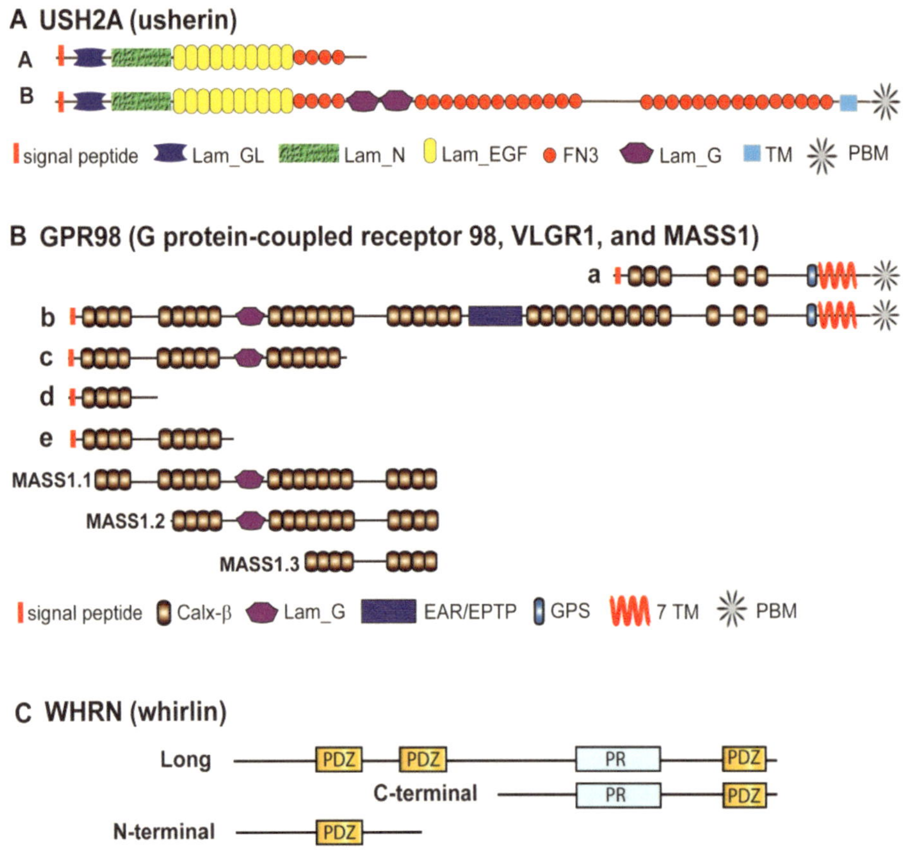

Fig. 2. Domain structures of USH2 proteins

USH2A is the most predominant causative gene in all USHs among different human ethnic populations (Eudy et al., 1998; Dreyer et al., 2000; Weston et al., 2000; Aller et al., 2004; van Wijk et al., 2004; Adato et al., 2005a; Hartong et al., 2006; Baux et al., 2007; Kaiserman et al., 2007; Dreyer et al., 2008; Nakanishi et al., 2009; Yan et al., 2009; McGee et al., 2010). Its mutations lead to a wide spectrum of vision and hearing defects in patients. Some *USH2A* mutations, such as p.C759F and p.G4674R, are known to cause only nonsyndromic retinitis pigmentosa (Rivolta et al., 2002; Seyedahmadi et al., 2004; Kaiserman et al., 2007). *USH2A* has 72 exons and is expressed as isoforms A and B (Figure 2A). Isoform B, the major isoform in the retina (Liu et al., 2007), is an extremely large transmembrane protein with 5202 amino acids (aa) in humans (van Wijk et al., 2004). Its long extracellular region has repeated various laminin (Lam) and fibronectin III (FN3) functional domains common in cell adhesion proteins and extracellular matrix proteins. Its cytoplasmic region has a PBM. Isoform A is an N-terminal 1546-aa fragment of isoform B. USH2A is thought to be involved in cell adhesion.

The *GPR98* gene, also known as *VLGR1* (Very Large G protein-coupled Receptor 1) and *MASS1* (Monogenic Audiogenic Seizure Susceptibility 1), exists only in the vertebrate (Gibert et al., 2005) and is one of the largest genes, with 90 exons (McMillan et al., 2002). Its mRNA is present mostly in the brain and spinal cord during development (McMillan et al., 2002; Weston et al., 2004), but it can also be found in many other tissues (Nikkila et al., 2000; Skradski et al., 2001; McMillan et al., 2002; Weston et al., 2004). *GPR98* expresses multiple mRNA transcripts, including isoforms a, b and c in humans and isoforms b, d, e and Mass1 in rodents (Figure 2B) (Nikkila et al., 2000; Skradski et al., 2001; McMillan et al., 2002; Yagi et al., 2005). Mutations in the longest isoform, isoform b, have been identified in patients with USH2C (Weston et al., 2004; Ebermann et al., 2009; Hilgert et al., 2009). Additionally, different mutations along the murine *Gpr98* gene share common phenotypes in vision and hearing (Skradski et al., 2001; McMillan and White, 2004; Johnson et al., 2005; Yagi et al., 2005; McGee et al., 2006; Michalski et al., 2007; Yagi et al., 2007). These findings suggest that isoform b is the major isoform in both the retina and the inner ear and is essential for vision and hearing. This isoform is 6306 aa long in humans. It has signature domains of family B of G protein-coupled receptors (GPCRs), i.e., a GPCR proteolytic site (GPS) and a 7-transmembrane domain (7TM). Therefore, GPR98 may function in signal transduction. GPR98 also has a PBM at its C-terminus. Along its long extracellular region, it has a laminin globular-like domain (LamG_L), an epilepsy associated repeat (EAR)/epitempin (EPTP) domain, and multiple tandem-arranged Calxβ domains. While the function of EAR/EPTP is unknown, LamG_L is a cell adhesion domain, and the Calxβ domain is able to bind to Ca^{2+} with low affinity in vitro (Nikkila et al., 2000; McMillan and White, 2011).

Mutations of whirlin cause either USH2D or nonsyndromic deafness, *DFNB31*. Interestingly, mutations at the N-terminal half of the gene, such as p.P246HfxX13 and compound heterozygosity of p.Q103X and c.837+1G>A, are manifested as USH2D (Ebermann et al., 2006; Audo et al., 2011), while mutations at the C-terminal half, such as p.R778X and c.2423delG, were found in patients with *DFNB31* (Mburu et al., 2003; Tlili et al., 2005). Whirlin has multiple mRNA transcripts in the inner ear and the retina (Mburu et al., 2003; Belyantseva et al., 2005; van Wijk et al., 2006; Yang et al., 2010), which can be conceptually translated into three groups of proteins, the long, N-terminal, and C-terminal isoforms (Figure 2C). The long isoform contains three PDZ domains and a proline-rich region (PR). Thus, whirlin is a homolog of harmonin. At the protein level, whirlin mainly expresses the long isoform in the retina and the long and C-terminal isoforms in the inner ear (Yang et al., 2010). Because both the PDZ domain and PR region are protein interaction modules, whirlin is believed to be implicated in the assembly of multi-protein complexes at specific subcellular locations, similar to harmonin.

2.3 USH3 and USH related genes

The only gene currently identified in USH3 is clarin-1 for the *USH3A* locus (Joensuu et al., 2001; Adato et al., 2002; Fields et al., 2002). Like other USH genes, clarin-1 has multiple transcript variants due to different splicings and usages of transcription start sites (Vastinsalo et al., 2010). The primary transcript encodes a protein with four predicted transmembrane domains and a C-terminal potential PBM (Figure 3). Clarin-1 shows a sequence homologous to stargazin, an auxiliary subunit of ion channels in the synapse (Osten and Stern-Bach, 2006; Tomita et al., 2007). Presently, several research groups are intensively focusing on understanding this gene (Aarnisalo et al., 2007; Geller et al., 2009; Geng et al., 2009; Tian et al., 2009; Zallocchi et al., 2009). However, the biological function and cellular expression of clarin-1 still remain elusive.

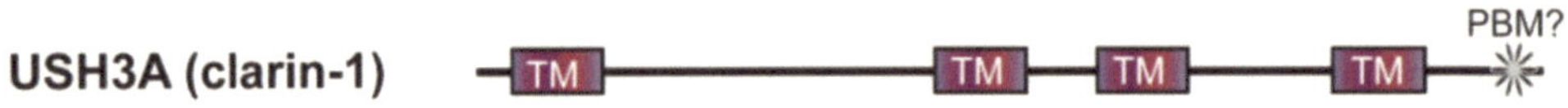

Fig. 3. Domain structure of USH3A

Recently, *PDZD7* was shown to be a modifier gene for the retinal symptom in USH2A patients and, together with *USH2A* or *GPR98*, to contribute to a digenic USH form (Ebermann et al., 2010). Interestingly, this newly identified USH modifier and contributor gene is also a homolog of harmonin. It has several isoforms (Schneider et al., 2009; Ebermann et al., 2010). The long isoform has three PDZ domains and one PR region. The two short isoforms are the N-terminal fragments of the long isoform with only two PDZ domains. However, the short isoforms have not been confirmed at the protein level. Similar to both harmonin and whirlin, different mutations in *PDZD7* are involved in either USH or nonsyndromic deafness. A homozygous reciprocal translocation, 46,XY,t(10;11)(q24;q23), was found to disrupt the *PDZD7* gene at intron 10, which causes nonsyndromic congenital hearing impairment (Schneider et al., 2009). A heterozygous p.R56PfsX mutation of *PDZD7* was found to exacerbate retinal degeneration in an USH2A patient, compared to her sibling carrying the same *USH2A* mutation. Additionally, the heterozygous mutations of *PDZD7*, c.1750-2A>G and p.C732LfsX, are present in USH patients with a heterozygous *USH2A* mutation, p.R1505SfsX, and with a heterozygous *GPR98* mutation, p.C732LfsX, respectively (Ebermann et al., 2010).

3. Animal models

Numerous spontaneous and transgenic USH animal models are now available. Table 1 lists the detailed information about the mouse models. The majority of these models show congenital hearing loss as expected. However, only a few of them, *Ush1c* knockin, *Ush2a* knockout, and whirlin knockout mice, manifest obvious widespread retinal degeneration. $Ush1c^{dfcr}$ mice on some specific genomic background and $Myo7a^{4626SB}$ and $Cdh23^{V}$ double mutant mice show only slight retinal degeneration (Johnson et al., 2003; Lillo et al., 2003; Williams et al., 2009). Among the rest of the USH mouse models, some *Myo7a, Cdh23, Pcdh15, and Grp98* mutant strains show abnormal electroretinogram (ERG) responses but no retinal degeneration (Libby and Steel, 2001; Libby et al., 2003; Haywood-Watson et al., 2006; McGee et al., 2006), indicating that the function of photoreceptors is compromised. The reasons for the discrepancy between USH patient symptoms and USH mutant mouse phenotypes are largely unclear. Many factors could contribute to this, such as the gene isoform composition, mutation type and position in the genes, genomic background, redundant protein compensation, photoreceptor structure and physiology, influence of non-genetic factors, sensitivity of diagnostic measures, etc. (El-Amraoui and Petit, 2005). Additionally, although retinitis pigmentosa in USH is characterized to have an onset before or during puberty (Smith et al., 1994; Petit, 2001), more and more atypical USH patients have been found (Edwards et al., 1998; Sadeghi et al., 2006; Cohen et al., 2007; Fishman et al., 2007; Sandberg et al., 2008; Malm et al, 2010.; Bashir et al., 2011). These patients have relatively late onset vision loss, which may explain the lack of retinal phenotype in most USH mutant mice, whose lifespan is only about two years.

Zebrafish models for several USH genes have also been reported, including mariner (*myo7a*), *ush1c*, sputnik (*cdh23*), and orbiter (*pcdh15*) (Phillips et al., 2011; Nicolson et al., 1998; Ernest et al., 2000; Sollner et al., 2004; Seiler et al., 2005). Defects in hearing, balance, and vision are manifested during the early life in two *ush1c* mutants. Interestingly, zebrafish has two orthologs of *PCDH15*. Disruption of one leads to the auditory and vestibular dysfunction, while disturbance of the other results in defects in the photoreceptor structure and retinal function. Mariner exhibits similar phenotypes to *Myo7a* mice in hearing, balance and vision. Sputnik has problems with the auditory and vestibular system, but its vision phenotype has not been reported. Currently, studies on other USH genes in zebrafish using the morpholino knockdown technique are being actively pursued (Ebermann et al., 2010). Moreover, a rat model with a point mutation leading to premature truncation of *Myo7a* was generated by N-ethyl-N-nitrosourea mutagenesis and named Tornado (Smits et al., 2005). In this model, hearing but not vision defects have been characterized. Therefore, exploration of USH genes in more vertebrate organisms will provide additional ways to understand the biological functions of these genes, in particular, in the retina.

Model name	Mutations	Phenotypes	References
USH1			
Myo7a			
$Myo7a^{sh1}$	p.R502P	Circling, head tossing, hearing impairment	(Mburu et al., 1997; Libby and Steel, 2001)
$Myo7a^{6J}$	p.R241P	Circling, head tossing, deafness	(Mburu et al., 1997; Libby and Steel, 2001)
$Myo7a^{26SB}$	p.F1762I	Circling, head tossing, deafness	(Mburu et al., 1997; Libby and Steel, 2001)
$Myo7a^{816SB}$	p.L646_Q655del	Circling, head tossing, deafness, reduced ERG	(Mburu et al., 1997; Libby and Steel, 2001)
$Myo7a^{3336SB}$	p.C2144X	Circling, head tossing, deafness	(Mburu et al., 1997; Libby and Steel, 2001)
$Myo7a^{4494SB}$	p.A246fs?X5	Circling, head tossing, deafness	(Mburu et al., 1997; Liu et al., 1999; Libby and Steel, 2001)
$Myo7a^{4626SB}$	p.Q720X	Circling, head tossing, deafness, reduced ERG	(Mburu et al., 1997; Libby and Steel, 2001)

Model name	Mutations	Phenotypes	References
Myo7a^{7J}	p.A1363AfsX27	Circling, head tossing, deafness, reduced ERG	(Mburu et al., 1997; Libby and Steel, 2001; Yang et al., 2011)
Myo7a^{Hdb}	p.I178F	Circling, head tossing, low-frequency hearing impairment	(Rhodes et al., 2004)
Myo7a^{8J}	Not known	Circling, head tossing, deafness, reduced ERG	(Mburu et al., 1997; Libby and Steel, 2001)
Myo7a^{9J}	Not known	Circling?, head tossing?, deafness?, reduced ERG	(Mburu et al., 1997; Libby and Steel, 2001)
Harmonin			
Ush1c knockout	Replacement of exons 1-4 with β-gal/neo cassette	Circling, head tossing, deafness	(Tian et al., 2010)
Ush1c^{dfcr}	A deletion involving exons 12-15, A-D	Circling, head tossing, deafness, slight retinal degeneration at 9 months of age	(Johnson et al., 2003)
Ush1c$^{dfcr-2J}$	One bp deletion in exon C	Circling, head tossing, deafness	(Johnson et al., 2003)
Ush1c$^{tm1.1Ugds}$	Exon 1 deletion	Circling, head tossing, deafness	(Lefevre et al., 2008)
Ush1c knockin	c.216G>A	Circling, head tossing, deafness, retinal degeneration	(Lentz et al., 2007; Lentz et al., 2010)
Ush1c-PDZ2^{AAA}	Replacement of GLG (221-223aa) in PDZ2 with AAA	Hair bundle defect	(Grillet et al., 2009)
Cdh23			
jera	p.V2360E	deafness	(Manji et al., 2011)
erlong	p.S70P	Circling, head tossing, deafness	(Han et al., 2010)
salsa	p.E737V	Circling, head tossing, deafness	(Schwander et al., 2009)
Cdh23^{V}	p.N279EfsX39	Circling, head tossing, deafness, reduced ERG responses	(Wilson et al., 2001; Libby et al., 2003)
Cdh23^{V-J}	p.E1169NfsX7	Circling, head tossing, deafness	(Wilson et al., 2001)
Cdh23^{V-2J}	c.4104 + 1G>A	Circling, head tossing, deafness, faster ERG responses	(Di Palma et al., 2001b; Libby et al., 2003)

Model name	Mutations	Phenotypes	References
Cdh23$^{V\text{-}3J}$	p.W1764X	Circling, head tossing, deafness	(Di Palma et al., 2001a)
Cdh23^{V4J}	p.N2718del3	Circling, head tossing, deafness	(Di Palma et al., 2001a)
Cdh23^{V5J}	p.R2935X	Circling, head tossing, deafness	(Di Palma et al., 2001a)
Cdh23$^{V\text{-}6J}$	p.E302X	Circling, head tossing, deafness	(Di Palma et al., 2001b)
Cdh23$^{V\text{-}7J}$	p.Y1197MfsX47	Circling, head tossing, deafness	(Di Palma et al., 2001a)
Cdh23$^{V\text{-}ngt}$	p.G49VfsX3	Circling, head tossing, deafness	(Wada et al., 2001)
Cdh23$^{V\text{-}Alb}$	c.1635C>Tdel119	Circling, head tossing, deafness, normal ERG responses	(Di Palma et al., 2001b; Libby et al., 2003)
Cdh23^{Vbus}	c.9633 + 1G>A	Circling, head tossing, deafness	(Yonezawa et al., 2006)
Cdh23^{Ahl}	c.753G>A	Susceptibility to age-related hearing loss	(Noben-Trauth et al., 2003)
Pcdh15			
Pcdh15$^{av\text{-}J}$	p.A645_K922del	Circling, head tossing, deafness, normal retinal function	(Alagramam et al., 2001a; Ball et al., 2003)
Pcdh15$^{av\text{-}2J}$	p.D31_N57del	Circling, head tossing, deafness, normal retinal function	(Alagramam et al., 2001a; Ball et al., 2003)
Pcdh15$^{av\text{-}3J}$	p.E1373RfsX36	Circling, head tossing, deafness, normal retinal function	(Alagramam et al., 2001a; Ball et al., 2003)
Pcdh15$^{av\text{-}5J}$	IVS14-2A>G	Circling, head tossing, deafness, reduced ERG responses	(Washington et al., 2005; Haywood-Watson et al., 2006)
Pcdh15$^{av\text{-}6J}$	p.G962_K1008del	Circling, head tossing, deafness	(Alagramam et al., 2011)
Pcdh15$^{av\text{-}Jfb}$	p.D701GfsX17	Circling, head tossing, deafness, reduced ERG responses	(Hampton et al., 2003; Haywood-Watson et al., 2006)
Pcdh15$^{av\text{-}TgN2742Rpw}$	A large insertion	Circling, head tossing, deafness, normal retinal function	(Alagramam et al., 2001a; Ball et al., 2003)
Sans			
Ush1g^{js}	p.E228RfsX8	Circling, head tossing, deafness	(Kikkawa et al., 2003)

Model name	Mutations	Phenotypes	References
Ush1g$^{js\text{-}2J}$	p.L81GfsX103	Circling, head tossing, deafness	*
Ush1g^{F1}	Exon 2 flanked with FRT sites	Hearing defects after deletion of exon 2	(Caberlotto et al., 2011)
USH2			
Ush2a			
Ush2a knockout	replacement of exon 5 with a neomycin^{r} cassette	hearing impairment, retinal degeneration	(Liu et al., 2007)
Gpr98			
Gpr98 knockout	replacement of exons 2-4 with a neomycin^{r} cassette	audiogenic seizure susceptibility, hearing impairment	(Yagi et al., 2005; Michalski et al., 2007)
Gpr98-EYFP knockin	replacement of exons 2-4 with a EYFP-neomycin^{r} cassette	defects in hair cell stereocilia	(Yagi et al., 2007)
Frings & BUB/BnJ	a G deletion at 6864 bp (NM_054053) causing a p.V2250X mutation	audiogenic seizure susceptibility, hearing impairment	(Skradski et al., 2001; Johnson et al., 2005)
Gpr98/del7TM	replacement of exon 82 with a HA-neomycin^{r} cassette	audiogenic seizure susceptibility, hearing impairment, mildly abnormal ERG responses	(McMillan and White, 2004; McGee et al., 2006)
Whrn			
Whrn knockout	partial replacement of exon 1 with a neomycin^{r} cassette	hearing impairment, retinal degeneration	(Yang et al., 2010)
whirler	a 592-bp deletion causing a p.H433fsX58 mutation	hearing impairment, no retinal degeneration	(Lane, 1963; Holme et al., 2002; Mburu et al., 2003; Yang et al., 2010)
USH3			
Ush3a			
Ush3a knockout	Disruption and deletion of promoter and exon 1	Circling, head tossing, deafness	(Geller et al., 2009)

MYO7A: NP_032689, CDH23: NP_075859, PCDH15: NP_075604, SANS: NP_789817

*: our unpublished data.

Table 1. USH mutant mouse models

4. Cellular localization of USH proteins

Defects in USH proteins result in Usher syndrome, nonsyndromic deafness, or retinitis pigmentosa, indicating that these proteins are essential in the inner ear and the retina. Therefore, extensive efforts have been put to investigate the cellular location of these proteins in these two tissues. The cellular localization of USH proteins in other tissues is relatively unclear, although some USH proteins are known to be present in the kidney, colon, brain, lung, olfactory neuron, ovary, oviduct, testes and intestine (el-Amraoui et al., 1996; Hasson et al., 1997; Wolfrum et al., 1998; Kobayashi et al., 1999; Scanlan et al., 1999; Bhattacharya et al., 2002; Pearsall et al., 2002).

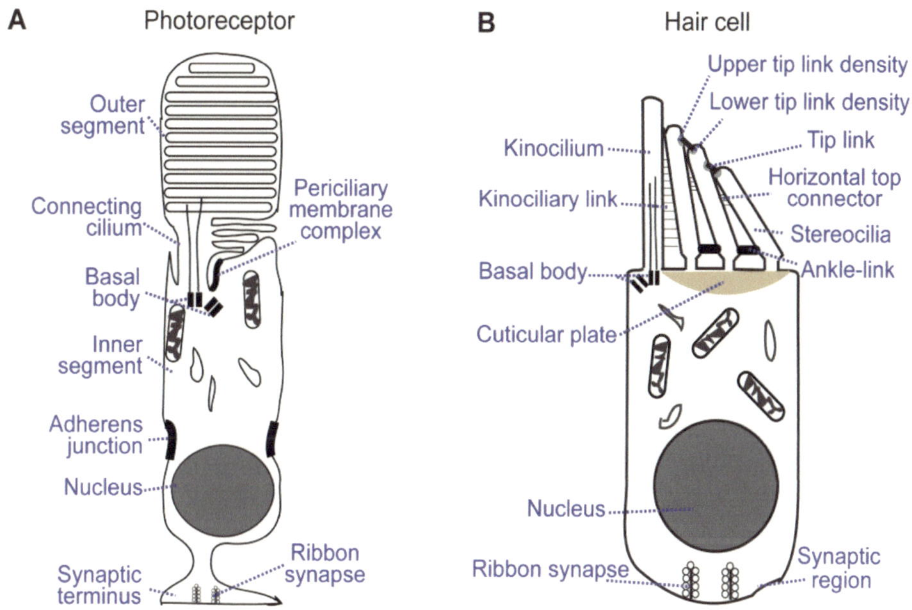

Fig. 4. Schematic diagrams of a rod photoreceptor and a hair cell

4.1 USH proteins in the inner ear

The inner ear is composed of the cochlea and vestibular system for hearing and balance, respectively. In the vestibular system, hair cells exist in the maculae of the saccule and utricle and the cristae ampullares of the semicircular canals. In the cochlea, one row of inner hair cells and three rows of outer hair cells exist in the organ of Corti. The inner hair cells are responsible for mechanoelectric transduction, whereas the electromotile outer hair cells also perform an electromechanical transduction, thereby amplifying the sound-evoked vibrations of the entire sensory epithelium (Leibovici et al., 2008). All types of hair cells have stereocilia on their apical surfaces, which are modified microvilli filled with bundles of actin filaments. The stereocilia are well-organized into rows of different lengths and form a staircase-like hair bundle (Figure 4). Along with the hair bundle, there exists a real cilium, called kinocilium, which is filled with microtubules. Various links have been discovered along the entire length of the stereocilia and the kinocilium during development and in adulthood (Goodyear and Richardson, 1999; Goodyear and Richardson, 2003; Goodyear et al., 2005).

The distribution of USH proteins in hair cells vary dramatically from the emergence of stereocilia to their maturation. All USH1 proteins are present either at the tip, the ankle links, the transient lateral links, or the kinociliary links of the stereocilia during the early stage of development. They are then restricted to the tip link and the accessory structures of the tip link, the upper (UTLD) and lower (LTLD) tip link densities, in mature hair cells (Figure 4) (Kussel-Andermann et al., 2000; Senften et al., 2006; Lefevre et al., 2008; Grillet et al., 2009; Bahloul et al., 2010; Caberlotto et al., 2011; Grati and Kachar, 2011). USH2 proteins are localized at the ankle links of the stereocilia (McGee et al., 2006; van Wijk et al., 2006; Michalski et al., 2007; Yang et al., 2010), which is a transient structure existing only during development (Goodyear et al., 2005). Whirlin is also present at the tip of stereocilia in the vestibular and cochlear hair cells all the time (Belyantseva et al., 2005; Delprat et al., 2005; Kikkawa et al., 2005). Clarin-1 was found at the stereocilia on postnatal day 0 (Zallocchi et al., 2009). Besides their location at the stereocilia, some USH proteins were found at the synaptic region of the outer and inner hair cells (Reiners et al., 2005b; van Wijk et al., 2006; Zallocchi et al., 2009), the cell body of the spinal ganglia (Alagramam et al., 2001b; Adato et al., 2002; van Wijk et al., 2006), the supporting cells (Alagramam et al., 2001b; Adato et al., 2005a; Adato et al., 2005b), various nervous fibers (van Wijk et al., 2006), and Reissner's membrane (Wilson et al., 2001; Lagziel et al., 2005). However, these distributions of USH proteins need to be further verified, because the specificity of antibodies used in the studies were not confirmed in their corresponding mutant mice.

4.2 USH proteins in the retina

In the retina, USH proteins are mainly localized in the photoreceptors (Kremer et al., 2006; Reiners et al., 2006; van Wijk et al., 2006; Liu et al., 2007; Maerker et al., 2008; Yang et al., 2010). The photoreceptor is a highly polarized sensory neuron converting light signals to electrical impulses. It consists of the outer segment, connecting cilium, inner segment, cell body, and synaptic terminus (Figure 4). It contacts Muller cells at the adherens junction (the outer limiting membrane in the retina). Its outer segment is immediately next to the retinal pigment epithelium (RPE) cells.

Compared with the studies in the inner ear, the cellular location of USH proteins is less well defined in the retina. All the USH proteins were once localized in the synaptic ends of photoreceptors (Reiners et al., 2005a; Reiners et al., 2005b; Maerker et al., 2008). However, these results are not conclusive (Williams, 2008; Saihan et al., 2009). They are not supported by the phenotypic analyses in USH mutant mice and the symptom manifestation in USH patients. For instance, ultrastructural abnormalities were not found at the synaptic terminus of photoreceptors in USH mice by electron microscopy (Self et al., 1998; Williams et al., 2009; Yang et al., 2010). No defective ERG waveforms typically resulting from abnormal photoreceptor synaptic transmission have been detected in USH mutant mice (Libby and Steel, 2001; Ball et al., 2003; Libby et al., 2003; Haywood-Watson et al., 2006; McGee et al., 2006; Liu et al., 2007; Yang et al., 2010) or in USH patients.

In addition to the synaptic distribution, MYO7A and SANS were shown to be present around the connecting cilium, harmonin at the outer segment, CDH23 in the inner segment, and PCDH15 at the base of the outer segment by one research group (Ahmed et al., 2003; Reiners et al., 2005a; Maerker et al., 2008). However, other research groups did not find harmonin in the outer segment (Williams et al., 2009), and MYO7A was demonstrated to be predominantly expressed in the RPE cells (Hasson et al., 1995; el-Amraoui et al., 1996; Lopes et al., 2011). USH2 proteins were initially localized to the inner segment, adherens junction, connecting cilium, basal bodies, and synaptic terminus in photoreceptors (Figure 4) (Kremer et al., 2006; Reiners et al., 2006; van Wijk et al., 2006; Maerker et al., 2008; Lagziel et al., 2009). With the antibodies whose specificities have been confirmed in their respective mutant mice, the three USH2 proteins were recently localized to the periciliary membrane complex (PMC) around the connecting cilium (Figure 4) (Liu et al., 2007; Yang et al., 2010; Yang et al., 2011; Zou et al., 2011). Finally, the distribution of clarin-1 in the retina is controversial. One report shows that it is present around the connecting cilium in photoreceptors (Zallocchi et al., 2009), while the other indicates that clarin-1 is restricted to the Muller cells but not photoreceptors (Geller et al., 2009).

The calycal processes in photoreceptors are thought as an analogous structure to the stereocilia in hair cells (Goodyear and Richardson, 1999). They are well developed in humans, frogs and other species. In mice, only cone photoreceptors have obvious calycal processes (Cohen, 1965; Fetter and Corless, 1987; Rana and Taraszka, 1991). GPR98 and CDH23 are localized at the calycal processes in mouse cone photoreceptors, while whirlin is not evident at this structure in frog photoreceptors (Goodyear and Richardson, 1999; Yang et al., 2010).

5. The USH protein complexes

The indistinguishable symptoms within the same USH clinical type and the similar symptoms across different USH clinical types indicate that various USH proteins probably participate in the same cellular pathway in a broad sense. Among the USH proteins, harmonin, whirlin and SANS possess multiple protein-protein interaction domains and are proposed to be scaffold proteins in multi-protein complexes. Biochemical assays have indeed revealed the existence of their self-interactions and interactions with most of other USH proteins in vitro (Table 2). Interestingly, the in vitro interactions among different USH1 and/or USH2 proteins exist extensively (Table 2). One USH protein is generally able to interact with at least three other USH proteins. In most cases, different regions of the same protein are involved in its binding to different USH proteins (Table 2). Although these interactions have not been individually confirmed in vivo, harmonin, MYO7A, and CDH23 were recently reported to form a ternary complex in hair cells (Bahloul et al., 2010). Based on these findings, it has been hypothesized that USH proteins form an interacting network, an interactome, in both hair cells and photoreceptors (Richardson et al.; Kremer et al., 2006; Reiners et al., 2006; Saihan et al., 2009; Millan et al., 2011).

The above hypothesis is supported by the facts that ablation of one USH protein in mice causes mislocation and/or disappearance of at least one other USH protein in hair cells (Table 3). This phenomenon occurs across USH1 and USH2 proteins. Normal distribution of the three USH2 proteins depends on MYO7A and the distribution of some CDH23 isoform at the tip of the stereocilia relies on GPR98 (Table 3). However, the USH1 and USH2 proteins are present at the different interstereociliary links in hair cells during development. Additionally, different USH proteins are localized at two distinct subcellular locations in photoreceptors, the PMC and the synapse. Due to these different cellular locations of USH proteins, it is reasonable to propose that more than one USH protein complex exist and they play different but highly related roles in a broad cellular process (Williams, 2008; Yang et al., 2011).

Proteins/domains	Interacting proteins/domains	References
MYO7A		
MyTH4-FERM	Harmonin/PDZ1	(Boeda et al., 2002)
Tail	CDH23/not determined	(Bahloul et al., 2010)
SH2	PCDH15	(Senften et al., 2006)
MyTH4-FERM	SANS/cen	(Wu et al., 2011; Adato et al., 2005b)
MyTH4-FERM	USH2A/cytoplasmic region	(Michalski et al., 2007)
MyTH4-FERM	GPR98/cytoplasmic region	(Michalski et al., 2007)
Not determined	Whirlin/not determined	(Delprat et al., 2005)
Harmonin		
PDZ1	MYO7A/MyTH4-FERM	(Boeda et al., 2002)
N-terminus, PDZ1/2	CDH23/PBMs	(Boeda et al., 2002; Siemens et al., 2002; Grillet et al., 2009; Pan et al., 2009; Bahloul et al., 2010)
PDZ2	PCDH15/CD1 PBM	(Adato et al., 2005b; Reiners et al., 2005b; Senften et al., 2006)
PDZ1/3	SANS/SAM, PBM	(Adato et al., 2005b; Yan et al., 2010)
PDZ1	USH2A/PBM	(Reiners et al., 2005b)
PDZ1	GPR98/PBM	(Reiners et al., 2005b)
PDZ1/2, CC2	Harmonin/PBM, CC2	(Siemens et al., 2002; Adato et al., 2005b)
CDH23		
not determined	MYO7A/tail	(Bahloul et al., 2010)
2 PBMs	Harmonin/N-terminus, PDZ1, PDZ2	(Boeda et al., 2002; Siemens et al., 2002; Grillet et al., 2009; Pan et al., 2009; Bahloul et al., 2010)
EC1-3	PCDH15/EC1	(Kazmierczak et al., 2007)
Cytoplasmic region	SANS/not determined	(Caberlotto et al., 2011)
ECs	CDH23/ECs	(Siemens et al., 2004; Kazmierczak et al., 2007)
PCDH15		
Cytoplasmic region	MYO7A/SH2	(Senften et al., 2006)
CD1 PBM	Harmonin/PDZ2	(Adato et al., 2005b; Reiners et al., 2005b; Senften et al., 2006)
EC1	CDH23/EC1-3	(Kazmierczak et al., 2007)
CD2/CD3	SANS/not determined	(Caberlotto et al., 2011)
ECs	PCDH15/ECs	(Kazmierczak et al., 2007)

Proteins/domains	Interacting proteins/domains	References
SANS		
cen	MYO7A/MyTH4-FERM	(Wu et al, 2011.; Adato et al., 2005b)
SAM, PBM	Harmonin/PDZ1	(Weil et al., 2003; Yan et al., 2010)
Not determined	CDH23/cytoplasmic region	(Caberlotto et al., 2011)
Not determined	PCDH15/CD2, CD3	(Caberlotto et al., 2011)
PBM	Whirlin/PDZ1-PDZ2	(Maerker et al., 2008)
cen	SANS/cen	(Adato et al., 2005b)
USH2A		
Cytoplasmic region	MYO7A/MyTH4-FERM	(Michalski et al., 2007)
PBM	Harmonin/PDZ1	(Reiners et al., 2005b)
PBM	Whirlin/PDZ1-PDZ2	(Adato et al., 2005a; van Wijk et al., 2006; Yang et al., 2010)
GPR98		
Cytoplasmic region	MYO7A/MyTH4-FERM	(Michalski et al., 2007)
PBM	Harmonin/PDZ1	(Reiners et al., 2005b)
PBM	Whirlin/PDZ1-PDZ2	(Adato et al., 2005a; van Wijk et al., 2006; Yang et al., 2010)
Whirlin		
Not determined	MYO7A/not determined	(Delprat et al., 2005)
PDZ1-PDZ2	SANS/PBM	(Maerker et al., 2008)
PDZ1-PDZ2	USH2A/PBM	(Adato et al., 2005a; van Wijk et al., 2006; Yang et al., 2010)
PDZ1-PDZ2	GPR98/PBM	(Adato et al., 2005a; van Wijk et al., 2006; Yang et al., 2010)
PDZ1-PDZ2, PR-PDZ3	Whirlin/PDZ1-PDZ2, PR-PDZ3	(Delprat et al., 2005; Yang et al., 2010)

Table 2. Interactions among USH proteins

In hair cells, the normal cellular localization of harmonin requires the presence of all other USH1 proteins, and loss of harmonin seems not to affect the localization of other USH1 proteins (Table 3), indicating that harmonin is dispensable for locating these USH1 proteins to their normal position in cells. In contrast, CDH23 is relatively independent on other USH1 proteins, and its loss results in mislocalization of the two putative scaffold proteins, harmonin and SANS (Table 3). Therefore, CDH23 may play a crucial role in anchoring/tethering USH1 proteins. Harmonin and SANS may help hold the USH1 proteins in the complex.

Besides the known USH proteins, many other putative components in the USH complexes has been identified. These components are able to interact with at least one of the USH proteins as shown by biochemical assays. For the currently known USH2-interacting proteins, please see the review (Yang et al., 2011). However, additional experiments are necessary to verify the existence of these putative components in the USH complexes in vivo and reveal their relationship with USH.

	MYO7A	USH1C	CDH23	PCDH15	SANS	USH2A	GPR98	WHRN
Myo7a$^{-/-}$		+ (Boeda et al., 2002; Lefevre et al., 2008)	- (Boeda et al., 2002; Senften et al., 2006)	+ (Senften et al., 2006)	- (Caberlotto et al., 2011)	+ (Michalski et al., 2007)	+ (Michalski et al., 2007)	+ (Michalski et al., 2007)
Ush1c$^{-/-}$	+/- (Lefevre et al., 2008; Yan et al., 2011)		- (Lefevre et al., 2008)	+/- (Lefevre et al., 2008; Yan et al., 2011)	+/- (Caberlotto et al., 2011; Yan et al., 2011)			
Cdh23$^{-/-}$	+ (Bahloul et al., 2010)	+ (Lefevre et al., 2008; Bahloul et al., 2010)		- (Senften et al., 2006)	+ (Caberlotto et al., 2011)			
Pcdh15$^{-/-}$	+ (Senften et al., 2006)	+ (Lefevre et al., 2008)	- (Senften et al., 2006)		+ (Caberlotto et al., 2011)			
Sans$^{-/-}$		+ (Lefevre et al., 2008)						
Ush2a$^{-/-}$							+ (Yang et al., 2010)	+ (Yang et al., 2010)
Gpr98$^{-/-}$			+ (Michalski et al., 2007)			+ (Michalski et al., 2007)		+ (Michalski et al., 2007)
Whrn$^{-/-}$						+ (Michalski et al., 2007; Yang et al., 2010)	+ (Michalski et al., 2007; Yang et al., 2010)	

+: existence of mislocalization, -: normal localization, +/-, contradictory results

Table 3. Interdependence of USH proteins in hair cells

6. Functions of the USH complexes

The severe and early-onset hearing phenotypes in various USH1 and USH2 mouse models make it relatively easier to decipher the functions of USH complexes in the inner ear than in the retina. The following will focus on the three main cellular processes generally believed to involve the USH complexes. Disruption of these USH functions is thought to be the molecular mechanisms underlying USH.

6.1 Hair bundle cohesion

During development, at the apex of hair cells, microvilli grow into stereocilia by recruiting more actin filaments. These stereocilia are bundled with transient lateral links and are connected with the kinocilium through kinociliary links. Following the establishment of the planar cell polarity, the kinocilium moves from the center to the periphery of the cell, and the stereocilia elongate differentially. The staircase-shape hair bundle is eventually formed. At the same time, the transient lateral links are gradually substituted by two distinct sets of interstereociliary links. They are the horizontal top connectors and the ankle links, close to the tip and base of the hair bundle, respectively (Figure 4). The tip links emerge, which are fibrous connections between the tip of medium and low stereocilia and the side of the neighboring taller stereocilia (Figure 4). Finally, the stereocilia grow both in length and in width and reach their mature size. In rodent mature cochlear hair cells, the ankle links and the kinociliary links disappear with the regression of the kinocilium (Frolenkov et al., 2004; Goodyear et al., 2005; Nayak et al., 2007).

CDH23 (Siemens et al., 2004; Lagziel et al., 2005; Michel et al., 2005; Rzadzinska et al., 2005; Lefevre et al., 2008) and PCDH15 (Goodyear et al., 2010; Webb et al., 2011; Lefevre et al., 2008) are localized at the transient lateral links and kinociliary links during early development of hair cells. In their mutant mice, hair bundles are usually splayed into several clumps; kinocilium is mispositioned and disconnected with the hair bundle (Lefevre et al., 2008), indicating that CDH23 and PCDH15, as components of the interstereociliary links, are important for hair bundle cohesion and that loss of the connection between the stereocilia and kinocilium causes the misorientation of the hair bundle. Interestingly, the mutant mouse models of all five USH1 genes share such similar phenotypes. This could be explained by the idea that the five USH1 proteins coordinate in this function. The PST domain of harmonin b binds to and bundles actin filaments (Boeda et al., 2002). MYO7A is a high duty ratio motor, which binds to actin filament strongly. Therefore, these two actin-binding proteins may anchor their interacting partners, CDH23 and PCDH15, to the actin bundle in the stereocilia of hair cells (Table 2). In *Ush1g*$^{-/-}$ mice, cohesion of stereocilia is disrupted. In *Ush1g*$^{fl/fl}$*Myo7a-cre*$^{+/-}$ mice, whose expression of SANS is disturbed only after birth, the stereocilia stay cohesive (Caberlotto et al., 2011). Therefore, SANS plays a role in stereocilia cohesion during the prenatal period. It may be involved in the organization of other USH1 proteins through directly interacting with them (Table 2).

All three USH2 proteins, USH2A, GPR98, and whirlin, are positioned at the ankle links of hair cells. Among these proteins, USH2A and GPR98 probably interact with each other or with some unidentified cell adhesion proteins to form the ankle links. Whirlin interacts with USH2A and GPR98 through the PDZ domain-mediated binding to anchor them at the base of the stereocilia. In the absence of GPR98, the ankle links are missing. Thus far, the dependence of the ankle links on USH2A and whirlin has not been examined. In the wild-type mouse, the stereocilia of outer hair cells are organized into a V-shaped staircase-like hair bundle. However, in all three *Ush2* mutant mice, the outer hair cells show various disorganized stereocilia and abnormal U-shape hair bundles (Mburu et al., 2003; McGee et al., 2006; Liu et al., 2007; Michalski et al., 2007; Yang et al., 2010). Accordingly, as components of the ankle links, the three USH2 proteins probably contribute to hair bundle cohesion as well.

6.2 Mechanotransduction

The stereocilia of hair cells are the cellular organelle conducting mechanotransduction. The vibration of the basilar membrane and tectorial membrane or the motion of endolymphatic fluid induces the hair bundle deflection. When the deflection is toward the longest stereocilia (the positive or excitatory direction), the transduction channels are open. The influx of Ca^{2+} and K^{+} through the channels elicits changes of the membrane potential and glutamate release at the ribbon synapse in hair cells. When the hair bundle moves away from the longest stereocilia (the negative or inhibitory direction), the transduction channels close, and the membrane potential and transmitter release resume their resting statuses. Although the molecular machinery of mechanotransduction is not well understood, the 'gating spring' model is popular in the field. In this model, the tip link, whose axis is parallel to the direction of the mechanical sensitivity of the hair bundle, is thought as a sensor to the stretch of the hair bundle. Alternatively, an unknown structure attached to the tip link fulfills this function (Vollrath et al., 2007; Gillespie and Muller, 2009). The transduction channel was recently localized to the plasma membrane at the lower end of the tip link in the stereocilia (Beurg et al., 2008).

In mature hair cells, CDH23 (Siemens et al., 2004; Sollner et al., 2004) and PCDH15 (Ahmed et al., 2006) were found associated with the tip links. CDH23 is mainly at the upper part and PCDH15 at the lower part of the links (Kazmierczak et al., 2007; Alagramam et al., 2011). In $Cdh23^{V\text{-}2J}$ and $Pcdh15^{av\text{-}6J}$ mice, the tip links are missing. Additionally, the response of the mechanotransduction is reduced. In the absence of stimulus, a fraction of transduction channels keep open in the wild-type hair cells, due to the resting tension of the tip links. However, the transduction channels in these two mutants do not open or take up the styryl dye FM1-43 at rest (Senften et al., 2006; Alagramam et al., 2011). Therefore, CDH23 and PCDH15 are believed to be components of the tip links and to participate in mechanotransduction in mature hair cells.

At the two ends of the tip link immediately beneath the stereocilia plasma membrane, there are electron-dense complexes, the UTLD and LTLD (Figure 4). Harmonin and MYO7A are present at the UTLD (Grillet et al., 2009; Michalski et al., 2009; Caberlotto et al., 2011; Grati and Kachar, 2011). In $Myo7a^{6J}$, $Myo7a^{4626SB}$, $Ush1c^{dfcr}$, and $Ush1c^{dfcr\text{-}2J}$ mice, the adaptation of mechanotransduction, a process for the hair cells to recover their sensitivity under sustained mechanical stimulation, was found consistently abnormal, while the amplitude of mechanotransduction responses is sometimes normal (Kros et al., 2002; Grillet et al., 2009; Michalski et al., 2009). These results suggest that harmonin and MYO7A are involved in the transduction adaptation. SANS may exist at both the LTLD and UTLD (Caberlotto et al., 2011; Grati and Kachar, 2011). Its loss in hair cells ($Ush1g^{-/-}$) causes elimination of the tip links and reduction in both the amplitude and sensitivity of the transduction currents

(Caberlotto et al., 2011). In *Ush1g^fl/fl^ Myo7a-cre^+/-^* mice, whose hair bundle morphology is intact, only the amplitude of transduction is affected. This finding indicates that SANS is implicated in mechanotransduction and plays a different role from harmonin or MYO7A.

Gpr98 knockout and *Gpr98^del7TM^* mice also show defects in mechanotransduction, though there are some discrepancies between them (McGee et al., 2006; Michalski et al., 2007). In general, the sensitivity to the stimulation direction is changed in both outer and inner hair cells. The amplitude and sensitivity of the transduction current decrease in the outer hair cells, but are normal in the inner hair cells and the utricular hair cells. It is suggested that the misorganization of hair bundles in *Gpr98* mutant mice accounts of the abnormal sensitivity direction. Alternatively, GPR98 could be indirectly related with the cellular process of mechanotransduction.

6.3 Protein and organelle transport

In photoreceptors, the outer segment is a large specialized cilium filled with many flat membrane disks, where phototransduction occurs (Figure 4). This cellular compartment undergoes continuous and rapid renewal (Young, 1967; LaVail, 1976; Young, 1976; Besharse and Hollyfield, 1979), which requires a large amount of proteins and membrane lipids to be synthesized in the inner segment and to be quickly transported to the base of the outer segment through the connecting cilium (Figure 4). The removal of the old outer segment is achieved through phagocytosis by RPE cells. In addition, in both photoreceptors and RPE cells, several proteins, involved in phototransduction and retinoid cycle, translocate between two different cellular compartments in response to light (Artemyev, 2008; Slepak and Hurley, 2008; Lopes et al., 2011).

Among USH proteins, MYO7A is an actin-based motor. In the retina, it is expressed in both RPE cells and photoreceptors. In RPE cells, MYO7A is essential for the transport of phagosomes to their degradation apparatus (Gibbs et al., 2003), tethering melanosomes during their movement (Gibbs et al., 2004), and the translocation of RPE65 responding to light exposure (Lopes et al., 2011). In photoreceptors, MYO7A is present along the connecting cilium. Loss of MYO7A was found to delay the transport of opsin from the inner to the outer segment (Liu et al., 1999) and the transducin translocation from the outer to the inner segment after light exposure (Peng et al., 2011). In hair cells, without MYO7A, all USH2 proteins are mislocalized from the ankle links (Table 3), suggesting that MYO7A may transport the USH2 proteins. These lines of evidence establish the notion that MYO7A may function in protein and organelle transport in various cells in the retina and the inner ear.

USH2 proteins are positioned at the PMC in mammalian photoreceptors, which is an analogous structure to the periciliary ridge complex (PRC) in frogs (Peters et al., 1983). The PRC is a morphologically-specialized structure with a symmetrical array of 9 ridges and 9 grooves. It has been proposed, based on immunocytochemistry and freeze-fracture electron microscopy, as the membrane fusion site for post-Golgi vesicles carrying opsin and docosahexaenoyl (DHA)-phospholipids before these cargos are transported from the inner to the outer segment (Peters et al., 1983; Papermaster et al., 1986; Rodriguez de Turco et al., 1997; Papermaster, 2002). Additionally, Rab8, rac1, Sec8, moesin, syntaxin 3 and SNAP-25 have been localized around the PRC in frog photoreceptors (Deretic et al., 2004; Mazelova et al., 2009). These proteins are proposed, though not verified using mouse genetics, to participate in and/or regulate the docking and membrane fusion of post-Golgi vesicles to the plasma membrane at the PRC. Therefore, the USH2 complex at the PMC might play either a direct or indirect role in the docking between the post-Golgi vesicles and plasma membrane at the base of the connecting cilium (Roepman and Wolfrum, 2007; Maerker et al., 2008). This proposed function can also be applied in hair cells. The ankle-links exist when stereocilia grow and differentiate from small microvilli. At this time, many vesicles are at the base of stereocilia (Forge et al., 1997; Hasson et al., 1997), which could be the post-Golgi vesicles carrying proteins and membrane lipids from the cell body to the growing stereocilia. Supportively, the *Gpr98* knockout mouse shows delocalization of some CDH23 long isoforms at the tip of the stereocilia and, possibly, loss of some apical links between the stereocilia (Michalski et al., 2007). However, solid evidence supporting this putative function of the USH2 complex is still scarce. For instance, obvious mislocalization of rhodopsin has not been observed in whirlin knockout and *Ush2a* knockout mice (Liu et al., 2007; Yang et al., 2010), and vesicles fused with the plasma membrane have not been demonstrated at the ankle links.

7. Therapeutic studies

Because of the widespread clinical application of the well-developed cochlear implant for hearing loss (Pennings et al., 2006; Liu et al., 2008), more attention is focused on seeking effective treatments for retinitis pigmentosa in USH. Next, I will address the current progress in studies on gene therapy, drug application, cell transplantation, and nutritional supplements (Yang et al., 2011).

Human neural progenitor cells from the post mortem fetal cortical brain have been tested in the *Ush2*a knockout mouse (Lu et al., 2009). The progenitor cells were transplanted between photoreceptors and RPE cells. There, they delayed the cellular changes in photoreceptors and alleviated retinal functional deterioration. However, due to the short follow-up time after the treatment, the study did not examine whether the treatment can rescue photoreceptor loss in this animal model.

Compared to the cell-based therapy, replacement of the mutant gene in the retina is straightforward. The efficiency and efficacy of a lentivirus-mediated gene replacement of MYO7A have been studied in the $Myo7a^{4626SB}$ mouse (Hashimoto et al., 2007). Although the delivery of MYO7A into photoreceptors and RPE cells is not quite efficient, the treated mutant retina does show correction of the histological phenotypes in these two cells. In addition, our laboratory utilized a combination of AAV and a photoreceptor-specific promoter to efficiently target the USH2D gene, whirlin, into both rod and cone photoreceptors. The transgenic whirlin was found to restore the changes of USH2A and GPR98 expression in the whirlin knockout retina (Zou et al., 2011). These encouraging progresses in the USH1B and USH2D mouse models lay a solid foundation for a further and detailed exploration of gene therapy for these and other USH subtypes.

Aminoglycosides and their derivatives can induce a read-through of nonsense mutations by inserting an amino acid at the stop codon. These drugs have been tested in vitro, in cell cultures and in retinal explants to suppress the nonsense mutations found in USH1F (PCDH15) and USH1C (harmonin) patients (Rebibo-Sabbah et al., 2007; Nudelman et al., 2009; Goldmann et al., 2010; Nudelman et al., 2010). However, the high cellular toxicity of these drugs and the low efficiency of their read-through activities set a hindrance for their further application to patients. A recent report has shown that PTC124, a drug unrelated to aminoglycosides, has a relatively low cellular toxicity and high read-through efficacy (Goldmann et al., 2011).

The nutritional supplementation, daily intakes of vitamin A at a dose of 15,000 international units (IU) and vitamin E less than 400 IU, is thought to be a potential effective therapy for retinitis pigmentosa (Berson et al., 1993; Berson, 2000). Although it has already been applied to patients, this vitamin A supplement therapy is still under debate and its underlying mechanism is unknown.

8. Summary and perspective

The research on USH has made tremendous progress since the discovery of its first causative gene, *MYO7A*, in 1995. Currently, nine genes have been identified responsible for this genetic disease. From the functional domain analysis, these genes have been proposed to participate in trafficking, scaffolding, cell adhesion, and signaling in cells. Many spontaneous and transgenic mouse, rat, and zebrafish models are available now. The majority of these animal models reproduce the hearing and balance problems in USH patients. However, not many of them manifest retinal degeneration, which is one of the typical symptoms in USH patients. The reason for this discrepancy is not clear. But lack of retinal phenotypes in these animal models hinders our studies on retinitis pigmentosa in USH patients. A large body of evidence from biochemical and cellular localization studies demonstrate that USH proteins are organized into multi-component complexes mainly in hair cells and photoreceptors. They play a role in hair bundle cohesion, mechanotransduction, and, possibly, protein/organelle transport in vivo. USH is an incurable disease. Effective treatments using different approaches are still being sought and explored.

9. References

Aarnisalo AA, Pietola L, Joensuu J, Isosomppi J, Aarnisalo P, Dinculescu A, Lewin AS, Flannery J, Hauswirth WW, Sankila EM, Jero J (2007) Anti-clarin-1 AAV-delivered ribozyme induced apoptosis in the mouse cochlea. Hear Res 230:9-16.

Adato A, Lefevre G, Delprat B, Michel V, Michalski N, Chardenoux S, Weil D, El-Amraoui A, Petit C (2005a) Usherin, the defective protein in Usher syndrome type IIA, is likely to be a component of interstereocilia ankle links in the inner ear sensory cells. Hum Mol Genet 14:3921-3932.

Adato A, Michel V, Kikkawa Y, Reiners J, Alagramam KN, Weil D, Yonekawa H, Wolfrum U, El-Amraoui A, Petit C (2005b) Interactions in the network of Usher syndrome type 1 proteins. Hum Mol Genet 14:347-356.

Adato A, Vreugde S, Joensuu T, Avidan N, Hamalainen R, Belenkiy O, Olender T, Bonne-Tamir B, Ben-Asher E, Espinos C, Millan JM, Lehesjoki AE, Flannery JG, Avraham KB, Pietrokovski S, Sankila EM, Beckmann JS, Lancet D (2002) USH3A transcripts encode clarin-1, a four-transmembrane-domain protein with a possible role in sensory synapses. Eur J Hum Genet 10:339-350.

Ahmed ZM, Riazuddin S, Khan SN, Friedman PL, Friedman TB (2009) USH1H, a novel locus for type I Usher syndrome, maps to chromosome 15q22-23. Clin Genet 75:86-91.

Ahmed ZM, Riazuddin S, Bernstein SL, Ahmed Z, Khan S, Griffith AJ, Morell RJ, Friedman TB, Wilcox ER (2001) Mutations of the protocadherin gene PCDH15 cause Usher syndrome type 1F. Am J Hum Genet 69:25-34.

Ahmed ZM, Smith TN, Riazuddin S, Makishima T, Ghosh M, Bokhari S, Menon PS, Deshmukh D, Griffith AJ, Friedman TB, Wilcox ER (2002) Nonsyndromic recessive deafness DFNB18 and Usher syndrome type IC are allelic mutations of USHIC. Hum Genet 110:527-531.

Ahmed ZM, Riazuddin S, Ahmad J, Bernstein SL, Guo Y, Sabar MF, Sieving P, Griffith AJ, Friedman TB, Belyantseva IA, Wilcox ER (2003) PCDH15 is expressed in the neurosensory epithelium of the eye and ear and mutant alleles are responsible for both USH1F and DFNB23. Hum Mol Genet 12:3215-3223.

Ahmed ZM, Goodyear R, Riazuddin S, Lagziel A, Legan PK, Behra M, Burgess SM, Lilley KS, Wilcox ER, Griffith AJ, Frolenkov GI, Belyantseva IA, Richardson GP, Friedman TB (2006) The tip-link antigen, a protein associated with the transduction complex of sensory hair cells, is protocadherin-15. J Neurosci 26:7022-7034.

Alagramam KN, Murcia CL, Kwon HY, Pawlowski KS, Wright CG, Woychik RP (2001a) The mouse Ames waltzer hearing-loss mutant is caused by mutation of Pcdh15, a novel protocadherin gene. Nat Genet 27:99-102.

Alagramam KN, Goodyear RJ, Geng R, Furness DN, van Aken AF, Marcotti W, Kros CJ, Richardson GP (2011) Mutations in protocadherin 15 and cadherin 23 affect tip links and mechanotransduction in mammalian sensory hair cells. PLoS One 6:e19183.

Alagramam KN, Yuan H, Kuehn MH, Murcia CL, Wayne S, Srisailpathy CR, Lowry RB, Knaus R, Van Laer L, Bernier FP, Schwartz S, Lee C, Morton CC, Mullins RF, Ramesh A, Van Camp G, Hageman GS, Woychik RP, Smith RJ (2001b) Mutations in the novel protocadherin PCDH15 cause Usher syndrome type 1F. Hum Mol Genet 10:1709-1718.

Aller E, Najera C, Millan JM, Oltra JS, Perez-Garrigues H, Vilela C, Navea A, Beneyto M (2004) Genetic analysis of 2299delG and C759F mutations (USH2A) in patients with visual and/or auditory impairments. Eur J Hum Genet 12:407-410.

Artemyev NO (2008) Light-dependent compartmentalization of transducin in rod photoreceptors. Mol Neurobiol 37:44-51.

Astuto LM, Weston MD, Carney CA, Hoover DM, Cremers CW, Wagenaar M, Moller C, Smith RJ, Pieke-Dahl S, Greenberg J, Ramesar R, Jacobson SG, Ayuso C, Heckenlively JR, Tamayo M, Gorin MB, Reardon W, Kimberling WJ (2000) Genetic heterogeneity of Usher syndrome: analysis of 151 families with Usher type I. Am J Hum Genet 67:1569-1574.

Audo I, Bujakowska K, Mohand-Said S, Tronche S, Lancelot ME, Antonio A, Germain A, Lonjou C, Carpentier W, Sahel JA, Bhattacharya S, Zeitz C (2011) A novel DFNB31 mutation associated with Usher type 2 syndrome showing variable degrees of auditory loss in a consanguineous Portuguese family. Mol Vis 17:1598-1606.

Bahloul A, Michel V, Hardelin JP, Nouaille S, Hoos S, Houdusse A, England P, Petit C (2010) Cadherin-23, myosin VIIa and harmonin, encoded by Usher syndrome type I genes, form a ternary complex and interact with membrane phospholipids. Hum Mol Genet 19:3557-3565.

Ball SL, Bardenstein D, Alagramam KN (2003) Assessment of retinal structure and function in Ames waltzer mice. Invest Ophthalmol Vis Sci 44:3986-3992.

Bashir R, Fatima A, Naz S (2011) A frameshift mutation in SANS results in atypical Usher syndrome. Clin Genet 78:601-603.

Baux D, Larrieu L, Blanchet C, Hamel C, Ben Salah S, Vielle A, Gilbert-Dussardier B, Holder M, Calvas P, Philip N, Edery P, Bonneau D, Claustres M, Malcolm S, Roux AF (2007) Molecular and in silico analyses of the full-length isoform of usherin identify new pathogenic alleles in Usher type II patients. Hum Mutat 28:781-789.

Belyantseva IA, Boger ET, Naz S, Frolenkov GI, Sellers JR, Ahmed ZM, Griffith AJ, Friedman TB (2005) Myosin-XVa is required for tip localization of whirlin and differential elongation of hair-cell stereocilia. Nat Cell Biol 7:148-156.

Ben Rebeh I, Benzina Z, Dhouib H, Hadjamor I, Amyere M, Ayadi L, Turki K, Hammami B, Kmiha N, Kammoun H, Hakim B, Charfedine I, Vikkula M, Ghorbel A, Ayadi H, Masmoudi S (2008) Identification of candidate regions for a novel Usher syndrome type II locus. Mol Vis 14:1719-1726.

Berson EL (2000) Nutrition and retinal degenerations. Int Ophthalmol Clin 40:93-111.

Berson EL, Rosner B, Sandberg MA, Hayes KC, Nicholson BW, Weigel-DiFranco C, Willett W (1993) A randomized trial of vitamin A and vitamin E supplementation for retinitis pigmentosa. Arch Ophthalmol 111:761-772.

Besharse JC, Hollyfield JG (1979) Turnover of mouse photoreceptor outer segments in constant light and darkness. Invest Ophthalmol Vis Sci 18:1019-1024.

Beurg M, Nam JH, Crawford A, Fettiplace R (2008) The actions of calcium on hair bundle mechanics in mammalian cochlear hair cells. Biophys J 94:2639-2653.

Bhattacharya G, Miller C, Kimberling WJ, Jablonski MM, Cosgrove D (2002) Localization and expression of usherin: a novel basement membrane protein defective in people with Usher's syndrome type IIa. Hear Res 163:1-11.

Bitner-Glindzicz M, Lindley KJ, Rutland P, Blaydon D, Smith VV, Milla PJ, Hussain K, Furth-Lavi J, Cosgrove KE, Shepherd RM, Barnes PD, O'Brien RE, Farndon PA, Sowden J, Liu XZ, Scanlan MJ, Malcolm S, Dunne MJ, Aynsley-Green A, Glaser B (2000) A recessive contiguous gene deletion causing infantile hyperinsulinism, enteropathy and deafness identifies the Usher type 1C gene. Nat Genet 26:56-60.

Boeda B, El-Amraoui A, Bahloul A, Goodyear R, Daviet L, Blanchard S, Perfettini I, Fath KR, Shorte S, Reiners J, Houdusse A, Legrain P, Wolfrum U, Richardson G, Petit C (2002) Myosin VIIa, harmonin and cadherin 23, three Usher I gene products that cooperate to shape the sensory hair cell bundle. Embo J 21:6689-6699.

Bok D, Galbraith G, Lopez I, Woodruff M, Nusinowitz S, BeltrandelRio H, Huang W, Zhao S, Geske R, Montgomery C, Van Sligtenhorst I, Friddle C, Platt K, Sparks MJ, Pushkin A, Abuladze N, Ishiyama A, Dukkipati R, Liu W, Kurtz I (2003) Blindness and auditory impairment caused by loss of the sodium bicarbonate cotransporter NBC3. Nat Genet 34:313-319.

Bolz H, von Brederlow B, Ramirez A, Bryda EC, Kutsche K, Nothwang HG, Seeliger M, del CSCM, Vila MC, Molina OP, Gal A, Kubisch C (2001) Mutation of CDH23, encoding a new member of the cadherin gene family, causes Usher syndrome type 1D. Nat Genet 27:108-112.

Bork JM et al. (2001) Usher syndrome 1D and nonsyndromic autosomal recessive deafness DFNB12 are caused by allelic mutations of the novel cadherin-like gene CDH23. Am J Hum Genet 68:26-37.

Boughman JA, Vernon M, Shaver KA (1983) Usher syndrome: definition and estimate of prevalence from two high-risk populations. J Chronic Dis 36:595-603.

Caberlotto E, Michel V, Foucher I, Bahloul A, Goodyear RJ, Pepermans E, Michalski N, Perfettini I, Alegria-Prevot O, Chardenoux S, Do Cruzeiro M, Hardelin JP, Richardson GP, Avan P, Weil D, Petit C (2011) Usher type 1G protein sans is a critical component of the tip-link complex, a structure controlling actin polymerization in stereocilia. Proc Natl Acad Sci U S A 108:5825-5830.

Chaib H, Kaplan J, Gerber S, Vincent C, Ayadi H, Slim R, Munnich A, Weissenbach J, Petit C (1997) A newly identified locus for Usher syndrome type I, USH1E, maps to chromosome 21q21. Hum Mol Genet 6:27-31.

Cohen AI (1965) New Details of the Ultrastructure of the Outer Segments and Ciliary Connectives of the Rods of Human and Macaque Retinas. Anat Rec 152:63-79.

Cohen M, Bitner-Glindzicz M, Luxon L (2007) The changing face of Usher syndrome: clinical implications. Int J Audiol 46:82-93.

Delprat B, Michel V, Goodyear R, Yamasaki Y, Michalski N, El-Amraoui A, Perfettini I, Legrain P, Richardson G, Hardelin JP, Petit C (2005) Myosin XVa and whirlin, two deafness gene products required for hair bundle growth, are located at the stereocilia tips and interact directly. Hum Mol Genet 14:401-410.

Deretic D, Traverso V, Parkins N, Jackson F, Rodriguez de Turco EB, Ransom N (2004) Phosphoinositides, ezrin/moesin, and rac1 regulate fusion of rhodopsin transport carriers in retinal photoreceptors. Mol Biol Cell 15:359-370.

Di Palma F, Pellegrino R, Noben-Trauth K (2001a) Genomic structure, alternative splice forms and normal and mutant alleles of cadherin 23 (Cdh23). Gene 281:31-41.

Di Palma F, Holme RH, Bryda EC, Belyantseva IA, Pellegrino R, Kachar B, Steel KP, Noben-Trauth K (2001b) Mutations in Cdh23, encoding a new type of cadherin, cause stereocilia disorganization in waltzer, the mouse model for Usher syndrome type 1D. Nat Genet 27:103-107.

Dreyer B, Tranebjaerg L, Rosenberg T, Weston MD, Kimberling WJ, Nilssen O (2000) Identification of novel USH2A mutations: implications for the structure of USH2A protein. Eur J Hum Genet 8:500-506.

Dreyer B, Brox V, Tranebjaerg L, Rosenberg T, Sadeghi AM, Moller C, Nilssen O (2008) Spectrum of USH2A mutations in Scandinavian patients with Usher syndrome type II. Hum Mutat 29:451.

Ebermann I, Wiesen MH, Zrenner E, Lopez I, Pigeon R, Kohl S, Lowenheim H, Koenekoop RK, Bolz HJ (2009) GPR98 mutations cause Usher syndrome type 2 in males. J Med Genet 46:277-280.

Ebermann I, Scholl HP, Charbel Issa P, Becirovic E, Lamprecht J, Jurklies B, Millan JM, Aller E, Mitter D, Bolz H (2006) A novel gene for Usher syndrome type 2: mutations in the long isoform of whirlin are associated with retinitis pigmentosa and sensorineural hearing loss. Hum Genet 121:203-211.

Ebermann I, Phillips JB, Liebau MC, Koenekoop RK, Schermer B, Lopez I, Schafer E, Roux AF, Dafinger C, Bernd A, Zrenner E, Claustres M, Blanco B, Nurnberg G, Nurnberg P, Ruland R, Westerfield M, Benzing T, Bolz HJ (2010) PDZD7 is a modifier of retinal disease and a contributor to digenic Usher syndrome. J Clin Invest 120:1812-1823.

Edwards A, Fishman GA, Anderson RJ, Grover S, Derlacki DJ (1998) Visual acuity and visual field impairment in Usher syndrome. Arch Ophthalmol 116:165-168.

El-Amraoui A, Petit C (2005) Usher I syndrome: unravelling the mechanisms that underlie the cohesion of the growing hair bundle in inner ear sensory cells. J Cell Sci 118:4593-4603.

El-Amraoui A, Petit C (2010) Cadherins as targets for genetic diseases. Cold Spring Harb Perspect Biol 2:a003095.

el-Amraoui A, Sahly I, Picaud S, Sahel J, Abitbol M, Petit C (1996) Human Usher 1B/mouse shaker-1: the retinal phenotype discrepancy explained by the presence/absence of myosin VIIA in the photoreceptor cells. Hum Mol Genet 5:1171-1178.

Ernest S, Rauch GJ, Haffter P, Geisler R, Petit C, Nicolson T (2000) Mariner is defective in myosin VIIA: a zebrafish model for human hereditary deafness. Hum Mol Genet 9:2189-2196.

Eudy JD, Weston MD, Yao S, Hoover DM, Rehm HL, Ma-Edmonds M, Yan D, Ahmad I, Cheng JJ, Ayuso C, Cremers C, Davenport S, Moller C, Talmadge CB, Beisel KW, Tamayo M, Morton CC, Swaroop A, Kimberling WJ, Sumegi J (1998) Mutation of a gene encoding a protein with extracellular matrix motifs in Usher syndrome type IIa. Science 280:1753-1757.

Fetter RD, Corless JM (1987) Morphological components associated with frog cone outer segment disc margins. Invest Ophthalmol Vis Sci 28:646-657.

Fields RR, Zhou G, Huang D, Davis JR, Moller C, Jacobson SG, Kimberling WJ, Sumegi J (2002) Usher syndrome type III: revised genomic structure of the USH3 gene and identification of novel mutations. Am J Hum Genet 71:607-617.

Fishman GA, Bozbeyoglu S, Massof RW, Kimberling W (2007) Natural course of visual field loss in patients with Type 2 Usher syndrome. Retina 27:601-608.

Forge A, Souter M, Denman-Johnson K (1997) Structural development of sensory cells in the ear. Semin Cell Dev Biol 8:225-237.

Frolenkov GI, Belyantseva IA, Friedman TB, Griffith AJ (2004) Genetic insights into the morphogenesis of inner ear hair cells. Nat Rev Genet 5:489-498.

Geller SF, Guerin KI, Visel M, Pham A, Lee ES, Dror AA, Avraham KB, Hayashi T, Ray CA, Reh TA, Bermingham-McDonogh O, Triffo WJ, Bao S, Isosomppi J, Västinsalo H, Sankila EM, Flannery JG (2009) CLRN1 is nonessential in the mouse retina but is required for cochlear hair cell development. PLoS Genet 5:e1000607.

Geng R, Geller SF, Hayashi T, Ray CA, Reh TA, Bermingham-McDonogh O, Jones SM, Wright CG, Melki S, Imanishi Y, Palczewski K, Alagramam KN, Flannery JG (2009) Usher syndrome IIIA gene clarin-1 is essential for hair cell function and associated neural activation. Hum Mol Genet 18:2748-2760.

Gerber S, Bonneau D, Gilbert B, Munnich A, Dufier JL, Rozet JM, Kaplan J (2006) USH1A: chronicle of a slow death. Am J Hum Genet 78:357-359.

Gibbs D, Kitamoto J, Williams DS (2003) Abnormal phagocytosis by retinal pigmented epithelium that lacks myosin VIIa, the Usher syndrome 1B protein. Proc Natl Acad Sci U S A 100:6481-6486.

Gibbs D, Azarian SM, Lillo C, Kitamoto J, Klomp AE, Steel KP, Libby RT, Williams DS (2004) Role of myosin VIIa and Rab27a in the motility and localization of RPE melanosomes. J Cell Sci 117:6473-6483.

Gibert Y, McMillan DR, Kayes-Wandover K, Meyer A, Begemann G, White PC (2005) Analysis of the very large G-protein coupled receptor gene (Vlgr1/Mass1/USH2C) in zebrafish. Gene 353:200-206.

Gillespie PG, Muller U (2009) Mechanotransduction by hair cells: models, molecules, and mechanisms. Cell 139:33-44.

Goldmann T, Overlack N, Wolfrum U, Nagel-Wolfrum K (2011) PTC124 mediated translational read-through of a nonsense mutation causing Usher type 1C. Hum Gene Ther 22:537-547.

Goldmann T, Rebibo-Sabbah A, Overlack N, Nudelman I, Belakhov V, Baasov T, Ben-Yosef T, Wolfrum U, Nagel-Wolfrum K (2010) Beneficial read-through of a USH1C nonsense mutation by designed aminoglycoside NB30 in the retina. Invest Ophthalmol Vis Sci 51:6671-6680.

Goodyear R, Richardson G (1999) The ankle-link antigen: an epitope sensitive to calcium chelation associated with the hair-cell surface and the calycal processes of photoreceptors. J Neurosci 19:3761-3772.

Goodyear RJ, Richardson GP (2003) A novel antigen sensitive to calcium chelation that is associated with the tip links and kinocilial links of sensory hair bundles. J Neurosci 23:4878-4887.

Goodyear RJ, Forge A, Legan PK, Richardson GP (2010) Asymmetric distribution of cadherin 23 and protocadherin 15 in the kinocilial links of avian sensory hair cells. J Comp Neurol 518:4288-4297.

Goodyear RJ, Marcotti W, Kros CJ, Richardson GP (2005) Development and properties of stereociliary link types in hair cells of the mouse cochlea. J Comp Neurol 485:75-85.

Grati M, Kachar B (2011) Myosin VIIa and sans localization at stereocilia upper tip-link density implicates these Usher syndrome proteins in mechanotransduction. Proc Natl Acad Sci U S A 108:11476-11481.

Grillet N, Xiong W, Reynolds A, Kazmierczak P, Sato T, Lillo C, Dumont RA, Hintermann E, Sczaniecka A, Schwander M, Williams D, Kachar B, Gillespie PG, Muller U (2009) Harmonin mutations cause mechanotransduction defects in cochlear hair cells. Neuron 62:375-387.

Grondahl J (1987) Estimation of prognosis and prevalence of retinitis pigmentosa and Usher syndrome in Norway. Clin Genet 31:255-264.

Hampton LL, Wright CG, Alagramam KN, Battey JF, Noben-Trauth K (2003) A new spontaneous mutation in the mouse Ames waltzer gene, Pcdh15. Hear Res 180:67-75.

Han F, Yu H, Tian C, Chen HE, Benedict-Alderfer C, Zheng Y, Wang Q, Han X, Zheng QY (2010) A new mouse mutant of the Cdh23 gene with early-onset hearing loss facilitates evaluation of otoprotection drugs. Pharmacogenomics J.

Hartong DT, Berson EL, Dryja TP (2006) Retinitis pigmentosa. Lancet 368:1795-1809.

Hashimoto T, Gibbs D, Lillo C, Azarian SM, Legacki E, Zhang XM, Yang XJ, Williams DS (2007) Lentiviral gene replacement therapy of retinas in a mouse model for Usher syndrome type 1B. Gene Ther 14:584-594.

Hasson T, Heintzelman MB, Santos-Sacchi J, Corey DP, Mooseker MS (1995) Expression in cochlea and retina of myosin VIIa, the gene product defective in Usher syndrome type 1B. Proc Natl Acad Sci U S A 92:9815-9819.

Hasson T, Walsh J, Cable J, Mooseker MS, Brown SD, Steel KP (1997) Effects of shaker-1 mutations on myosin-VIIa protein and mRNA expression. Cell Motil Cytoskeleton 37:127-138.

Haywood-Watson RJ, 2nd, Ahmed ZM, Kjellstrom S, Bush RA, Takada Y, Hampton LL, Battey JF, Sieving PA, Friedman TB (2006) Ames Waltzer deaf mice have reduced electroretinogram amplitudes and complex alternative splicing of Pcdh15 transcripts. Invest Ophthalmol Vis Sci 47:3074-3084.

Heissler SM, Manstein DJ (2011) Functional characterization of the human myosin-7a motor domain. Cell Mol Life Sci.

Hilgert N, Kahrizi K, Dieltjens N, Bazazzadegan N, Najmabadi H, Smith RJ, Van Camp G (2009) A large deletion in GPR98 causes type IIC Usher syndrome in male and female members of an Iranian family. J Med Genet 46:272-276.

Hmani-Aifa M, Benzina Z, Zulfiqar F, Dhouib H, Shahzadi A, Ghorbel A, Rebai A, Soderkvist P, Riazuddin S, Kimberling WJ, Ayadi H (2009) Identification of two new mutations in the GPR98 and the PDE6B genes segregating in a Tunisian family. Eur J Hum Genet 17:474-482.

Holme RH, Kiernan BW, Brown SD, Steel KP (2002) Elongation of hair cell stereocilia is defective in the mouse mutant whirler. J Comp Neurol 450:94-102.

Hope CI, Bundey S, Proops D, Fielder AR (1997) Usher syndrome in the city of Birmingham--prevalence and clinical classification. Br J Ophthalmol 81:46-53.

Joensuu T, Hamalainen R, Yuan B, Johnson C, Tegelberg S, Gasparini P, Zelante L, Pirvola U, Pakarinen L, Lehesjoki AE, de la Chapelle A, Sankila EM (2001) Mutations in a novel gene with transmembrane domains underlie Usher syndrome type 3. Am J Hum Genet 69:673-684.

Johnson KR, Zheng QY, Weston MD, Ptacek LJ, Noben-Trauth K (2005) The Mass1frings mutation underlies early onset hearing impairment in BUB/BnJ mice, a model for the auditory pathology of Usher syndrome IIC. Genomics 85:582-590.

Johnson KR, Gagnon LH, Webb LS, Peters LL, Hawes NL, Chang B, Zheng QY (2003) Mouse models of USH1C and DFNB18: phenotypic and molecular analyses of two new spontaneous mutations of the Ush1c gene. Hum Mol Genet 12:3075-3086.

Kaiserman N, Obolensky A, Banin E, Sharon D (2007) Novel USH2A mutations in Israeli patients with retinitis pigmentosa and Usher syndrome type 2. Arch Ophthalmol 125:219-224.

Kalay E, de Brouwer AP, Caylan R, Nabuurs SB, Wollnik B, Karaguzel A, Heister JG, Erdol H, Cremers FP, Cremers CW, Brunner HG, Kremer H (2005) A novel D458V mutation in the SANS PDZ binding motif causes atypical Usher syndrome. J Mol Med (Berl) 83:1025-1032.

Kazmierczak P, Sakaguchi H, Tokita J, Wilson-Kubalek EM, Milligan RA, Muller U, Kachar B (2007) Cadherin 23 and protocadherin 15 interact to form tip-link filaments in sensory hair cells. Nature 449:87-91.

Keats BJ, Corey DP (1999) The usher syndromes. Am J Med Genet 89:158-166.

Kikkawa Y, Mburu P, Morse S, Kominami R, Townsend S, Brown SD (2005) Mutant analysis reveals whirlin as a dynamic organizer in the growing hair cell stereocilium. Hum Mol Genet 14:391-400.

Kikkawa Y, Shitara H, Wakana S, Kohara Y, Takada T, Okamoto M, Taya C, Kamiya K, Yoshikawa Y, Tokano H, Kitamura K, Shimizu K, Wakabayashi Y, Shiroishi T, Kominami R, Yonekawa H (2003) Mutations in a new scaffold protein Sans cause deafness in Jackson shaker mice. Hum Mol Genet 12:453-461.

Kobayashi I, Imamura K, Kubota M, Ishikawa S, Yamada M, Tonoki H, Okano M, Storch WB, Moriuchi T, Sakiyama Y, Kobayashi K (1999) Identification of an autoimmune enteropathy-related 75-kilodalton antigen. Gastroenterology 117:823-830.

Kremer H, van Wijk E, Marker T, Wolfrum U, Roepman R (2006) Usher syndrome: molecular links of pathogenesis, proteins and pathways. Hum Mol Genet 15 Spec No 2:R262-270.

Kros CJ, Marcotti W, van Netten SM, Self TJ, Libby RT, Brown SD, Richardson GP, Steel KP (2002) Reduced climbing and increased slipping adaptation in cochlear hair cells of mice with Myo7a mutations. Nat Neurosci 5:41-47.

Kussel-Andermann P, El-Amraoui A, Safieddine S, Nouaille S, Perfettini I, Lecuit M, Cossart P, Wolfrum U, Petit C (2000) Vezatin, a novel transmembrane protein, bridges myosin VIIA to the cadherin-catenins complex. EMBO J 19:6020-6029.

Lagziel A, Ahmed ZM, Schultz JM, Morell RJ, Belyantseva IA, Friedman TB (2005) Spatiotemporal pattern and isoforms of cadherin 23 in wild type and waltzer mice during inner ear hair cell development. Dev Biol 280:295-306.

Lagziel A, Overlack N, Bernstein SL, Morell RJ, Wolfrum U, Friedman TB (2009) Expression of cadherin 23 isoforms is not conserved: implications for a mouse model of Usher syndrome type 1D. Mol Vis 15:1843-1857.

Lane PW (1963) Whirler Mice: A Recessive Behavior Mutation in Linkage Group Viii. J Hered 54:263-266.

LaVail MM (1976) Rod outer segment disk shedding in rat retina: relationship to cyclic lighting. Science 194:1071-1074.

Lefevre G, Michel V, Weil D, Lepelletier L, Bizard E, Wolfrum U, Hardelin JP, Petit C (2008) A core cochlear phenotype in USH1 mouse mutants implicates fibrous links of the hair bundle in its cohesion, orientation and differential growth. Development 135:1427-1437.

Leibovici M, Safieddine S, Petit C (2008) Mouse models for human hereditary deafness. Curr Top Dev Biol 84:385-429.

Lentz J, Pan F, Ng SS, Deininger P, Keats B (2007) Ush1c216A knock-in mouse survives Katrina. Mutat Res 616:139-144.

Lentz JJ, Gordon WC, Farris HE, MacDonald GH, Cunningham DE, Robbins CA, Tempel BL, Bazan NG, Rubel EW, Oesterle EC, Keats BJ (2010) Deafness and retinal degeneration in a novel USH1C knock-in mouse model. Dev Neurobiol 70:253-267.

Libby RT, Steel KP (2001) Electroretinographic anomalies in mice with mutations in Myo7a, the gene involved in human Usher syndrome type 1B. Invest Ophthalmol Vis Sci 42:770-778.

Libby RT, Kitamoto J, Holme RH, Williams DS, Steel KP (2003) Cdh23 mutations in the mouse are associated with retinal dysfunction but not retinal degeneration. Exp Eye Res 77:731-739.

Lillo C, Kitamoto J, Liu X, Quint E, Steel KP, Williams DS (2003) Mouse models for Usher syndrome 1B. Adv Exp Med Biol 533:143-150.
Liu X, Udovichenko IP, Brown SD, Steel KP, Williams DS (1999) Myosin VIIa participates in opsin transport through the photoreceptor cilium. J Neurosci 19:6267-6274.
Liu X, Bulgakov OV, Darrow KN, Pawlyk B, Adamian M, Liberman MC, Li T (2007) Usherin is required for maintenance of retinal photoreceptors and normal development of cochlear hair cells. Proc Natl Acad Sci U S A 104:4413-4418.
Liu XZ, Walsh J, Mburu P, Kendrick-Jones J, Cope MJ, Steel KP, Brown SD (1997) Mutations in the myosin VIIA gene cause non-syndromic recessive deafness. Nat Genet 16:188-190.
Liu XZ, Angeli SI, Rajput K, Yan D, Hodges AV, Eshraghi A, Telischi FF, Balkany TJ (2008) Cochlear implantation in individuals with Usher type 1 syndrome. International Journal of Pediatric Otorhinolaryngology 72:841-847.
Lopes VS, Gibbs D, Libby RT, Aleman TS, Welch DL, Lillo C, Jacobson SG, Radu RA, Steel KP, Williams DS (2011) The Usher 1B protein, MYO7A, is required for normal localization and function of the visual retinoid cycle enzyme, RPE65. Hum Mol Genet 20:2560-2570.
Lu B, Wang S, Francis PJ, Li T, Gamm DM, Capowski EE, Lund RD (2009) Cell transplantation to arrest early changes in an ush2a animal model. Invest Ophthalmol Vis Sci 51:2269-2276.
Maerker T, van Wijk E, Overlack N, Kersten FF, McGee J, Goldmann T, Sehn E, Roepman R, Walsh EJ, Kremer H, Wolfrum U (2008) A novel Usher protein network at the periciliary reloading point between molecular transport machineries in vertebrate photoreceptor cells. Hum Mol Genet 17:71-86.
Malm E, Ponjavic V, Moller C, Kimberling WJ, Andreasson S (2010) Phenotypes in Defined Genotypes Including Siblings with Usher Syndrome. Ophthalmic Genet.
Malm E, Ponjavic V, Moller C, Kimberling WJ, Stone ES, Andreasson S (2011) Alteration of rod and cone function in children with Usher syndrome. Eur J Ophthalmol 21:30-38.
Manji SS, Miller KA, Williams LH, Andreasen L, Siboe M, Rose E, Bahlo M, Kuiper M, Dahl HH (2011) An ENU-Induced Mutation of Cdh23 Causes Congenital Hearing Loss, but No Vestibular Dysfunction, in Mice. Am J Pathol 179:903-914.
Mazelova J, Ransom N, Astuto-Gribble L, Wilson MC, Deretic D (2009) Syntaxin 3 and SNAP-25 pairing, regulated by omega-3 docosahexaenoic acid, controls the delivery of rhodopsin for the biogenesis of cilia-derived sensory organelles, the rod outer segments. J Cell Sci 122:2003-2013.
Mburu P, Liu XZ, Walsh J, Saw D, Jr., Cope MJ, Gibson F, Kendrick-Jones J, Steel KP, Brown SD (1997) Mutation analysis of the mouse myosin VIIA deafness gene. Genes Funct 1:191-203.
Mburu P et al. (2003) Defects in whirlin, a PDZ domain molecule involved in stereocilia elongation, cause deafness in the whirler mouse and families with DFNB31. Nat Genet 34:421-428.
McGee J, Goodyear RJ, McMillan DR, Stauffer EA, Holt JR, Locke KG, Birch DG, Legan PK, White PC, Walsh EJ, Richardson GP (2006) The very large G-protein-coupled receptor VLGR1: a component of the ankle link complex required for the normal development of auditory hair bundles. J Neurosci 26:6543-6553.

McGee TL, Seyedahmadi BJ, Sweeney MO, Dryja TP, Berson EL (2010) Novel mutations in the long isoform of the USH2A gene in patients with Usher syndrome type II or non-syndromic retinitis pigmentosa. J Med Genet 47:499-506.

McMillan DR, White PC (2004) Loss of the transmembrane and cytoplasmic domains of the very large G-protein-coupled receptor-1 (VLGR1 or Mass1) causes audiogenic seizures in mice. Mol Cell Neurosci 26:322-329.

McMillan DR, White PC (2011) Studies on the very large g protein-coupled receptor: from initial discovery to determining its role in sensorineural deafness in higher animals. Adv Exp Med Biol 706:76-86.

McMillan DR, Kayes-Wandover KM, Richardson JA, White PC (2002) Very large G protein-coupled receptor-1, the largest known cell surface protein, is highly expressed in the developing central nervous system. J Biol Chem 277:785-792.

Michalski N, Michel V, Bahloul A, Lefevre G, Barral J, Yagi H, Chardenoux S, Weil D, Martin P, Hardelin JP, Sato M, Petit C (2007) Molecular characterization of the ankle-link complex in cochlear hair cells and its role in the hair bundle functioning. J Neurosci 27:6478-6488.

Michalski N, Michel V, Caberlotto E, Lefevre GM, van Aken AF, Tinevez JY, Bizard E, Houbron C, Weil D, Hardelin JP, Richardson GP, Kros CJ, Martin P, Petit C (2009) Harmonin-b, an actin-binding scaffold protein, is involved in the adaptation of mechanoelectrical transduction by sensory hair cells. Pflugers Arch 459:115-130.

Michel V, Goodyear RJ, Weil D, Marcotti W, Perfettini I, Wolfrum U, Kros CJ, Richardson GP, Petit C (2005) Cadherin 23 is a component of the transient lateral links in the developing hair bundles of cochlear sensory cells. Dev Biol 280:281-294.

Millan JM, Aller E, Jaijo T, Blanco-Kelly F, Gimenez-Pardo A, Ayuso C (2011) An update on the genetics of usher syndrome. J Ophthalmol 2011:417217.

Nakanishi H, Ohtsubo M, Iwasaki S, Hotta Y, Mizuta K, Mineta H, Minoshima S (2009) Identification of 11 novel mutations in USH2A among Japanese patients with Usher syndrome type 2. Clin Genet 76:383-391.

Nayak GD, Ratnayaka HS, Goodyear RJ, Richardson GP (2007) Development of the hair bundle and mechanotransduction. Int J Dev Biol 51:597-608.

Nicolson T, Rusch A, Friedrich RW, Granato M, Ruppersberg JP, Nusslein-Volhard C (1998) Genetic analysis of vertebrate sensory hair cell mechanosensation: the zebrafish circler mutants. Neuron 20:271-283.

Nikkila H, McMillan DR, Nunez BS, Pascoe L, Curnow KM, White PC (2000) Sequence similarities between a novel putative G protein-coupled receptor and Na+/Ca2+ exchangers define a cation binding domain. Mol Endocrinol 14:1351-1364.

Noben-Trauth K, Zheng QY, Johnson KR (2003) Association of cadherin 23 with polygenic inheritance and genetic modification of sensorineural hearing loss. Nat Genet 35:21-23.

Nudelman I, Glikin D, Smolkin B, Hainrichson M, Belakhov V, Baasov T (2010) Repairing faulty genes by aminoglycosides: development of new derivatives of geneticin (G418) with enhanced suppression of diseases-causing nonsense mutations. Bioorg Med Chem 18:3735-3746.

Nudelman I, Rebibo-Sabbah A, Cherniavsky M, Belakhov V, Hainrichson M, Chen F, Schacht J, Pilch DS, Ben-Yosef T, Baasov T (2009) Development of novel

aminoglycoside (NB54) with reduced toxicity and enhanced suppression of disease-causing premature stop mutations. J Med Chem 52:2836-2845.
Osten P, Stern-Bach Y (2006) Learning from stargazin: the mouse, the phenotype and the unexpected. Curr Opin Neurobiol 16:275-280.
Pakarinen L, Tuppurainen K, Laippala P, Mantyjarvi M, Puhakka H (1995) The ophthalmological course of Usher syndrome type III. Int Ophthalmol 19:307-311.
Pan L, Yan J, Wu L, Zhang M (2009) Assembling stable hair cell tip link complex via multidentate interactions between harmonin and cadherin 23. Proc Natl Acad Sci U S A 106:5575-5580.
Papermaster DS (2002) The birth and death of photoreceptors: the Friedenwald Lecture. Invest Ophthalmol Vis Sci 43:1300-1309.
Papermaster DS, Schneider BG, DeFoe D, Besharse JC (1986) Biosynthesis and vectorial transport of opsin on vesicles in retinal rod photoreceptors. J Histochem Cytochem 34:5-16.
Pearsall N, Bhattacharya G, Wisecarver J, Adams J, Cosgrove D, Kimberling W (2002) Usherin expression is highly conserved in mouse and human tissues. Hear Res 174:55-63.
Peng YW, Zallocchi M, Wang WM, Delimont D, Cosgrove D (2011) Moderate light induced degeneration of rod photoreceptors with delayed transducin translocation in shaker1 mice. Invest Ophthalmol Vis Sci.
Pennings RJ, Damen GW, Snik AF, Hoefsloot L, Cremers CW, Mylanus EA (2006) Audiologic performance and benefit of cochlear implantation in Usher syndrome type I. Laryngoscope 116:717-722.
Peters KR, Palade GE, Schneider BG, Papermaster DS (1983) Fine structure of a periciliary ridge complex of frog retinal rod cells revealed by ultrahigh resolution scanning electron microscopy. J Cell Biol 96:265-276.
Petit C (2001) Usher syndrome: from genetics to pathogenesis. Annu Rev Genomics Hum Genet 2:271-297.
Phillips JB, Blanco-Sanchez B, Lentz JJ, Tallafuss A, Khanobdee K, Sampath S, Jacobs ZG, Han PF, Mishra M, Williams DS, Keats BJ, Washbourne P, Westerfield M (2011) Harmonin (Ush1c) is required in zebrafish Muller glial cells for photoreceptor synaptic development and function. Dis Model Mech.
Rana MW, Taraszka SR (1991) Monkey photoreceptor calycal processes and interphotoreceptor matrix as observed by scanning electron microscopy. Am J Anat 192:472-477.
Rebibo-Sabbah A, Nudelman I, Ahmed ZM, Baasov T, Ben-Yosef T (2007) In vitro and ex vivo suppression by aminoglycosides of PCDH15 nonsense mutations underlying type 1 Usher syndrome. Hum Genet 122:373-381.
Reiners J, Marker T, Jurgens K, Reidel B, Wolfrum U (2005a) Photoreceptor expression of the Usher syndrome type 1 protein protocadherin 15 (USH1F) and its interaction with the scaffold protein harmonin (USH1C). Mol Vis 11:347-355.
Reiners J, Nagel-Wolfrum K, Jurgens K, Marker T, Wolfrum U (2006) Molecular basis of human Usher syndrome: deciphering the meshes of the Usher protein network provides insights into the pathomechanisms of the Usher disease. Exp Eye Res 83:97-119.

Reiners J, Reidel B, El-Amraoui A, Boeda B, Huber I, Petit C, Wolfrum U (2003) Differential distribution of harmonin isoforms and their possible role in Usher-1 protein complexes in mammalian photoreceptor cells. Invest Ophthalmol Vis Sci 44:5006-5015.

Reiners J, van Wijk E, Marker T, Zimmermann U, Jurgens K, te Brinke H, Overlack N, Roepman R, Knipper M, Kremer H, Wolfrum U (2005b) Scaffold protein harmonin (USH1C) provides molecular links between Usher syndrome type 1 and type 2. Hum Mol Genet 14:3933-3943.

Rhodes CR, Hertzano R, Fuchs H, Bell RE, de Angelis MH, Steel KP, Avraham KB (2004) A Myo7a mutation cosegregates with stereocilia defects and low-frequency hearing impairment. Mamm Genome 15:686-697.

Richardson GP, de Monvel JB, Petit C (2011) How the genetics of deafness illuminates auditory physiology. Annu Rev Physiol 73:311-334.

Rivolta C, Berson EL, Dryja TP (2002) Paternal uniparental heterodisomy with partial isodisomy of chromosome 1 in a patient with retinitis pigmentosa without hearing loss and a missense mutation in the Usher syndrome type II gene USH2A. Arch Ophthalmol 120:1566-1571.

Rodriguez de Turco EB, Deretic D, Bazan NG, Papermaster DS (1997) Post-Golgi vesicles cotransport docosahexaenoyl-phospholipids and rhodopsin during frog photoreceptor membrane biogenesis. J Biol Chem 272:10491-10497.

Roepman R, Wolfrum U (2007) Protein networks and complexes in photoreceptor cilia. Subcell Biochem 43:209-235.

Rosenberg T, Haim M, Hauch AM, Parving A (1997) The prevalence of Usher syndrome and other retinal dystrophy-hearing impairment associations. Clin Genet 51:314-321.

Rzadzinska AK, Derr A, Kachar B, Noben-Trauth K (2005) Sustained cadherin 23 expression in young and adult cochlea of normal and hearing-impaired mice. Hear Res 208:114-121.

Sadeghi AM, Eriksson K, Kimberling WJ, Sjostrom A, Moller C (2006) Longterm visual prognosis in Usher syndrome types 1 and 2. Acta Ophthalmol Scand 84:537-544.

Saihan Z, Webster AR, Luxon L, Bitner-Glindzicz M (2009) Update on Usher syndrome. Curr Opin Neurol 22:19-27.

Sandberg MA, Rosner B, Weigel-DiFranco C, McGee TL, Dryja TP, Berson EL (2008) Disease course in patients with autosomal recessive retinitis pigmentosa due to the USH2A gene. Invest Ophthalmol Vis Sci 49:5532-5539.

Scanlan MJ, Williamson B, Jungbluth A, Stockert E, Arden KC, Viars CS, Gure AO, Gordan JD, Chen YT, Old LJ (1999) Isoforms of the human PDZ-73 protein exhibit differential tissue expression. Biochim Biophys Acta 1445:39-52.

Schneider E, Marker T, Daser A, Frey-Mahn G, Beyer V, Farcas R, Schneider-Ratzke B, Kohlschmidt N, Grossmann B, Bauss K, Napiontek U, Keilmann A, Bartsch O, Zechner U, Wolfrum U, Haaf T (2009) Homozygous disruption of PDZD7 by reciprocal translocation in a consanguineous family: a new member of the Usher syndrome protein interactome causing congenital hearing impairment. Hum Mol Genet 18:655-666.

Schwander M, Xiong W, Tokita J, Lelli A, Elledge HM, Kazmierczak P, Sczaniecka A, Kolatkar A, Wiltshire T, Kuhn P, Holt JR, Kachar B, Tarantino L, Muller U (2009) A mouse model for nonsyndromic deafness (DFNB12) links hearing loss to defects in tip links of mechanosensory hair cells. Proc Natl Acad Sci U S A 106:5252-5257.

Seiler C, Finger-Baier KC, Rinner O, Makhankov YV, Schwarz H, Neuhauss SC, Nicolson T (2005) Duplicated genes with split functions: independent roles of protocadherin15 orthologues in zebrafish hearing and vision. Development 132:615-623.

Self T, Mahony M, Fleming J, Walsh J, Brown SD, Steel KP (1998) Shaker-1 mutations reveal roles for myosin VIIA in both development and function of cochlear hair cells. Development 125:557-566.

Senften M, Schwander M, Kazmierczak P, Lillo C, Shin JB, Hasson T, Geleoc GS, Gillespie PG, Williams D, Holt JR, Muller U (2006) Physical and functional interaction between protocadherin 15 and myosin VIIa in mechanosensory hair cells. J Neurosci 26:2060-2071.

Seyedahmadi BJ, Rivolta C, Keene JA, Berson EL, Dryja TP (2004) Comprehensive screening of the USH2A gene in Usher syndrome type II and non-syndromic recessive retinitis pigmentosa. Exp Eye Res 79:167-173.

Sheng M, Sala C (2001) PDZ domains and the organization of supramolecular complexes. Annu Rev Neurosci 24:1-29.

Siemens J, Kazmierczak P, Reynolds A, Sticker M, Littlewood-Evans A, Muller U (2002) The Usher syndrome proteins cadherin 23 and harmonin form a complex by means of PDZ-domain interactions. Proc Natl Acad Sci U S A 99:14946-14951.

Siemens J, Lillo C, Dumont RA, Reynolds A, Williams DS, Gillespie PG, Muller U (2004) Cadherin 23 is a component of the tip link in hair-cell stereocilia. Nature 428:950-955.

Skradski SL, Clark AM, Jiang H, White HS, Fu YH, Ptacek LJ (2001) A novel gene causing a mendelian audiogenic mouse epilepsy. Neuron 31:537-544.

Slepak VZ, Hurley JB (2008) Mechanism of light-induced translocation of arrestin and transducin in photoreceptors: interaction-restricted diffusion. IUBMB Life 60:2-9.

Smith RJ, Berlin CI, Hejtmancik JF, Keats BJ, Kimberling WJ, Lewis RA, Moller CG, Pelias MZ, Tranebjaerg L (1994) Clinical diagnosis of the Usher syndromes. Usher Syndrome Consortium. Am J Med Genet 50:32-38.

Smits BM, Peters TA, Mul JD, Croes HJ, Fransen JA, Beynon AJ, Guryev V, Plasterk RH, Cuppen E (2005) Identification of a rat model for usher syndrome type 1B by N-ethyl-N-nitrosourea mutagenesis-driven forward genetics. Genetics 170:1887-1896.

Sollner C, Rauch GJ, Siemens J, Geisler R, Schuster SC, Muller U, Nicolson T (2004) Mutations in cadherin 23 affect tip links in zebrafish sensory hair cells. Nature 428:955-959.

Spandau UH, Rohrschneider K (2002) Prevalence and geographical distribution of Usher syndrome in Germany. Graefes Arch Clin Exp Ophthalmol 240:495-498.

Tian C, Liu XZ, Han F, Yu H, Longo-Guess C, Yang B, Lu C, Yan D, Zheng QY (2010) Ush1c gene expression levels in the ear and eye suggest different roles for Ush1c in neurosensory organs in a new Ush1c knockout mouse. Brain Res 1328:57-70.

Tian G, Zhou Y, Hajkova D, Miyagi M, Dinculescu A, Hauswirth WW, Palczewski K, Geng R, Alagramam KN, Isosomppi J, Sankila EM, Flannery JG, Imanishi Y (2009) Clarin-1, encoded by the Usher Syndrome III causative gene, forms a membranous microdomain: possible role of clarin-1 in organizing the actin cytoskeleton. J Biol Chem 284:18980-18993.

Tlili A, Charfedine I, Lahmar I, Benzina Z, Mohamed BA, Weil D, Idriss N, Drira M, Masmoudi S, Ayadi H (2005) Identification of a novel frameshift mutation in the DFNB31/WHRN gene in a Tunisian consanguineous family with hereditary non-syndromic recessive hearing loss. Hum Mutat 25:503.

Tomita S, Shenoy A, Fukata Y, Nicoll RA, Bredt DS (2007) Stargazin interacts functionally with the AMPA receptor glutamate-binding module. Neuropharmacology 52:87-91.

Usher CH (1914) On the inheritance of retinitis pigmentosa, with notes of cases. R Lond Ophthalmol Hosp Rep 19:130-236.

van Wijk E, Pennings RJ, te Brinke H, Claassen A, Yntema HG, Hoefsloot LH, Cremers FP, Cremers CW, Kremer H (2004) Identification of 51 novel exons of the Usher syndrome type 2A (USH2A) gene that encode multiple conserved functional domains and that are mutated in patients with Usher syndrome type II. Am J Hum Genet 74:738-744.

van Wijk E, van der Zwaag B, Peters T, Zimmermann U, Te Brinke H, Kersten FF, Marker T, Aller E, Hoefsloot LH, Cremers CW, Cremers FP, Wolfrum U, Knipper M, Roepman R, Kremer H (2006) The DFNB31 gene product whirlin connects to the Usher protein network in the cochlea and retina by direct association with USH2A and VLGR1. Hum Mol Genet 15:751-765.

Vastinsalo H, Jalkanen R, Dinculescu A, Isosomppi J, Geller S, Flannery JG, Hauswirth WW, Sankila EM (2010) Alternative splice variants of the USH3A gene Clarin 1 (CLRN1). Eur J Hum Genet 19:30-35.

Verpy E, Leibovici M, Zwaenepoel I, Liu XZ, Gal A, Salem N, Mansour A, Blanchard S, Kobayashi I, Keats BJ, Slim R, Petit C (2000) A defect in harmonin, a PDZ domain-containing protein expressed in the inner ear sensory hair cells, underlies Usher syndrome type 1C. Nat Genet 26:51-55.

Vollrath MA, Kwan KY, Corey DP (2007) The micromachinery of mechanotransduction in hair cells. Annu Rev Neurosci 30:339-365.

von Graefe A (1858) Vereinzelte Beobachtungen und Bemerkungen. Exceptionelles Verhalten des Gesichtsfeldes bei Pigmententartung des Netzhaut. Albrecht Graefes Arch Klin Ophthalmol 4:250-253.

Wada T, Wakabayashi Y, Takahashi S, Ushiki T, Kikkawa Y, Yonekawa H, Kominami R (2001) A point mutation in a cadherin gene, Cdh23, causes deafness in a novel mutant, Waltzer mouse niigata. Biochem Biophys Res Commun 283:113-117.

Washington JL, 3rd, Pitts D, Wright CG, Erway LC, Davis RR, Alagramam K (2005) Characterization of a new allele of Ames waltzer generated by ENU mutagenesis. Hear Res 202:161-169.

Webb SW, Grillet N, Andrade LR, Xiong W, Swarthout L, Della Santina CC, Kachar B, (2011) Muller U Regulation of PCDH15 function in mechanosensory hair cells by alternative splicing of the cytoplasmic domain. Development 138:1607-1617.

Weil D, Kussel P, Blanchard S, Levy G, Levi-Acobas F, Drira M, Ayadi H, Petit C (1997) The autosomal recessive isolated deafness, DFNB2, and the Usher 1B syndrome are allelic defects of the myosin-VIIA gene. Nat Genet 16:191-193.

Weil D, Blanchard S, Kaplan J, Guilford P, Gibson F, Walsh J, Mburu P, Varela A, Levilliers J, Weston MD, et al. (1995) Defective myosin VIIA gene responsible for Usher syndrome type 1B. Nature 374:60-61.

Weil D, El-Amraoui A, Masmoudi S, Mustapha M, Kikkawa Y, Laine S, Delmaghani S, Adato A, Nadifi S, Zina ZB, Hamel C, Gal A, Ayadi H, Yonekawa H, Petit C (2003) Usher syndrome type I G (USH1G) is caused by mutations in the gene encoding SANS, a protein that associates with the USH1C protein, harmonin. Hum Mol Genet 12:463-471.

Weston MD, Luijendijk MW, Humphrey KD, Moller C, Kimberling WJ (2004) Mutations in the VLGR1 gene implicate G-protein signaling in the pathogenesis of Usher syndrome type II. Am J Hum Genet 74:357-366.

Weston MD, Eudy JD, Fujita S, Yao S, Usami S, Cremers C, Greenberg J, Ramesar R, Martini A, Moller C, Smith RJ, Sumegi J, Kimberling WJ (2000) Genomic structure and identification of novel mutations in usherin, the gene responsible for Usher syndrome type IIa. Am J Hum Genet 66:1199-1210.

Williams DS (2008) Usher syndrome: animal models, retinal function of Usher proteins, and prospects for gene therapy. Vision Res 48:433-441.

Williams DS, Aleman TS, Lillo C, Lopes VS, Hughes LC, Stone EM, Jacobson SG (2009) Harmonin in the murine retina and the retinal phenotypes of Ush1c-mutant mice and human USH1C. Invest Ophthalmol Vis Sci 50:3881-3889.

Wilson SM, Householder DB, Coppola V, Tessarollo L, Fritzsch B, Lee EC, Goss D, Carlson GA, Copeland NG, Jenkins NA (2001) Mutations in Cdh23 cause nonsyndromic hearing loss in waltzer mice. Genomics 74:228-233.

Wolfrum U, Liu X, Schmitt A, Udovichenko IP, Williams DS (1998) Myosin VIIa as a common component of cilia and microvilli. Cell Motil Cytoskeleton 40:261-271.

Wu L, Pan L, Wei Z, Zhang M (2011) Structure of MyTH4-FERM domains in myosin VIIa tail bound to cargo. Science 331:757-760.

Yagi H, Takamura Y, Yoneda T, Konno D, Akagi Y, Yoshida K, Sato M (2005) Vlgr1 knockout mice show audiogenic seizure susceptibility. J Neurochem 92:191-202.

Yagi H, Tokano H, Maeda M, Takabayashi T, Nagano T, Kiyama H, Fujieda S, Kitamura K, Sato M (2007) Vlgr1 is required for proper stereocilia maturation of cochlear hair cells. Genes Cells 12:235-250.

Yan D, Kamiya K, Ouyang XM, Liu XZ (2011) Analysis of subcellular localization of Myo7a, Pcdh15 and Sans in Ush1c knockout mice. Int J Exp Pathol 92:66-71.

Yan D, Ouyang X, Patterson DM, Du LL, Jacobson SG, Liu XZ (2009) Mutation analysis in the long isoform of USH2A in American patients with Usher Syndrome type II. J Hum Genet 54:732-738.

Yan J, Pan L, Chen X, Wu L, Zhang M (2010) The structure of the harmonin/sans complex reveals an unexpected interaction mode of the two Usher syndrome proteins. Proc Natl Acad Sci U S A 107:4040-4045.

Yang J, Wang L, Song H, Sokolov M (2011) Current understanding of usher syndrome type II. Frontiers in Bioscience 17:1165-1183.

Yang J, Liu X, Zhao Y, Adamian M, Pawlyk B, Sun X, McMillan DR, Liberman MC, Li T (2010) Ablation of whirlin long isoform disrupts the USH2 protein complex and causes vision and hearing loss. PLoS Genet 6:e1000955.

Yonezawa S, Yoshizaki N, Kageyama T, Takahashi T, Sano M, Tokita Y, Masaki S, Inaguma Y, Hanai A, Sakurai N, Yoshiki A, Kusakabe M, Moriyama A, Nakayama A (2006) Fates of Cdh23/CDH23 with mutations affecting the cytoplasmic region. Hum Mutat 27:88-97.

Young RW (1967) The renewal of photoreceptor cell outer segments. J Cell Biol 33:61-72.

Young RW (1976) Visual cells and the concept of renewal. Invest Ophthalmol Vis Sci 15:700-725.

Zallocchi M, Meehan DT, Delimont D, Askew C, Garige S, Gratton MA, Rothermund-Franklin CA, Cosgrove D (2009) Localization and expression of clarin-1, the Clrn1 gene product, in auditory hair cells and photoreceptors. Hear Res 255:109-120.

Zou J, Luo L, Shen Z, Chiodo VA, Ambati BK, Hauswirth WW, Yang J (2011) Whirlin Replacement Restores the Formation of the USH2 Protein Complex in Whirlin Knockout Photoreceptors. Invest Ophthalmol Vis Sci 52:2343-2351.

Part 5

Treatment

15

Cochlear Implants in Children: A Review

Julia Sarant
The University of Melbourne
Australia

1. Introduction

In 1980, the first child in the world was implanted with the single-channel House cochlear implant device (Eisenberg & House, 1982). Children who initially received cochlear implants during this first paediatric clinical trial were quite old compared to current ages (the average age in the first House clinical trial was 8 years, whereas children are now being implanted as young as 6 months of age), and the majority communicated using sign language (Eisenberg & Johnson, 2008). It is now known that implanting older children who do not communicate orally gives little chance of speech perception or spoken language development. In 1985, the first children received a multichannel cochlear implant in Australia (Clark et al., 1987). This clinical trial selected children who had a higher potential for success, including shorter duration of deafness and a commitment to oral communication both at home and in their educational programs. At this time, it was unknown whether the speech processing schemes used with adults who had lost their hearing after developing language (ie. post-lingually deafened) would be appropriate for facilitating the speech perception and language development of young children with immature auditory systems. It is important also to note that the desired outcomes for adults and children differed; while the goal for adults was to improve auditory skills and communication using previously acquired cognitive, spoken language, and social skills, the goal for children was to develop these skills using the auditory information provided by the cochlear implant, having had no useful auditory experience (and therefore presumably no neural development of their auditory system) until they received their cochlear implant. The implantation of children was also highly controversial. For many years, cochlear implantation in children was opposed by the Deaf Community, on the grounds that deafness in children should be considered as a cultural and linguistic difference rather than as a disability that could be remediated by a cochlear implant. Over time, this view has changed such that in 2000, a position paper of the National Association of the Deaf in the U.S. stated that "cochlear implantation is a technology that represents a tool to be used in some forms of communication, and not a cure for deafness" (National Association of the Deaf, 2000).

It is now well documented that children with severe-profound hearing loss receive significant benefits from cochlear implants in terms of speech perception and language development (Blamey et al., 2006; Geers et al., 2008; Moog, 2002; Nicholas & Geers 2007). Cochlear implants are becoming the standard of care for children with severe-profound hearing loss, with increasing uptake of simultaneous bilateral implants over recent years. There is a large variation in implementation of cochlear implant technology around the world, and also within regions in some countries. Bilateral implantation is becoming the standard of care for children in developed countries, such as Germany, England and the United States, while in developing countries it is very infrequent. In less developed countries, many children are still receiving unilateral single-channel cochlear implants, which are cheaper to manufacture, and many are not able to access the technology at all due to high cost. For example, of the estimated 1 million children with profound hearing loss in India, only approximately 5000 are reported to have cochlear implants. It is difficult to estimate how many children worldwide have received cochlear implants to date, as reports vary widely. However, in December 2010, the U.S. Food and Drug Administration (FDA) reported that approximately 219,000 people worldwide had received implants (National Institute on Deafness and other Communication Disorders, 2011). Despite variations in estimates, it is generally accepted that approximately half of the number of cochlear implant recipients are children.

2. Suitability for a cochlear implant

2.1 Criteria for candidature

In the early days of cochlear implantation in children, children were only considered as suitable recipients for a cochlear implant when they had no useable aided hearing, and therefore had nothing to lose if the outcome were not good, as cochlear implantation damages the inner ear such that acoustic hearing is not usually possible post-operatively. As technological improvements in electrode design, speech processing strategies, receiver/stimulator design and programming have gradually facilitated improving outcomes with cochlear implants, the clinical perspective has changed.

Determining suitability in children is a more complicated process than it is for post-lingually deafened adults, whose speech production and language skills are fully developed. Whereas for adults it can be assumed that the ability to perceive speech is limited by hearing ability alone, for children, speech perception is limited by language knowledge and speech production skills as well as by residual hearing quality and quantity (DesJardin et al., 2009; Sarant et al., 1997). Unsurprisingly, speech perception scores (obtained from measuring the number of sounds, words, or sentences perceived correctly on a test) in children are more highly correlated with spoken language abilities than with any other factor (Blamey et al., 2001a), and are also influenced by speech production skills (Paatsch et al., 2004). Therefore, basing decisions about cochlear implant candidature for children on speech perception scores alone could risk implanting some children who have sufficient aided hearing to develop spoken language through hearing aids, but who are limited in their speech perception ability by their undeveloped spoken language skills. This risk has increased over time as the age at which children receive cochlear implants has decreased. Further, as speech perception results with cochlear implants have improved, the amount of hearing being risked in order to achieve the potential benefits of a cochlear implant has increased. Given this increasing risk, accurate prediction of a particular child's potential to benefit from a cochlear implant has become even more important.

Blamey and Sarant (2002) proposed a method of combining speech perception and language assessment scores to calculate an objective criterion for cochlear implant suitability, so that a child's pre-operative aided speech perception performance is compared to a distribution of speech perception scores for children with cochlear implants who are matched according to language ability (Blamey & Sarant, 2002). While this approach is helpful for older children with some language ability, it is not suitable for use with very young children whose speech perception, production and language skills are undeveloped, independent of their degree of hearing loss, and for whom, due to behavioural and cognitive developmental issues, it is very difficult to assess speech perception ability.

Since the 1990's, several researchers have proposed alternate methods of determining suitability for a cochlear implant in children. Osberger et al. (1991) classified children using hearing aids into 'gold', 'silver' and 'bronze' categories, based on their unaided pure tone thresholds (PTA) averaged across 0.5, 1, and 2 kHz. Initially, it was predicted that only children in the 'bronze' category (mean >110dbHL and >110dbHL at two of the three frequencies) were suitable candidates for a cochlear implant. These categories were revised when it became apparent that children with cochlear implants were outperforming not only hearing aid users in the bronze, but also in the silver (mean = 104dbHL and 101-110 dbHL at two of the three frequencies) and gold (mean = 94dbHL and 90-100 dbHL in two of the three frequencies) categories. A further methodology that compared speech perception results for children using hearing aids and cochlear implants in order to determine criteria for suitability used the concept of 'equivalent hearing loss' (EHL). Boothroyd and Eran (1994) compared the abilities of children using hearing aids with those using a cochlear implant on an imitative test of phonetic (speech sound) contrasts, and derived EHL by plotting speech perception results against the three-frequency unaided PTA for each ear. Linear regression statistical analysis was used to transform the speech perception scores of the children into EHL values. Although the EHL for the children using cochlear implants suggested that their potential for speech perception was similar to that of children with a severe hearing loss using hearing aids, there were still children using cochlear implants whose speech perception skills were no better than those of children with a profound hearing loss using hearing aids. In 1997, Boothroyd reported that children with cochlear implants who were educated mostly in oral communicative environments achieved speech perception scores equivalent to those of children using hearing aids with a hearing loss in the 70-89 dbHL (severe) range (Boothroyd, 1997). Similar results have been reported more recently (Davidson, 2006; Eisenberg et al., 2004).

Throughout the current decade, several studies of large numbers of children with cochlear implants have reported speech perception results that are comparable to those achieved by post-lingually deafened adults using cochlear implants, and even to those achieved by children with a moderate hearing loss using hearing aids (Geers et al., 2003; Svirsky et al., 2004; Tajudeen et al. 2010; Wie et al. 2007). In response to these achievements, the criteria for suitability have again changed such that even very young children with a severe to severe-profound hearing loss are now deemed suitable recipients for cochlear implants, and children with significant, or useable, residual hearing are currently being implanted in centers not under the jurisdiction of the United States FDA (Geers & Moog, 1994; Leigh et al., 2011; Svirsky & Meyer, 1999; Zwolan et al., 1997). Currently, the more conservative FDA guidelines approve cochlear implantation in children aged 12-23 months with bilateral profound sensorineural hearing loss (>90dbHL) and in children aged 2 years and older with severe-profound hearing loss (greater than or equal to 90dBHL in the better hearing ear).

The introduction of neonatal hearing screening programs in developed countries over the past decade has meant that hearing loss is now identified in babies as young as a few days or months old, and there is earlier referral and diagnosis than ever before (Dalzell, 2000; White & Maxon, 1995; Yoshinaga-Itano, 2003a). Very young infants and toddlers now represent the majority of paediatric cochlear implant candidates in these countries, and for these children, decisions about candidacy must currently be based solely or primarily on audiometric information if cochlear implants are to be given early, as there are limited tools available to measure speech perception or language abilities in this age group. The audiometric information is usually objective data obtained from the transient evoked auditory brainstem response (ABR) used in hearing screening, otoacoustic emissions, or auditory steady state responses (ASSR). These results may be combined with behavioural data derived from testing conducted by audiologists, depending on the protocol of individual cochlear implant programs. Most recently, an "equivalent PTA" model was derived to be applied to audiometric data for very young children from a comparison of the open-set speech perception scores of preschool and elementary school-aged children using cochlear implants and hearing aids. The model gives equivalent PTA for a 75% through to 95% chance of improvement in speech perception outcomes in 5% steps. Using a less conservative 75% chance of improvement criterion (as opposed to the 95% criterion that has until now been applied), the model recommends that children with bilateral profound hearing loss through to children with unaided pure tone average thresholds of 75 to 90 dBHL are suitable recipients for cochlear implants, while children with lesser hearing loss than 75dbHL are encouraged to continue with hearing aid use (Leigh et al., 2011).

2.2 Children with additional disabilities: Implications for candidacy

It is well established that 30-40% of children with severe-profound hearing loss also have an additional physical and/or cognitive disability, such as visual impairment, cognitive impairment, learning disabilities, autistic spectrum disorders (ASD) or developmental delay (Archbold & O'Donoghue, 2009; Edwards, 2007; Holt et al., 2005). Often, the additional disability is related to the cause of deafness, and is part of a syndrome or other grouping of disabilities. Children with additional disabilities present a further challenge with regard to determining suitability for cochlear implants, because the degree of benefit derived by the 'average' child with hearing loss is unlikely to be experienced by these children due to the effects of their additional disabilities. For this reason, children with additional disabilities were not considered suitable cochlear implant candidates for many years. Although excluded from FDA clinical trials in the past (Holt et al., 2005), small numbers of children with additional disabilities have received cochlear implants. Little is known about the degree of benefit children with hearing loss and additional disabilities derive from cochlear implants with regard to speech perception and spoken language development, for several reasons. Firstly, much of the research effort around cochlear implants has been directed at identifying outcomes and predictive factors for the majority of children with cochlear implants who do not have additional disabilities. Secondly, due to the fact that there are smaller numbers of children with additional disabilities, and many are unable to complete standardised assessment procedures, quantitative analysis of outcomes has been difficult. A further challenge is that there are a large number of additional disabilities spread across a relatively small population of children, therefore obtaining sufficient numbers to define the aspects of each disability and its impact on communication development after implantation has been difficult.

The few studies of children with cochlear implants and additional disabilities have generally reported poorer performance on speech perception, production and language assessments, particularly when higher level speech processing abilities are required. For example, in one of the first studies of these children, (Pyman et al., 2000) found that although 90% of 75 children with motor and/or cognitive delays could discriminate consonants and vowels after four years of cochlear implant use, only around 60% of the children were able to use this information to perceive open-set sentences (those presented with no context), compared to over 80% of children without additional disabilities. Similarly, a further study of children with a variety of disabilities, such as attention-deficit disorder, cerebral palsy, central auditory processing disorder, dyspraxia and autism, showed some speech perception skill development at a slower rate than for the general population (Waltzman et al., 2000). Children whose additional disability is mild can derive significant benefit from cochlear implants, whereas children with more severe disabilities have much less favourable outcomes, with some showing almost no progress (Edwards, Frost & Witham, 2006; Filipo et al., 2004; Hamzavi et al., 2000; Holt & Kirk, 2005; Meinzen-Derr et al., 2011; Vlahovic & Sindija, 2004). Most studies have highlighted that children with additional disabilities require longer periods of implant use before demonstrating any benefit, and as for children in the general cochlear implant population, variation in outcomes is wide for children with additional disabilities (Hamzavi et al., 2000; Waltzman et al., 2000). It was reported for some children that the assessment tasks were too difficult to complete (Donaldson et al., 2004; Waltzman et al., 2000), which is a factor that has added to the difficulty of determining outcomes for this population.

Children with autistic spectrum disorders (ASD) have historically been considered poor cochlear implant candidates, but as the age at which children are being implanted has decreased, there are now a number of children who have been implanted before their diagnosis of ASD. The single published study of progress in a group of children with ASD reported that smaller gains on tests of speech perception and language had been made in comparison to those reported for the cochlear implant general population, but that parent reports suggested positive improvements in their children's functioning and responsiveness (Donaldson et al., 2004).

In summary, although the degree of benefit obtained from cochlear implants is often lower for children with additional disabilities, many children still receive measurable benefit from their devices, and this benefit adds to their quality of life. Some of the observed benefits cannot be quantified on standardised tests, and have been instead reported anecdotally, with observations of improvements in social interaction and responsiveness to the environment, behaviour, vocalization, self-help skills, motor skills and the ability to follow instructions (Donaldson et al., 2004; Filipo et al., 2004; Fukuda et al., 2003; Waltzman et al., 2000; Wiley et al., 2005). There is still a need to determine the impact of additional disabilities on post-operative benefit with cochlear implants, and to define more clearly what benefits might reasonably be expected for children with different additional disabilities. The point at which a cochlear implant will not be beneficial also needs to be determined with regard to the degree of severity of additional disabilities, and the definition of benefit should be carefully explored, with improved psychological well-being, children's maximum potential, and quality of life being taken into consideration in addition to quantitative outcomes on tests.

2.3 Candidacy and selected aetiologies/pathologies of deafness

A further group of children for whom candidacy issues are more complex are those with selected pathologies that not only cause severe-profound hearing loss but may also impact on outcomes with cochlear implants. Although there are many such pathologies, the most common of these will be discussed as examples of the impact aetiology, or cause of hearing loss, may have on post-implantation outcomes.

In the 1990's, auditory neuropathy (AN) was defined as a distinct type of hearing disorder that disrupts neural activity in the central and peripheral auditory pathways (Starr et al., 1996). Auditory neuropathy is characterised by normal outer hair cell function in the cochlea (which enables many babies to pass newborn hearing screening if otoacoustic emission testing is used), and a retro cochlear lesion (dysfunction in the inner hair cells or auditory [eighth] nerve), which manifests as an absent or abnormal response to auditory brainstem response (ABR) testing. Features of this pathology include poorer than expected speech perception abilities in relation to degree of hearing loss in the majority of children, with some children who have only a mild hearing loss demonstrating a severely impaired ability to use their hearing for speech understanding (Rance et al., 2007). This pathology affects approximately 0.23% of at-risk children (Rance et al., 1999). Given the unusual pattern of perceptual deficits that characterises AN, much of the research in this area has focused on whether or not a cochlear implant can assist these children to understand speech through their hearing. The few published investigations on speech perception have varied widely, reporting no benefit (Miyamoto et al., 1999; Teagle et al., 2010) through to benefit comparable to that received by the general population of children with cochlear implants (Buss et al., 2002; Peterson et al., 2003; Rance & Barker, 2008; Trautwein et al., 2000). For the children who demonstrated significant benefit, it was noted that electrical stimulation via the cochlear implant elicited ABR responses, which suggests that the implant was able to enable greater neural synchrony and therefore to overcome the desynchronization thought to underlie AN. Studies of language and speech production outcomes for these children are again limited, and results are similar to those for speech perception, with wide variation in outcomes, but also with some children demonstrating the same level of development as the general population of children with cochlear implants (Jeong et al., 2007; Madden, 2002; Rance et al., 2007). For parents of children with this pathology, there is reasonable evidence to suggest that children may benefit from a cochlear implant, although expectations may need to be lower than for the general population of children with sensorineural hearing loss.

Usher syndrome is the most common condition that affects both hearing and vision, and its major symptoms are congenital or progressive deafness resulting in severe-profound hearing loss, and progressive loss of vision due to retinitis pigmentosa, an eye disorder which causes night blindness and a loss of peripheral vision. Many children with Usher syndrome also have significant balance problems, which can delay walking in very young children. Approximately 6-12% of children with hearing loss, or 4 in every 100,000 births in the United States (Boughman et al., 1983) and 6 per 100,000 births in England (Hope et al., 1997) have Usher Syndrome, which is a genetic condition. Once children have lost their vision, the auditory information provided by a cochlear implant is their only means of connecting and communicating with the world, so it is very important that these children are diagnosed and receive their cochlear implants early in order to establish communication through audition prior to the loss of vision. Usher syndrome is one of the 20% of causes of deafness that involve abnormalities in cochlea-vestibular anatomy. These abnormalities increase the potential for surgical difficulties and complications, such as damage to the facial nerve and incomplete insertion of the implant electrode array in the cochlea (Bauer et al., 2002; Chadha et al., 2009).

Some other children with congenital deafness also have cochlear abnormalities, often due to a range of genetic causes, another of which is CHARGE syndrome. Children with this rare genetic syndrome have deafness, visual problems, and a variety of other physical abnormalities, including serious heart defects, colobomas (or holes) in one or both eyes, growth retardation, genital abnormalities and external and internal ear malformations. Anatomical abnormalities in the structure of the cochlea can also create difficulties for programming, with reduced dynamic ranges for children with more severe cochlear abnormalities (Papsin, 2005). For these reasons, malformation of the cochlea was considered a contra-indication to cochlear implant surgery in the early years of cochlear implantation in children, and it is still not possible to implant some of these children (Bamiou et al., 2001). Despite these difficulties, initial results for small numbers of children with cochlear anomalies have shown that implantation is possible, with some children achieving speech perception and language results similar to those without anatomical abnormalities (Chadha et al., 2009; Dettman et al., 2011). Children with a common cavity anomaly (a single cavity in the cochlea) and other more severe syndromic anomalies have achieved much poorer results (Bauer et al., 2002; Chadha et al., 2009; Lanson et al., 2007; Loundon et al., 2003; Young et al., 1995).

Children with viral causes of deafness such as rubella, cytomegalovirus (CMV), toxoplasmosis and meningitis also require special consideration, as these viruses can cause developmental neurological deficits, including learning and cognitive difficulties (Edwards, 2007; Grimwood et al., 2000; Isaacson et al., 1996). A significant difference between children with deafness caused by meningitis and that caused by the other viruses is that while CMV, toxoplasmosis and rubella are contracted perinatally, children who have had meningitis will have experienced sound prior to infection and may have developed some spoken language skills. A further complication of meningitis is ossification (bone growth) within the cochlea, which is usually bilateral and can commence within four weeks of the illness (Durisin et al., 2010). This makes it imperative that children who have had meningitis are diagnosed with hearing loss and receive cochlear implants as soon as possible, before ossification limits both the potential for a full insertion and for benefit. Again, limited reports of post-operative benefit for children with these causes of deafness show a wide range of speech perception skills, intelligibility and language outcomes, with some children doing well (Francis et al., 2004; Lee et al., 2005) and others doing poorly (Isaacson et al., 1996; Ramirez Inscoe & Nikolopoulos, 2004; Wie et al., 2007).

3. Benefits of unilateral cochlear implants

3.1 Environmental awareness

At the most basic level, cochlear implants provide children with an auditory awareness of their environment. Through their cochlear implant, children can hear many environmental sounds that would not be audible to them through hearing aids. These include high frequency sounds such as water running, birds singing, the kettle whistling, the car indicators ticking and the phone ringing. Being able to hear what is going on in their environment gives children a feeling of connectedness with the world, and also provides them with a greater degree of safety, although localization of sound sources is usually not achieved by most children with only one cochlear implant. Children are more easily able to hear their name being called, to determine when someone is speaking to them, and even to enjoy music. In the early days of cochlear implantation, when only older children received implants, and before it was realised that children could use cochlear implants to develop spoken language, environmental awareness was a prime motivating factor in the decision to implant some children (Sarant et al., 1994).

3.2 Speech perception

The cochlear implant assists children to process spoken auditory information in their environment both as an aid to lip reading, which is particularly useful in noisy educational environments, and also as a source of auditory information that can be relied upon without lip reading in appropriate listening conditions. As briefly mentioned earlier, speech perception results for children have steadily improved over time with advances in device hardware and software, surgical techniques, and experience with programming speech processors and habilitation. Initially, it was not expected that children with congenital hearing loss would be able to achieve the speech perception abilities shown by post-lingually deafened adults, but many children have exceeded these levels of perceptual ability. By the mid 1990's, 60 to 80% of children with unilateral implants achieved open-set word and sentence speech perception abilities comparable to those achieved by adults using audition only (Dowell et al., 1995; Dowell et al., 1997; Geers et al., 2003; Sarant et al., 2001).

More recent studies of children implanted at younger ages and using more recent technologies report even better speech perception abilities. While it has been suggested for some time that children with cochlear implants perform at a level equivalent to that of a child with a severe hearing loss using hearing aids (Blamey et al., 2001a; Boothroyd, 1997; Svirsky & Meyer, 1999), it has recently been reported that very young children can perform on tests of speech recognition at a level equivalent to that of children with a moderate hearing loss using hearing aids (Leigh et al., 2008b). Recent long-term studies have also shown that high proportions of children (79% and 60%) can use the telephone (Beadle et al., 2005; Uziel et al., 2007). These are considerable achievements for children who have been profoundly deaf since birth, and who have developed their auditory processing abilities through the reduced and fragmented sound provided by cochlear implants. It is also worth noting that a meta-analysis of 1916 reports on speech perception performance in children with cochlear implants suggested that, rather than levelling out, speech perception benefits continue to increase as children grow older (Cheng et al., 1999).

The assessment of speech perception abilities in adults and older children is relatively straightforward. It may involve an individual listening to a sound or word and pointing to a picture that best represents that sound or word (closed-set testing) or could involve the individual listening to and repeating a sound, word or sentence spoken by the assessor with no context (open-set testing). Children with age-appropriate cognitive abilities are able to complete these sorts of tasks from the age of around 3 to 4 years, when they have developed the ability to label sounds, letters or words (Spencer et al., 2011). With the introduction of earlier diagnosis of hearing loss through newborn hearing screening, a need to assess very young children has developed in order to determine their suitability for cochlear implants. There are several methods of doing this, but these are less objective, and are much more reliant on the expertise and judgement of professionals in observing behavioural responses in very young children, and also on parent reports of responses to speech sounds and specific familiar words. Reports using these modified forms of speech perception testing in very young children have suggested that speech perception skills can develop rapidly within the first two years of cochlear implantation for children implanted before 4 years of age (Robbins et al., 2004a; Svirsky et al., 2004; Tajudeen et al., 2010; Wie et al., 2007).

As previously mentioned, much of the improvement in speech perception scores is attributable to advancements in technology, and particularly to the development of more effective speech processing strategies for the three commercially available cochlear implant devices (the Nucleus/Cochlear device, the Clarion device, and the Med-El device). The development of speech processing technology in the Cochlear device, which retains a dominant international market share of around 70% (Patrick et al., 2006) will be discussed as an example of this progress. In the early Nucleus 22-channel cochlear implant device, speech feature extraction schemes that presented only the fundamental frequency of speech and the first two formants (or bursts of energy) of speech (F0F2 and F0F1F2) were used (Clark et al., 1983). These strategies provided an aid to lip reading and very limited speech perception ability (Dowell et al., 1985). They had several disadvantages, such as not discriminating between speech and non-speech sounds, causing some environmental noises to sound quite unnatural, and providing no information above 3kHz, which made it impossible for users to perceive unvoiced information about consonants (such as 's', 'sh', 'f',' th' etc.).

In the early 1990's, a new strategy, known as Multipeak (MPEAK), was introduced with the goal of improving consonant recognition scores. MPEAK still used feature extraction algorithms, but also provided information about high frequency sounds on three fixed bands of the implant electrode array. The MPEAK strategy represented an improvement in that it distinguished between voiced and unvoiced sounds, and some electrodes were allocated to the representation of high frequency consonant information, which is extremely important for speech perception. The additional information provided through this speech processing strategy led to improved speech perception scores, particularly for fricatives (eg. 's', 'sh'), in both quiet and noise conditions (Clark, 1989; Dowell et al., 1991). Despite the improvements in benefit with MPEAK, an ongoing disadvantage of formant extraction strategies was that in background noise the speech processor made errors.

By 1995, improvements in electronics technology had allowed a new approach to speech processing to be adopted, using bandpass filtering principles in order to provide more information about the speech spectrum. The Spectral (SPEAK) speech processing strategy used bandpass filters to select 6 to 10 of the largest spectral components in each analysis time period and assigned these to particular electrodes in the cochlea. In this strategy, groups of electrodes, rather than single electrodes, were stimulated to represent particular speech features such as vowels, and stimulation occurred at a much higher rate than for previous strategies, which meant that more information could be presented more quickly. The selection of the highest amplitude information increased the chance of presenting only the most salient speech information, and of suppressing lower amplitude background noise. The SPEAK strategy resulted in large increases in speech perception benefit for children and adults, particularly in background noise (Cowan et al., 1995; McKay et al., 1991), and probably contributed to the largest increase in speech perception benefit of all the technological advancements made before or since that time. Other significant technological improvements in cochlear implants over the last decade have included new receiver-stimulators, smaller, body-worn and behind-the-ear digital speech processors, and further high-rate speech processing strategies. These have facilitated further improvements in speech perception benefit, particularly in very young children who have had access to all of the recent technology.

One of the most challenging findings of research on speech perception ability in children with cochlear implants is the enormous variation in performance between individuals (Cowan et al., 1997; Pyman et al., 2000; Sarant et al., 2001; Staller et al., 1991). While many reports describe 'average' performance, this concept minimises and perhaps even disguises the fact that while many children do reasonably well, and some do as well as their peers with normal hearing, there are still children who derive very little benefit from their cochlear implant. This variation in outcomes makes it difficult to predict how a particular child will perform after implantation, and therefore to determine which children are suitable for a cochlear implant, particularly when they risk losing useable residual hearing in order to have one. Several factors that have been identified as predictive of post-operative performance will be discussed in section 4 of this chapter.

3.3 Speech production

The development of speech production has always been a significant problem for children with severe-profound hearing loss, as they do not have the auditory capacity to monitor their own speech or to hear the speech of normal-hearing individuals. For many years, most children using hearing aids with this degree of hearing loss have been rated as unintelligible, or as having very low intelligibility, to adult listeners unfamiliar with the speech of children with hearing loss (Bamford & Saunders, 1992; Gold, 1980; Spencer et al., 2011). Cochlear implants can provide children with auditory information that makes their own speech and that of others audible, so that they can learn from speakers with normal hearing, and self-monitor their own speech production. As with speech perception, children with cochlear implants show a wide range of speech production abilities, with many children performing at a very high level, and others showing low levels of performance (Connor et al., 2006; Spencer & Oleson, 2008; Tobey et al., 2003), but even children implanted at relatively late ages and with only a few years of implant use are generally rated as much more intelligible than their peers with a similar degree of hearing loss using hearing aids (Connor et al., 2006; Flipsen, 2008; Tobey & Hasenstab, 1991; Tye-Murray et al., 1995). Speech production outcomes have improved over time, as a result of longer periods of implant experience and improved hardware and speech processing strategies, although for many children they are still not equivalent to those of children with normal hearing (Chin et al., 2003; Peng et al., 2004).

Speech production skills and speech intelligibility ratings equivalent to those of 'gold' hearing aid users have been reported after less than 3 years of implant use (Blamey et al., 2001b; Svirsky et al., 2000). Children who are implanted at younger ages and use more recent technology demonstrate the greatest achievements, with intelligibility ratings of 60-75% and much higher rates of speech production accuracy reported for children implanted as preschoolers (Ertmer et al., 2007; Flipsen, 2008; Peng et al., 2004; Tobey et al., 2003). More recent reports of children followed for longer post-operative periods of up to ten years have reported speech intelligibility rates of 77%, 90%, and 67% respectively, and suggest that the development of intelligibility does not plateau after a few years, but increases over time with chronological age and increased length of cochlear implant use (Beadle et al., 2005; Blamey et al., 2001c; Chin et al., 2003; Uziel et al., 2007). Beadle and colleagues showed that although 48% of the children in their study had developed connected speech that was intelligible to the average listener after 5 years of cochlear implant use, after 10 years this figure had increased to 77% (Beadle et al. 2005).

It was initially unknown whether children with cochlear implants would follow the same pattern of sound acquisition as their peers with normal hearing, or what their rate of progress would be compared to the former. In children with normal hearing, speech acquisition generally takes between 4 to 7 years (Chin et al., 2003). Studies of consonant and vowel acquisition in children with cochlear implants suggest that, on average, these children demonstrate a pattern of phoneme (or speech sound) acquisition similar to that of children with normal hearing (Ertmer et al., 2007; Serry et al., 1997), although their rate of development is often slower (Blamey et al., 2001b). This has meant that the speech acquisition process has still been incomplete at the age at which children with normal hearing have mastered speech production, but with little or no evidence that a plateau in development has been reached for children implanted between 2 and 5 years of age (Blamey et al., 2001c). Initial investigations of a small number of children implanted before the age of 12 months have yielded conflicting results, with one study reporting that the rate of speech production development for children implanted under the age of 12 months matched that of children with normal hearing (Leigh et al., 2008c), and another finding that children implanted before age 12 months and those implanted between 12-24 months showed no difference in their speech production development (Holt & Svirsky, 2008). Future research will hopefully clarify the critical period during which children should receive cochlear implants in order to facilitate speech production outcomes that are similar to those of children with normal hearing.

3.4 Language development

Language development is generally measured using standardised assessments of vocabulary and grammatical knowledge. In the early 1990s, most reports on language were case studies demonstrating changes thought to be associated with cochlear implantation, but knowledge in this area has grown over time, and there is now solid evidence for large numbers of children regarding language outcomes. Initial research concentrated on whether children with cochlear implants developed language more quickly than their peers with hearing aids, or compared development to predictions based on pre-operative language development with hearing aids. One of the earlier studies compared language development in three groups of children with cochlear implants, hearing aids and tactile aids (body-worn aids that provide vibratory or electrical stimulation) over 3 years (Geers & Moog, 1994). On average, the language growth of children with cochlear implants in this study was equal to or exceeded that for the other groups of children, and even approached that of children with hearing aids who had 20dB better hearing. Earlier this decade, children with cochlear implants were reported to be developing at a rate similar to that of children with a severe hearing loss of around 78dbHL (Blamey et al., 2001a), and it is now well established that on average, children with cochlear implants demonstrate significantly faster spoken language development than their peers with similar levels of hearing loss who use hearing aids (Connor et al., 2000; Miyamoto et al., 1999; Svirsky et al., 2000; Tomblin et al., 1999). Given these promising results, the focus changed to comparing the progress of children with cochlear implants to that of their normally-hearing peers.

By the late 1990's, although language outcomes for children with cochlear implants had improved compared to those for children with similar degrees of loss using hearing aids, on average, children with cochlear implants were still demonstrating language growth rates of only 50-60% of the rate of children with normal hearing (Blamey et al., 2001a; Davis & Hind, 1999; Geers, 2002; Ramkalawan & Davis, 1992; Wake et al., 2004). Given the fact that these children were already delayed in their language development by the amount of time it had taken for diagnosis and implantation to occur, this slower rate of growth meant that by the time they were of school age, many children were delayed by at least 1 year, and approximately half had a severe language delay (ie. greater than 2 standard deviations below the mean for children with normal hearing). This rate of progress clearly has severe implications for academic achievement and functional literacy outcomes.

Over the past decade, with a decreasing average age at implantation and improved cochlear implant speech processing technology and hardware, language outcomes have further improved for children with cochlear implants, such that some children now acquire spoken language as do children with mild to moderate hearing loss (Spencer et al., 2011). More recently, several studies have shown that children who have received their cochlear implants at very young ages (and have had several years of experience) can achieve spoken language development at similar rates to children with normal hearing (Connor et al., 2006; Duchesne et al., 2009; Geers, 2006b; Schorr et al., 2008; Svirsky et al., 2004; Tomblin et al., 2005). For example, Dettman et al. 2008 reported that children implanted before the age of 2.5 years showed an average vocabulary development rate of 85% of that of children with normal hearing. This means that the gap between chronological age and language age for these children remains more constant, and for some diminishes instead of growing, as has commonly been reported in the past.

Greater proportions of children are showing age-appropriate development in receptive and expressive vocabulary (50% & 58%; Geers et al., 2009) and receptive and expressive language (47% & 39%; Nicholas & Geers, 2008) than previously. It has also been observed that some children with cochlear implants are even able to learn language more quickly than the average child with normal hearing and therefore 'catch up' some of the delay in language acquisition incurred before they received a cochlear implant, with reports of language development at age-appropriate levels between the ages of 4 and 7 years (Yoshinaga-Itano et al., 2010). As with speech perception and speech production, there is still enormous variation in language skills between individuals and between different populations of children (Spencer et al., 2003), with recent reports still documenting many children with significant language delays (Ching, 2010; Connor et al., 2000; Nikolopoulos et al., 2004; Sarant et al., 2009; Young & Killen, 2002).

The capacity for learning language in children with normal hearing is so great that they are not only able to develop fluency in their native language, but can also become fluent speakers of more than three other languages without specific instruction. However, there have long been concerns that language delay in bilingual children is due to simultaneously learning two languages, due to the fact that learning a second language delays the learning process with the first language. It seemed logical that, for children with impaired auditory systems who are facing even greater challenges in language acquisition, learning two languages simultaneously would further delay the acquisition of the first language. More recently, it has been found that delays in vocabulary and slower progress in learning the second language dissipate in the early primary school years, and are likely to be due to the amount of exposure children have to each language (ie. the language that is used the most develops more quickly). It has also been demonstrated that language impairments found in bilingual children are due to individual children's innate capacity to learn language, and are not caused by simultaneous language learning (Genesee, 2001).

Despite the significant challenge inherent in mastering one spoken language with a cochlear implant, there is emerging evidence that it is also possible for children with cochlear implants to develop competence in a second spoken language. Robbins et al (2004b) reported on 12 children implanted before age 3 years, who not only demonstrated exceptional proficiency in their first language (almost all children had age-appropriate first language) but also solid progress in their second language over the 2 years during which they were followed. The children who were most proficient in their second language development had parents who spoke the second language at home, had opportunities to use the second language outside home, and had extensive cochlear implant experience. It was noted that, as a group, many of these children were 'ideal' cochlear implant recipients; half had hereditary deafness without additional disabilities, none had less than a full electrode array insertion, all had received intensive auditory-oral therapy prior to and after implantation, and none had meningitis-caused deafness. Two other studies have documented the ability of children with cochlear implants to develop competency in a second language. Of 18 children who received their cochlear implants by the age of 5 years and had a mean usage time of 4.5 years, the majority had achieved age-appropriate receptive and/or expressive language skills in their primary language, although their second language skills were still in the early stages of development (Waltzman et al., 2003). Uziel and colleagues (2007) also documented that some of the children in their study showed some ability to develop competency in a second language.

3.5 Social and emotional development

Children with profound hearing loss, including children with cochlear implants, are at increased risk for adverse life outcomes such as loneliness, poorer quality personal relationships, behaviour problems, drug and alcohol problems, and generally poorer quality of life than their normally hearing peers (Meadow, 1980; Watson et al., 1990). These problems can be attributed to a reduced ability to acquire many of the skills that underpin social functioning due to hearing loss (Marschark, 1993), despite their improved auditory capabilities. It is also important to note, however, that not all children with profound hearing loss and/or cochlear implants develop these problems. The impact of hearing loss on children's social and emotional development is also affected by several factors external to the children themselves, such as parental acceptance of and adaptation to their child's hearing loss, quality of family life, the ability of the family to cope, school and community support, and resources (Calderon, 2000; Montanini-Manfredi, 1993). Of course, a child's personality and method of interacting with their social environment also contributes significantly. The few studies that examine the psychosocial development of children with cochlear implants show mixed results (Martin et al., 2011).

It has been reported that children with cochlear implants often have limited pragmatic skills, which can lead to poor social integration (Bat-Chava et al., 2005). Pragmatic skills include using language for different purposes (eg. greeting people, requesting information, demanding information), being able to change language according to the situation or listener (eg. speaking to an adult versus a toddler), and following conversational rules (eg. turn-taking in conversations, using facial expressions and eye contact, rephrasing when misunderstood). Children with poor pragmatic skills may say inappropriate things during conversations, may show little variety in the language they use, or may relate stories in a disorganised, illogical way. These behaviours often lead to a higher incidence of communication breakdown, and can lower social acceptance, as many children may choose to avoid having uncomfortable interactions with others who have pragmatic difficulties. Pragmatic problems are often related to delayed language development, which may include a limited vocabulary, and deficits in knowledge of grammar and age-appropriate slang.

It is not uncommon for children with severe-profound deafness to demonstrate significantly reduced emotional development and social maturity (Bat-Chava et al., 2005; Hintermair, 2006). These children also report loneliness, a lack of close friendships and other psychosocial difficulties more frequently than do their normally-hearing peers (Most, 2007; Stinson & Whitimire, 2000), and some studies show that this is the same for some children with cochlear implants (Boyd et al.,2000; Dammeyer, 2010; Leigh et al., 2009). Older children with cochlear implants (aged 9-14 years) are generally more affected by loneliness than younger children (aged 5-9 years), with children who receive their implants when older being most affected (Schorr, 2006). This may reflect the fact that social interaction becomes increasingly complex in adolescence, and peer group size tends to increase at this time, making communication more difficult due to increased acoustic and social challenges (Bat-Chava & Deignan, 2001; Martin et al., 2011).

Unsurprisingly, loneliness and psychosocial difficulties are greatest for children with additional disabilities, particularly those with low speech intelligibility and poor communication skills, as this increases communication breakdown and results in poorer peer attitudes towards children with these difficulties, who may be rejected or ignored by their peers (Dammeyer, 2010; Hintermair, 2007; Most, 2007; van Gent et al., 2007). Conversely, other studies have found no increased incidence of loneliness and psychosocial difficulties in children with cochlear implants compared to children with normal hearing (Percy-Smith et al., 2008a; Schorr, 2006), and children have been observed by parents to have improved communication skills and social relationships as a result of cochlear implantation (Archbold et al., 2008b; Bat-Chava & Deignan, 2001; Bat-Chava et al., 2005; Huber, 2005; Huttunen & Valimaa, 2010). Children with cochlear implants have been reported to be more likely to be acculturated to hearing society than those with a severe-profound hearing loss using hearing aids (Leigh et al., 2008a).

A statistically significant association has also been found between the level of social well-being in children with cochlear implants and their speech perception, production and language skills (Dammeyer, 2010; Percy-Smith et al., 2008b). Social development usually follows language skill development, and improvements in both have been observed to occur more quickly for children with cochlear implants than for children with severe-profound hearing loss using hearing aids (Bat-Chava et al., 2005). It has been suggested that improved spoken language and communication skills facilitate psychosocial development through an ability to communicate and a subsequent increase in confidence (Bat-Chava & Deignan, 2001). Children with severe-profound deafness have historically been found to have lower levels of self-esteem than their peers with normal hearing (Nicholas & Geers, 2003), with the self-esteem of adolescents being lower than that of younger children (Schorr, 2006). It has been suggested that unless their language skills match those of their hearing peers, children with cochlear implants cannot fully integrate into the hearing community and develop positive self-esteem (Crouch, 1997; Lane & Grodin, 1997). However, as with many recent outcomes for children with cochlear implants, more recent research has shown equivalent levels of self esteem in children with cochlear implants and children with normal hearing (Loy et al., 2010; Martin et al., 2011; Sahli & Belgin, 2006).

Recent studies have also used measures of health-related quality of life (QOL) to investigate psychosocial development in children with cochlear implants, using both parental and child reports. QOL is considered to be an assessment of well-being across various areas of life such as social interaction, school adjustment, friendships, communication, and listening ability. Although a potential limitation of QOL measures can be that although parents are well-informed of their children's level of physical functioning, they have a tendency to underestimate their psychosocial functioning (Zaidman-Zait, 2011), QOL assessments are still regarded as a useful method of obtaining a more holistic measure of benefit. Loy and colleagues (2010) found no significant differences between overall reported QOL for children with cochlear implants compared to their peers with normal hearing, in either younger (8-11 years) or older (12-16 years) groups, although the younger group rated QOL more highly than did the adolescent group. Others have reported similar findings for children of various ages (Huber, 2005; Warner-Czyz et al., 2009).

Several factors have been found to influence psychosocial development in children with cochlear implants. Children who are implanted earlier and therefore have a longer duration of implant use are reported to be more socially competent (Leigh et al., 2008a; Martin et al., 2011), with girls outperforming boys (Martin et al., 2011; Nicholas & Geers, 2003; Percy-Smith et al., 2008b). As mentioned earlier, children implanted at older ages appear to be at greater risk of loneliness (Schorr, 2006), and it has been suggested that this may be due to the fact that they do not develop feelings of belonging and inclusion at a young age, as do children with normal hearing, due to their delayed language prior to implantation. It is also reported that children with cochlear implants in mainstream educational settings who are exposed to spoken, rather than signed, language at home have a higher level of social well-being (Percy-Smith et al., 2008b; van Gent et al., 2007). This may be because children in these settings are more likely to have hearing parents, and therefore are continuing to speak their first language in these settings, rather than using sign language at home and spoken language at school, as would children of many deaf parents. There is also no evidence that children with cochlear implants in mainstream educational settings, where speech is used exclusively for communication, have an increased incidence of social or emotional difficulties compared to children in special educational settings (Filipo et al., 1999; Nicholas & Geers, 2003; Percy-Smith et al., 2008b).

Once again, there is enormous variability between individuals in their communication and social development after cochlear implantation, with some children progressing at, or even above, the average rate of children with normal hearing, and others who lag behind their peers. Although there appear to be no negative reports on social/emotional development of children as a result of cochlear implantation, a cochlear implant will not guarantee that the social difficulties experienced by many children with severe-profound hearing loss are avoided (Punch & Hyde, 2011). The research does offer hope, however, that an early cochlear implant may not only facilitate the development of speech and language skills, but can also give children the potential to develop a healthy and positive social identity and competent interactional skills.

3.6 Literacy and academic outcomes

With documented improvements in speech perception, production and language outcomes clearly attributable to the improved auditory access provided by cochlear implants, there has been an expectation that academic outcomes for children with cochlear implants would also improve, with implanted children showing significantly better performance than their peers with hearing aids. However, although the proportion of children with cochlear implants who are enrolled in mainstreamed education settings is increasing steadily (Geers & Brenner, 2003), the degree to which cochlear implants have impacted on academic outcomes in children with severe-profound hearing loss is not yet clear. Much of the research on children with hearing loss is limited mainly to studies of reading ability, and few children who have received cochlear implants at a young age are currently old enough for longer-term outcomes to be measured.

Many children with severe-profound hearing loss, including those with cochlear implants, have 4 to 5 year delays in spoken language development by the time they enter secondary school (Blamey et al., 2001a; Dahl et al., 2003; Davis & Hind, 1999; Ramkalawan & Davis, 1992; Sarant et al., 2009). Generally, the greater the degree of hearing loss, the larger the language delay (Boothroyd et al., 1991). It is well known that poor spoken language ability is a primary cause of difficulty in learning to read for children with normal hearing, and it is therefore unsurprising that literacy achievement for children with hearing loss has historically been low, with many children failing to progress in reading beyond the identification of a limited number of words, or the fourth grade level of primary school (Geers et al., 2008; Moeller et al., 2007). Reported rates of progress have varied from 1 to 6 months for every year of education, with the delay in reading widening in adolescence (Geers et al., 2008; Thoutenhoofd, 2006). A significant proportion of graduating students with hearing loss are functionally illiterate (Helfand, 2001; Moeller et al., 2007; Traxler, 2000; Walker et al., 1998), having not even acquired mastery of spoken language, which is necessary not only for the development of literacy but also for the development of literate thought (Paul 1998). Low literacy achievement and low academic outcomes have seriously impacted on the ability of many children with hearing loss to obtain employment as adults, with resulting low skill employment and reduced income for some, and others simply not having sufficient literacy skills to succeed in the workplace at all.

One of the key language skills required for learning to read is vocabulary, which is often limited in children with hearing loss due to phonetic and phonological delays (Connor & Zwolan, 2004; James et al., 2008; Johnson & Goswami, 2010; Moeller et al., 2007; Moores &

Sweet, 1990). Phonological processing occurs when a child analyses words into their constituent parts, repeats strings of syllables that form new words, or quickly names common words. These processing abilities enable word decoding to occur, which in turn facilitates word recognition and comprehension of word meaning. Delayed phonological awareness, and a subsequently delayed vocabulary, makes it difficult to learn to read. Further compounding this difficulty is the fact that reading is a skill that must be learned through explicit instruction, some of which may be 'missed' due to compromised perceptual abilities caused by hearing loss, and also through an inability to understand some of the instruction due to poorer language skills (Moeller et al., 2007). It has been shown, however, that vocabulary development accelerates after cochlear implantation (Connor et al., 2006; Dawson, 1995; Geers et al., 2007; Johnson & Goswami, 2010; Nicholas & Geers, 2008), although there are conflicting reports regarding whether vocabulary growth rates slow over time, particularly for children who received their cochlear implants at older ages (El-Hakim et al., 2001) or remain constant (James et al., 2007). There is wide variability in vocabulary development between children (Connor et al., 2000), and long-term follow up of some children in their teen or early adult years still documents many children not having attained age-appropriate vocabulary (Uziel et al., 2007).

Reading outcomes to date for children with cochlear implants are promising, with evidence that children with cochlear implants are often achieving better reading outcomes at a faster rate than their peers with hearing loss who use hearing aids (Marschark et al., 2007), although many children are still significantly delayed. The number of children with cochlear implants who achieve age-appropriate reading skills is increasing (Geers, 2002; 2003). It has also been documented that almost 4 times as many children who have used a cochlear implant for at least 2 years have achieved a reading level beyond that of fourth grade compared to children with severe-profound hearing loss of similar ages using hearing aids (Spencer et al., 2003; Vermeulen et al., 2007). Higher levels of reading performance have been documented for girls than for boys (Moog & Geers, 2003), as has been observed in children with normal hearing. As with normally-hearing children, the factor that most affects reading outcome is language ability (Connor & Zwolan, 2004; Geers, 2003; Johnson & Goswami, 2010; Spencer et al., 2003), with children who are more competent in producing an oral narrative attaining better reading comprehension skills (Crosson & Geers, 2001). Cognitive ability (Geers & Hayes, 2011), speech intelligibility and speech perception ability have also been shown to be strong predictive factors of reading outcomes (Geers, 2003; Johnson & Goswami, 2010; Spencer & Oleson, 2008).

There is increasing evidence that some children with cochlear implants can not only acquire better reading outcomes than their peers with hearing aids, but can even achieve similar outcomes to their peers with normal hearing (Archbold et al., 2008a; Spencer et al., 2003; Spencer & Oleson, 2008). James and colleagues (2008) reported that children implanted between the ages of 2 to 3.6 years achieved reading scores that were within one standard deviation of the hearing normative mean, scoring higher than children implanted between ages 5 and 7 years. Geers and Hayes (2011) also documented 47-66% of adolescents who received their implants as pre-schoolers achieving reading abilities within the average range for their hearing peers. Other studies have reported similar results, with 70%, 61%, and 51% of children reading within age-appropriate levels (Moog, 2002; Geers, 2003, Johnson & Goswami, 2010 respectively).

Other studies have shown that although early cochlear implantation facilitates improved reading outcomes in terms of both decoding and reading comprehension, a significant number of children are still not reading at the same level as their normally-hearing peers, and are falling behind over time (Archbold et al., 2008a; Connor & Zwolan, 2004). Geers and colleagues showed that only 44% of secondary school students showed age-appropriate reading performance, compared to 56% of the same group when in primary (elementary) school (Geers et al., 2008). Although the group of children was reading, on average, at an age-appropriate level when aged 8-9 years, the same children were delayed on average by almost 2 years in their reading by age 15-16 years. More recently, Geers and Hayes (2011) also reported that although 72% of the adolescents in the same sample had retained their reading standing in comparison with hearing peers since primary school, (demonstrating age-appropriate growth in reading skills over that time), 60% were still delayed overall. For many children, the reading gap between children with cochlear implants and their peers with normal hearing still widens as they grow older. Some studies still report that some children still do not make any progress at all (James et al., 2008).

Studies of writing in children with hearing loss have evaluated syntax (or grammar), looking specifically at complexity, productivity and grammaticality. The writing of children with hearing loss has generally been found to be composed of shorter sentences than those used by their hearing peers (Kretchmer & Kretchmer, 1986), repetitive phrasing, and many subject-object-verb constructions (Lichtenstein, 1998; Wilbur, 1977). There are also many errors of omission, substitution and word addition (Myklebust, 1964), including the omission of articles, prepositions, copulas, pronouns and conjunctions (Crosson & Geers, 2001). Lichtenstein also noted many errors of morphology such as plurality, verb agreement and tense in the writing of children with hearing loss. It has been concluded that children with hearing loss have even greater difficulties with writing than with learning to read (Paul, 1998).

During the primary (or elementary) school years, early writing patterns appear to follow those of spoken language development (ie. children write as they would speak). As their writing skills develop, they use more sophisticated forms of language so that their writing becomes more "detached" from their spoken language (Spencer et al., 2003). Children with cochlear implants are reported to persist in the documented pattern of immature writing skills, with shorter, less complex sentences containing more errors reported for a group of 9-year-old children using cochlear implants (Spencer et al., 2003). In this study, correlations between language abilities and writing productivity suggested that the children had not yet 'detached' their written from their spoken language. Geers and Hayes (2011) also documented the poor spelling and writing skills of children with cochlear implants compared to their peers with normal hearing. Children in this study continued to struggle with phonological processing tasks, and performed at delayed levels on measures of phonological awareness, expository writing, and spelling.

Academic success relies on reading and writing abilities, and there is now a body of work focused on literacy in children with cochlear implants. However, information on overall academic performance of these children is scarce. Spencer and colleagues (2004) examined academic achievement in science, social studies and humanities in young adults with cochlear implants, finding that consistent users of cochlear implants performed comparably to their hearing peers, achieving an overall mean standard score of 103.88 on the relevant subtests of the Woodcock-Johnson Tests of Achievement (the expected average score for children with normal hearing would be 100). This study is novel because it is the only report of fully comparable academic performance for children with cochlear implants. A more recent report on educational and employment achievements in France showed that although 42-61% of the children had failed one grade (or year level) at school (a higher rate of failure than for children with normal hearing), over 60% of those aged 18 years and over either held a university degree and/or were employed at levels similar to those of their peers with normal hearing. These figures were reported as being very similar to those for the general population of France, where 53% of individuals have at least a high school diploma (Venail et al., 2010). A third study of Malaysian children reported that for children implanted relatively late (aged 3-4 years), 56% performed below the average level academically, with greatest achievement in mathematics rather than language (Mukari et al., 2007).

As with other areas of development, wide variability in literacy and academic outcomes has been reported. As children are implanted at younger ages and enter school with better language skills, it is likely that future research will show a further narrowing of the gap in literacy and academic performance between children with cochlear implants and children with normal hearing. However, although many younger children are reported to be performing at age appropriate levels, some studies suggest that this level of performance is not sustained long-term by all children. Currently, the effect of cochlear implants on the long-term academic outcomes of children appears promising, but unclear.

4. Factors affecting speech perception, production and language outcomes

Despite the significant improvements made in cochlear implant technology, and the large body of clinical knowledge gained over time regarding likely benefits for children with cochlear implants, one of the remaining significant challenges is to identify predictors of post-implant outcomes, as there is great variation in benefits between individuals. Several factors have currently been identified as influential in children's speech perception, speech production, language and academic development after implantation, and the most important of these are discussed below.

4.1 Age at diagnosis

With the establishment of newborn hearing screening in many developed countries around the world, the average age of diagnosis of hearing loss in these countries has dropped to 12-25 months, with many babies identified as young as 3 months of age (Dalzell et al., 2000; Harrison et al., 2003; Watkin et al., 2007). As mentioned previously, the earlier identification of hearing loss has resulted in a rapid rise in the numbers of children receiving cochlear implants at younger ages (ASHA, 2004). It was estimated that the number of children receiving cochlear implants before the age of 2 years between 1991 and 2002 increased forty fold (Drinkwater, 2004), and it is likely that this growth rate has not declined. However, there are still many children in developed countries who are not receiving cochlear implants early in life. It is disappointing to note that despite earlier identification of hearing loss through newborn hearing screening programs, many families (and almost half of the families in the U.S. who are referred for further hearing assessment of their newborn babies) still do not receive early intervention services by the age of 6 months, as is recommended by the 2007 Position Statement of the Joint Committee on Infant Hearing (JCIH, 2007). The reasons for this are varied, and include a lack of understanding of the importance of early identification and intervention, problems with follow-up systems, lack of access to appropriate services and other issues related to babies' health (Sass-Lehrer, 2011). It is also reported that around one third of pediatric implant recipients who passed the newborn hearing screening assessment subsequently become implant candidates through progressive hearing loss in the first years of life due to genetic causes such as the Connexin 26 mutation, Usher Syndrome, or to other causes such as auditory neuropathy or congenital Cytomegalovirus (CMV) (Young et al., 2011), and these children also receive cochlear implants when older.

Although age at diagnosis has been reported by many studies to be an influential factor in outcomes for children with cochlear implants, some studies have not found this link (Geers et al., 2009; Geers, 2004; Harris & Terlektsi 2011; Sarant et al., 2009; Wake et al., 2005). Two of these studies included a greater proportion of children who were diagnosed late and were therefore implanted at older ages, reporting poorer performance than other studies of children whose hearing loss was identified earlier. Nicholas and Geers (2006) reported that age at diagnosis was not a significant predictive factor in language outcomes unless it led to children receiving a cochlear implant before 24 months of age. Evidence that age at diagnosis is an important factor has become stronger as children receive cochlear implants at younger ages. Several studies have reported excellent speech perception abilities and age-appropriate language outcomes for many young children who were diagnosed with hearing loss in the first six months of life (Apuzzo, 1995; Yoshinaga-Itano, 2003b; Yoshinaga-Itano et al., 1998), and there is mounting evidence that early-diagnosed children are developing language at a faster rate than their later-diagnosed peers (Connor & Zwolan, 2004; Kennedy et al., 2006).

4.2 Age at implant/duration of profound deafness

Age at implantation is often quite close to time of diagnosis early in life due to newborn screening. For children with congenital hearing loss, 'age at implant' is equal to 'duration of deafness'. Many human and animal studies of the development of the neurosensory pathways of the primary auditory cortex in the brain have suggested that the plasticity, or potential for development, of neural pathways is greatest during early development, and that there is therefore a 'critical period', during which auditory stimulation must occur in order for neural maturation to occur (Kral et al., 2001; Sharma et al., 2002). If stimulation does not occur within this timeframe, the auditory system degenerates (Kral et al., 2001; Shepherd, 1997). In humans with normal hearing, maturation of the central auditory system continues throughout childhood through to adolescence. Research with humans has shown that the central auditory system can retain its plasticity for some years without auditory input, and when stimulated by a cochlear implant will commence maturation at the same rate as for children with normal hearing, with the maturational sequence delayed by the period of sensory deprivation (Ponton et al., 1996).

It has been found, however, that after long periods of deprivation, such as in children who have used a unilateral implant for several years and have then received a second, bilateral implant, that there were abnormalities in spatial patterns of cortical activity in the brain not observed in children who received a second cochlear implant after a shorter time (Gordon et al., 2010). Further physiological studies suggest that in the absence of normal auditory stimulation there is a period of about 3.5 years during which the central auditory system retains its maximum plasticity. This can extend in some children up to the age of approximately 7 years, after which it is significantly reduced (Sharma et al., 2005; Sharma et al., 2002). Harrison and colleagues (2005), who examined the speech perception performance of children implanted at different ages, argue that the situation is not quite as simple as this. They hypothesize that although central auditory plasticity is limited for children implanted at older ages, there is no age at which there is a clear cut-off, but instead there is an age-related plasticity effect that depends to some extent on the tests used to assess performance.

Early research on cochlear implantation in children supported the biological plasticity theory, showing a strong negative relationship between duration of deafness (or age at implant) and speech perception outcomes (Apuzzo, 1995; Nikolopoulos et al., 1999; Osberger, 1991; Staller et al., 1991). Initially, speech perception results for children who were not congenitally deaf, received their cochlear implant relatively quickly, and therefore had a shorter period of deafness, were superior to those for children with congenital deafness and later implantation (Pisoni et al., 1999; Staller et al., 1991). As Marshark (2007) noted, children who have later onset hearing loss have usually developed better language skills prior to implantation, and therefore show better achievement afterwards (for example, Moog & Geers, 2003). For children with congenital deafness, a significant correlation between age at implantation and outcomes has also been documented in many recent studies. Children implanted earlier show faster growth of speech perception (Tajudeen et al., 2010; Uziel et al., 2007), language (Connor et al., 2000; Nikolopoulos et al., 2004; Schorr et al., 2008; Tomblin et al., 2005) and reading abilities (Archbold et al., 2008a; Geers et al., 2008; James et al., 2008; Johnson & Goswami, 2010), and also have improved psychosocial outcomes (Schorr, 2006). Development of speech production is also associated with age at implantation, with slower rates of development shown by children who received their implants later (Flipsen, 2008; Peng et al., 2004; Tye-Murray et al., 1995). Interestingly, for children implanted very early, early age at implantation and speech production have been observed to have the opposite association, with one study documenting slower vocal development for children implanted when younger. Greater physical, cognitive, and social maturity were thought to provide children implanted at older ages with an advantage for early speech development (Ertmer et al., 2007).

More recently, there have been reports of even better outcomes in children implanted around the age of 2 years or younger, with higher proportions of children achieving speech perception, language and reading skills commensurate with those of their hearing peers (Duchesne et al., 2009; Geers, 2004; Niparko et al,. 2010; Svirsky et al., 2004). These results have been observed to be "consistent with the existence of a 'sensitive period' for language development, and a gradual decline in language acquisition skills as a function of age" (Svirsky et al., 2004). Svirsky and colleagues qualify this observation by suggesting that the auditory information provided by a cochlear implant is significantly inferior to that received by children with normal hearing, and that it is possible that sensitive periods for speech and language development may exist for cochlear implant users and not for children with normal hearing because of the diminished auditory signal the former receive.

Nicholas and Geers (2007) studied the language development of 76 children who had received a cochlear implant by their third birthday. They concluded that children who received an implant by 12-16 months, before substantial spoken language delay had developed, were more likely to achieve age-appropriate spoken language. These children 'caught up' with their hearing peers by 4.5 years of age, whereas children implanted after 24 months of age did not. Both Nicholas and Geers (2007) and Tomblin and colleagues (2005) observed an early burst of language growth in children implanted before the age of 18 months which was not seen in children implanted after this age. More recent studies suggest implanting children as early as before 12 months of age, with strong development of speech perception and language skills reported at age-appropriate rates for many or all of the children (Svirsky et al., 2004; Tajudeen et al., 2010; Waltzman & Roland, 2005; Wie, 2010).

A review of recent studies concluded that the evidence suggests that cochlear implantation before the age of 2 years is more effective than after this time, but that it is not yet clear whether implantation of children under 12 months of age provides greater benefit (Ali & O'Connell, 2007). As implantation of children under the age of 2 years is a relatively recent practice, limited evidence has been obtained for short-term outcomes (only up to approximately 5-8 years post-implantation) and the effect of implantation at a very young age on longer-term outcomes is still unknown (Ali & O'Connell, 2007). It is also not yet known whether children implanted at older ages, who have been shown to develop more slowly, will eventually reach equivalent long-term milestones to those implanted earlier. Some more recent longer term studies support this view, showing that although age at implantation strongly influences outcomes in younger children, the effect of this factor appears to wane with increasing age and implant experience (Geers, 2004; Hay-McCutcheon et al., 2008; Moog & Geers, 2003). Finally, when considering these reports, it is also important to remember that children implanted at younger ages are more likely to use oral communication, a factor that has also been shown to improve speech perception and spoken language outcomes.

4.3 Degree of hearing loss

There is conflicting evidence regarding the influence of degree of hearing loss on outcomes for children with cochlear implants. This factor has been reported as highly predictive of outcomes for children with cochlear implants in many studies. Speech perception abilities, language development and reading in children with hearing loss and those with cochlear implants have been found to decrease with increasing severity of hearing loss (Boothroyd et al., 1991; El-Hakim et al., 2001; Holt & Svirsky, 2008; Wake et al., 2005; Zwolan et al., 1997). Nicholas and Geers (2007) observed that children with better hearing prior to implantation showed faster language growth with increasing implant experience than did children with less pre-implant hearing. Conversely, some other studies that included more children who were older when implanted and at testing have not found a significant correlation between degree of hearing loss and speech perception, vocabulary or speech production outcomes (Blamey et al. 2001a; Harris & Terlektsi, 2011). The majority of published evidence supports a significant influence of degree of hearing loss on outcomes.

4.4 Cognitive ability

Non-verbal cognitive ability has been identified as one of the most influential factors on language outcomes in preschool children with hearing loss. The influence of cognitive skills is no less important for outcomes in children with cochlear implants, and several studies have reported it to be one of the most significant factors of all those examined, having much greater influence than other variables (Geers et al., 2009; Geers, 2003). Non-verbal IQ has been shown to have a significant effect on the development of vocabulary (Mayne, 2000), language (Geers et al., 2009; Geers et al., 2008; Sarant et al., 2009; Sarant, Hughes, & Blamey, 2010), reading (Moog & Geers, 2003), and speech production (Tobey et al., 2003). Although, after adjusting for the effect of language, cognitive ability usually has no direct effect on speech perception performance, it does have an indirect effect on this outcome. This is because language is strongly influenced by cognitive ability, and is the medium through which speech perception assessments are conducted; children have to comprehend the language used in speech perception tests and respond using spoken language (Sarant et al., 2010). Many studies have demonstrated a strong association between language and speech perception ability (for example, Blamey et al., 2001; Niparko et al., 2010).

Cognitive delay has been associated with reduced development of speech perception and production skills in populations of children with diagnosed additional disabilities (Holt & Kirk, 2005; Pyman et al., 2000; Waltzman et al., 2000), but is also a predictive factor for children who are in the average range for non-verbal cognitive abilities (Moog & Geers, 2003). Pisoni and colleagues emphasized the importance of cognitive factors such as memory, attention, and verbal rehearsal speed in determining outcomes after implantation (Pisoni & Cleary, 2003; Pisoni et al., 1999), and postulated that 'central' cognitive factors might explain some of the previously unexplained variance in outcomes for children with cochlear implants (Pisoni & Cleary, 2003; Pisoni et al., 1999). Geers and Sedey (2011) added credence to this theory with their recent observation that faster verbal rehearsal speed contributed to better language outcomes in children implanted between 2 and 5 years of age with more than 10 years of cochlear implant experience. In further support of Pisoni and colleagues' theory, it has recently been reported that when compared to children of the same age and cognitive ability, children with cochlear implants still demonstrate language delays that are disproportionate to their cognitive potential (Meinzen-Derr et al., 2011). The cognitive processes underlying this performance-functional gap need to be investigated and understood in order to implement appropriate intervention strategies to close the gap and improve outcomes for a greater proportion of children with cochlear implants.

4.5 Communication mode

Communication mode, often dichotomized into oral communication and total communication (signing plus speaking), has long been investigated as a source of variance in outcomes for children with cochlear implants, with mixed results. Proponents of oral communication maintain that maximal auditory benefit from cochlear implants can only be gained if hearing and speech are the only media for communication. There are several reports of children attending oral communication programs achieving higher speech perception and language scores than children in total communication programs (Archbold et al., 2000; El-Hakim et al., 2001; Geers et al., 2003; Meyer et al., 1998; Moog & Geers, 2003). Similarly, speech production outcomes are reported to be better for children in oral education settings. Tobey et al (2003) found oral-aural communication and teaching methods that emphasized speaking and listening to be the most influential factors in determining speech production development in children implanted by age 5 years. These environments were found to enhance speech production development, regardless of whether the environment was a mainstream school or a special school, although children in mainstream environments outperformed those in special education environments.

Proponents of the total communication approach maintain that children will obtain maximal information through the use of both speech and some form of manually coded English, as the latter will provide information that may be missed due to insufficient auditory abilities. Improved vocabulary development has been documented for children implanted early and enrolled in total communication educational programs over those in oral programs (Connor et al., 2000). There are also reports that mode of communication does not significantly influence some outcomes. Yoshinaga-Itano and Snyder (1996) found that mode of communication and learning did not significantly affect students' performance in the lexical/semantic characteristics of their written language. They hypothesized that written language is acquired in such a way that students need only one well-established language in order to acquire the written form of their language, and that both oral and signed communication methods may provide students with sufficient bases from which to learn written English. Similarly, several studies of speech perception, production, language, reading and later academic outcomes of children with cochlear implants have not found oral or total communication modes to be predictive of better results (Geers, 2003; Miyamoto et al., 1993; Niparko et al., 2010; Robbins et al., 1999; Uziel et al., 2007).

The absence of overwhelming evidence of the superiority of one communication method over the other may be due to differences in the characteristics of the children studied. Children who are implanted at younger ages are more likely to use an oral communication method, and particular educational programs may also have selection biases towards children with characteristics such as greater preoperative residual hearing or higher cognitive ability (Geers, 2006a). Some non-government funded educational programs are not accessible to families of lower socioeconomic status, and in this way only children from families with greater financial means and likely higher educational achievements will be enrolled in particular programs. When considering the effect of mode of communication, it is unclear in many cases whether children use oral communication after cochlear implantation because they are progressing well, or whether their rate of progress is due to their use of oral communication.

4.6 Family characteristics

Several family characteristics have been found to contribute to various outcomes for children with hearing loss, including those with cochlear implants. Family size has been observed to impact on speech production outcomes, with children from smaller families making faster progress (Moog & Geers, 2003; Tobey et al., 2003). This is presumably due to the fact that parents of smaller families may have more time and/or resources to devote to assisting their children's communication development. Similarly, children from families of higher socioeconomic status have achieved better speech production, language and literacy outcomes (Connor & Zwolan, 2004; Dollaghan et al., 1999; Holt & Svirsky, 2008; Niparko et al., 2010; Tobey et al., 2003). Greater parental involvement in children's intervention programs has also been associated with improved language development (Moeller, 2000; Sarant et al., 2009; Watkin et al., 2007). This is presumably due to increased follow-up and improved communication at home, as parents who become involved in intervention have been shown to demonstrate better communication skills and make higher contributions to children's progress than non-participating parents (Fallon & Harris, 1991).

Unsurprisingly, maternal communication skills are also a significant indicator for language development, early reading skills, and psychosocial development, with children of mothers who are better communicators developing better reading and language skills and having fewer behaviour problems (Calderon, 2000; Niparko et al., 2010). Children with a more highly educated parent caregiver have been reported to have better language, even in studies where the average educational level was relatively high (Geers et al., 2009; Sarant et al., 2009). It has been suggested that the relationship between socioeconomic status and language outcomes is actually mediated solely by properties of maternal speech that differ as a function of socioeconomic status (Hoff, 2003; Hoff & Tian, 2005). Gender also contributes to the variation in outcomes between children, with females consistently achieving better results with regard to speech production (Tobey et al., 2003), reading (Moog & Geers, 2003) and language development (Geers et al., 2009).

4.7 Other factors

Cochlear implant and speech characteristics such as the number of active electrodes in the implant array, larger dynamic ranges in speech processor maps, greater growth of loudness and length of time using the latest speech processing strategies have been found to significantly influence speech production and language outcomes in children implanted by age 5 years (Connor et al., 2000; Moog & Geers, 2003; Peng et al., 2004; Tobey et al., 2003). The number of surviving nerves has also been postulated to contribute to outcomes (Pyman et al., 2000).

5. Limitations in outcomes with unilateral cochlear implants

Historically, the consequences of unilateral hearing loss (UHL) have been underestimated, both for children with normal hearing and those with a unilateral cochlear implant, as spoken language can still be developed with one hearing ear. Prior to the introduction of neonatal hearing screening, many children with UHL were undiagnosed until they attended school, where communication difficulties in noisy educational environments or failure to progress academically at the expected rate raised suspicions of hearing loss. Although there has been limited research on the effect of UHL on the development of spoken language, mild through to significant delays have been reported in several studies of children with UHL and normal hearing in the unimplanted ear, although there has been insufficient follow-up to determine whether the reported delays persisted through childhood (Cho Lieu, 2004). A review of the literature in this area also found that school-aged children with UHL have increased rates of academic failure (22-35% rate of repeating at least one grade), additional needs for educational assistance (12-41%), and behavioural problems in the classroom (Cho Lieu, 2004).

Despite the fact that many children with a unilateral implant demonstrate excellent speech perception abilities in the controlled testing environment of a sound proof booth (Cheng et al., 1999; Leigh et al. 2008c; Sarant et al., 2001), this performance does not represent their speech perception abilities in the real world. The difficulties experienced by children with one normal hearing ear and one ear with UHL are similar (but worse) for children with a single cochlear implant and a severe-profound or profound hearing loss in the non-implanted ear. These include difficulty understanding speech that is soft, or speech in noisy environments, such as the playground or classroom, and difficulty locating sound sources, such as their peers in a group conversation, or their teachers in the classroom. These auditory challenges can limit their ability to follow or take part in a group conversation, or to focus in the correct direction when the teacher begins to speak. The amount and quality of speech heard by children with one cochlear implant and a significant hearing loss in the other ear is greatly reduced and fragmented compared to what is heard by children with normal hearing. Further, understanding what they do hear is made difficult by their often delayed language skills. With poor language knowledge, many of these children are unable to piece together poorly heard or overheard information, and therefore to learn incidentally (without direct teaching), as do children with normal hearing. The inability to 'overhear' spoken conversations limits the access of these children to many avenues of incidental learning, and therefore restricts their acquisition of knowledge of language, social interaction, and how the world works, stifling their development in many areas.

A unilateral cochlear implant does not guarantee the development of language, speech production, academic or social skills comparable to those of children with normal hearing. Although there are many children with a unilateral cochlear implant who are able to develop these skills at an age-appropriate rate, there also remain many who show delayed development in these areas, some of whom maintain or increase their delay through to adulthood. Given the difficulties of unilateral hearing loss, giving children bilateral cochlear implants could potentially improve outcomes.

6. Bilateral cochlear implants

A recent report on worldwide trends in bilateral cochlear implantation estimated that 59%of bilateral cochlear implant recipients in the U.S., and 78% of recipients in other countries are currently children (Peters et al., 2010). It was observed that by the end of 2007, 70% of all bilateral cochlear implants had been received by children, with children aged 3-10 years being most highly represented in this group (33% of all bilateral surgeries; Peters et al., 2010). 70% of children received 2 cochlear implants in sequential operations (2 separate operations). Of the remaining 30%, children aged less than 3 years were the only group for whom the majority (58%) received bilateral cochlear implants simultaneously (during the same operation). Bilateral cochlear implantation in children is a growing trend worldwide; in 2010, implant manufacturers' databases indicated that there were 4986 children with bilateral implants (Peters et al., 2010).

6.1

6.1.1 Decision making

The decision to give a child one or two cochlear implants is a difficult one for parents, despite the growing trend toward implanting children at a young age with simultaneous bilateral cochlear implants. Until recently, there has been a lack of strong evidence to support bilateral implantation, particularly with regard to longer term outcomes (Hyde et al., 2010). For parents of children with no useable residual hearing, the decision is more straightforward, as binaural hearing offers significant benefits over monaural hearing. However, parents of children with useable aided residual hearing face a more difficult decision, as loss of functional and useful hearing is being risked for a probable, but not guaranteed, benefit. Parents usually take into account their child's degree of hearing loss in both ears (if the child has no cochlear implants) or in the non-implanted ear, professional recommendations, costs (typically between $US40,000 -$US60,000 (Papsin & Gordon, 2007), their own attitudes and desires for their child, and surgical/medical and other risks (see section 6.1.4). Parents of children who are deemed eligible by an implant team for bilateral cochlear implants may still choose to give their child a unilateral implant. Reasons for this decision have included a desire to see what the benefits of one implant are before proceeding with another, concerns about the appearance of children wearing two speech processors, saving an ear for future technological developments (see 6.1.3), and difficulty accepting children's hearing loss.

6.1.2 Physiological and functional arguments for bilateral cochlear implantation

The arguments for bilateral cochlear implantation include stimulation of both auditory nerves to ensure that the better ear is stimulated, as the benefits of cochlear implantation are not necessarily symmetrical for each ear. As previously discussed, many factors influence outcomes, and although some factors will be the same for both ears in a particular individual (for example, communication mode, cognitive ability etc.), others may not. These could include the anatomical structure and physiology of the ears, effects of the pathology that caused the hearing loss, and in the case of children who receive two cochlear implants separated in time (sequential implantation), the duration of deafness will differ between the ears. A further reason for bilateral cochlear implantation is to prevent the neural degeneration that has been documented in humans and animal studies as a result of auditory deprivation (Hardie, 1998; Sharma et al., 2002; Shepherd, 1997). Bilateral implantation also ensures that children still have hearing in the case of speech processor or device failure in one ear, which can significantly reduce stress for children and their families if these events occur. Finally, having bilateral cochlear implants may facilitate binaural hearing, which requires the perception of auditory information in both ears. As discussed earlier, children with unilateral cochlear implants experience the difficulties associated with unilateral deafness, such as an inability to localize sounds, and difficulty perceiving speech in background noise. For the relatively small number of children who have sufficient hearing to use a hearing aid in their non-implanted (or contralateral) ear, the literature shows that binaural benefit is gained through use of the cochlear implant and hearing aid together (Frush Holt et al., 2005; Mok et al., 2007). However, for many children with a bilateral profound or severe-profound hearing loss, the use of a contralateral hearing aid in the non-implanted ear is not a viable option, due to a lack of residual hearing. For these children, bilateral cochlear implantation is the only means of providing binaural hearing.

6.1.3 Access to future technology

Arguments against bilateral implantation include 'saving' an ear for future technology while using a hearing aid with residual hearing (if there is sufficient residual hearing). Although it is known that changes in the cochlea occur after implantation, and that these are permanent, it is not known whether repeated re-implantation with cochlear implants or with other future technology is possible after many years of cochlear implant use (although re-implantation is usually successful in the case of device failure). It is also unknown if or when future technologies such as gene therapy or neural regeneration will become available for clinical use, and it is accepted that there is a critical time period for central auditory brain and language development, beyond which future technology may not be beneficial. Without knowing what form future technologies may take, it is not possible to predict how useful they may be for individuals who have 'waited' and not proceeded with the current cochlear implant technology.

6.1.4 Risks

Many parents have concerns about the risks of cochlear implant surgery, and some of these risks are increased with two separate implant operations, as is the case with sequential implant procedures. Simultaneous implant operations require less than double the surgery time and eliminate the need for, and risks of, two anaesthetics and recovery periods. Complications as a result of cochlear implant surgery can be categorised as major and minor, and most occur very close to the time of surgery, although some have been reported up to 14 years post-surgery, and can recur. Major complications include infections or skin flap breakdown in the area around the implant, extrusion of the end of the electrode array outside the cochlea, device failure (requiring explantation of the device), cholesteatoma, permanent facial nerve damage, persistent eardrum perforation, cerebrospinal fluid leak with subsequent meningitis, and magnet displacement. For children with anatomical deformities of the cochlea (such as Mondini deformity, in which there are less than the normal two and a half turns in the cochlea), the risk of facial nerve damage is greater. However, reported major complication rates are very low, ranging from 2 - 5% (Bhatia et al., 2004; Cohen et al., 1989; Loundon et al., 2010).

Minor complications are those which can be resolved without surgery, and include vertigo with or without nausea, persistent otitis media (middle ear infection), facial palsy, tinnitus, mild skin flap infection, flap swelling, hematoma (bruising), taste disturbance, and pain around the operation site. The incidence of minor complications is higher and more subject to variation between cochlear implant centers; studies of large numbers of patients ranging from 4% - 20% (Bhatia et al., 2004; Dutt et al., 2005; Loundon et al., 2010). Other risks include those of any surgical procedure, including the risks associated with an anaesthetic and blood loss. Some risks are increased for younger children, including an increased risk of anaesthetic complications. A further risk is due to the relatively small size of their skulls. Although their cochleae are adult-sized at birth, their small skull size increases the risk of displacement of the electrode array with subsequent significant skull growth. There is also a high prevalence of otitis media in this age group, which raises the risk of significant infection in the implant area as a result of infection spread from the middle ear. Due to these concerns, the FDA currently approves cochlear implantation in children only from the age of 2 years and older (ASHA, 2004). In summary, although there are several possible complications of cochlear implant surgery, the incidence of life-threatening complications is extremely low, and the rates of major and minor post-operative complications are also low, making cochlear implant surgery in children a reliable and safe procedure.

Longer term risks of cochlear implantation include device failure. Although cochlear implants are designed to last for a lifetime, about 2% of devices do fail (ASHA, 2004). Device failure can result in a changed auditory percept or a total lack of function, and re-implantation is the only solution. Fortunately, most re-implants function as well as, or better than, the original implants, but the risks, costs, and inconvenience of surgery must be undertaken. Another longer-term risk is the increased risk of bacterial meningitis, due to the fact that the cochlear implant is a foreign body, and can act as a nidus for infection when there is a bacterial illness (ASHA, 2004). This risk is highest for children with malformed cochleae, those who contract meningitis prior to cochlear implantation, children aged less than five years, and children with otitis media or immunodeficiency. A further longer-term complication is facial nerve stimulation, which can occur at any time after cochlear implantation, but is rare. Children most at risk of this are those with malformed cochleae. Fortunately, it is a simple procedure for an audiologist to switch off the electrode/s causing the unwanted sensation.

A final and important risk that is unique to sequential bilateral cochlear implantation is that some (usually older) children may not like the sound of their second cochlear implant, and will eventually become non-users. While many children, particularly those who have had one cochlear implant and have another after a significant period of time, may not initially like the sound of their second implant, most adapt to it over time with encouragement and support. However, some children never adapt, and show a pattern of inconsistent use over several years that culminates in rejection when they are older. There have been no reports in the literature to date about adaptation and non-user rates for either large groups of children with bilateral implants or for simultaneously implanted children. Factors thought to contribute to this outcome in children with a unilateral cochlear implant include older age at implantation, dislike of the auditory percept, facial nerve pain or twitching, peer pressure in secondary school, family issues, non-mainstream school settings, use of signed communication, lack of involvement in the decision-making process (older children), and poor speech intelligibility after several years of cochlear implant use (Archbold et al., 2009; Ray et al., 2006; Watson & Gregory, 2005).

Published information on the current non-user rate for children with unilateral cochlear implants suggests the risk of rejection is low; the reported non-user rate is currently around 3% (Archbold et al. 2009; Uziel et al. 2007). However, for children receiving a second, sequential cochlear implant, the situation is entirely different, as they must adapt to a second, different sound percept; one that may not compare favourably with that provided by their first cochlear implant. In the first study to be published on adaptation in children with bilateral implants, Galvin and Hughes (in press) noted that a higher proportion of children who were implanted simultaneously adapted to full-time use of their devices (95%) than those implanted sequentially (70%), and that adaptation to bilateral implant use was not easy for almost 20% of the 46 children studied. Both Galvin and colleagues, and Archbold (2009; in a study of long term use of unilateral cochlear implants in children) noted that children who eventually become non-users often first demonstrate a pattern of inconsistent use. Archbold also noted that children who became non-users usually had disabilities additional to their hearing loss. The possibility of this eventuality should be taken into account by parents, and also by children old enough to participate in the decision-making process.

6.2 Benefits of bilateral cochlear implants

When a person with normal hearing listens with two ears (rather than just one) sound quality is improved, it is easier to locate the source of a sound, and it is easier to understand speech, particularly in background noise. The improved sound quality with two ears is commonly described as fuller, more spacious, and more natural. To locate sound sources, the listener primarily uses the differences in timing and level of sound arriving at each ear, with sound arriving later and being softer at the ear furthest from the sound source. This localization ability allows the listener to locate sounds in the environment, to find the speaker in a group conversation, and to be more aware of changes in their auditory environment. Speech perception is improved with two ears because the brain has two opportunities to process the same signal (binaural redundancy), and because the combined signal is slightly louder (binaural summation). The benefits of two ears are particularly significant when speech and noise are coming from different directions. Firstly, due to the physical barrier of the head (the head-shadow effect), the noise level will be lower at the ear that is furthest from the noise source. Given that speech will usually be arriving from in front of the head, the level of the speech signal is equal at both ears. The listener is therefore better able to perceive speech by attending primarily to the ear at which the noise level is lower. Secondly, with speech and noise coming from different directions, each ear receives a different balance of speech and noise. The brain is able to compare these two different signals and reduce the impact of the noise to increase the salience of the speech signal (binaural unmasking).

6.2.1 Speech perception

The speech perception abilities of children with bilateral cochlear implants have been explored using both standardized measures and a variety of study-specific measures in quiet conditions and in various noise conditions (for example, Galvin et al., 2007a, b; Scherf et al., 2007; van Deun et al., 2010). A review of the research found that 11/13 of the studies reported significant improvement in children's speech perception in noise abilities (Johnston et al., 2009). Some of these improvements were due simply to the head shadow effect, or to the ability to concentrate on the sound from one ear over another (Galvin et al., 2008a; Galvin et al., 2007a; Litovsky et al., 2006a). A recent study found that although they did not perform as well as children with normal hearing, bilaterally implanted children performed significantly better than unilaterally implanted children on tests of speech perception performance in noise (Lovett et al., 2010). As with outcomes for children with unilateral cochlear implants, the degree of improvement varies widely between individuals. Improved speech perception in noise has been associated with shorter periods of hearing loss in the second ear in some studies (Litovsky et al., 2004; Peters et al., 2007; Steffens et al., 2008), but not all have found this link (Kuhn-Inacker et al., 2004; Litovsky et al., 2006a; Wolfe et al., 2007). Two studies that did not find improvements in speech perception in noise included children who had a long time period between their first and second cochlear implants. There have also been reports of improved speech perception performance in quiet conditions with bilateral implants (Scherf et al., 2007; Zeitler et al., 2008).

6.2.2 Localization of sound

Bilateral cochlear implantation has not yet shown a clear benefit for sound localization. In assessments of localization performance for long-term users to date, some children can localize sounds well (Litovsky et al., 2006b; Lovett et al., 2010). Bilateral implantation has been associated with increases of 18.5% in the accuracy of sound localization (Lovett et al.,

2010). Other children are more limited in their localization ability; able to lateralize sounds from the left or right side of their heads confidently and with high accuracy, but unable to determine the direction of the sound source (as occurs with true binaural processing) as the stimulus is presented closer to the front and centre of their heads (Galvin et al., 2008b; Grieco-Calub & Litovsky, 2010). Many other bilaterally implanted children (particularly older children) have shown no ability at all to locate sound sources (Galvin et al., 2007a). Of the children who show some spatial awareness, many do not differ significantly in their ability to children with bimodal stimulation (a cochlear implant plus hearing aid), and none have the abilities of children with normal hearing (Sparreboom et al., 2010). Although overall the best performers are younger, not all young children demonstrate an ability to locate sound sources (Galvin et al., 2010; Galvin et al., 2007a).

6.2.3 Broader outcomes of bilateral implantation

Most of the research on outcomes for children with bilateral cochlear implants has focused on speech perception in noise and sound localization abilities. There is little research to date comparing broader outcomes of children with unilateral versus bilateral cochlear implants, and at the time of writing, there were no reports of speech production or academic outcomes. An initial theoretical analysis of the cost effectiveness of bilateral implantation suggested that it "is possibly a cost-effective use of resources", but that further data on the costs and benefits of bilateral implantation compared with unilateral implantation are required to reach a definitive conclusion (Summerfield et al., 2010). To date, two studies using standardized quality-of-life measures have attempted to determine whether bilateral implants facilitate improved quality of life in children, however neither reported a significant improvement for children with bilateral implants (Beijen, 2007; Lovett et al., 2010).

Information on the impact of bilateral cochlear implantation on language is currently limited. A recent study comparing the preverbal communication of children implanted before age 3 years (27 bilaterally; 42 unilaterally) reported that children with bilateral cochlear implants were significantly more likely to use vocalisation to communicate and to use hearing when interacting with an adult than were children with unilateral implants (Tait et al., 2010). After statistically controlling for the influence of age at implantation and length of deafness, it was found that bilateral implantation contributed to 51% of the variance in outcomes. A multi-center study of 91 children with unilateral (n=60) and bilateral (n=31) implants reported that bilateral implantation was not associated with improved expressive or receptive language development (Niparko et al., 2010). Similarly, Nittrouer & Chappman (2009) examined the vocabulary, receptive and expressive language abilities of 58 children tested at age 3.5 years and also found no differences in outcomes between 15 children with unilateral and 26 with bilateral cochlear implants. Both of these studies provide no support, in terms of language development, for providing young children with bilateral cochlear implants.

However, recent initial results of another prospective, multicentre study comparing outcomes for children with unilateral and bilateral cochlear implants showed a significant advantage for bilaterally implanted children with regard to language development (Sarant et al., in press). The groups of unilaterally (n= 11) and bilaterally (n=17) implanted 5-year-old children in this study did not differ with regard to average non-verbal cognitive ability, parent involvement in intervention or parent stress levels, and children with bilateral cochlear implants achieved significantly higher expressive and total language scores than did children with unilateral cochlear implants. Initial results of a Belgian study of 25 bilaterally implanted children matched for 10 factors with 25 unilaterally implanted children also reported significantly better receptive and expressive language outcomes for the bilaterally implanted children (Boons et al., in press).

Considering other benefits of bilateral implants, Galvin and colleagues' research and clinical experience with older children and young adults indicates that there are more general benefits, such as ease of listening, awareness of the auditory environment, and increased confidence in social situations, that are of great functional value to children with bilateral implants (Galvin & Hughes, in press). For this group, self-motivation and external support and encouragement were particularly important, as adapting to a second implant at a later age is a more difficult process. Parent questionnaire data from this study for 38 children and young adults showed that 79% of children were using two cochlear implants more than 60% of the time, and 68% reported using bilateral implants more than 90% of the time. Reports of perceived benefit in everyday life also indicated that there was no upper age limit beyond which additional benefit could not be gained from bilateral implants. When considering the risks, time and effort required to obtain bilateral implants versus any additional benefit gained, 79% of the families reported that the second cochlear implant was worthwhile, 16% were unsure, and only 5% felt that obtaining bilateral implants had not been worthwhile (Karyn Galvin, personal communication, August 16th, 2011).

6.3 Timing of first and second cochlear implants; sequential and simultaneous implantation

It is reasonable to assume that children who receive a second cochlear implant early in life will have greater neural plasticity of the central auditory system, and that the first implant will have dominated the auditory neural pathways for a shorter period of time also. Electrophysiological studies of auditory brainstem responses in children with early onset of deafness support this view, showing prolonged wave latencies in the second implanted ear for children implanted sequentially compared to those implanted simultaneously (Gordon, 2008; Gordon et al., 2010). Follow up of children has shown that wave latencies improve over time, particularly for children implanted under 3 years of age (Gordon et al., 2007), and that cortical evoked responses are fundamentally different for children implanted before and after age 3.5 years in terms of wave morphology and latency (Bauer et al., 2006; Sharma et al., 2005). These studies suggest that the shortest delay possible (ie. simultaneous bilateral implantation) will maximise the chance of developing true binaural auditory processing. The clinical evidence reported to date supports the electrophysiological findings. Children who receive bilateral implants sequentially when younger adapt more quickly (Dowell et al., 2011; Galvin & Hughes, in press; Scherf et al., 2009) and generally have better speech perception and sound localization outcomes than those implanted when older (Galvin et al., 2007a).

There appears to be a consensus that children receiving a second implant over the age of 4 years perform much more poorly on speech recognition and sound localization tasks, and do not show evidence of true binaural processing (for example, Galvin et al., 2007a; Johnston et al., 2009; Wolfe et al., 2007). Current evidence suggests that simultaneous bilateral implantation is a safe surgical procedure, and may also offer advantages to ease of adaptation, although there may be greater challenges associated with programming and managing two devices in younger children (Ramsden et al., 2009).

6.4 Factors affecting outcomes

Outcomes with bilateral implants are influenced by many of the same interacting factors as with unilateral implants (see section 4). As with unilateral implants, factors such as age at time of first implant and amount of pre-operative auditory stimulation in the ear implanted second contribute to outcomes, with younger children and those with pre-implant hearing aid use achieving better results (Galvin et al., 2007a; Peters et al., 2007; Wolfe et al., 2007; Zeitler et al., 2008) . Consistency of device use also influences outcomes, with most children implanted at younger ages adapting more quickly and with greater ease to using bilateral implants, whether they are simultaneously or sequentially implanted (Galvin et al., 2008a; Scherf et al., 2009). Older sequentially implanted children and young adults (who are responsible for their own consistency of device use) must be highly self-motivated in order to persist with learning to use their second cochlear implant; this can be particularly difficult for children aged 7-12 years, especially if they have not been involved in the decision-making process (Galvin et al., 2009). Children implanted at younger ages are also more likely to achieve similar listening abilities with either device, and appear to have greater potential for the development of localization abilities.

For children implanted sequentially, greater improvements in speech perception and localization abilities are demonstrated when there is a shorter time period between the first and second implants (Galvin et al., 2008a; Schafer & Thibodeau, 2006). Factors associated with poor outcomes include poorer than expected outcomes with the first implant, a long time delay between the first and second implants, and limited experience and/or habilitation using the second implant on its own (Dowell et al., 2011). Given the limited information about outcomes for bilaterally implanted children to date, it is not currently possible to accurately predict outcomes for individuals.

6.5 Limitations in current knowledge of outcomes with bilateral implants

The early literature is limited in showing what is possible for bilaterally implanted children. Many studies have included children with very little experience at the time of assessment (as low as 6-12 months for many studies; Sparreboom et al., 2010). We know from the experience of both adults and children with unilateral implants that speech perception and other skills can improve over a period of years, and from bilateral studies that localization skills also require time to develop, therefore it is reasonable to expect that results could improve over time. The evidence is also limited in terms of the number of children who have been followed. A review of paediatric bilateral implant research noted that over half of the published studies reviewed had only 10 or fewer participants (Johnston et al., 2009). Although there are no reports to date on outcomes for children who have received bilateral cochlear implants aged under one year, it would not be unreasonable to expect that very early bilateral implantation would also further optimize outcomes, given the electrophysiological and other evidence collected to date (Peters et al., 2010). There is also currently a lack of evidence regarding quality of life, language, literacy and academic outcomes for children with bilateral compared to unilateral implants. As more children receive bilateral implants, studies with larger numbers of participants observed over longer periods of time will be conducted, as has occurred with unilateral implants. These studies will no doubt provide further information on which the magnitude of the effect of bilateral implants on outcomes can be measured.

7. Conclusion

Enormous progress has been made over the past three decades in the development of cochlear implants. We have progressed from uncertainty and controversy around whether children could use the incomplete auditory information provided by a unilateral cochlear implant to develop spoken language, to documenting outstanding and life-transforming success for many children with unilateral or bilateral cochlear implants. Cochlear implants are now accepted as the standard of care for children with severe-profound hearing loss. They have allowed many children to attend regular schools, and to develop their language, social and academic skills to levels that exceed those for their peers with severe-profound hearing loss using hearing aids. For some children, cochlear implants have facilitated outcomes such as those their hearing peers achieve, including post-secondary school study, fulfilling employment, and rich social relationships in the hearing world. However, there are still a significant number of children with cochlear implants whose speech intelligibility, speech perception, spoken language, academic and social development are far below that of children with normal hearing. There remains enormous variation in outcomes between individuals with both unilateral and bilateral cochlear implants. Other influences related to neural maturation and development, and also to complex interactions between demographic variables, environmental factors, intervention and learning processes, are not yet understood. A challenge for the future will be to make progress in our understanding of these factors and processes in order to improve outcomes for a greater proportion of children with cochlear implants. Further follow-up of children with unilateral and bilateral cochlear implants is required in the future to determine what the best outcomes will be.

8. References

Ali, W. & O'Connell, R. 2007. The effectiveness of early cochlear implantation for infants and young children with hearing loss. *NZHTA Technical Brief*, Vol. 6, No.5, Christchurch, New Zealand.

Apuzzo, M. & Yoshinaga-Itano, C. 1995. Early identification of infants with significant hearing loss and the Minnesota Child Development Inventory. *Seminars in Hearing*, Vol. 16, pp. 124-39.

Archbold, S., Harris, M., O'Donoghue, G., Nikolopoulos, T., White, A. & Lloyd Richmond, H. 2008a. Reading abilities after cochlear implantation: The effect of age at implantation on outcomes at 5 and 7 years after implantation. *International Journal of Pediatric Otorhinolaryngology*, Vol 72, pp. 1471-78.

Archbold, S., Nikolopoulos, T. Tait, M. O'Donoghue, G. Lutman, M.E. & Gregory, S. 2000. Approach to communication, speech perception and intelligibility after paediatric cochlear implantation. *British Journal of Audiology*, Vol. 34, No. 4, pp. 257-64.

Archbold, S., Sach, T., O'Neill, C., Lutman, M. & Gregory, S. 2008b. Outcomes from cochlear implantation for child and family: parental perspectives. *Deafness & Education International*, Vol 10, No. 3, pp. 120-42.

Archbold, S.M., Nikolopoulos, T.P. & Lloyd-Richmond, H. 2009. Long-term use of cochlear implant systems in paediatric recipients and factors contributing to non-use. *Cochlear Implants International*, Vol. 10, No.1, pp. 25-40.

Archbold, S.M. & O'Donoghue, G.M. 2009. Cochlear implantation in children: current status. *Paediatrics & Child Health*, Vol. 19, No.10, pp. 457-63.

American Speech and Hearing Association(ASHA). 2004. Technical Report: Cochlear Implants. *ASHA Supplement*, Vol 24, pp. 1-52. Rockville, MD.

Bamford, J. & Saunders, E. 1992. *Hearing Impairment, Auditory Perception & Language Disability*. Whurr Publishers Ltd., London, UK; Baltimore, MD, USA.

Bamiou, D. E., Worth, S., Phelps, P., Sirimanna, T. & Rajput, K. 2001. Eighth nerve aplasia and hypoplasia in cochlear implant candidates: The clinical perspective. *Otology & Neurotology*, Vol. 22, No. 4, pp. 492-96.

Bat-Chava, Y. & Deignan, E. 2001. Peer relationships of children with cochlear implants. *Journal of Deaf Studies & Deaf Education*, Vol. 6. No. 3, pp. 186-99.

Bat-Chava, Y., Martin, D., & Kosciw, J. 2005. Longitudinal improvements in communication and socialization of deaf children with cochlear implants and hearing aids: evidence from parental reports. *The Journal of Child Psychology & Psychiatry*, Vol. 46, No. 12, pp. 1287-96.

Bauer, P.W., Sharma, A., Martin, K., & Dorman, M. 2006. Central auditory development in children with bilateral cochlear implants. *Archives of Otolaryngology, Head & Neck Surgery*, Vol. 132, No. 10, pp. 1133-36.

Bauer, P.W., Wippold F.J., Goldin, J., & Lusk, R.P. 2002. Cochlear implantation in children with CHARGE Association. *Archives of Otolaryngology, Head & Neck Surgery*, Vol. 128, No. 9, pp. 1013-17.

Beadle, E. A. R., McKinley, D. J., Nikolopoulos, T. P., Brough, J.G., O'Donoghue, M., & Archbold, S.M. 2005. Long-term functional outcomes and academic-occupational status in implanted children after 10 to 14 years of cochlear implant use. *Otology & Neurotology*, Vol. 26, No. 6, pp. 1152-60.

Beijen, J.W. 2007. Sound localization ability of young children with bilateral cochlear implants. *The American Journal of Otology, Vol.* 28, No.4, pp. 479-485.

Bhatia, K., Gibbin, K.P., Nikolopoulos, T.P., & O'Donoghue, G.M. 2004. Surgical complications and their management in a series of 300 consecutive pediatric cochlear implantations. *Otology & Neurotology*, Vol. 25, No.5, pp. 730-39.

Blamey, P., Barry, J., Bow, C., Sarant, J., Paatsch, L., & Wales, R. 2001. The development of speech production following cochlear implantation. *Clinical Linguistics & Phonetics*, Vol 15, No.5, pp. 363-82.

Blamey, P., Barry, J., & Jacq, P. 2001. Phonetic inventory development in young cochlear implant users 6 years post operation. *Journal of Speech, Language & Hearing Research*, Vol. 44, No.1, pp. 73-79.

Blamey, P. & Sarant, J., 2002. Speech perception and language criteria for paediatric cochlear implant candidature. *Audiology & Neuro-Otology*, Vol. 7, No. 2, pp. 114-21.

Blamey, P., Sarant, J., & Paatsch, L. 2006. Relationships among speech perception and language measures in hard-of-hearing children. In: *Advances in the spoken language development of deaf and hard-of-hearing children*, P. E. Spencer,. M. Marshark, pp. 85-102, Oxford University Press Inc., New York.

Blamey, P., Sarant, J., Paatsch, L., Barry, J., Bow, C., Wales, R., Wright, M., Psarros, C., Rattigan, K., & Tooher, R. 2001a. Relationships among speech perception, production, language, hearing loss, and age in children. *Journal of Speech, Language and Hearing Research,* Vol. 44, pp.264-85.

Boons, T., van Wieringen, A., Brokx, J.P.L., Frijns J.H.M., Peeraer, L., Philips, B.A., Vermeulen, M., & Wouters, J. In press. Benefit of paediatric bilateral cochlear implantation on language outcomes. Proceedings of *10th European Symposium on Pediatric Cochlear Implantation,* Athens, Greece, May 12-15, 2011.

Boothroyd, A. 1997. Auditory capacity of hearing-impaired children using hearing aids and cochlear implants: Issues of efficacy and assessment. *Scandinavian Audiology Supplementum,* Vol. 46, pp. 17-25.

Boothroyd, A., Geers, A., & Moog, J. 1991. Practical implications of cochlear implants in children. *Ear & Hearing,* Vol 12, No. 4, pp. 81S-89S.

Boughman, J.A., Vernon, M., & Shaver, K.A. 1983. Usher syndrome: Definition and estimate of prevalence from two high-risk populations. *Journal of Chronic Diseases,* Vol. 36, No. 8, pp. 595-603.

Boyd, R.C., Knutson, J.F., & Dahlstrom, A.J. 2000. Social interaction of pediatric cochlear implant recipients with age-matched peers. *Annals of Otology Rhinology & Laryngology,* Vol. 109, No. 12, pp. 105-09.

Buss, E., Labadie, R.F., Brown, C.J., Gross, A.J., Grose, J.H., & Pillsbury, H.C. 2002. Outcome of Cochlear Implantation in Pediatric Auditory Neuropathy. *Otology & Neurotology,* Vol. 23, No.3, pp. 328-32.

Calderon, R. 2000. Parental involvement in deaf children's education programs as a predictor of child's language, early reading, and social-emotional development. *Journal of Deaf Studies & Deaf Education,* Vol.5, No. 2, pp. 140-55.

Chadha, N.K., James, A.L., Gordon, K.A., Blaser, S., & Papsin B.C. 2009. Bilateral cochlear implantation in children with anomalous cochleovestibular anatomy. *Archives of Otolaryngology, Head & Neck Surgery,* Vol. 135, No. 9, pp. 903-09.

Cheng, A., Grant, G.D., & Niparko, J. 1999. Meta-analysis of pediatric cochlear implant literature. *The Annals of Otology, Rhinology & Laryngology,* Vol. 108, No. 4, pp. 124-28.

Chin, S.B., Tsai, P.L., & Gao, S. 2003. Connected speech intelligibility of children with cochlear Implants and children with normal hearing. *American Journal of Speech-Language Pathology,* Vol.12, No. 4, pp. 440-451.

Ching, T. 2010. Language develoment and everyday functioning of children with hearing loss assessed at 3 years of age. *International Journal of Speech Language Pathology,* Vol. 12, No. 2, pp. 124-31.

Cho Lieu, J. 2004. Speech-language and educational consequences of unilateral hearing loss in children. *Archives of Otolaryngology Head & Neck Surgery,* Vol. 130, pp. 524-30.

Clark, G.M. 1989. The bionic ear and beyond. *Journal of the Otolaryngological Society of Australia,* Vol. 6, No. 4, pp. 244-249.

Clark, G.M., Blamey, P. Busby, P.A. Dowell, R.C. Franz, B.K.-H. Musgrave, G.N. Nienhuys, T.G. Pyman, B.C. Roberts, S.A. Tong, Y.C. Webb, R.L., Kuzma, J.A., Money, D.K., Patrick, J.F., & Seligman P.M., 1987. A multiple-electrode intracochlear implant for children. *Archives of Otolaryngology Head & Neck Surgery,* Vol. 113, No. 8, pp. 825-28.

Clark, G. M., Tong, Y. C., & Dowell, R. C. 1983. Clinical results with a multichannel pseudobipolar system. *Annals of the New York Academy of Science*, Vol. 404, pp. 370-77.

Cohen, N.L., Hoffman, R.A., & Stroschein, M. 1989. Medical or surgical complications related to the Nucleus multichannel cochlear implant. *Annals of Otology Rhinology & Laryngology Supplement*, Vol. 135, pp. 8-13.

Connor, C.M., Craig, H.K., Raudenbush, S.W., Heavner, K., & Zwolan T.A. 2006. The age at which young deaf children receive cochlear implants and their vocabulary and speech-production growth: Is there an added value for early implantation? *Ear & Hearing*, Vol. 27, pp. 628-44.

Connor, C.M., Hieber, S., Arts, H.A., & Zwolan T.A., 2000. Speech, vocabulary, and the education of children using cochlear implants: Oral or total communication? *Journal of Speech, Language & Hearing Research*, Vol. 43, No. 5, pp. 1185-203.

Connor, C. M., & Zwolan, T. A. 2004. Examining multiple sources of influence on the reading comprehension skills of children who use cochlear implants. *Journal of Speech, Language & Hearing Research*, Vol. 47, pp. 509-26.

Cowan, R. S., Brown, C., Whitford, L. A., Galvin, K. L., Sarant, J. Z., Barker, E. J., Shaw, S. , King, A., Skok, M. , Seligman, P. M., Dowell, R.C., Everingham, C., Gibson, W.P.R., & Clark, G.M. 1995. Speech perception in children using the advanced Speak speech-processing strategy. *Annals of Otology, Rhinology, & Laryngology - Supplement* 166, pp. 318-21.

Cowan, R.S., DelDot, J., Barker, E.J., Sarant, J.Z., Pegg, P., Dettman, S., Galvin, K.L., Rance, G., Hollow, R., Dowell, R.C., Pyman, B., Gibson, W.P., & Clark G.M. 1997. Speech perception results for children with implants with different levels of preoperative residual hearing. *American Journal of Otology*, Vol. 18, No. 6 Suppl, pp. S125-S126.

Crosson, J., & Geers, A. 2001. Analysis of Narrative Ability in Children with Cochlear Implants. *Ear & Hearing* Vol. 22, No. 5, pp. 381-94.

Crouch, R.A. 1997. Letting the deaf be deaf. *Hastings Center Report* Vol. 27, No.4, pp 14-21.

Dahl, H.H., Wake, M., Sarant, J., Poulakis, Z., Siemering, K., & Blamey, P. 2003. Language and speech perception outcomes in hearing-impaired children with and without connexin 26 mutations. *Audiology & Neuro-Otology*, Vol. 8, No.5, pp. 263-268.

Dalzell L., Orlando, M., MacDonald, M,. Berg, A., Bradley M., Cacace, A., Campbell, D., DeCristofaro, J., Gravel, J., Greenberg, E., Gross, S., Pinheiro, J., Regan, J., Spivak, L., Stevens, F., & Prieve, B. 2000. The New York State Universal Newborn Hearing Screening Demonstration Project: Ages of hearing loss identification, hearing aid fitting, and enrolment in early intervention." *Ear & Hearing*, Vol.21, No. 2, pp. 118-30.

Dammeyer, J. 2010. Psychosocial development in a Danish population of children with cochlear implants and deaf and hard-of-hearing children. *Journal of Deaf Studies & Deaf Education*, Vol.15, No. 1, pp. 50-58.

Davidson, L.S. 2006. Effects of stimulus level on the speech perception abilities of children using cochlear implants or digital hearing aids. *Ear & Hearing*, Vol.27, No. 5, pp. 493-507.

Davis, A., & Hind,S. 1999. The impact of hearing impairment: A global health problem. *International Journal of Pediatric Otorhinolaryngology*, Vol. 49, Suppl. 1, pp. S51-S54.

Dawson, P., Blamey P.J., Barker, E.J., & Clark, G.M. 1995. A clinical report on receptive vocabulary skills in cochlear implant users. *Ear & Hearing*, Vol. 16, No. 3, pp. 287-294.

DesJardin, J.L., Ambrose, S. E., Martinez, A S., & Eisenberg L.S. 2009. Relationships between speech perception abilities and spoken language skills in young children with hearing loss. *International Journal of Audiology*, Vol. 48, pp.248-59.

Dettman, S., Hoenig, N., Dowell, R., Leigh, J. 2008. Long term language outcomes for children using cochlear implants: Are we still failing to close the gap? *10th International Conference on Cochlear Implants and other Implantable Technologies.* San Diego, CA.

Dettman, S., Sadeghi-Barzalighi, A., Ambett, R., Dowell, R., Trotter, M., & Briggs. R. 2011. Cochlear implants in forty-eight children with cochlear and/or vestibular abnormality. *Audiology & Neurotology*, Vol.16, No.4, pp. 222-322.

Dollaghan, C.A., Campbell, T.F., Paradise, J.L., Feldman, H.M., Janosky, J.E., Pitcairn, D. N., & Kurs-Lasky, M. 1999. Maternal education and measures of early speech and language. *Journal of Speech, Language & Hearing Research*, Vol. 42, pp.1432-1443.

Donaldson, A.I., Heavner, K.S., & Zwolan, T.A. 2004. Measuring progress in children with autism spectrum disorder who have cochlear implants. *Archives of Otolaryngology, Head & Neck Surgery*, Vol. 130, No. 5, pp. 666-671.

Dowell, R., Blamey, P., & Clark, G. 1995. Potential and limitations of cochlear implants in children. *Annals of Otology, Rhinology & Laryngology*, Vol. 104, No. 9 (Part 2), pp. 324-327.

Dowell, R.C., Blamey, P.J., & Clark, G.M. 1997. Factors affecting outcomes in children with cochlear implants. *Cochlear Implants: Proceedings of XVI World Congress of Otorhinolaryngology, Head & Neck Surgery*, Bologna, 1997, pp. 297-303.

Dowell, R.C., Brown, A., Seligman, P.M., & Clark, G.M. 1985. Patient results for a multiple-channel cochlear prosthesis. R. A. Schindler, M. M. Merzenich, Raven Press, New York, pp. 421-431.

Dowell, R.C., Dawson, P.W., Dettman, S.J., Shepherd, R.K., Whitford, L.A., Seligman, P.M., & Clark, G.M. 1991. Multichannel cochlear implantation: A summary of current work. *The American Journal of Otology*, Vol. 12, Suppl., 137-143.

Dowell, R.C., Galvin, K.L., Dettman, S.J., Leigh, J.R., Hughes, K.C., & Van Hoesel, R. 2011. Bilateral cochlear implants in children. *Seminars in Hearing*, Vol. 32, No. 1, pp. 53-72.

Drinkwater, T. 2004. The benefits of cochlear implantation in young children. *White paper.* Sydney, Australia: Cochlear Ltd.

Duchesne, L., Sutton, A., & Bergeron, F. 2009. Language achievement in children who received cochlear implants between 1 and 2 years of age: Group trends and individual patterns. *Journal of Deaf Studies & Deaf Education*, Vol.14, pp. 465-485.

Durisin, M., Bartling, S., Arnoldner, C., Ende, M., Prokein, J., Lesinski-Schiedat, A., Lanfermann, H., Lenarz, T., & Stöver. T., 2010. Cochlear osteoneogenesis after meningitis in cochlear implant patients: A retrospective analysis. *Otology & Neurotology*, Vol. 31, No. 7, pp. 1072-1078.

Dutt, S.N., Ray, J., Hadjihannas, E., Cooper, H., Donaldson, I., & Proops D., W. 2005. Medical and surgical complications of the second 100 adult cochlear implant patients in Birmingham. *Journal of Laryngology & Otology*, Vol.119, No. 10, 759-764.

Edwards, L. 2007. Children with cochlear implants and complex needs: A review of outcomes research and psychological practice. *Journal of Deaf Studies & Deaf Education*, Vol. 12, No. 3, pp. 258-267.

Edwards, L.C., Frost, R., & Witham, F. 2006. Developmental delay and outcomes in paediatric cochlear implantation: Implications for candidacy. *International Journal of Pediatric Otorhinolaryngology*, Vol. 70, No. 9, pp. 1593-1600.

Eisenberg, L.S., & House W.F. 1982. Initial experience with the cochlear implant in children. *Annals of Otology, Rhinology & Laryngology*, Vol. 91, No. 2, Part 3, Suppl., pp. 67-73.

Eisenberg, L.S., & Johnson K.C. 2008. Audiologic contributions to pediatric cochlear implants. *The ASHA Leader*, Vol. 13, No.4, pp. 10-13.

Eisenberg, L. S., Kirk, K.I., Martinez, A.S., Ying E.A., & Miyamoto, R.T. 2004. Communication Abilities of Children With Aided Residual Hearing: Comparison With Cochlear Implant Users. *Archives of Otolaryngology Head & Neck Surgery*, Vol. 130, pp. 563-569.

El-Hakim, H., Levasseur, J., Papsin, B.C., Panesar, J., Mount, R.J., Stevens, D., & Harrison R.V. 2001. Assessment of Vocabulary Development in Children After Cochlear Implantation. *Archives of Otolaryngology Head & Neck Surgery*, Vol. 127, No. 9, pp. 1053-1059.

Ertmer, D.J., Young, N.M., & Nathani, S. 2007. Profiles of vocal development in young cochlear implant recipients. *Journal Of Speech, Language, & Hearing Research*, Vol. 50, No. 2, pp. 393-407.

Fallon, M.A., & Harris, M. 1991. Training parents to interact with their young children with handicaps: professional directed and parent-oriented approaches. *Infant Toddler Intervention*, Vol. 1, pp. 297-313.

Filipo, R., Bosco, E., Barchetta, C., & Mancini, P. 1999. Cochlear implantation in deaf children and adolescents:effects on family schooling and personal well-being. *International Journal of Pediatric Otorhinolaryngology*, Vol. 49, No 1, Suppl., pp. S183-S87.

Filipo, R., Bosco, E., Mancini, P., & Ballantyne, D. 2004. Cochlear implants in special cases: deafness in the presence of disabilities and/or associated problems. *Acta Oto-Laryngologica*, Vol. 124, No. 552, Suppl. pp. 74-80.

Flipsen, P. 2008. Intelligibility of spontaneous conversational speech produced by children with cochlear implants: A review. *International Journal of Pediatric Otorhinolaryngology*, Vol. 72, No. 5, pp. 559-64.

Francis, H.W., Pulsifer, M.B., Chinnici, J., Nutt, R., Venick, H.S., Yeagle, J.D., & Niparko, J.K. 2004. Effects of Central Nervous System Residua on Cochlear Implant Results in Children Deafened by Meningitis. *Archives of Otolaryngology Head & Neck Surgery*, Vol. 130, No.5, pp. 604-611.

Fukuda, S., Fukushima, K., Maeda, Y., Tsukamura, K., Nagayasu, R., Toida, N., Kibayashi, N., Kasai, N., Sugata, A., & Nishizaki, K. 2003. Language development of a multiply handicapped child after cochlear implantation. *International Journal of* Pediatric Otorhinolaryngology , Vol. 67, No. 6, pp. 627-633.

Galvin, K., & Hughes, K. In press. Adapting to bilateral cochlear implants: early post-operative device use by children receiving sequential or simultaneous implants at or before 3.5 years. *Cochlear Implants International.* DOI: 10.1179/1754762811Y.0000000001

Galvin, K., Hughes, K., & Mok, M. 2010. Can adolescents and young adults with prelingual hearing loss benefi t from a second, sequential cochlear implant? *International Journal of Audiology*, Vol. 49, pp. 368-377.

Galvin, K., Mok, M., Dowell, R., & Briggs, R. 2008a. Speech detection and localization results and clinical outcomes for children receiving sequential bilateral cochlear implants before 4 years. *International Journal of Audiology*, Vol. 47, pp. 636-646.

Galvin, K.L., Hughes, K.C., & Mok, M. 2009. Documenting progress with sequential, bilateral cochlear implants: reported device use and performance milestones achieved by toddlers, children and young adults. *9th European Symposium on Pediatric Cochlear Implantation,* Warsaw, Poland, 2009.

Galvin, K.L., Mok, M., & Dowell. R.C. 2007a. Perceptual benefit and functional outcomes for children using sequential bilateral cochlear implants. *Ear & Hearing*, Vol. 28, No. 4, pp. 470-482.

Galvin, K.L., Mok, M., Dowell, R.C., & Briggs R.J. 2007b. 12-Month Post-Operative Results for Older Children Using Sequential Bilateral Implants. *Ear & Hearing*, Vol. 28, No. 2, Suppl., pp. S19-S21.

Galvin, K.L., Mok, M., Dowell, R.C., & Briggs, R.J. 2008b. Speech detection and localization results and clinical outcomes for children receiving sequential bilateral cochlear implants before four years of age. *International Journal of Audiology*, Vol. 47, pp. 636-646.

Geers, A. 2006a. Spoken language in children with cochlear implants. In: *Advances in the spoken language development of deaf and hard-of-hearing children*, P.E. Spencer, M. Marshark, pp. 244-270. Oxford University Press Inc., New York.

Geers, A., & Brenner, C. 2003. Background and Educational Characteristics of Prelingually Deaf Children Implanted by Five Years of Age. *Ear & Hearing*, Vol. 24, No. 1, pp. 2S-14S.

Geers, A., Brenner, C., & Davidson, L. 2003. Factors Associated with Development of Speech Perception Skills in Children Implanted by Age Five. *Ear & Hearing*, Vol. 24, No. 1, pp. 24S-35S.

Geers, A., & Hayes, H.. 2011. Reading, Writing, and Phonological Processing Skills of Adolescents With 10 or More Years of Cochlear Implant Experience. *Ear & Hearing*, Vol. 32, pp. 49S-59S.

Geers, A., Moog, J., Biedenstein, J., Brenner, C., & Hayes, H. 2009. Spoken Language Scores of Children Using Cochlear Implants Compared to Hearing Age-Mates at School Entry. *Journal of Deaf Studies & Deaf Education*, Vol. 14, pp. 371-385.

Geers, A., Nicholas, J.G. & Moog, J. 2007. Estimating the influence of cochlear implantation on language development in children. *Audiological Medicine*, Vol. 5, No. 4, pp. 262-273.

Geers, A., Tobey, E.A., Moog, J., & Brenner, C. 2008. Long-term outcomes of cochlear implantation in the preschool years: From elementary grades to high school. *International Journal of Audiology*, Vol. 47, pp. S21-S30.

Geers, A.E. 2002. Factors affecting the development of speech, language, and literacy in children with early cochlear implantation. *Language, Speech, & Hearing Services in Schools.* Vol. 33, No. 3, pp. 172-183.

Geers, A.E. 2003. Predictors of Reading Skill Development in Children with Early Cochlear Implantation. *Ear & Hearing* Vol. 24, No. 1, pp. 59S-68S.

Geers, A.E. 2004. Speech, language, and reading skills after early cochlear implantation. *Archives of Otolaryngology Head & Neck Surgery*, Vol. 130, pp. 634-638.

Geers, A.E. 2006b. Factors influencing spoken language outcomes in children following early cochlear implantation. *Advances in Oto Rhino Laryngology*, Vol. 64, pp. 50-65.

Geers, A.E., & Moog, J.S. 1994. Effectiveness of cochlear implants and tactile aids for deaf children - The sensory aids study at the Central Institute for the Deaf - Foreword. *Volta Review*, Vol. 96, No. 5, pp. R5-R6.

Genesee, F. 2001. Bilingual first language acquisition: exploring the limits of the language faculty. *Annual Review of Applied Linguistics*, Vol. 21, pp. 153-168.

Gold, T. 1980. Speech Production in Hearing-Impaired Children. *Journal of Communication Disorders*, Vol. 13, No. 6, pp.397-418.

Gordon, K.A. 2008. Abnormal timing delays in auditory brainstem responses evoked by bilateral cochlear implant use in children. *The American Journal of Otology*, Vol. 29, No. 2, pp. 193-198.

Gordon, K.A., Valero, J., & Papsin, B.C. 2007. Auditory brainstem activity in children with 9-30 months of bilateral cochlear implant use. *Hearing Research*, Vol. 233, No.1-2, pp. 97-107.

Gordon, K.A., Wong, D.D.E, & Papsin, B.C. 2010. Cortical function in children receiving bilateral cochlear implants simultaneously or after a period of interimplant delay. *Otology & Neurotology*, Vol. 31, No. 8, pp. 1293-1299.

Grieco-Calub, T.M., & Litovsky, R.Y. 2010. Sound localization skills in children who use bilateral cochlear implants and in children with normal acoustic hearing. *Ear & Hearing*, Vol 31, No. 5, pp. 645-656.

Grimwood, K., Anderson, P., Anderson, L., Tan, L., & Nolan, T. 2000. Twelve year outcomes following bacterial meningitis: further evidence for persisting effects. *Archives of Disease in Childhood*, Vol. 83, No. 2, pp. 111-116.

Hamzavi, J., Baumgartner, W.D., Egelierler, B., Franz, B., Schenk, B., & Gstoettner, W. 2000. Follow up of cochlear implanted handicapped children. *International Journal of Pediatric Otorhinolaryngology*, Vol. 56, No. 3, pp. 169-174.

Hardie, N.A. 1998. Neonatal sensorineural hearing loss affects synaptic density in the auditory midbrain. *Neuroreport*, Vol. 9, No. 9, pp. 2019-2021.

Harris, M., & Terlektsi, E. 2011. Reading and spelling abilities of deaf adolescents with cochlear Implants and hearing aids. *Journal of Deaf Studies & Deaf Education*, Vol. 16, No. 1, pp. 24-34.

Harrison, R.V., Gordon, K.A., & Mount, R.J. 2005. Is there a critical period for cochlear implantation in congenitally deaf children? Analyses of hearing and speech perception performance after implantation. *Developmental Psychobiology*, Vol. 46, No. 3, pp. 252-261.

Harrison, M., Roush, J., & Wallace, J. 2003. Trends in age of identification and intervention in infants with hearing loss. *Ear & Hearing*, Vol. 24, No. 1, pp. 89-95.

Hay-McCutcheon, M.J., Iler Kirk, K., Henning, S.C., Gao, S., & Rong, Q. 2008. Using early language outcomes to predict later language ability in children with cochlear implants. *Audiology & Neurotology*, Vol. 13, pp. 370-378.

Helfand, M., Thompson, D., Davis, R., McPhillips, H., Homer, C., & Lieu, T. 2001. Newborn hearing screening. Systematic evidence review number 5 (Contract 290-97-0018 to the Oregon Health & Science University Evidence-based Practice Center, Portland, Oregon). Rockville, MD: Agency for Healthcare Research & Quality.

Hintermair, M. 2006. Parental resources, parental stress, and socioemotional development of deaf and hard of hearing children. *Journal of Deaf Studies & Deaf Education*, Vol. 11, No. 4., pp. 493-513.

Hintermair, M. 2007. Prevalence of socioemotional problems in deaf and hard of hearing children in Germany. *American Annals of the Deaf*, Vol. 152, No. 3, pp. 320-330.

Hoff, E. 2003. The specificity of environmental influence: Socioeconomic status affects early vocabulary development via maternal speech. *Child Development*, Vol. 74, No. 5, pp. 1368-1378.

Hoff, E., & Tian, C. 2005. Socioeconomic status and cultural influences on language. *Journal of Communication Disorders*, Vol. 38, pp. 271-278.

Holt, F.R., Iler-Kirk, K., Eisenberg, L.S., Martinez, A.S., & Campbell, W. 2005. Spoken word recognition development in children with residual hearing using cochlear implants and hearing aids in opposite ears. *Ear & Hearing*, Vol. 26, No. 4, pp. 82S-91S.

Holt, R F., & Kirk. K.I. 2005. Speech and language development in cognitively delayed children with cochlear implants. *Ear & Hearing*, Vol. 26, No. 2., pp. 132-148.

Holt, R.F., & Svirsky, M. 2008. An exploratory look at pediatric cochlear implantation: Is earliest always best? *Ear & Hearing*, Vol. 29, pp. 492-511.

Hope, C.I., Fielder, A.R., Bundey, S., & Proops, D. 1997. Usher syndrome in the city of Birmingham--prevalence and clinical classification. *British Journal of Ophthalmology*, Vol. 81, No. 1, pp.46-53.

Huber, M. 2005. Health-related quality of life of Austrian children and adolescents with cochlear implants. *International Journal of Paediatric Otorhinolaryngology*, Vol. 69, pp. 1089-1101.

Huttunen, K., & Valimaa, T. 2010. Parents' views on changes in their child's communication and linguistic and socioemotional development after cochlear implantation. *Journal of Deaf Studies & Deaf Education*, Vol. 15, No. 4, pp. 383-404.

Hyde, M., Punch, R., & Komesaroff, L. 2010. Coming to a Decision About Cochlear Implantation: Parents Making Choices for their Deaf Children. *Journal of Deaf Studies & Deaf Education*, Vol. 15, No. 2, pp. 162-178.

Isaacson, J.E., Hasenstab, M.S., Wohl, D.L., & Williams, G.H. 1996. Learning Disability in Children With Postmeningitic Cochlear Implants. *Archives of Otolaryngology, Head & Neck Surgery* , Vol. 122, No. 9, pp. 929-936.

James, D., Rajput, K., Brinton, J., & Goswami, U. 2008. Phonological awareness, vocabulary, and word reading in children who use cochlear implants: Does age of implantation explain individual variability in performance outcomes and growth? *Journal of Deaf Studies & Deaf Education*, Vol. 13, No. 1, pp. 117-137.

Jeong, S.-W., Kim, L.-S., Kim, B.-Y., Bae, W.-Y., & Kim, J.-R. 2007. Cochlear implantation in children with auditory neuropathy: outcomes and rationale. *Acta Oto-Laryngologica*, Vol. 558, Suppl., pp. 36-43.

Johnson, C., & Goswami, U. 2010. Phonological awareness, vocabulary, and reading in deaf children with cochlear implants. *Journal of Speech, Language & Hearing Research*, Vol. 53, pp. 237-261.

Johnston, J.C., Durieux-Smith, A., Angus, D., O'Connor, A., & Fitzpatrick, E.M. 2009. Bilateral padiatric cochlear implants: A critical review. *International Journal of Audiology*, Vol. 48, pp. 601-617.

Kennedy, C.R., McCann, D.C., Campbell, M.J., Law, C.M., Mullee, M., Petrou, S., Watkin, P., Worsfold, S., Yuen, H.M., & Stevenson, J. 2006. Language ability after early detection of permanent childhood hearing impairment. *New England Journal of Medicine*, Vol. 354, No. 20, pp. 2131-2141.

Kral, A., Hartmann, R., Tillein, J., Heid, S., Klinke, R. 2001. Delayed maturation and sensitive Periods in the auditory cortex. Audiology & Neurotology, Vol. 6, No. 6, pp. 346-362.

Kretchmer, R., & Kretchmer, L. 1986. Language in Perspective. In: *Deafness In Perspective*, D. Luterman, pp. 131-165, College-Hill Press, San Diego.

Kuhn-Inacker, H., Shehata-Dieler,W., Muller, J., & Helms, J. 2004. Bilateral cochlear implants: a way to optimize auditory perception abilities in deaf children? *International Jpurnal of Pediatric Otorhinolaryngology*, Vol. 68, No.10, pp. 1257-1266.

Lane, H., & Grodin, M. 1997. Ethical issues in cochlear implant surgery: An exploration into disease, disability, and the best interests of the child. *Kennedy Institute of Ethics Journal*, Vol. 7, No. 3, pp. 231-251.

Lanson, B.G., Green, J.E., Roland, J.T., Lalwani, A.K., & Waltzman, S.B. 2007. Cochlear implantation in children with CHARGE syndrome: Therapeutic decisions and outcomes. *Laryngoscope*, Vol. 117, No. 7, pp. 1260-66.

Lee, D.J., Lustig, L., Sampson, M., Chinnici, J., & Niparko, J.K. 2005. Effects of Cytomegalovirus (CMV) related deafness on pediatric cochlear implant outcomes. *Otolaryngology, Head & Neck Surgery*, Vol. 133, No. 6, pp. 900-905.

Leigh, I. W., Maxwell-McCaw, D., Bat-Chava, Y., & Christiansen, J.B. 2008a. Correlates of Psychosocial Adjustment in Deaf Adolescents With and Without Cochlear Implants: A Preliminary Investigation. *Journal of Deaf Studies & Deaf Education*, Vol. 14, No. 2, pp. 244-259.

Leigh, J., Dettman, S., Dowell, R., & Sarant, J. 2011. Evidence-Based Approach for Making Cochlear Implant Recommendations for Infants with Residual Hearing. *Ear & Hearing*, Vol. 32, No. 1, pp. 1-10.

Leigh, J.S., Dettman, S., Dowell, R., Sarant, J., Hollow, R., & Briggs, R.J. 2008b. Evidence based approach for making cochlear implant recommendations for infants with significant residual hearing. *Beyond Newborn Hearing Screening: Infant & Childhood Hearing in Science & Clinical Practice.* Cernobbio (Como Lake) , Italy, 2008.

Leigh, J., Dettman, S., Holland, J., Dowell, R., & Briggs, R.J. 2008c. Long-term language, speech production, and speech perception outcomes for children who received a cochlear implant at or before 12 months of age. *Reflecting Connections: A Joint Conference Between New Zealand Speech-Language Therapists Association and Speech Pathology Australia.* Auckland, New Zealand, 2008.

Lichtenstein, E.H. 1998. The relationships between reading processes and English skills of deaf college students. *Journal of Deaf Studies and Deaf Education*, Vol. 3, No.2, pp. 80-134.

Litovsky, R., Johnstone, P., Parkinson, A., Peters,R., & Lake, J. 2004. Bilateral cochlear implants in children. *International Congress Series*, Vol. 1273, pp. 451-54.

Litovsky, R.Y., Johnstone, P.M., Godar, S. Agrawal, S., Parkinson, A.J., Peters, R., & Lake, J. 2006a. Bilateral cochlear implants in children: Localization acuity measured with minimum audible angle. *Ear & Hearing*, Vol. 27, No. 1, pp. 43-59.

Litovsky, R.Y., Johnstone, P.M., & Godar, S. 2006b. Benefits of bilateral cochlear implants and/or hearing aids in children. *International Journal of Audiology*, Vol. 45, No 1, Suppl, pp. S78-S91.

Loundon, N., Blanchard, M., Roger, G., Denoyelle, F., & Garabedian, E.N. 2010. Medical and surgical complications in pediatric cochlear implantation." *Archives of Otolaryngology, Head & Neck Surgery*, Vol. 136, No. 1, pp. 12-15.

Loundon, N., Marlin, S., Busquet, D., Denoyelle, F., Roger, G., Renaud, F., & Garabedian, E.N. 2003. Usher syndrome and cochlear implantation. *Otology & Neurotology*, Vol. 24, No. 2, pp. 216-221.

Lovett, R.E.S., Kitterick, P.T., Hewitt, C.E., & Summerfield, A.Q. 2010. Bilateral or unilateral cochlear implantation for deaf children: an observational study. *Archives of Disease in Childhood*, Vol. 95, pp. 107-112.

Loy, B., Warner-Czyz, A.D., Tong, L., Tobey, E.A., & Roland, P.S. 2010. The children speak: an examination of the quality of life of pediatric cochlear implant users. *Otolaryngology, Head & Neck Surgery*, Vol 142, No. 2, pp. 247-253.

Madden, C. 2002. Pediatric cochlear implantation in auditory neuropathy. *The American Journal of Otology*, Vol. 23, No. 2, pp. 163-168.

Marschark, M. 1993. *Psychological development of deaf children*. Oxford University Press, New York.

Marschark, M., Rhoten, C., & Fabich, M. 2007. Effects of cochlear implants on children's reading and academic achievement. *The Journal of Deaf Studies & Deaf Education*, Vol. 12, No. 3, pp. 269-282.

Martin, D., Bat-Chava, Y., & Waltzman, S.B. 2011. Peer relationships of deaf children with cochlear implants: Predictors of peer entry and peer interaction success. *Journal of Deaf Studies & Deaf Education*, Vol. 16, No. 1, pp. 108-120.

Mayne, A., Yoshinaga-Itano, C., Sedey, A., & Carey, A. 2000. Expressive vocabulary development of infants and toddlers who are deaf or hard of hearing. *The Volta Review*, Vol. 100, No. 5, pp. 1-28.

McKay, C.M., McDermott, H.J., Vandali, A.E., & Clark, G.M. 1991. Preliminary results with a six spectral maxima sound processor for the University of Melbourne/Nucleus multiple-electrode cochlear implant. *Journal of the Otolaryngological Society of Australia*, Vol. 6, No. 5, pp. 354-359.

Meadow, K. P. 1980. *Deafness and child development*. University of California Press, Berkeley.

Meinzen-Derr, J., Wiley, S. Grether, S., & Choo, D.I. 2011. Children with cochlear implants and developmental disabilities: A language skills study with developmentally matched hearing peers. *Research in Developmental Disabilities*, Vol. 32, No. 2, pp. 757-767.

Meyer, T.A., Svirsky, M.A., Kirk, K.I., & Miyamoto, R.T. 1998. Improvements in speech perception by children with profound prelingual hearing loss: effects of device, communication mode, and chronological age. *Journal Of Speech, Language, & Hearing Research*, Vol. 41, No. 4, pp. 846-858.

Miyamoto, R.T., Kirk, K.I., Svirsky, M., & Sehgal, S.T. 1999. Communication Skills in Pediatric Cochlear Implant Recipients. *Acta Otolaryngology*, Vol. 119, pp. 219-224.

Miyamoto, R.T., Osberger, M.J., Robbins, A.M., Myres, W.A., & Kessler, K. 1993. Prelingually deafened children's performance with the nucleus multichannel cochlear implant. *American Journal of Otology*, Vol. 14, No. 5, pp. 437-445.

Moeller, M.P. 2000. Early intervention and language development in children who are deaf and hard of hearing. *Pediatrics*, Vol. 106, No. 3, pp. E43-E60.

Moeller, M.P., Tomblin, J.B., Yoshinaga-Itano, C., Connor, C., & Jerger, S. 2007. Current state of knowledge: language and literacy of children with hearing impairment. *Ear & Hearing*, Vol. 28, No. 6, pp. 740-753.

Mok, M., Galvin, K.L., Dowell, R.C., & McKay, C.M. 2007. Spatial unmasking and binaural advantage for children with normal hearing, a cochlear implant and a hearing aid, and bilateral implants. *Audiology & Neuro-Otology*, Vol. 12, No. 5, pp. 295-306.

Montanini-Manfredi, M. 1993. The emotional development of deaf children. *Psychological Perspectives on Deafness*. M. Marshark, M.D. Clark, pp. 49-63, Lawrence Erlbaum Associates, Hillsdale, New Jersey.

Moog, J.S. 2002. Changing expectations for children with cochlear implants. *Annals of Otology, Rhinology & Laryngology*, Vol. 189, pp. 138S-42S.

Moog, J.S. & Geers, A.E. 2003. Epilogue: Major findings, conclusions and implications for deaf education. *Ear & Hearing*, Vol. 24, No. 1, pp. 121S-125S.

Moores, D., & Sweet, C. 1990. Relationships of english grammar and communicative fluency to reading in deaf adolescents. *Exceptionality*, Vol. 1, pp. 97-106.

Most, T. 2007. Speech intelligibility,loneliness, and sense of coherence among deaf and hard-of-hearing children in individual inclusion and group inclusion. *Journal of Deaf Studies & Deaf Education*, Vol. 12, No. 4, pp. 495-503.

Mukari, S. Z., Ling, L.N., & Ghani, H.A. 2007. Educational performance of pediatric cochlear implant recipients in mainstream classes. *International Journal of Pediatric Otorhinolaryngology*, Vol. 71, No. 2, pp. 231-240.

Myklebust, H. 1964. *The Psychology of Deafness*. Grune and Stratton, New York, USA.

National Association of the Deaf. 2000. *NAD Position Statement*. Accessed August 9, 2011, at http://www.nad.org/site

Nicholas, J.G., & Geers, A. 2007. Will they catch up? The role of age at cochlear implantation in the spoken language development of children with severe to profound hearing loss. *Journal of Speech Language & Hearing Research*, Vol. 50, pp. 1048-1062.

Nicholas, J.G., & Geers, A.E. 2003. Personal, social, and family adjustment in school-aged children with a cochlear implant. *Ear & Hearing*, Vol. 24, No. 1, pp. 69S-81S.

Nicholas, J.G., & Geers, A.E. 2008. Expected test scores for preschoolers with a cochlear implant who use spoken language. *American Journal of Speech-Language Pathology*, Vol. 17, No. 2, pp. 121-138.

National Institute on Deafness and other Communication Disorders. 2011. *Cochlear Implants*. Bethesda, MD USA.

Nikolopoulos, T.P., Dyar, D., Archbold, S., & O'Donoghue, G. 2004. Development of spoken language grammar following cochlear implantation in prelingually deaf children. *Archives of Otolaryngology Head & Neck Surgery*, Vol. 130, pp. 629-633.

Nikolopoulos, T.P., O'Donoghue, G.M., & Archbold, S. 1999. Age at implantation: Its importance in pediatric cochlear implantation. *The Laryngoscope*, Vol. 109, No. 4, pp. 595-599.

Niparko, J., Tobey, E .A., Thal, D., Eisenberg, L.S., Wang, N.Y., Quittner, A.L., & Fink, N.E. 2010. Spoken language development in children following cochlear implantation. *Journal of the American Medical Association*, Vol. 303, No. 15, pp. 1498-1506.

Nittrouer, S. & Chappman, C. 2009. The effects of bilateral electric and bimodal electric–acoustic stimulation on language development. *Trends In Amplification*, Vol. 13, No. 3, pp. 190-205.

Osberger, M.J. 1991. Effect of age at onset of deafness on children's speech perception abilities with a cochlear implant. *Annals of Otology, Rhinology & Laryngology*, Vol. 100, No. 11, pp. 883-888.

Paatsch, L.E., Blamey, P.J., Sarant, J.Z., Martin, L.F., & Bow, C.P. 2004. Separating contributions of hearing, lexical knowledge, and speech production to speech-perception scores in children with hearing impairments. *Journal of Speech Language & Hearing Research*, Vol. 47, No. 4, pp. 738-750.

Papsin, B.C. 2005. Cochlear implantation in children with anomalous cochleovestibular anatomy. *The Laryngoscope*, Vol. 115, No. 106, Suppl., pp. 1-26.

Papsin, B. C., & K. A. Gordon. 2007. Cochlear Implants for Children with Severe-to-Profound Hearing Loss. *The New England Journal of Medicine*, Vol. 357, No. 23, pp. 2380-2387.

Patrick, J. F., Busby, P.A., & Gibson, W. 2006. The development of the Nucleus FreedomTM cochlear implant system. *Trends In Amplification*, Vol. 10, pp. 175-200.

Paul, P. 1998. *Literacy and Deafness: The Development of Reading, Writing, and Literate Thought.* Allyn & Bacon, Needham Heights, MA.

Peng, S.-C., Spencer, L.J., & Tomblin, J.B. 2004. Speech intelligibility of pediatric cochlear implant recipients with 7 years of device experience. *Journal Of Speech, Language, & Hearing Research*, Vol. 47, No. 6, pp. 1227-1236.

Percy-Smith, L., Caye´-Thomasen, P., Gudman, M, Hedegaard Jensen, J., & Thomsen, J. 2008a. Self-esteem and social well-being of children with cochlear implant compared to normal-hearing children. *International Journal of Pediatric Otorhinolaryngology*, Vol. 72, pp.1113-1120.

Percy-Smith, L., Jensen, J.H., Caye-Thomasen, P., Thomsen, J., Gudman, M., & Lopez, A.G. 2008b. Factors that affect the social well-being of children with cochlear implants. *Cochlear Implants International*, Vol. 9, No. 4, pp. 199-214.

Peters, B., Litovsky, R., Parkinson, A.J., & Lake, J. 2007. Importance of age and postimplantation experience on speech perception measures in children with sequential bilateral cochlear implants. *Otology & Neurotology*, Vol. 28, pp. 649-657.

Peters, B., Wyss, J., & Manrique, M. 2010. Worldwide trends in bilateral cochlear implantation. *The Laryngoscope*, Vol. 120, No. 2, Suppl., pp. S17-S44.

Peterson, A., Shallop, J., Driscoll, C., Breneman, A., Babb, J., Stoeckel, R., & Fabry, L. 2003. Outcomes of cochlear implantation in children with auditory neuropathy. *Journal of the American Academy of Audiology*, Vol. 14, No. 4, pp. 188-201.

Pisoni, D.B., & Cleary, M. 2003. Measures of working memory span and verbal rehearsal speed in deaf children after cochlear implantation. *Ear & Hearing*, Vol. 24, No. 1, pp. 106S-120S.

Pisoni, D.B., Cleary, M., Geers, A., & Tobey, E.A. 1999. Individual differences in effectiveness of cochlear Implants in children who are prelingually deaf. *Volta Review*, Vol. 101, No. 3, pp. 111-165.

Ponton, C.W., Don, M., Eggermont, J.J., Waring, M.D., Kwong, B., & Masuda, A. 1996. Auditory system plasticity in children after long periods of complete deafness. *Neuroreport*, Vol. 8, pp. 61-65.

Punch, R., & Hyde, M. 2011. Social participation of children and adolescents with cochlear implants: A qualitative analysis of parent, teacher, and child interviews. *Journal of Deaf Studies & Deaf Education*, Vol. 16, No. 4, pp. 474-493.

Pyman, B., Blamey, P., Lacy, P., Clark, G., & Dowell, R. 2000. The development of speech perception in children using cochlear implants: effects of etiologic factors and delayed milestones. *The American Journal of Otology*, Vol. 21, No. 1, pp. 57-61.

Ramirez Inscoe, J.M., & Nikolopoulos, T.P. 2004. Cochlear implantation in children deafened by cytomegalovirus: Speech perception and speech intelligibility outcomes. *Otology & Neurotology*, Vol. 25, No. 4, pp. 479-82.

Ramkalawan, T., & Davis, A. 1992. The effects of hearing loss and age of intervention on some language metrics in young hearing-impaired children. *British Journal of Audiology*, Vol. 26, No. 97-107.

Ramsden, J.D., Papsin, B.C., Leung, R., James, A., Gordon, K.A. 2009. Bilateral Simultaneous Cochlear Implantation in Children: Our first 50 cases. *The Laryngoscope*, Vol 119, No. 12, pp. 2444-2448.

Rance, G., & Barker, E.J. 2008. Speech perception in Children with auditory neuropathy/dyssynchrony managed with either hearing aids or cochlear implants. *Otology & Neurotology*, Vol. 29, No. 2, pp. 179-182.

Rance, G., Barker, E.J., Sarant, J.Z., & Ching, T.Y.C. 2007. Receptive language and speech production in children with auditory neuropathy/dyssynchrony type hearing loss. *Ear & Hearing*, Vol. 28, No. 5, pp. 694-702.

Rance, G., Beer, D.E., Cone-Wesson, B., Shepherd, R.K., Dowell, R.C., King, A.M., Rickards, F.W., & Clark, G.M. 1999. Clinical findings for a group of infants and young children with auditory neuropathy. *Ear & Hearing*, Vol. 20, No. 3, pp. 238-252.

Ray, J., Wright, T., Fielden, C., Cooper, H., Donaldson, I., & Proops, D.W. 2006. Non-users and limited users of cochlear implants. *Cochlear Implants International*, Vol. 7, No. 1, pp. 49-58.

Robbins, A.M., Bollard, P.M., & Green, J. 1999. Language development in children implanted with the CLARION cochlear implant. *The Annals Of Otology, Rhinology & Laryngology*, Vol. 177, Suppl., pp. 113-118.

Robbins, A., Green, J.E., & Waltzman, S.B. 2004b. Bilingual oral language proficiency in children with cochlear implants. *Archives of Otolaryngology, Head & Neck Surgery*, Vol. 130, No. 5, pp. 644-647.

Robbins, A., Koch, D.B., Osberger, M.J., Zimmerman-Phillips, S., & Kishon-Rabin, L. 2004a. Effect of age at cochlear implantation on auditory skill development in infants and toddlers. *Archives of Otolaryngology, Head & Neck Surgery*, Vol. 130, No. 5, pp. 570-574.

Sahli, S., & Belgin, E. 2006. Comparison of self-esteem level of adolescents with cochlear implant and normal hearing. *International Journal of Pediatric Otorhinolaryngology*, Vol. 70, No. 9, pp. 1601-1608.

Sarant, J., Galvin, K., Holland, J., Bant, S., Blamey, P., Wales, R., Busby, P., & Moran, M. In press. Bilateral versus unilateral cochlear implants for children: Early language findings of a 5-year study of language, academic, psychosocial and other outcomes.

Proceedings of 10th European Symposium on Peadiatric Cochlear Implantation, Athens, Greece, May 12-15, 2011.

Sarant, J., Holt, C., Dowell, R., Rickards, F., & Blamey, P. 2009. Spoken language development in oral preschool children with permanent childhood hearing impairment. *Journal of Deaf Studies & Deaf Education*, Vol. 14, No. 2, pp. 205-217.

Sarant, J., Hughes, K., & Blamey, P. 2010. The effect of IQ on spoken language and speech perception development in children with impaired hearing. *Cochlear Implants International*, Vol. 11, No. 1, Suppl. pp. 370-374.

Sarant, J.Z., Blamey, P.J., Cowan, R.S., & Clark, G.M. 1997. The effect of language knowledge on speech perception: what are we really assessing? *American Journal of Otology*, Vol. 18, No. 6, Suppl., pp. S135-137.

Sarant, J.Z., Blamey, P.J., Dowell, R.C., Clark, G.M., & Gibson, W.P. 2001. Variation in speech perception scores among children with cochlear implants. *Ear & Hearing*, Vol. 22, No. 1, pp. 18-28.

Sarant, J.Z., Cowan, R.S., Blamey, P.J., Galvin, K.L., & Clark, G.M. 1994. Cochlear implants for congenitally deaf adolescents: is open-set speech perception a realistic expectation? *Ear & Hearing*, Vol. 15, No. 5, pp. 400-403.

Sass-Lehrer, M. 2011. Early intervention: Birth to three. *The Oxford handbook of Deaf Studies, Language, and Education.* M. Marshark, P. E. Spencer, pp. 63-81. Oxford University Press Inc., New York.

Schafer, E.C. & Thibodeau, LM. 2006. Speech recognition in noise in children with cochlear implants while listening in bilateral, bimodal, and FM-system arrangements. *American Journal of Audiology*, Vol. 15, pp. 114-126.

Scherf, F., van Deun, L., van Wieringen, A., Wouters, J., Desloovere, C., Dhooge, I., Offeciers, E., Deggouj, N., De Raeve, L., De Bodt, M., & Van de Heyning, P.H. 2007. Hearing benefits of second-side cochlear implantation in two groups of children. *International Journal of Pediatric Otorhinolaryngology*, Vol. 71, No. 12, pp. 1855-1863.

Scherf, F., van Deun, L., van Wieringen, A., Wouters, J., Desloovere, C., Dhooge, I., Offeciers, E., Deggouj, N., De Raeve, L., De Bodt, M., & Van de Heyning, P.H. 2009. Three-year postimplantation auditory outcomes in children with sequential bilateral cochlear implantation. *The Annals Of Otology, Rhinology, & Laryngology*, Vol. 118, No. 5, pp. 336-344.

Schorr, E.A. 2006. Early cochlear implant experience and emotional functioning during childhood: Loneliness in middle and late childhood. *Volta Review*, Vol. 106, No. 3, pp. 365-379.

Schorr, E.A., Roth, F., & Fox, N. 2008. A Comparison of the Speech and Language Skills of Children With Cochlear Implants and Children With Normal Hearing. *Communication Disorders Quarterly*, Vol. 29, No. 4, pp. 195-210.

Serry, T., Blamey, P., & Grogan, M. 1997. Phoneme acquisition in the first 4 years of implant use. *The American Journal of Otology*, Vol. 18, Suppl., pp. S122-S24.

Sharma, A., Dorman, M.F., & Kral, A. 2005. The influence of a sensitive period on central auditory development in children with unilateral and bilateral cochlear implants. *Hearing Research*, Vol. 203, pp. 134-143.

Sharma, A., Dorman, M.F., & Spahr, A.J. 2002. A sensitive period for the development of the central auditory system in children with cochlear implants: Implications for age of implantation. *Ear & Hearing*, Vol. 23, No. 6, pp. 532-538.

Shepherd, R.K. 1997. The central auditory system and auditory deprivation: experience with cochlear implants in the congenitally deaf. *Acta Oto-Laryngologica,* Vol. 117, No. 532, pp. 28-33.

Sparreboom, M., van Schoonhoven, J., van Zanten, B.G.A., Scholten, R.J.P.M., Mylanus, E.A.M., Grolman, W., Maat, B. 2010. The effectiveness of bilateral cochlear implants for severe-to-profound deafness in children: A systematic review. *Otology & Neurotology,* Vol. 31, pp. 1062-1071.

Spencer, L.E., & Oleson, J.J. 2008. Early listening and speaking skills predict later reading proficiency in pediatric cochlear implant users. *Ear & Hearing,* Vol. 29, pp. 270-280.

Spencer, L.J., Barker, B.A., & Tomblin, J.B. 2003. Exploring the Language and Literacy Outcomes of Pediatric Cochlear Implant Users. *Ear & Hearing,* Vol. 24, No. 3, pp. 236-247.

Spencer, L.J., Gantz, B., & Knutson, J.F. 2004. Outcomes and achievement of students who grew up with access to cochlear implants. *The Laryngoscope,* Vol. 114, No. 9. pp. 1576-1581.

Spencer, P.E., Marschark, M., & Spencer, L.J. 2011. Cochlear Implants: Advances, Issues, and Implications. In: *The Oxford Handbook of Deaf Studies, Language, and Education,* M. Marshark, P. Spencer, pp. 452-470, Oxford University Press, New York.

Staller, S.J., Beiter, A.L., Brimacombe, J.A., & Arndt, P.L. 1991. Pediatric performance with the Nucleus 22-channel cochlear implant system. *American Journal of Otology,* Vol 12, Suppl., pp. 126-136.

Starr, A., Picton, T.W., Sininger Y.S., Hood, L.J., Berlin, C.I. 1996. Auditory Neuropathy. *Brain,* Vol. 119, pp. 741-753.

Steffens, T., Lesinski-Schiedat, A., Strutz, J., Aschendorff, A., Klenzner, T., Ruhl, S., Voss, B., Wesarg, T., Laszig, R., & Lenarz, T. 2008. The benefits of sequential bilateral cochlear implantation for hearing-impaired children. *Acta Oto-Laryngologica,* Vol. 128, No. 2, pp. 164-176.

Stinson, M.S., & Whitimire, K.A. 2000. Adolescents who are deaf or hard of hearing: A communication perspective on educational placement. *Topics in Language Disorders,* Vol. 20, No. 2, pp. 58-72.

Summerfield, A.Q., Lovett, R.E.S., Bellenger, H., & Batten, G. 2010. Estimates of the cost-effectiveness of pediatric bilateral cochlear implantation. *Ear & Hearing,* Vol. 315, pp. 611-624.

Svirsky, M., & Meyer, T.A. 1999. Comparison of speech perception abilities in pediatric Clarion cochlear implant and hearing aid users. *The Annals of Otology, Rhinology & Laryngology,* Vol. 108, No. 4, pp. 104-109.

Svirsky, M.A., Robbins, A.M., Kirk, K I., Pisoni, D.B., & Miyamoto, R.T. 2000. Language development in profoundly deaf children with cochlear implants. *Psychological Science,* Vol. 11, No. 2, pp. 153-158.

Svirsky, M.A., Teoh, S.-W., & Neuburger, H. 2004. Development of language and speech perception in congenitally, profoundly deaf children as a function of age at cochlear implantation. *Audiology & Neurotology,* Vol. 9, No. 4, pp. 224-233.

Tait, M., Nikolopoulos, T.P., De Raeve, L., Johnson, S., Datta, G., Karltorp, E., Ostlund, E., Johansson, U., van Knegsel, E., Mylanus, E.A.M., Gulpen, P.M.H., Beers, M., & Frijns, J.H.M. 2010. Bilateral versus unilateral cochlear implantation in young children. *International Journal of Pediatric Otorhinolaryngology,* Vol. 74, pp. 206-211.

Tajudeen, B.A., Waltzman, S.B., Jethanamest, D., & Svirsky, M.A. 2010. Speech perception in congenitally deaf children receiving cochlear implants in the first year of life. *Otology & Neurotology, Vol.* 8, pp. 1254-1260.

Teagle, H.F.B., Roush, P.A., Woodard, J.S., Hatch, D.R., Zdanski, C.J., Buss, E., & Buchman, C.A. 2010. Cochlear implantation in children with Auditory Neuropathy Spectrum Disorder. *Ear & Hearing*, Vol. 31, No. 3, pp. 325-335.

Thoutenhoofd, E. 2006. Cochlear implanted pupils in scottish schools: 4-year school attainment data (2000–2004). *Journal of Deaf Studies & Deaf Education*, Vol. 11, No. 2, 171-188.

Tobey, E.A., Geers, A.E., Brenner, C., Altuna, D., & Gabbert, G. 2003. Factors associated with development of speech production skills in children implanted by age five. *Ear & Hearing*, Vol. 24, No. 1, pp. 36S-45S.

Tobey, E.A., & Hasenstab, M.S. 1991. Effects of a Nucleus multichannel cochlear implant upon speech production in children. *Ear & Hearing* 12, No. 4, Suppl., pp. 48S-54S.

Tomblin, J., Spencer, L., Flock, S., Tyler, R., Gantz, B., & Rockville, J. 1999. A comparison of language achievement in children with Cochlear implants and children using hearing aids. *Journal of Speech, Language, & Hearing Research*, Vol. 42, No. 2, pp. 497-510.

Tomblin, J. B., Barker, B.A., Spencer, L.J., Zhang, X., & Gantz, B.J. 2005. The effect of age at cochlear implant initial stimulation on expressive language growth in infants and toddlers. *Journal of Speech, Language, & Hearing Research*, Vol. 48, No. 4, pp. 853-867.

Trautwein, P.G., Sininger, Y.S., & Nelson, R. 2000. Cochlear implantation of auditory neuropathy. *Journal of the American Academy of Audiology*, Vol. 11, No. 6, pp. 309-315.

Traxler, C.B. 2000. The Stanford Achievement Test, 9th Edition: National norming and performance standards for deaf and hard-of-hearing students. *Journal of Deaf Studies & Deaf Education*, Vol. 5, pp. 337-348.

Tye-Murray, N., Spencer, L., & Woodworth, G.G. 1995. Acquisition of speech by children who have prolonged cochlear implant experience. *Journal of Speech & Hearing Research*, Vol. 38, No. 2, pp. 327-337.

Uziel, A. S., M. Sillon, A. Vieu, F. Artieres, J.-P. Piron, J.-P. Daures, & Mondain, M. 2007. Ten-year follow-up of a consecutive series of children with multichannel cochlear implants. *Otology & Neurotology*, Vol. 28, No.5, pp. 615-628.

van Deun, L., van Wieringen, A., & Wouters, J. 2010. Spatial speech perception benefits in young children with normal hearing and cochlear implants. *Ear & Hearing*, Vol. 31, No. 5, pp. 702-713.

van Gent, T., Goedhart, A.W., Hindley, P.A., & Treffers, P.D.A. 2007. Prevalence and correlates of psychopathology in a sample of deaf adolescents. *Journal Of Child Psychology & Psychiatry, & Allied Disciplines*, Vol. 48, No. 9, pp. 950-958.

Venail, F., Vieu, A., Artieres, F., Mondain, M., & Uziel, A. 2010. Educational and employment achievements in prelingually deaf children who receive cochlear implants. *Archives of Otolaryngology Head & Neck Surgery*, Vol. 136, No. 4, pp. 366-372.

Vermeulen, A., van Bon,W., Schreuder, R., Knoors, H., & Snik, A. 2007. Reading comprehension of deaf children with cochlear implants. *The Journal of Deaf Studies & Deaf Education*, Vol. 12, No. 3, pp. 283-302.

Vlahovic, S. & Sindija, B. 2004. The influence of potentially limiting factors on paediatric outcomes following cochlear implantation. *International Journal of Pediatric Otorhinolaryngology*, Vol. 68, No. 9, pp. 1167-1174.

Wake, M., Hughes, E.K., Poulakis, Z., Collins, C., & Rickards, F.W. 2004. Outcomes of children with mild-profound congenital hearing loss at 7 to 8 years: A population study. *Ear & Hearing*, Vol. 1, No. 25, pp. 1-8.

Wake, M., Poulakis, Z, Hughes, E.K., Carey-Sargeant, C., & Rickards, F.W. 2005. Hearing impairment: a population study of age at diagnosis, severity, and language outcomes at 7-8 years. *Archives of Disease in Childhood*, Vol. 3, No. 90, pp. 238-244.

Walker, L., Munro, J, & Rickards, F.W. 1998. Literal and inferential reading comprehension of students who are deaf or hard of hearing. *Volta Review*, Vol. 100, No. 2, pp. 87-103.

Waltzman, S.B., Robbins, A.M., Green, J.E., & Cohen, N.L. 2003. Second oral language capabilities in children with cochlear implants. *Otology & Neurotology*, Vol. 24, No. 5, pp. 757-763.

Waltzman, S.B., & Roland, J.T. 2005. Cochlear Implantation in Children Younger Than 12 Months. *Pediatrics*, Vol. 116, No. 4, pp. e487-e493.

Waltzman, S. B., V. Scalchunes, & N. L. Cohen. 2000. Performance of multiply handicapped children using cochlear implants. *Otology & Neurotology*, Vol. 21, No. 3, pp. 329-335.

Warner-Czyz, A. D., Loy, B., Roland, P.S., Tong, L., & Tobey, E.A. 2009. Parent versus child assessment of quality of life in children using cochlear implants. *International Journal of Paediatric Otorhinolaryngology*, Vol. 73, pp. 1423-1429.

Watkin, P., McCann, D., Law, C., Mullee, M., Petrou, S., Stevenson, J., Worsfold, S., Yuen, H. M., & Kennedy, C. 2007. Language Ability in Children With Permanent Hearing Impairment: The Influence of Early Management and Family Participation. *Pediatrics*, Vol. 120, No. 3, pp. e694-e701.

Watson, L. M., & Gregory, S. 2005. Non-use of cochlear implants in children: child and parent perspectives. *Deafness Education International*, Vol. 7, No. 1, pp. 43-58.

Watson, S. M., Henggler, S. W., & Whelan, J. P. 1990. Family functioning and the social adaptation of hearing-impaired youths. *Journal of Abnormal Child Psychology*, Vol. 18, No. 2, pp. 143-163.

White, K. R., & Maxon, A. B. 1995. Universal screening for infant hearing impairment: simple, beneficial, and presently justified. *International Journal of Pediatric Otorhinolaryngology*, Vol. 32, pp. 201-211.

Wie, O. B. 2010. Language development in children after receiving bilateral cochlear implants between 5 and 18 months. *International Journal of Paediatric Otorhinolaryngology*, Vol. 74, pp. 1258-1266.

Wie, O. B., Falkenberg, E. S., Tvete, O., & Tomblin, J. B. 2007. Children with a cochlear implant: Characteristics and determinants of speech recognition, speech-recognition growth rate, and speech production. *International Journal of Audiology* , Vol 46, pp. 232-243.

Wiley, S., Jahnke, M., Meinzen-Derr, J., & Choo, D. 2005. Perceived qualitative benefits of cochlear implants in children with multi-handicaps. *International Journal of Pediatric Otorhinolaryngology*, Vol 69, No. 6, pp. 791-798.

Wolfe, J., Baker, S., Caraway, T., Kasulis, H., Mears. A., Smith, J., Swim, L., & Wood, M. 2007. 1-year postactivation results for sequentially implanted bilateral cochlear implant users. *Otology & Neurotology*, Vol. 28, pp. 589-596.

Yoshinaga-Itano, C. 2003a. Early intervention after universal neonatal hearing screening: Impact on outcomes. *Mental Retardation & Developmental Disabilities Research Reviews*, Vol. 9, No. 4, pp. 252-266.

Yoshinaga-Itano, C. 2003b. From screening to early identification and intervention: Discovering predictors to successful outcomes for children with significant hearing loss. *Journal of Deaf Studies & Deaf Education*, Vol. 8, No.1, pp.11-30.

Yoshinaga-Itano, C., Baca, R. L., & Sedey, A. 2010. Describing the trajectory of language development in the presence of severe-profound hearing loss: A closer look at children with cochlear implants. *Otology & Neurotology*, Vol. 31, No. 8, pp. 1268-1274.

Yoshinaga-Itano, C., Sedey, A. L., Coulter, D. K., & Mehl, A. L. 1998. Language of early- and later-identified children with hearing loss. *Pediatrics*, Vol. 102, 5, pp.1161-1171.

Yoshinaga-Itano, C., & Snyder, L. S. 1996. Can lexical/semantic skills differentiate deaf or hard-of-hearing readers and non readers? *Volta Review*, Vol. 98, No. 1, pp. 39-62.

Young, G. A., & Killen, D. H. 2002. Receptive and expressive language skills of children with five years of experience using a cochlear implant. *Annals of Otology, Rhinology & Laryngology,* Vol 111, No. 9, pp. 802-810.

Young, N. M., Johnson, J. C., Mets, M. B., & Hain, T. C. 1995. Cochlear implants in young children with Usher's syndrome. *The Annals of Otology, Rhinology & Laryngology,* Vol 166, Suppl., pp. 342-345.

Young, N. M., Reilly, B. K., & Burke L. 2011. Limitations of universal newborn hearing screening in early identification of pediatric cochlear implant candidates. *Archives of Otolaryngology, Head & Neck Surgery*, Vol. 137, No. 3, pp. 230-234.

Zaidman-Zait, A. 2011. Quality of Life Among Cochlear Implant Recipients. In: *International Encyclopedia of Rehabilitation,* J.H. Stone, M Blouin, Center for International Rehabilitation Research Information and Exchange (CIRRIE).Retrieved from http://cirrie.buffalo.edu/encyclopedia/en/article/293/

Zeitler, D. M., Kessler, M. A. Terushkin, V. Roland, J. T., Svirsky, M. A., Lalwani, A. K., & Waltzman, S. B. 2008. Speech perception benefits of sequential bilateral cochlear implantation in children and adults: A retrospective analysis. *Otology & Neurotology*, Vol. 29, pp. 314-325.

Zwolan, T. A., ZimmermanPhillips, S., Ashbaugh, C. J., Hieber, S. J., Kileny, P. R., & Telian, S. A. 1997. Cochlear implantation of children with minimal open-set speech recognition skills. *Ear & Hearing*, Vol. 18, No. 3, pp. 240-251.

16

Intratympanic Corticosteroid for Neurosensorial Hearing Loss Treatment

Malek Mnejja, Bouthaina Hammami, Amine Chakroun, Adel Chakroun, Ilheme Charfeddine and Abdelmonem Ghorbel
Department of ENT and Head Neck Surgery, CHU Habib Bourguiba, Sfax Tunisia

1. Introduction

The application of drugs through the eardrum and into the middle ear to treat various otologic disorders, such as Meniere's disease and sudden sensorineural hearing loss has recently gained widespread popularity. The intratympanic treatment modality can provide also a chemoprotection strategy for exposure to noise (1) cisplatin (2), and aminoglycosides (3).

Inflammatory processes may play a role in the etiology of various inner ear pathologies of which the pathogenesis is poorly understood. Intratymapanic corticosteroid may be a promising therapy for several ear disorders.

Neurosensorial hearing loss therapy to date has consisted mostly of the systemic administration of steroids and has been limited by their side effects and low therapeutic concentrations within the fluids and tissues of the inner ear. It has been shown in animals and humans that systemically applied glucocorticoids reach only low drug concentrations in the perilymph. The local application of drugs to treat inner ear diseases is expected to provide advantages as compared with systemic treatments, namely: 1) bypassing the blood-labyrinthine barrier, 2) resulting in higher concentrations in the inner ear fluids 3) avoiding major unwanted effects of systemically administered medications.

Despite some successes, the local medical treatment of inner ear conditions, is often frustrating to patients and physicians. We review the status of the intratympanic corticosteroids treatment.

2. History

The delivery of medications to the inner ear through the transtympanic route dates back to 1935, when Barany (4) used intratympanic lidocaine for treatment of tinnitus. Since then, other molecules have been used and the indications have expanded. In 1948, streptomycin was used to treat patients with unilateral Meniere's disease specifically on the basis of its vestibulotoxic effects (5). It was Harold Schuknecht who proposed the use of streptomycin as an alternative to surgical unilateral labyrinthine ablation (6). Francis Bauer, in 1969 and 1971 reported on the treatment of "Glue Ear" by using intratympanic urea (7). Another interesting application of intratympanic medication was reported by Bryan in 1973, when he described the use of intratympanic steroids in a patient with facial paralysis (8). Itoh (9), in 1991, used steroids for Meniere's disease. Silverstein (10) in 1996, used steroids for Sensorineural Hearing Loss.

3. Anatomy

The cochlea can be thought of as a long coiled tube looking much like a snail shell (11). It is composed of three compartments. The middle compartment is the scala media, which is filled with endolymph. The lower and upper fluid compartments respectively are the scala tympani and scala vestibuli, both of which are filled with perilymph. These two compartments communicate with each other at the apex of the cochlea through the helicotrema. The round window is a membranous opening in the bone within the scala tympani. It sits at the base of the scala tympani and is very compliant, capable of bulging into the middle ear. It separates perilymph from the middle ear space. The oval window, in the scala vestibuli, contains the footplate of the stapes, one of the middle ear bones, that transmits acoustic vibrations from eardrum to the inner ear.

4. Physiology

Most of the structures of the cochlea are protected from the systemic circulation by the presence of a blood-cochlear barrier (or blood-labyrinthine barrier), similar to the blood-brain barrier. There is exchange between the different compartments of the inner ear: between tympanic perilymph and vestibular perilymph and between endolymph and perilymph. But also between the inner ear fluids and cerebrospinal fluid and between the inner ear fluid and plasma (12) (13). Exchanges between endolymph and plasma are through the stria vascularis and between perilymph and plasma through the capillaries perilymphatic. At this level makes a pass filtering products: blood-labyrinthine barrier (13).

This blood–inner ear barrier consist of tight junctions and other mechanisms that limit access of molecules to inner ear targets. In fact the endothelial cells are connected with tight junctions and without fenestrations (14). This network of tightly coupled endothelial cells is the dominant component of the blood-cochlear barrier which make this solid barrier impermeable to macromolecules. In addition to this physical barrier, there is a chemical barrier between blood and endolymph/perilymph wich has a selectivity to electrolytes and water-soluble molecules (15).

In the fluid of the inner ear, there are other obstacles to the spread of drugs administered systemically: Because the scala media has a relatively high positive charge due to the endocochlear potential, the charge the drug carries will be a significant factor in its ability to enter the scala media, with positively charged drugs at a disadvantage (13).

The relatively high protein content of perilymph will tend to bind drugs (16). Protein interactions with drugs are as important in the perilymph as in blood. Albumin levels are high and can bind acidic drugs, and acid glycoproteins can bind basic drugs (16). Partition coefficients of drugs with these proteins will determine free concentration of the drug. The free fraction of the drug binds to the sensory cells and exerts its effect (13).

The cochlea is surrounded by the petrous bone. It was shown that there is a direct exchange between the extracellular space of the petrous bone and perilymph through the lacuna canaliculi which are canals or holes in the bone in free communication with the scala tympani (17).

5. Pharmacokinetics and pharmacodynamics

Treatment given by intratympanic will diffuse in liquid of the inner ear. There are 3 practical entry points: 1) through round window membrane RWM (at the base of the cochlea on the scala tympani side), 2) through or near the oval window (at the base of the cochlea on the scala vestibuli side), 3) through the bone of the cochlea via application in the middle ear. This infusion is mainly through the round window.

The RWM has three layers (18): an outer epithelial layer on the middle ear side, a middle fibrous layer, and another epithelial layer facing the inner ear. The outer epithelial layer contains some microvilli and abundant mitochondria, suggesting that it may be able to absorb substances and carry out metabolic activities. The inner epithelial layer has areas of discontinuous basement membrane that may provide space for substances to traverse the membrane.

Plontke (19), and colleagues have extensively modeled the distribution of drugs applied at the RWM. They suggest that in addition to diffusion along the length of the cochlea, diffusion through the tissue of the cochlea from one scala to another must be considered as well.

Some factors facilitate the passage of molecules through the round window membrane: low molecular weight, water-soluble nature, the ionic charge, histamine, prostaglandins, leukotrienes, endotoxin of E. coli, Staphylococcus exotoxins (20). The contact time with the round window membrane has the most important effect. Wang (21) demonstrates that the inner ear pharmacokinetic profile of steroids administered intratympanically is dependent upon the nature of the vehicle as well as the physicochemical properties of the steroid drug itself. In fact the degree of aqueous solubility of the drug has a major impact on its residence time and exposure in the inner ear (21).

Glucocorticoid receptors have been identified in the inner ear and are more abundant in the cochlea (22). The presence of glucocorticoid receptors in the inner ear provides a cellular means by which circulating glucocorticoids can directly affect the inner ear physiology. Corticosteroids have been used extensively for inner ear disease because of their anti-inflammatory effects but also affect the vascularity of the inner ear. Corticosteroids have many effects : they prevent a decrease in cochlear blood flow, reduce degeneration of the stria vascularis and have an antioxidant effect (23).

6. Choice of drug

Two corticosteroids are used by the majority of the researchers: dexamethasone and methylprednisolone. The concentration is varied between 4 mg/ ml and 25 mg/ml for dexamethasone and between 32 mg/ ml and 62,5 mg/ml for methylprednisolone.

Parnes in pharmacokinetic animal study compared intracochlear levels of three glucocortiocoids: dexamethasone (Dexa), methylprednisolone (MP), and hydrocortisone

(24). When correcting for the lower Dexa concentration (4 mg/mL) compared to MP (40 mg/mL) in their study and for the higher potency, dexamethasone is expected to reach higher effective levels in perilymph after application to the round window membrane. In addition, contrary to Dexa, MP solution is not stable but hydrolyzed after some days in the pump cartridge (19) (25).

7. Intratympanic delivery methods

There is no standard protocol for IT corticosteroid injections; the frequency of injections, concentration and type of corticosteroid. Method of injection is determined by the individual surgeon.

Multiple intratympanic delivery methods are descripted:

Syringe delivery is a simple method. However, direct injections do not allow for prolonged delivery. We can anesthetize the tympanic membrane with 10 percent Xylocaine. A drop of phenol on the ear drum is one method. Another is a topical anesthetic such as "Emla" cream. The drug is injected, left in the middle ear for 30 minutes.

The myringotomy is placed in the most superior and anterior location to allow maximal filling of the middle ear space with the corticosteroid solution while the patient is supine. Placement of the tube eliminates the need for a new myringotomy for each subsequent injection. For injection, we use a 25-gauge spinal needle attached to a 1-mL tuberculin-type syringe. To equalize pressure, two needle punctures were made in the anterior superior quadrant of the tympanic membrane, the first for injection and the second (superior) for air escap. The initial injection was followed by a second injection about 15 minutes later for a total volume of approximately 0.5 mL. The patient remained supine for 30 to 40 minutes, with the head turned to the side and the injected ear upright, and was instructed to swallow as little as possible to help maintain the fluid in the middle ear space for longer duration.

Microwick is the polyvinyl acetate wick (1 mm diameter by 9 mm length). It absorbs medication and transports it directly to the RWM. It's placed through a tube, at the round window niche. It allows instillation by the patient himself at home. The MicroWick should be removed or replaced after 4 weeks of treatment to prevent it from becoming adherent to the mucosa of the round window (26).

Microcatheter is composed of two tubes: one for injection and the other for the return of excess liquid. It ends with a bulge that is placed at the round window niche under general anesthesia. Some researchers propose to link the catheter to a pump. This would allow continuous irrigation and delivery of the product constantly at the round window.

8. Indications

Corticosteroids are indicated in several types of sensorineural affects. Indications are : sudden deafness, autoimmune Deafness, Deafness and Dizziness related to Meniere's disease and Tinnitus.

They are also available for otoprotection against physical and chemical aggressions of the inner ear. It seems that corticosteroids will respond to inner ear hair cells and nerve cells. They may prevent, limit and recover the damage caused by noise trauma (27). They may be given in anticipation of ototoxicity that could be associated with systemic aminoglycoside antibiotic or cisplatinum and other chemotherapeutic agents. They can also be used after injuries (28).

9. Results

Intratympanic corticosteroids for sudden hearing loss and Meniere's disease has been the subject of retrospective, uncontrolled studies and a few controlled studies with small numbers of subjects. Hamid in 2001 with a single injection of high concentration of Dexamethasone (24mg/ml) for patients with Meniere's disease, was able to get control of vertigo in 90% of cases with an improvement of hearing threshold, the percentage of discrimination and sensation of fullness (29) (26). In his study, 90% of patients had vertigo control, 90% had improved speech discrimination, and 90% had decreased aural pressure.

Garduno (30), compared intra tympanic Dexamethasone versus placebo in Meniere disease. He obtained full control of vertigo in 82% of cases against 57% with placebo with significant differences. He also noted a reduction of tinnitus in 48% of cases and hearing improvement in 35% of cases.

In sudden deafness, Ahn (31) compared two groups: systemic corticosteroids alone versus intratympanic corticosteroids associated with systemic treatment. He found no significant difference in overall response, but noted a significant improvement on the low frequencies in intratympanic treatment group. HONG (32) compared intratympanic corticosteroids alone versus systemic corticosteroids alone also found no difference, but noted a significant improvement over the low frequencies. Alatas (33) concluded that intratympanic dexamethasone is an effective therapy for low frequency hearing loss. Hunchaisri (34) concluded that it may have benefits for patients with sudden sensorineural hearing loss who failed systemic steroid therapy.

In diabetic patients with sudden sensorineural hearing loss, intratympanic corticoid injection is as effective as systemic steroid treatment and it can avoid undesirable side effects (35). Han studied three groups of diabetics and compared prednisolone administered by oral, intravenous and intra tympanic Dexamethasone. He noted a better outcome with intratympanic treatment without significant difference. However, systemic treatment was discontinued in 6 patients due to problems of hyperglycemia. This disadvantage is not observed with the intratympanic treatment.

Many studies concluded that using the continuous intratympanic dexamethasone by MicroWick is effective, safe and efficient for treatment of sudden idiopathic sensorineural hearing loss (26) (19).

There is an increasing number of series evaluating intratympanic (IT) steroids as first line or salvage therapy in ISSHL with some studies presenting control groups and randomized controlled trials (Table 1).

The effect of intratympanic corticosteroids on tinnitus is difficult to assess due to limited work. Shulman (37) treated tinnitus with intratympanic dexamethasone and obtained control of tinnitus in 50% cases (for 1 year and over).

Author	Type of study	Steroid used	Protocol	Results
Gianoli (48)	prospective		salvage treatment Steroids through a ventilation tube 4 separate occasions over the course of 10 to 14 days	Hearing improvement in 44%
Xenellis (49)	Randomized controlled study	Methylprednisolone	salvage treatment 40 mg/mL 4 times within a 15-day period	Significant improvement
Haynes (36)	retrospective	Dexamethasone	24 mg/mL	27.5% showed improvement (≥20dB)
Ahn (31)	controlled study	Dexamethasone	0.3 mL on days 1, 3, and 5	Total recovery rate was 73.3% and 70.0% in the control group better hearing improvement at 250 Hz than the control group
Hong (50)	Randomized controlled study	Dexamethosone	Primary treatment 5mg/ml once a day for eight days	hearing recovery rate compared with patients treated with oral steroids improvement at low frequencies
Han (35)	Prospective, nonrandomized multicenter clinical trial	Dexamethasone	SNHL with diabetes four times within a two-week period	no significant difference with systemic treatment no patients who failed to control their blood sugar level
Lee (51)	retrospective	Dexamethasone	salvage treatment 5 mg/mL, six injections over 2 weeks	significant improvement for severe SNHL

Author	Type of study	Steroid used	Protocol	Results
Kara (52)	Prospective control	Dexamethasone	5 intratympanic injections with the dose of 4 mg/ml,	Intratympanic steroids gave better hearing results than systemic steroids with no systemic side effects
Plontke (19)	Randomized, double-blind, placebo controlled multicenter trial.	Dexamethasone	4 mg/ml continuously applied for 14 days	better hearing improvement in the treatment group absence of serious adverse events

Table 1. Review of Literature on Intratympanic steroid Therapy for sudden neurosensorial hearing loss

The effectiveness of steroids in reducing noise induced hearing loss has been inconclusive (13). Many types of steroids, antioxidants and growth factors have been studied to protect the ear from trauma or to minimize or reverse damage (38) (39). Some researchers have used antioxidants such as D-methionine and N-acetylcysteine to prevent noise induced hearing loss (40). A variety of growth factors and peptides, are being introduced to combat the effects of Noise induced hearing loss : Insulin-like growth factor-1 (IGF-1), neurotrophic factor-3 (NT-3) , AM-111 and D-JNKI-1 peptides (41) (42) (40).

Steroids have also been tested for their otoprotective attributes during antibiotic treatment. The intracochlear infusion of dexamethasone before and after kanamycin delivery protected hearing (43). Hill (44) concluded that IT dexamethasone may be a safe, simple and effective intervention that minimizes cisplatin ototoxicity without interfering with the chemotherapeutic actions of cisplatin.

A sudden or progressive hearing loss can occur during radiation treatment of head and neck tumors (45). Patients are commonly given steroids to reduce inflammation, but their local delivery would reduce the side effects associated with systemic steroid treatment (13). Inflammation often results from inner ear surgical trauma, as well (46).

10. Complications

Complications of intratympanic injections of corticosteroids are uncommon and banal (19). Those most often reported in the literature are: 1) some individuals experience intense pain during injection, 2) vertigo and tinnitus, 3) Other complications are rare and include acute otitis media and mastoiditis.

Patients who undergone trans-tympanic aerator to avoid multiple injections or to put in the microwick have an increasing risk of persistent eardrum perforation (47). In fact, 20% of these patients had non healing perforations that needed repair using a fat graft (26).

11. Conclusion

The intratympanic treatment has several advantages. It is an effective procedure for the control of cochleovestibular disorders such as sudden deafness and Ménière's disease. Up till now, there is no consensus on the IT protocol. Future studies will define the best prtocole. The perspective is the development of the gene therapy and the intracochlear treatment.

12. References

[1] Yamashita D, Jiang HY, Le Prell CG, et al. Postexposure treatment attenuates noise-induced hearing loss. *Neuroscience.* 2005, 134 : 633-642.
[2] Dickey DT, Muldoon L L, Doolittle ND, et al. Effect of N-acetylcysteine route of administration on chemoprotection against cisplatin-induced toxicity in rat models. *Cancer Chemother Pharmacol* . 2007, 62: 235-241.
[3] Chen Y, Huang WG, Zha DJ, et al. Aspirin attenuates gentamicin ototoxicity: From the laboratory to the clinic. *Hear Res.* 2007, 226: 178-182.
[4] Barany, R. Die Beinflussung des Ohrensausens durch intravensˇs injizierte Lokal anaestetica. *Acta Otlaryngol.* 1935, 23: 201-3.
[5] Fowler, E. Streptomycin treatment of vertigo. *Trans Am Acad Ophth Otolaryngol* . 1948, 52: 239-301.
[6] Schuknecht, H. Ablation therapy for the relief of Meniere's disease. *Laryngoscope.* 1956, 66: 859-70.
[7] Bauer, F. Intratympanic injection of urea in the treatment of "Glue Ear". *Acta Otorhinolaryngol Belg* . 1971, 25: 811-6.
[8] Bryant, FL. Intratympanic injection of steroid for treatment of facial paralysis. *Laryngoscope.* 1973,83: 700-6.
[9] Itoh A, Sakata E. Treatment of vestibular disorders. *Acta Otolaryngol Suppl.* . 1991, 481: 617-23.
[10] Silverstein H, Choo D, Rosenberg SI, Kuhn J, Seidman M, Stein I. Intratympanic steroid treatment of inner ear disease and tinnitus (preliminary report). *Ear Nose Throat J.* 1996, 75, 8: 468-71.
[11] Schuknecht, H. *Pathology of the ear.* s.l. : Lea and Febiger, Malvern, PA, ., 1993.
[12] Juhn, S. Barrier systems in the inner ear. *Acta Otolaryngol.* 1988, Suppl. 458: 79-83.
[13] Swan EE, Mescher MJ, Sewell WF, Tao SL, Borenstein JT. Inner ear drug delivery for auditory applications. *Adv Drug Deliv Rev.* 2008, 60, 15: 1583-99.
[14] Kimura, R. Ota, C. Ultrastructure of the cochlear blood vessels. *Acta Otolaryngol.* 1974, 77: 231-250.
[15] Jahnke, K. The fine structure of freeze-fractured intercellular junctions in the guinea pig inner ear. *Acta Otolaryngol.* 1975, Suppl. 336: 1-40.
[16] Thalmann, I. Kohut,R. Ryu,J. Comegys, T. Senarita,M. Thalmann,R. Protein profile of human perilymph: in search of markers for the diagnosis of perilymph fistula and other inner ear disease. *Otolaryngol. Head Neck Surg.* 1994, 111: 273-280.
[17] Shepherd, R. Colreavy, M. Surface microstructure of the perilymphatic space:implications for cochlear implants and cell- or drug-based therapies,. *Arch.Otolaryngol. Head Neck Surg.* 2004, 130: 518-523.

[18] Carpenter AM, Muchow D, Goycoolea MV. Ultrastructural studies of the human round window membrane. *Arch Otolaryngol Head Neck Surg.* 1989, 115, 5: 585–90.

[19] Plontke, et al. Randomized, Double Blind, Placebo Controlled Trial on the Safety and Efficacy of Continuous Intratympanic Dexamethasone Delivered Via a Round Window Catheter for Severe To Profound Sudden Idiopathic Sensorineural Hearing Loss after Failure of Systemic The. *Laryngoscope.* 2009, 119: 359-369.

[20] Goycoolea, MV. Clinical aspects of round window membrane permeability under normal and pathological conditions. *Acta Otolaryngol.* 2001, 121, 4: 437–47.

[21] Wang, et al. Vehicle and Drug-Dependent Inner Ear Sustained Release. *Laryngoscope.* 2011, 121: 385–391.

[22] Rarey KE, Curtis LM, ten Cate WJ. Tissue specific levels of glucocorticoid receptor within the rat inner ear. *Hear Res.* 1993, 64: 205–10.

[23] Nagura M, Iwasaki S, Wu R, Mizuta K, Umemura K, Hoshino T. Effects of corticosteroid, contrast medium and ATP on focal microcirculatory disorders of the cochlea. *Eur J Pharmacol.* 1999, 366: 47–53.

[24] Parnes LS, Sun AH, Freeman DJ. Corticosteroid pharmacokinetics in the inner ear fluids: an animal study followed by clinical application. *Laryngoscope.* 1999, 109, 7 Pt 2: 1–17.

[25] Nahata MC, Morosco RS, Hipple TF. Stability of diluted methylprednisolone sodium succinate injection at two temperatures. *Am J Hosp Pharm.* 1994, 51, 17: 2157–2159.

[26] Rauch, SD. Intratympanic steroids for sensorineural hearing loss. *Otolaryngol Clin North Am.* 2004, 37, 5: 1061-74.

[27] Kujawa SG, Liberman MC. Adding insult to injury:cochlear nerve degeneration after "temporary" noise-induced hearing loss. *J Neurosci.* 2009, 29: 14077–14085.

[28] Poe, DS.Pyykko,I. Nanotechnology and the treatment of inner ear diseases. *WIREs Nanomedicine and Nanobiotechnology.* 2011 .

[29] Hamid, MA. Intratympanic dexamethasone perfusion in Meniere's disease. *Presented at the Spring Meeting of The American Neurotology Society.* Palm Desert (CA), May 12,2001.

[30] Garduño-Anaya, MA, Couthino De Toledo H, Hinojosa-González R, Pane-Pianese C, Ríos-Castañeda LC. Dexamethasone inner ear perfusion by intratympanic injection in unilateral Ménière's disease: a two-year prospective, placebo-controlled, double-blind, randomized trial. *Otolaryngol Head Neck Surg.* 2005, 133, 2: 285-94.

[31] Ahn JH, Yoo MH, Yoon TH, et al. Can intratympanic dexamethasone added to systemic steroids improve hearing outcome in patients with sudden deafness? *Laryngoscope .* 2008, 118: 279–82.

[32] Hong SM, Park CH, Lee JH. Hearing outcomes of daily intratympanic dexamethasone alone as a primary treatment modality for ISSHL. *Otolaryngol Head Neck Surg.* 2009, 141, 5: 579-83.

[33] Alatas, N. Use of intratympanic dexamethasone for the therapy of low frequency hearing loss. *Eur Arch Otorhinolaryngol.* 2009, 266, 8: 1205-12.

[34] Hunchaisri N, Chantapant S, Srinangyam N. Intratympanic dexamethasone for refractory sudden sensorineural hearing loss. *J Med Assoc Thai.* 2010, 93, 12: 1406-14.

[35] Han CS, Park JR, Boo SH, Jo JM, Park KW, Lee WY, Ahn JG, Kang MK, Park BG, Lee H. Clinical efficacy of initial intratympanic steroid treatment on sudden sensorineural hearing loss with diabetes. *Otolaryngol Head Neck Surg.* 2009, 141, 5: 572-8.

[36] Haynes DS, O'Malley M, Cohen S, Watford K, Labadie RF. Intratympanic dexamethasone for sudden sensorineural hearing loss after failure of systemic therapy. *Laryngoscope.* 2007, 117, 1: 3–15.
[37] Shulman A, Goldstein B. Intratympanic drug therapy with steroids for tinnitus control: a preliminary report. *Int Tinnitus J.* 2000, 6, 1: 10-20.
[38] Henderson, D. McFadden, S.L. Liu, C.C. Hight, N. Zheng, X.Y. The role of antioxidants in protection from impulse noise. *Ann. N. Y. Acad. Sci.* 1999, 28: 368–380.
[39] Takemura K, Komeda M, Yagi M, Himeno C, Izumikawa M, Doi T, Kuriyama H, Miller JM, Yamashita T. Direct inner ear infusion of dexamethasone attenuates noise-induced trauma in guinea pig. *Hear Res.* 2004, 196, 1-2: 58-68.
[40] Coleman JK, Kopke RD, Liu J, Ge X, Harper EA, Jones GE, Cater TL, Jackson RL. Pharmacological rescue of noise induced hearing loss using N-acetylcysteine and acetyl-L-carnitine. *Hear Res.* 2007, 226, 1-2: 104-13.
[41] Iwai K, Nakagawa T, Endo T, Matsuoka Y, Kita T, Kim TS, Tabata Y, Ito J. Cochlear protection by local insulin-like growth factor-1 application using biodegradable hydrogel. *Laryngoscope.* 2006, 116, 4: 529-33.
[42] Shoji F, Miller AL, Mitchell A, Yamasoba T, Altschuler RA, Miller JM. Differential protective effects of neurotrophins in the attenuation of noise-induced hair cell loss. *Hear Res.* 2000, 146, 1-2: 134-42.
[43] Himeno C, Komeda M, Izumikawa M, Takemura K, Yagi M, Weiping Y, Doi T, Kuriyama H, Miller JM, Yamashita T. Intra-cochlear administration of dexamethasone attenuates aminoglycoside ototoxicity in the guinea pig. *Hear Res.* 2002, 167, 1-2: 61-70.
[44] Hill GW, Morest DK, Parham K. Cisplatin-induced ototoxicity: effect of intratympanic dexamethasone injections. *Otol Neurotol.* 2008, 29, 7: 1005-11.
[45] Bhandare N, Antonelli PJ, Morris CG, Malayapa RS, Mendenhall WM. Ototoxicity after radiotherapy for head and neck tumors. *Int J Radiat Oncol Biol Phys.* 2007, 67, 2: 469-79.
[46] Ye Q, Tillein J, Hartmann R, Gstoettner W, Kiefer J. Application of a corticosteroid (Triamcinolon) protects inner ear function after surgical intervention. *Ear Hear.* . 2007, 28, 3: 361-9.
[47] Rutt AL, Hawkshaw MJ, Sataloff RT. Incidence of tympanic membrane perforation after intratympanic steroid treatment through myringotomy tubes. *Ear Nose Throat J.* 2011, 90, 4: E21-7.
[48] Gianoli GJ, Li JC. Transtympanic steroids for treatment of sudden hearing loss. *Otolaryngol Head Neck Surg.* 2001, 125, 3: 142-6.
[49] Xenellis J, Papadimitriou N, Nikolopoulos T, Maragoudakis P, Segas J, Tzagaroulakis A, Ferekidis E. Intratympanic steroid treatment in idiopathic sudden sensorineural hearing loss: a control study. *Otolaryngol Head Neck Surg.* 2006, 134, 6: 940-5.
[50] Hong SM, Park CH, Lee JH. Hearing outcomes of daily intratympanic dexamethasone alone as a primary treatment modality for ISSHL. *Otolaryngol Head Neck Surg.* 2009, 141, 5: 579-83.
[51] Lee JD, Park MK, Lee CK, Park KH, Lee BD. Intratympanic steroids in severe to profound sudden sensorineural hearing loss as salvage treatment. *Clin Exp Otorhinolaryngol.* 2010, 3, 3: 122-5.
[52] Kara E, Cetik F, Tarkan O, Sürmelioğlu O. Modified intratympanic treatment for idiopathic sudden sensorineural hearing loss. *Eur Arch Otorhinolaryngol.* . 2010, 267, 5: 701-7.

17

Effects and Prognostic Factors of Acupuncture Treatment for Idiopathic Sudden Sensorineural Hearing Loss

Kyu Seok Kim and Hae Jeong Nam
Department of Ophthalmology & Otorhinolaryngology,
College of Oriental Medicine, Kyung Hee University, Seoul
Republic of Korea

1. Introduction

Idiopathic sudden sensorineural hearing loss (ISSHL), sometimes called sudden sensorineural hearing loss (SSHL) is usually defined as loss of at least 30 dB in 3 contiguous frequencies over a period of 3 days or less.

It is difficult to estimate the efficacy of the various treatments and impact of prognostic factors for ISSHL because the natural history of ISSHL is still unknown (Fetterman et al., 1996). There have been many studies reported the effect of various treatment including systemic corticosteroids, tympanic corticosteroids injection, antiviral, anticoagulant, and vitamin etc. on ISSHL, but the results were controversial (Eisenman D., 2000).

There also have been several studies reported the prognostic factors of ISSHL (Mattox & Simmons, 1977; Shikowitz, 1991; Byl, 1984; Ceylan et al., 2007). However, the rate of spontaneous recovery of ISSHL is 45 to 65 percent (Mattox & Simmons, 1977; Eisenman D., 2000) and there is no improvement criterion that was universally accepted. Thus, the results of several studies for prognostic factors were also controversial.

Traditional Chinese Medicine (TCM) has long been widely used in East Asia. Acupuncture is frequently used for the treatment of neurological conditions (Lee et al., 2007). Since 1970s, there have been some studies which reported effect of acupuncture on ISSHL. Some studies reported positive results (Yoon et al., 2003; Ha & Choi, 2003), while the others reported the opposite trend (Vincent & Richardson, 1987; Borton, 1976).

In previous study, we demonstrated that the acupuncture treatment (AT) has some effect on ISSHL patients who did not respond to conventional therapy (Yin et al., 2010). However, the efficacy and prognostic factors of AT on ISSHL are still unclear.

This study was conducted to evaluate the effects and prognostic factors of AT for ISSHL. We analyzed variables which related to improvement in ISSHL by AT; these included gender, age, location of lesion, presence of vertigo, presence of disease (hypertension and diabetes mellitus), the time interval from the onset of hearing loss to the start of AT and severity of hearing loss on the day of the initial visit. We also analyzed our data to search the prognostic factors affecting the improvement of ISSHL using feature selection analysis and decision tree model.

2. Materials and methods

2.1 Patients and eligibility

We reviewed the medical records of ISSHL patients who visited 'Tinnitus & Hearing loss clinic' in Kyung Hee Oriental Medical Hospital, Seoul, Korea from June 2006 to February 2011. Patients who met the definition of ISSHL, which is defined as an abrupt or rapidly progressing hearing loss of at least 25 dB in 3 contiguous frequencies over a period of no more than 3 days, were eligible to participate in this study. We excluded patients with sensorineural hearing loss caused by trauma, noise, tumors, otitis media or Meniere's disease. Additionally, patients were ineligible if they have hearing loss in both ears.

Of a total 117 patients, ten had Meniere's disease, two had senile progressive hearing loss, four had hearing loss in both ears, one had otitis media and twenty-eight failed to undergo a follow up audiogram. Therefore, 72 patients (40 males, 32 females) were enrolled in this study (Fig. 1). This study was approved by the Institutional Review Board of Kyung Hee Oriental Medical Hospital (KOMCIRB-2011-09).

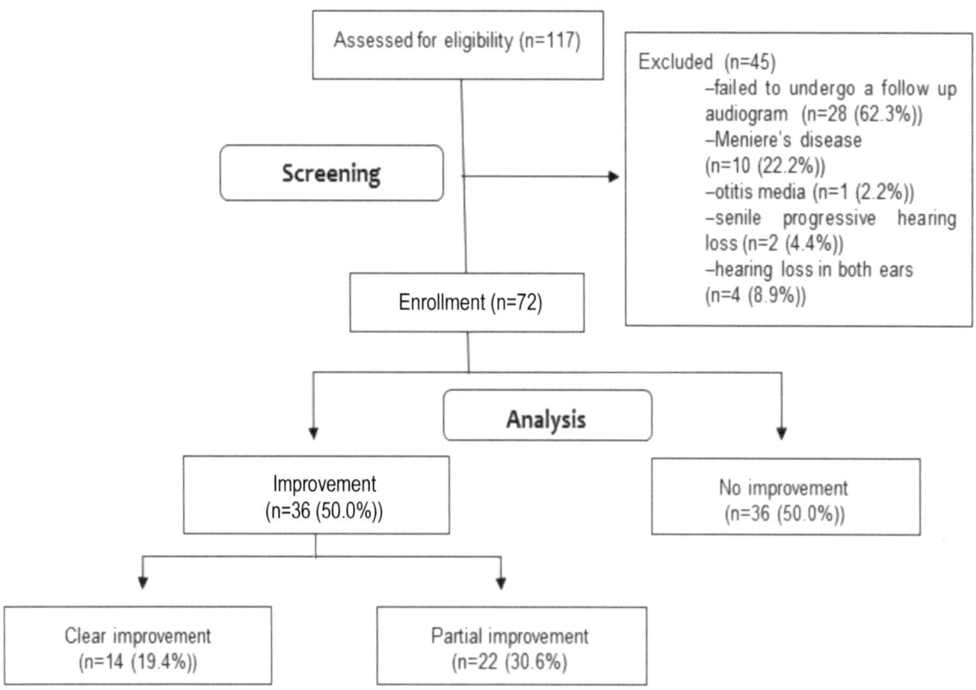

Fig. 1. Flow chart of the study

2.2 Audiological assessment

All patients underwent a full physical exam as well as a routine audiological evaluation and otolaryngologic history was also recorded. Magnetic resonance images were acquired if necessary. Pure tone audiograms were conducted using a *GSI 61 audiogram (Grason-Stadler, Inc., WI, USA)* on the day of the initial visit and the day of the follow-up measurement, which was usually after 10 rounds (1st follow-up) and 20 rounds (2nd follow-up) of AT. However, the follow-up measurement was performed before 10 or 20 rounds of acupuncture for some patients who request an earlier audiogram because they felt clear improvement. If partial improvement in the audiogram was observed at the time of the first follow-up measurement, AT was continued until the second follow-up measurement. The hearing results were evaluated based on the pure tone average (PTA) of 4 frequencies (250, 500, 1000, 2000 Hz). A clear improvement of hearing was defined as a final hearing level less than 25 dB and a partial improvement of hearing was defined as a final hearing level not less than 25dB but decreased in PTA of 10 dB or more.

2.3 Acupuncture treatment

All patients received the same method of AT from one TCM doctor. It was typically performed two times a week and the frequency was increased or decreased as necessary. The sterile acupuncture needles (length: 40 mm and diameter: 0.25 mm, Dondbang Co. Korea) were inserted to a depth of 10 - 30 mm until the patient felt the characteristic needling sensation of soreness, numbness or distension around the acupuncture point. Stimulated acupuncture points included GV14, GV15, GV16, GB20, GB21, BL10, SI4, SI15 and additional local points (TE21, TE22, SI19, GB2, ST7, BL2, LI20, GV20, EX-HN3) as necessary in the prone position, right after the 1st stimulated acupuncture were removed, and the liver tonification formula of Saam acupuncture theory (KI10, LR8, LU8 and LR4) (Yin CS et al., 2007) which were combined with contralateral LI4, LR3, and ST36 in the supine position. The needles were retained at each position for 10 minutes. Most patients were also administered herbal medicine individually to improve their body condition.

2.4 Statistical analysis

All continuous variables represented in this study were expressed as the means ± the standard deviation and all categorical variables were expressed as patient number and percentage (%). The differences between improvement and no improvement groups were analyzed by the independent-samples T test for all continuous variables if the distribution was normal. If the distribution was abnormal, the differences between groups were analyzed by the Mann-Whitney U test. In addition, categorical variables were analyzed using a Chi-square test or Fisher's exact test. These statistical analyses were conducted using SPSS 17.0 statistical software for windows.

We also analyzed our data using the feature selection model to classify the important variables. Then, based on these important variables, we analyzed our data using a decision tree model to identify and rank prognostic factors affecting the improvement of ISSHL by AT. These calculations were performed using SPSS Clementine version 12.0 statistical software for windows.

Probability values of 0.05 or less were considered statistically significant.

3. Results

3.1 Patient population

Seventy-two patient charts were reviewed (40 males, 32 females). The average age of the patients was 49.4 years (range, 8 to 76) and the average time interval from the onset of hearing loss to the start of AT was 109.1 days (range, 1 to 1460).

3.2 PTA changes before and after acupuncture treatment

Before acupuncture, mean PTA scores of improvement and no improvement groups were 63.92 ± 22.82 dB and 63.78 ± 17.99 dB, respectively and there was no statistical difference between groups (P = 0.977). After AT, mean PTA of improvement and no improvement groups were 39.55 ± 21.77 dB and 62.64 ± 18.23 dB, respectively and a significant difference between groups was evident (P = 0.000) (Fig. 2).

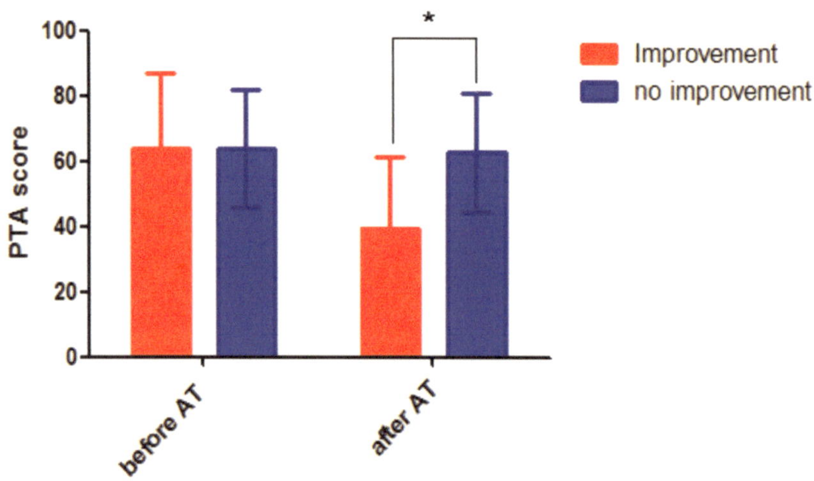

* : Statistically significant difference, P<0.05 using independent-samples T test

Fig. 2. Mean PTA before and after AT between Improvement and No Improvement Groups

3.3 Overall improvement rate

Overall, after completing the treatment, 36 patients (50.0%) showed improvement including a clear (14 patients, 19.4%) and partial (22 patients, 30.6%) improvement. In improvement group, the average age was 51.2 years (range, 19 to 76), the average time interval from the onset of hearing loss to the start of AT was 51.06 ± 69.39 days (range, 1 to 330) and the average improvement in PTA was 24.47 ± 14.85 dB (range, 9 to 63) including two cases which the average improvement in PTA was less than 10dB, but PTA was within 25dB.

3.4 Gender, age, location of lesion, vertigo, hypertension and diabetes mellitus

There was no significant difference in the gender distribution between improvement and no improvement groups. Also, no significant difference between groups was observed in regards to the occurrence of vertigo, the location of lesion, presence of hypertension and diabetes mellitus (Table 1).

	improvement			P^*
	Yes	No	Total	
Gender				
Male	20 (27.8%)	20 (27.8%)	40 (55.6%)	
Female	16 (22.2%)	16 (22.2%)	32 (44.4%)	1.000
Total	36 (50.0%)	36 (50.0%)	72 (100%)	
Age				
≤60	27 (37.5%)	31 (43.1%)	58 (80.6%)	
>60	9 (12.5%)	5 (6.9%)	14 (19.4%)	0.234
Total	36 (50.0%)	36 (50.0%)	72 (100%)	
Location of lesion				
Left	22 (30.6%)	24 (33.3%)	46 (63.9%)	
Right	14 (19.4%)	12 (16.7%)	27 (36.1%)	0.624
Total	36 (50.0%)	36 (50.0%)	72 (100%)	
Vertigo				
Yes	9 (12.5%)	7 (9.7%)	16 (22.2%)	
No	27 (37.5%)	29 (40.3%)	56 (77.8%)	0.571
Total	36 (50.0%)	36 (50.0%)	72 (100%)	
Hypertension				
Yes	11 (15.3%)	10 (13.9%)	21 (29.2%)	
No	25 (34.7%)	26 (36.1%)	51 (70.8%)	0.795
Total	36 (50.0%)	36 (50.0%)	72 (100%)	
Diabetes Mellitus				
Yes	0 (0%)	1 (1.4%)	1 (1.4%)	
No	36 (50.0%)	35 (48.6%)	73(98.6%)	1.000
Total	36 (50.0%)	36 (50.0%)	72 (100%)	

* Statistically significant difference, $P<0.05$ using χ^2 test or Fisher's Exact test

Table 1. Relationship of Character of Patients and Improvement of ISSHL

3.5 Time interval from the onset of hearing loss to the start of acupuncture treatment

The time intervals from the onset of hearing loss to the start of AT for improvement and no improvement groups were 51.06 days (±69.39 SD) and 167.22 days (±265.01 SD), respectively, which differed significantly (P=0.013) (Table 2).

	Improvement		P^*
	Yes	No	
Time interval from the onset of hearing loss to the start of acupuncture treatment	51.06 ± 69.39	167.22 ± 265.01	0.013*

* Statistically significant difference, $P<0.05$ using independent-samples T test

Table 2. Differences in the Time Interval from the Onset of Hearing Loss to the Start of Acupuncture Treatment between Improvement and No Improvement Groups

To analyze the relationship between ISSHL improvement and the time interval, we divided 72 patients into four groups (within 2 weeks, 2 – 6 weeks, 6 weeks – 6 months and over 6 months groups). In this analysis, 9 of 10 patients (90%) and 15 of 25 patients (60%) showed improvement with the time interval within 2 weeks and 2 - 6 weeks, respectively. Only 10 of 26 patients (38.5%) and 2 of 11 patients (18.2%) showed improvement with the time interval of 6 weeks – 6 months and greater than 6 months, respectively (Table 3).

Time interval	ISSHL improvement				
	Yes		No		*P*
	Clear	Partial		Total	
Within 2 weeks	5 (6.9%)	4 (5.6%)	1 (1.4%)	10 (13.9%)	
2 - 6 weeks	4 (5.6%)	11 (15.3%)	10 (13.9%)	25 (34.7%)	
6 weeks – 6 months	4 (5.6%)	6 (8.3%)	16 (22.2%)	26 (36.1%)	0.004*
6months or more	1 (1.4%)	1 (1.4%)	9 (12.5%)	11 (15.3%)	
Total	14 (19.4%)	22 (30.6%)	36 (50.0%)	72 (100%)	

* Statistically significant difference, P<0.05 using χ^2 test

Table 3. Relationship between the Time Interval and ISSHL Improvement

3.6 Severity of hearing loss on the day of initial visit as a prognostic factor

As mentioned earlier, there was no difference in mean PTA before and after AT between improvement and no improvement groups (Fig. 2).
To evaluate the co-relationship between severity of hearing loss and time interval with improvement, we divided patients with 2 groups; within 6 weeks and over 6 weeks. Within 6 weeks, there was no difference of severity of hearing loss on the day of initial between improvement and no improvement groups (P = 0.145). On the other hand, over 6 weeks, severity of hearing loss on the day of initial in no improvement group was higher than in improvement group. However, there was no statistical significance (P = 0.055) (Table 4).

Time interval from the onset of hearing loss to the start of acupuncture treatment	Improvement		*P**
	Yes	No	
Within 6 weeks	69.74 ± 22.03 (n = 24)	59.20 ± 18.36 (n = 11)	0.145
Over 6 weeks	52.29 ± 20.52 (n =12)	65.60 ± 17.82 (n = 25)	0.055

* Statistically significant difference, P<0.05 using Mann-Whitney U test

Table 4. Severity of Hearing Loss on the Day of Initial Visit as a Prognostic Factor

3.7 Important variables for ISSHL improvement

In the feature selection analysis to classify the most important variables to the improvement of ISSHL by AT, pure tone at each frequency (250, 500, 1000, 2000 Hz), PTA on the day of the initial visit and time interval (categorical variable) were determined to be important variables (Table 5).

Rank	Field	Importance	Value
1	pure tone at 500Hz (middle-low frequency range) on the day of the initial visit	Important	1.0
2	pure tone average on the day of the initial visit	Important	1.0
3	pure tone at 1000Hz (middle-high frequency range) on the day of the initial visit	Important	1.0
4	pure tone at 250Hz (low frequency range) on the day of the initial visit	Important	1.0
5	pure tone at 2000Hz (high frequency range) on the day of the initial visit	Important	0.993
6	time interval from the onset of hearing loss to the start of acupuncture treatment (categorical)	Important	0.988
7	age	Unimportant	0.727
8	presence of vertigo	Unimportant	0.217
9	location of lesion (right / left)	Unimportant	0.18
10	presence of hypertension	Unimportant	0.166
11	Gender	Unimportant	0.133

* 1 screened field: presence of diabetes mellitus

Table 5. Results of Feature Selection of Important Variables Contributing to the Improvement of ISSHL

3.8 Prognosis factors for ISSHL improvement

Based on the results of feature selection model, we identified the prognosis factors that affect ISSHL improvement by AT using a decision tree model. In patients who started AT within 2 weeks and over 6 months, the improvement was not affected by PTA on the day of the initial visit. Otherwise, in patients who started treatment 6 weeks - 6 months PTA on the day of the initial visit were found to be important variables to the prognosis for ISSHL improvement. Especially, in patients who started treatment between 2 and 6 weeks, pure tones at 500Hz (middle-low frequency range) were found to be important variables to the prognosis for ISSHL improvement (Fig. 3).

4. Discussion

Acupuncture is one of the most important tools in traditional Chinese Medicine (TCM). There are meridian and acupuncture point theory in TCM, and according this theory TCM doctors usually choose multiple acupuncture points and combine them for treatment. Since early 1970s, people have paid attention to acupuncture as a complementary therapy of western treatment (Eisenberg DM et al., 1998).

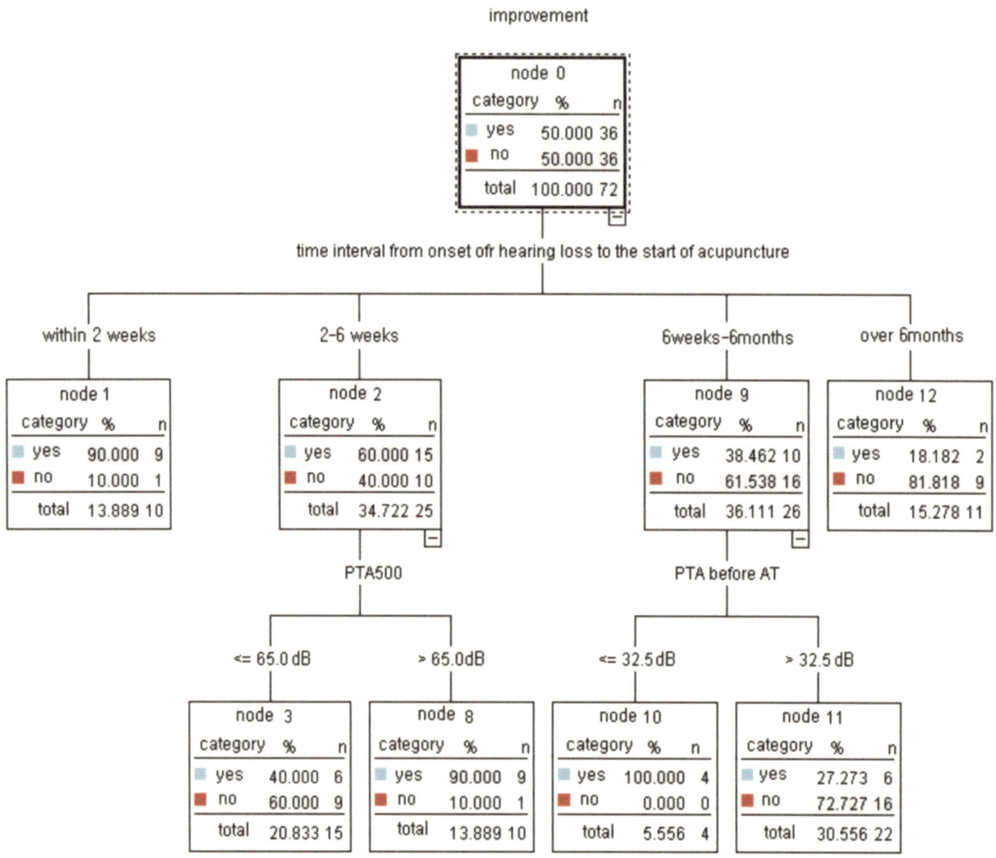

Abbreviation: PTA500=pure tone at 500 Hz on the day of the initial visit; PTA before AT=pure tone audiogram before acupuncture treatment

Fig. 3. Decision Tree Model of Important Variables as Prognosis Factors of ISSHL

Although there have been several studies about AT, it has not been fully explained how acupuncture works. Since gate-control theory, basic scientific research has focused on acupuncture theory from a neurobiologic perspective. Therefore, several studies have reported the effect of acupuncture on neurologic diseases, like seizure, cerebrovascular disorders, Parkinson's disease, etc. According to these studies, there is no evidence which is conclusive to support the use of acupuncture for a range of neurological disorders. (Lee H et al., 2007). The other study suggested that acupuncture have some effect on psychosomatic diseases, like pain, headache and smoking (Vincent CA., 1987).

Even though there was no strong scientific and clinical evidence, people have tried AT on the diseases which have unknown causes, for example, ISSHL.

There have been several studies to evaluate the effects of AT on ISSHL (Abel SM et al., 1976; Madell JR, 1975; Zhang CY & Wang Y, 2006; Zhang XZ et al., 2009; Yin CS et al., 2010; Yoon HS et al., 2003; Ha MK & Choi IH, 2003). Some studies have demonstrated that AT did not produce significant shifts in hearing compared with sham groups (Abel SM et al., 1976) or there were no clinically important differences during and post treatment (Madell JR, 1975). However, other studies have reported that AT was effective to patients with ISSHL (Yin CS et al., 2010; Yoon HS et al., 2003; Ha MK & Choi IH, 2003).

In spite of these results, the efficacy of AT on ISSHL is still unknown, because these studies often lacked definite diagnostic standards. Therefore, we excluded patients who had sensorineural hearing loss not from ISSHL but from other diseases even if the patients had a good response to make strict diagnostic standards.

The acupuncture points, methods and depth of acupuncture methods and the depth of acupuncture are regarded as important things for the better effect.

On SSHL including ISSHL, common acupuncture points are as follows; GB20, TE21, SI19, GB2, TE17, LI4, GB43, TE3, GB20, GV23, GV20, EX-HN 1, TE5, KI1 and so on (Zhang CY & Wang Y, 2006; Zhang XZ et al., 2009; Yin CS et al., 2010; Yoon HS et al., 2003; Ha MK & Choi IH, 2003). Especially, TE21, SI19 and GB2 are main points on ISSHL. We combined with these acupuncture points with Samm acupuncture points. Saam acupuncture is a traditional Korean acupuncture theory that originated in the 17th century. This acupuncture system applies a five-phase theory in which each of five transport points in 12 meridians correspond to one of the five phases. Saam acupuncture also simultaneously modulates other relative channels, which are selected based on the theory of nourishing or suppressing cycle relationships, to ensure whole-body balance (Hwang DS et al., 2011; Yin CS et al., 2007).

Some studies revealed that deep needling is more significantly effective than shallow needling at TE21, SI19 and GB2 combined with body acupuncture (Zhang CY & Wang Y, 2006). According to these studies, acupuncture needles in our trial were inserted to a deep depth of 20-30 mm at TE21, SI19 and GB2 until the patient felt the characteristic needling sensation of soreness, numbness or distension around the acupuncture points.

ISSHL is one of the tough problems in ear diseases area because there is no definite answer for this disease. There is not even universally acceptable standard definition of ISSHL. Although many studies define ISSHL as loss of at least 30 dB in 3 contiguous frequencies over a period of 3 days (Shemirani et al., 2009, Xenellis J., 2006, etc), some studies defined as a >20 dB (Haberkamp & Tanyeri, 1999), and others defined ISSHL as a >25 dB loss. (BYL FM, 1984). We defined ISSHL as hearing loss of at least 25 dB in 3 contiguous frequencies over a period of no more than 3 days, because there were some patients who complained hearing disturbance even if they had PTA lower than 30 dB.

ISSHL is thought to be the clinical manifestation of diverse pathologic processes: viral infection, circulatory disorders, labyrinthine membrane rupture, and autoimmune reactions have been suggested to be possible causative factors (Eisenman D & Arts HA, 2000). Because of the multifactorial etiopathology, a number or different regimens have been used as therapy, including vasodilators, anticoagulants, corticosteroids, vitamins, plasma expander, histamine, antiviral agents, batroxobin, contrast media, stellate ganglion block, hyperbaric oxygen, and carbogen (Suzuki H et al., 2011).

Antiviral was selected because ISSHL is regarded as one of the viral infection diseases. However, use of antivirals had no impact on recovery time or improvement in hearing

(Shaikh JA & Roehm PC, 2011). Vasodilators which widen blood vessels and thus improve blood flow were selected because it has been frequently considered that ISSHL may have a vascular origin. However, the effectiveness of vasodilators in the treatment of ISSHL could not be proven (Agarwal L & Pothier DD, 2010). Usually, early use of high-dose systemic steroid therapy improves hearing recovery. However, persistent hearing losses after 2 weeks of oral treatment with steroids have a poorer prognosis (Ito et al., 2002). There have been several reports regarding the benefits of intratympanic steroids for the treatment of refractory ISSHL, but the efficacy of intratympanic steroids is still controversial (Haynes et al., 2007).

On the one hand, the controversial results for various therapies would be reasonable because the rate of spontaneous recovery of ISSHL is 45 to 65 percent (Mattox & Simmons, 1977; Eisenman D., 2000). On the other, the lack of universally accepted standard criterion of effect would make this controversial result. The standard criterion is very important factor for study, because the results on effectiveness and prognostic factors could be changed by this. Unfortunately, each study of ISSHL used different criterion of effect.

We decided the criterion valuation basis for effectiveness at least 10 dB decrease in PTA of contiguous 4 frequencies (250, 500, 1000, 2000 Hz) because most of patients visited our clinic after they failed to conventional therapies, so we considered that 10 dB was reasonable comparing other studies (Xenellis J et al., 2006; Rauch SD et al., 2011; Wu HP et al., 2011)

After completing the AT, 50% patients (36/72) showed clear or partial improvement. If the 10 patients within 2 weeks from the onset were excluded to eliminate the effect from nature spontaneous recovery, 43.5% patients (27/62) showed clear or partial improvement. These results were similar to or higher than average recovery rate of other studies especially considering the time interval from onset of ISSHL to start treatment(Xenellis J et al., 2006; Haynes DS et al., 2007; Raymundo IT et al., 2010; Wu HP et al., 2011; Rauch SD et al., 2011; Park MK et al., 2011).

Commonly, the time interval from onset to treatment was regarded as the most important factor for improvement of ISSHL. Therefore, most of studies of ISSHL were conducted with the patients within 2 weeks from onset. Even the studies that conducted with patients who failed to conventional therapy, the periods of ISSHL were only a few months. Haynes et al. (Haynes DS et al., 2007) conducted a retrospective review of 40 SSHL patients who failed systemic therapy and underwent intratympanic dexamethasone. They found that 27.5 % (11 patients) patients recovered (criteria for improvement: 20 -dB PTA or 20 % improvement in SDS), and that the average duration from onset of symptoms to intratympanic therapy was 40 days with a range of 7 days to 310 days. However, even in this study, no patient receiving intratympanic corticosteroids after 36 days recovered their hearing. Psifidis AD et al. (Psifidis AD et al., 2006) conducted a review of 15-year retrospective series of 80 patients diagnosed with SSHL and they concluded that any additional treatment after 2 months should not affect the outcome of the hearing.

In our study, 37 out of 72 (51.3%) patients started AT 6 weeks after onset of ISSHL, and 13 patients (35.1%) showed improvement, even 5 patients showed complete recovery. Yeo SW et al (Yeo SW et al., 2007) conducted retrospective study of 156 SSHL patients who were treated by 10-day course of admission therapy and followed for at least months. They concluded that delayed recovery occurred later than 1 month after discharge. The result of this study is very interesting because this study was conducted in Korea, also. Almost of patients in our study visited our clinic after they had failed conventional therapies. Even though, Yeo SW et al hypothesized that conventional therapies for ISSHL might have long term effects, they didn't check if their patients had oriental medicine as the 2nd treatment or not. So, we hypothesized cautiously that the reason of delayed recovery in Yeo's study might be Oriental medicine, including acupuncture. Of course, we admit that our hypothesis is too much jump because there is no other study like Yeo's. From now, further studies were necessary to certify our hypothesis.

There have been several studies reported about the prognostic factors of ISSHL. Several factors, including gender, age, presence of vertigo, time interval from the onset to the start of treatment, severity of hearing loss, etc. have been suggested. Some studies have reported that the female gender was suggested to be poor prognostic factor for recovery of hearing loss (Ceylan et al., 2007) and male gender was related to better hearing outcomes (Xenellis J et al., 2006). In our study, correlation between gender and prognosis for recovery of hearing loss was not evident.

Standard age of prognosis on ISSHL is different according to each study. Wang L et al (Wang L et al., 2009) reported that the prognosis of patients under the age of 55 was better and Lee HN & Ban JH (Lee HN & Ban JH, 2010) proposed that the prognosis of patients under the age of 60 was better. In our finding, age was not a prognostic factor for recovery of hearing loss.

Location of lesion is regarded as an important factor in TCM. According to the TCM theory, the left side is controlled by *Blood-Liver* and the right side is controlled by *Qi-Lung*. From this theory, TCM doctors usually consider that the main reason of disease in left side is the stress and in right side is the deficiency of body-energy. However, location of lesion was not a prognostic factor for recovery of ISSHL in our study.

The presence of vertigo is one of important prognostic factors for recovery of hearing loss which many studies recommended (Kang D & Wan L, 2005; Suzuki H et al., 2011; Cvorović L et al., 2008). Some studies reported that BPPV in patients with SSHL, representing definitive vestibular damage, was closely related to poor prognosis (Lee NH & Ban JH, 2010). Other study revealed that the presence of vertigo was found to be significantly correlated with the lack of improvement in hearing, but only at the 8-kHz frequency (Ben-David J et al., 2002). But, our findings showed that the presence of vestibular damage such as vertigo or tinnitus was not related to improvement of ISSHL. These results were consistent with Wang L et al (Wang L et al., 2009).

Luo Y et al (Luo Y et al., 2010) reported that diabetes, hypertension, hyperlipidemia, high blood viscosity, cerebral blood supply insufficiency and liver disease were the risk factors of sudden hearing loss. Our findings showed that diabetes and hypertension was not related to recovery rate of hearing loss in accordance with some studies (Wang L et al., 2009; Kang D & Wan L, 2005).

Some studies have reported that the prognosis for recovery from hearing loss was better when the patients begin treatment within 2 weeks (Shikowitz, 1991; Byl, 1984; Wang L et al., 2009). In consistent with these findings, the most important prognosis variable in our study was also the time interval from the onset of hearing loss to the start of AT. Nine of 10 patients (90%) who started treatment for ISSHL within 2 weeks showed clear or partial improvement.

Many studies regarded the severity of hearing loss is one of the important prognostic factors for improvement of ISSHL(Byl FM., 1984; Fetterman BL et al., 1999; Psifidis AD et al, 2006; Cvorovic L et al., 2008; Ceylan A et al., 2007) However, the standard of severity which could affect the prognosis, was different in each study Moreover, some studies have reported that the initial hearing level had no statistical point on prognosis (Suzuki H et al., 2011; Wang L et al., 2009). In our study, there was no difference in severity of hearing loss between improvement and no improvement groups. However, in patients who started AT after 6 weeks of onset, no improvement group showed higher severity of hearing loss on the day of initial than improvement group. Even if there was no statistical significance, the difference was considerably high (P=0.055). Moreover, in feature selection analysis, PTA on the day of initial visit was one of the important variables contributing the improvement of ISSHL by AT.

Several studies reported that an upward-sloping audiogram pattern was related to better hearing outcomes (Xenellis J et al., 2006; Wu J et al, 2011). Wu J et al suggested that concave audiogram pattern as well as upward-sloping may be a favorable prognostic factor (Wu J et al, 2011). Cvorović L et al demonstrated that flat audometric curves had worse prognosis. To analysis of audiogram patterns, we divided frequency into low (250 Hz), middle-low (500 Hz), middle-high (1000 Hz), high (2000 Hz) frequency and analyzed each pure tone level according to each frequency. In patients who started treatment within 2 weeks, the improvement rate was not related to PTA on the day of the initial visit. Otherwise, in patients who started acupuncture treatment after 2 weeks, pure tones at 500Hz (middle-low frequency range) were found to be important variables to the prognosis for ISSHL improvement. These findings are very unique and our analysis method is the first trial combined to the time interval from the onset of hearing loss and audiogram.

In conclusion, our findings indicate that AT have some effects on ISSHL even for the patients who failed to respond to conventional therapies. It also demonstrated that favorable prognosis was directly related to the time interval from the onset of hearing loss to the start of AT. The severity of hearing loss, especially at middle-low frequency was also considerable as an important factor.

5. References

Abel SM, Barber TD, Briant TD. (1976). A study of acupuncture in adult sensorineural hearing loss. *J Otolaryngol*. Vol.6, pp.166-172

Agarwal L, Pothier DD. (2009). Vasodilators and vasoactive substances for idiopathic sudden sensorineural hearing loss. *Cochrane Database Syst Rev*. Vol.7, CD003422

Ben-David J, Luntz M, Podoshin L, Sabo E, Fradis M. (2002). Vertigo as a prognostic sign in sudden sensorineural hearing loss. *Int Tinnitus J*, Vol.8, pp.127-128

Borton TE. Acupuncture and sensorineural hearing loss: a review. (1976). *South Med J*,Vol. 69, pp.600-601

Byl. FM. (1984). Sudden hearing loss: eight years experience and suggested prognostic table. *Laryngoscope*, Vol. 94, pp.647-661

Ceylan A, Celenk F, Kemaloğlu YK, Bayazit YA, Göksu N, Ozbilen S. (2007). Impact of prognostic factors on recovery from sudden hearing loss. *J Laryngol & Otol*, Vol. 121, pp.1035-1040

Cvorović L, Deric D, Probst R, Hegemann S. (2008). Prognostic model for predicting hearing recovery in idiopathic sudden sensorineural hearing loss. *Otol Neurotol*, Vol. 29, pp.464-469

Eisenberg DM, Davis RB, Ettner SL, Appel S, Wilkey S, Van Rompay M, Kessler RC. (1998) Trends in alternative medicine use in the United States, 1990-1997: Results of follow-up national survey. *JAMA*, Vol. 280, pp.1569-1575

Eisenman D, Arts HA. (2000). Effectiveness of treatment for sudden sensorineural hearing loss. *Arch Otolaryngol Head Neck Surg*, Vol. 126, pp.1161-1164

Fetterman BL, Saunders JE, Luxford WM. (1996). Prognosis and treatment of sudden sensorineural hearing loss. *Am J Otolaryngol*, Vol. 17, pp.529-536

Haberkamp TJ, Tanyeri HM. (1999). Management of idiopathic sudden sensorineural hearing loss. *AM J Otol*, Vol. 20, pp.587-595

Ha MK, Choi IH. (2003). A clinical study of sudden sensorineural hearing loss. *J Oriental Med Surg, Ophthalmol & Otolaryngol*, Vol. 16, pp.141-153

Haynes DS, O'Malley M, Cohen S, Watford K, Labadie RF. (2007). Intratympanic dexamethasone for sudden sensorineural hearing loss after failure of systemic therapy. *Laryngoscope*. Vol. 117, pp.3-15.

Hwang DS, Kim HK, Seo JC, Shin IH, Kim DH, Kim YS. (2011). Sympathomodulatory effects of Saam acupuncture on heart rate variability in night-shift-working nurses. *Complement Ther Med*,19, pp.S33-40

Ito S, Fuse T, Yokota M, Watanabe T, Inamura K, Gon S, Aoyagi M. (2002). Prognosis is predicted by early hearing improvement in patients with idiopathic sudden sensorineural hearing loss. *Clin Otolaryngol*, Vol. 27, pp.501-504

Kang D, Wan L. (2005). Analysis of factors influencing therapeutic results of idiopathic sudden hearing loss. *J Med Theor & Prac*. Vol. 18, pp.144-145

Lee H, Park HJ, Park J, Kim MJ, Hong M, Yang J, Choi S, Lee H. (2007). Acupuncture application for neurological disorders. *Neurol Res*, Vol. 29, pp.S49-S54

Lee NH, Ban JH. (2010). Is BPPV a Prognostic Factor in Idiopathic Sudden Sensory Hearing Loss? *Clin Exp Otorhinolaryngol*, Vol. 3, pp.199-202

Luo Y, Qian L, Zhou X, Jiang Z, Li H, Yang X.(2010). Conditional logistic analysis on the risk factors of sudden hearing loss. *Clin Remedies & Clin*, Vol. 10, pp.1101-1102

Madell JR. (1975). Acupuncture for sensorineural hearing loss. *Arch Otolaryngol*, Vol. 101, pp.441-445

Mattox DE, Simmons FB. (1977). Natural history of sudden sensorineural hearing loss. *Ann otol Rhinol Laryngol*, Vol. 86, pp.463-480

Park MK, Lee CK, Park KH, Lee JD, Lee CG, Lee BD. (2011). Simultaneous versus Subsequent Intratympanic Dexamethasone for Idiopathic Sudden Sensorineural Hearing Loss. *Otolaryngol Head Neck Surg*. Epub ahead of print

Psifidis AD, Psillas GK, Daniilidis J Ch. (2006). Sudden sensorineural hearing loss: Long-term follow-up results. *Otolaryngol Head Neck Surg* Vol. 134, pp.809-815

Rauch SD, Halpin CF, Antonelli PJ, Babu S, Carey JP, Gantz BJ, Goebel JA, Hammerschlag PE, Harris JP, Isaacson B, Lee D, Linstrom CJ, Parnes LS, Shi H, Slattery WH, Telian SA,

Vrabec JT, Reda DJ. (2011). Oral vs intratympanic corticosteroid therapy for idiopathic sudden sensorineural hearing loss: a randomized trial. *JAMA*, Vol. 305, pp.2071-2079

Raymundo IT, Bahmad F Jr, Barros Filho J, Pinheiro TG, Maia NA, Oliveira CA. (2010). Intratympanic methylprednisolone as rescue therapy in sudden sensorineural hearing loss. *Braz J Otorhinolaryngol*, Vol. 76, pp.499-509

Shaikh JA, Roehm PC. (2011). Does addition of antiviral medication to high-dose corticosteroid therapy improve hearing recovery following idiopathic sudden sensorineural hearing loss? *Laryngoscope*. doi: 10.1002/lary.21963.

Shemirani NL, Schmidt M, Friedland DR. (2009). Sudden sensorineural hearing loss: an evaluation of treatment and management approaches by referring physicians. *Otolaryngol Head Neck Surg*, Vol. 140, pp.86-91

Shikowitz MJ. (1991). Sudden sensorineural hearing loss. Med. *Clinics North Am*, Vol. 75, pp.1239-1250

Spear SA, Schwartz SR. (2011). Intratympanic steroids for sudden sensorineural hearing loss: a systematic review. *Otolaryngol Head Neck Surg*, Vol. 145, pp.534-543

Suzuki H, Mori T, Hashida K, Shibata M, Nguyen KH, Wakasugi T, Hohchi N. (2011.) Prediction model for hearing outcome in patients with idiopathic sudden sensorineural hearing loss. *Eur Arch Otorhinolaryngol*, Vol. 268, pp.497-500

Vincent CA, Richardson PH. (1987). Acupuncture for some common disorders: a review of evaluative research. *J R Coll Gen Pract*, Vol. 37, pp.77-81

Wang L, Li H, Jiang L, Zhang L. (2009). Analysis of prognosis factors of idiopathic sudden hearing loss. *J Clin Otorhinolaryngol Head Neck Surg*, Vol. 23, pp.1030-1031

Wu HP, Chou YF, Yu SH, Wang CP, Hsu CJ, Chen PR. (2011). Intratympanic Steroid Injections as a Salvage Treatment for Sudden Sensorineural Hearing Loss: A Randomized, Double-Blind, Placebo-Controlled Study. *Otol Neurotol*, Vol. 32, pp.774-779.

Wu J, Liu Y, Huang X, Zhu W, Duan M. (2011). Audiogram patterns and prognosis in sudden deafness. *Chin J Otol*. Vol. 9, pp.34-37

Xenellis J, Karapatsas I, Papadimitriou N, Nikolopoulos T, Maragoudakis P, Tzagkaroulakis M, Ferekidis E. (2006). Idiopathic sudden sensorineural hearing loss: prognostic factors. *J Laryngol Otol*, Vol. 120, pp.718-724

Yin CS, Park HJ, Nam HJ. (2010). Acupuncture for refractory cases of sudden sensori-neural hearing loss. *J Altern Complement Med*, Vol. 16, pp.1-6

Yin CS, Park HJ, Chae Y, Ha E, Park HK, Lee HS. (2007). Korean acupuncture: the individualized and practical acupuncture. *Neurol Res*, Vol. 29, pp.S10-S15

Yoon HS, Lee SE, Han EJ, Kim YB. (2003). Six cases of sudden sensorineural hearing loss. *J Oriental Med Ophthalmol & Otolaryngol & Dermatol*, Vol. 16, pp221-43

Zhang CY, Wang Y. (2006). Comparison of therapeutic effects of deep needling and shallow needling on sudden deafness. *Zhongguo Zhen Jiu*, Vol. 26, pp.256-258

Zhang XZ, Wang RM, Qian J. (2009). Observation on therapeutic effects of different treatments for sudden deafness. *Zhongguo Zhen Jiu*, 2 Vol. 9, pp.525-528